Nephrology

Volume 7 of
THE SCIENCE AND PRACTICE OF CLINICAL MEDICINE

John M. Dietschy, M.D.

Editor-in-Chief

Professor of Internal Medicine
University of Texas
Southwestern Medical School
Attending Staff
Parkland Memorial Hospital
Dallas, Texas

Nephrology

Edited by

Jay H. Stein, M.D.

Professor and Chairman
Department of Medicine
University of Texas Health Science Center
at San Antonio
San Antonio, Texas

GRUNE & STRATTON
A Subsidiary of Harcourt Brace Jovanovich, Publishers
New York   London   Toronto   Sydney   San Francisco

Library of Congress Cataloging in Publication Data

Main entry under title:

Nephrology.

   (The Science and practice of clinical medicine;
v. 7)
   Bibliography: p.
   Includes index.
   1. Nephrology. I. Stein, Jay H., 1937–
II. Series: Science and practice of clinical
medicine; v. 7. [DNLM: 1. Kidney diseases. WJ300
N4373]
RC902.N419   616.6′1   80-13568
ISBN 0-8089-1246-1

Grune & Stratton, Inc.
111 Fifth Avenue
New York, New York 10003

Distributed in the United Kingdom by
Academic Press, Inc. (London) Ltd.
24/28 Oval Road, London NW 1

Library of Congress Catalog Number 80-13568
International Standard Book Number 0-8089-1246-1

Printed in the United States of America

To Susan, Phillip, Karen, Barbara, and David

Contents

Preface

This volume of *The Science and Practice of Clinical Medicine* has been designed to describe systematically the various electrolyte disorders and renal diseases seen in clinical practice. This has been done in a manner which emphasizes basic physiologic and immunologic principles and their alteration in pathophysiologic states.

The book has been divided into nine sections. The first three sections review the anatomy and various physiologic functions of the kidney with a broad discussion of the effect of various hormones on renal function. The fourth section is designed to describe in detail the procedures available to the clinician for diagnosis of renal functional impairment. The next two sections describe the symptoms of renal disease and the various clinical syndromes that occur. Emphasis is given to the workup of a patient with these problems and the differential diagnosis.

Section Seven discusses disorders of water, sodium, potassium, and acid–base balance with emphasis on the basic pathophysiologic mechanisms involved in these specific disorders.

The initial chapter of Section Eight discusses the current immunologic aspects of renal injury. This is followed by a series of chapters that consider specific renal diseases. The clinical course, histopathology, and treatment of these various entities are described in detail.

Finally, a section is devoted to the general principles of treatment for the patient with renal disease. Medical management as well as dialysis and transplantation are discussed and compared.

It is hoped that this approach to the subject of renal and electrolyte disorders will be well received. We have attempted to emphasize both basic concepts and practical aspects of patient management. The breadth of subject coverage is neither superficial nor encyclopedic and should be useful to students, house officers, and practicing physicians.

Jay H. Stein, M.D.

2

Contributors

Edward A. Alexander, M.D.
Professor and Chief
Renal Section
Boston City Hospital
Thorndike Memorial Laboratory
Boston, Massachusetts

Allen I. Arieff, M.D.
Chief, Nephrology Section
Veterans Administration Medical Center
San Francisco, California

Jose A. L. Arruda, M.D.
Associate Professor of Medicine
Associate Professor of Physiology
Chief, Nephrology Service
Veterans Administration Hospital
Chicago, Illinois

George A. Bannayan, M.D.
Professor of Pathology
Department of Pathology
University of Texas Health Science Center at San
   Antonio
San Antonio, Texas

L. H. Banowsky, M.D.
Professor
Division of Urology
University of Texas Health Science Center at San
   Antonio
San Antonio, Texas

John J. Bardgette, M.D.
Assistant Instructor
Department of Medicine
Division of Renal Diseases
University of Texas Health Science Center at San
   Antonio
San Antonio, Texas

Larry D. Barnes, Ph.D.
Assistant Professor
Department of Biochemistry
University of Texas Health Science Center at San
   Antonio
San Antonio, Texas

Nama Beck, M.D.
Associate Professor of Medicine
Department of Medicine
Division of Renal Diseases
University of Texas Health Science Center at San
   Antonio
San Antonio, Texas

William M. Bennett, M.D.
Professor of Medicine
Head, Division of Nephrology
University of Oregon Health Sciences Center
Portland, Oregon

Jacques J. Bourgoignie, M.D.
Professor Medicine
Director, Division of Nephrology
Investigator, Howard Hughes Medical Institute
University of Miami School of Medicine
Miami, Florida

John D. Conger, M.D.
Associate Professor of Medicine
University of Colorado Medical Center
Denver, Colorado

P. C. Chauvenet, Ph.D.
Assistant Professor
Department of Surgery
University of Texas Health Science Center at San
   Antonio
San Antonio, Texas

Andrew K. Diehl, M.D.
Assistant Professor of Medicine
Department of Medicine
University of Texas Health Science Center at San
   Antonio
San Antonio, Texas

James V. Donadio, Jr., M.D.
Professor of Medicine
Mayo Medical School
Consultant, Nephrology and Internal Medicine
Mayo Clinic
Rochester, Minnesota

Steven Z. Fadem, M.D.
Clinical Instructor in Medicine
University of Texas Health Science Center
Houston, Texas

Thomas F. Ferris, M.D.
Professor and Chairman
Department of Medicine
University of Minnesota
Minneapolis, Minnesota

Alfred J. Fish, M.D.
Associate Professor of Medicine
Pediatric Nephrology
University of Minnesota Medical School
Minneapolis, Minnesota

Marvin Forland, M.D.
Professor and Deputy Chairman
Department of Medicine
University of Texas Health Science Center at San
  Antonio
San Antonio, Texas

Marvin R. Garovoy, M.D.
Assistant Professor of Medicine
Department of Medicine
Peter Bent Brigham Hospital
Boston, Massachusetts

Thomas A. Golper, M.D.
Assistant Professor of Medicine
University of Oregon Health Science Center
Veterans Administration Hospital
Portland, Oregon

Robert A. Gutman, M.D.
Associate Professor of Medicine
Duke University Medical Center
Durham, North Carolina

Michael J. Hanley, M.D.
Assistant Professor of Medicine
Department of Medicine
Division of Renal Diseases
University of Texas Health Science Center at San
  Antonio
San Antonio, Texas

Michael H. Humphreys, M.D.
Assistant Professor of Medicine
University of California Medical Center
Chief, Renal Service
San Francisco General Hospital
San Francisco, California

Allan I. Jacob, M.D.
Fellow in Nephrology
University of Miami School of Medicine
Miami, Florida

J. Daniel Johnson, M.D.
Chief Resident, Urology
University of Texas Health Science Center at San
  Antonio
San Antonio, Texas

Michael M. Kaplan, M.D.
Clinical Assistant Professor of Medicine
University of Miami School of Medicine
Miami, Florida

Robert T. Kunau, Jr., M.D.
Associate Professor of Medicine
Department of Medicine
Division of Renal Diseases
University of Texas Health Science Center at San
  Antonio
San Antonio, Texas

Neil A. Kurtzman, M.D.
Professor of Medicine
Chief, Section of Nephrology
University of Illinois Hospital
Chicago, Illinois

N. Lameire, M.D.
Associate Professor of Medicine
Renal Division
Department of Medicine
University Hospital
Ghent, Belgium

Meyer D. Lifschitz, M.D.
Associate Professor
Department of Medicine
Division of Renal Diseases
University of Texas Health Science Center at San
  Antonio
San Antonio, Texas

David A. McCarron, M.D.
Assistant Professor of Medicine
Chief, Hypertension Clinic
University of Oregon Health Sciences Center
Portland, Oregon

Allan E. Nickel, M.D.
Assistant Instructor
Division of Renal Diseases
Department of Medicine
University of Texas Health Science Center at San
  Antonio
San Antonio, Texas

Martin L. Nusynowitz, M.D.
Professor and Head
Division of Nuclear Medicine
Department of Radiology
University of Texas Health Science Center at San
  Antonio
San Antonio, Texas

Charles Y. C. Pak, M.D.
Professor of Internal Medicine
Department of Internal Medicine
University of Texas Health Science Center at Dallas
Dallas, Texas

Richard Parker, M.D.
Fellow, Division of Nephrology
Department of Medicine
University of Oregon Health Sciences Center
Portland, Oregon

Charles E. Plamp, III, M.D.
Fellow, Division of Nephrology
University of Oregon Health Sciences Center
Portland, Oregon

George A. Porter, M.D.
Professor and Chairman
Department of Medicine
University of Oregon Health Sciences Center
Portland, Oregon

Howard M. Radwin, M.D.
Professor and Chairman
Division of Urology
Department of Surgery
University of Texas Health Science Center at San
  Antonio
San Antonio, Texas

H. John Reineck, M.D.
Assistant Professor of Medicine
Department of Medicine
Division of Renal Diseases
University of Texas Health Science Center at San
  Antonio
San Antonio, Texas

Mark S. Schiffer, M.D.
Assistant Professor of Pediatrics
La Rabida Children Hospital
University of Chicago
Chicago, Illinois

Domenic A. Sica, M.D.
Renal Fellow
Department of Medicine
Division of Renal Diseases
University of Texas Health Science Center at San
  Antonio
San Antonio, Texas

Peter Smolens, M.D.
Assistant Instructor
Department of Medicine
Division of Renal Diseases
University of Texas Health Science Center at San
  Antonio
San Antonio, Texas

Terry B. Strom, M.D.
Assistant Professor of Medicine
Department of Medicine
Peter Bent Brigham Hospital
Boston, Massachusetts

Michael J. Sweeney, M.D.†
Professor and Head
Division of Nephrology
Department of Pediatrics
University of Texas Health Science Center at San
  Antonio
San Antonio, Texas

Manjeri A. Venkatachalam, M.D.
Professor
Departments of Pathology and Medicine
University of Texas Health Science Center at San
  Antonio
San Antonio, Texas

Richard E. Weitzman, M.D.
Assistant Professor of Medicine
UCLA School of Medicine
Head, Section on Hypertension
LA County Harbor-UCLA Medical Center
Torrance, California

Curtis B. Wilson, M.D.
Member, Department of Immunopathology
Research Institute of Scripps Clinic
La Jolla, California

Marsha Wolfson, M.D.
Assistant Professor of Medicine
Chief, Nephrology Section
Hemodialysis Unit
Veterans Administration
Portland, Oregon

† Deceased February 18, 1979

Nephrology

Anatomy and Histology of the Kidney

Manjeri A. Venkatachalam

This chapter highlights the structural characteristics of the mammalian kidney that are most relevant to normal and altered function. The overall consideration will be that of the human kidney; however, many descriptions of nephron structure and vascular anatomy are derived from observations made in the rat and dog. Among the three species, there is a generality in structural features that are most relevant to renal function. Where appropriate, pertinent differences between species are outlined.

GROSS FEATURES

The kidneys, bean-shaped paired organs, are located retroperitoneally on either side of the vertebral column. In the adult male, normal kidney weights range between 120 and 170 g; the weights in females are slightly lower. They measure approximately 11 × 6 × 2.5 cm and possess loosely adherent fibrous capsules. Their medial aspects are sharply concave, forming an open cavity called the hilus. In the hilus are situated the renal pelvis, blood vessels, lymphatics, and a nerve plexus. The blood vessels, lymphatics, and nerves are loosely embedded in fibrofatty tissue in the space between the pelvis and the fibrous capsule lining the inner wall of the hilus, which they pierce to enter or emerge from the parenchyma. There is usually a single renal artery that divides in the hilus into anterior and posterior branches that subsequently subdivide into five segmental branches. The segmental arteries give rise to interlobar arteries, which pierce the renal parenchyma. The renal vein, situated anterior to the artery, receives tributaries that generally follow the distribution of the arterial branches.

ZONATION OF THE KIDNEY

From the kidney surface inwards, the parenchyma exhibits a characteristic zonation (Figs. 1 and 2). There is a peripheral band of tissue, the cortex; the inner renal mass or the medulla is divided into many conical bodies, the pyramids. The bases of the pyramids are at the corticomedullary junction. The apices or the papillae protrude medially towards the pelvis. The rat kidney is unipapillate and has one pyramid only. Each pyramid has an outer medulla and an inner medulla or papilla. The outer medulla is divided into an outer stripe

and an inner stripe. In the human kidney, the cortex is about 1 cm thick, and extends between the renal pyramids to form the columns of Bertin (Fig. 1). Radially oriented bundles of tubules, called medullary rays, extend from the base of each pyramid through the cortex towards the renal surface. (See Fig. 2.)

NEPHRON SUBUNIT

Kidneys consist of several subunits or nephrons (Figs. 3 and 4). Human kidneys each have approximately 1.3 million nephrons, the corresponding figure for the rat being 30,000. In sequence, the nephron is composed of the glomerulus and Bowman's capsule, the proximal tubule, the thin limbs of the loop of Henle, the distal tubule, and the initial portion of the cortical collecting duct. The proximal and distal tubules each have convoluted and straight segments. Several initial cortical collecting ducts unite: these ducts traverse the length of the medulla, receiving further tributaries, and find their terminus at the papillary tips as the papillary ducts of Bellini. The ducts of Bellini, being formed by the union of collecting ducts from several nephrons, are relatively few in number, between 10 and 25 per pyramid in the human kidney. Each nephron has a loop of Henle consisting of a descending proximal straight tubule, a thin limb segment, and an ascending thick limb segment. Based on the length of Henle's loops, nephrons may be classified as short or long looped. Outer cortical nephrons have short loops whose descending thin segments turn back as ascending thick limbs within the inner stripe of the outer medulla. Juxtamedullary nephrons have longer loops with well developed descending and ascending thin segments that extend variable distances into the inner medulla. Mid-cortical nephrons have Henle's loops with lengths that are intermediate. In the human kidney, there are seven times as many nephrons with short loops than nephrons with long loops.

The anatomic zones of the kidney correspond to the distribution of nephron segments within them. Glomeruli are located in the cortex exclusively. Proximal convoluted tubules are present in the cortex between the medullary rays; upon transition to the proximal straight tubule, the nephron enters a medullary ray and

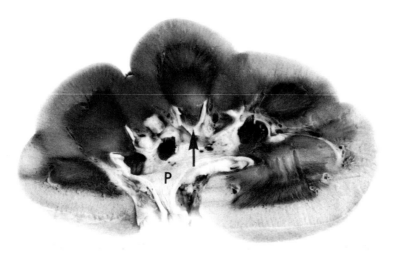

Fig. 1. Bisected human kidney from a 4-yr-old child. The cortex forms a peripheral pale band of tissue and extends in between the pyramids as the columns of Bertin. The outer medulla is dark in color, whereas the inner medulla or papilla is pale. The pelvis (P) and the calyces are shown as white structures. Each papilla protrudes into a minor calyx in a characteristic fashion (arrow). [Reprinted with permission from Tisher CC: Anatomy of the kidney, in Brenner BM, Rector FC (eds): The Kidney, vol I. Philadelphia, W.B. Saunders, 1976, p 5.]

courses towards the medulla. The proximal straight tubule undergoes a transition at the junction of the outer and inner stripes of the outer medulla and continues as the descending thin limb of Henle. Short Henle's loops turn back as ascending thick limbs within the inner stripe and thus possess no ascending thin limb segments. In long loops, ascending thin limbs undergo transition at the inner medulla–outer medulla boundary to ascending thick limbs of Henle. Ascending thick limbs of Henle of both short and long loops course upwards through the outer medulla and the cortical medullary rays and make contact with the vascular poles of their parent glomeruli at a specialized epithelial zone known as the macula densa. Following the macula densa, the distal tubule follows a convoluted course in the cortex before joining the cortical collecting duct.

EXTERNAL COLLECTING SYSTEM

The external collecting system of the kidney is formed by the renal pelvis and its outpouchings, the major and minor calyces. In the human kidney, there are two or three major calyces. From each major calyx, several minor calyces extend towards the renal mass. The renal papillae protrude into the minor calyces in a characteristic fashion. The urine formed by each pyramid drains into a minor calyx through the ducts of Bellini. The inner surfaces of the collecting system are lined by transitional epithelium. At the upper ends of the calyces, the epithelial layer is reflected on to the renal parenchyma as a less differentiated cuboidal epithelium. The latter continues on to line the urinary surface of the medulla. The external fibrous wall of the pelvis and calyces are fused with the fibrous capsule of the kidney. There is smooth muscle within the walls of the collecting system, the periodic contraction of which aids the onward transport of urine.

INTRARENAL VASCULATURE

The branches of the renal artery are end arteries; i.e., there is no collateral circulation between them (Figs. 4–6). The interlobar arteries pierce the renal parenchyma and give rise to arcuate arteries at the corticomedullary junction. The arcuate arteries, in turn, give off radially oriented interlobular arteries. Afferent arterioles branch off from the interlobular arteries and supply the glomeruli. Afferent arterioles vary in length between 100 and 1000 Å and have a mean internal diameter of 13 μm in superficial as well as juxtamedullary regions of the dog kidney. Deep or juxtamedullary glomeruli are larger than superficial cortical glomeruli. Within the glomeruli, each afferent arteriole progressively subdivides into 20–40 capillary loops arranged in several units or lobules. The capillary loops ultimately merge to form the efferent arterioles. Anastomotic connections are present between the capillaries that make up the lobule and between afferent and efferent ends of the loops.

After emerging from the glomeruli, efferent arterioles empty into the network of capillaries that surround the tubules of the nephron. These efferent vascular tubular relationships have been well studied in the dog. In the superficial cortex, the capillary network around proximal and distal convoluted tubules is supplied by efferent arterioles derived from parent glomeruli, and capillaries surrounding straight nephron segments are perfused by efferent arterioles from deeper glomeruli. Going from the superficial to the mid and deep cortex, there is a progressive dissociation of the vascular supply of tubular segments from the efferent vessel of parent glomeruli. Thus convoluted tubules of juxtamedullary nephron segments are fed by efferent vessels from more superficial glomeruli, and most efferent arterioles of juxtamedullary glomeruli are destined to break up into many descending arterial vasa recta that supply the outer and inner medulla. Descending arterial vasa recta and corresponding ascending venous vasa recta run parallel and countercurrent to each other and are segregated into distinct regions of the outer medulla called vascular bundles. Tubular segments in the interbundle region are perfused by a dense capillary network, which is fed by arterial vasa recta and drained by veins that join the arcuate veins at the corticomedullary junction. Ascending venous vasa recta also drain ultimately into the arcuate veins.

Most descending vasa recta leave the vascular bundles to enter the outer medullary capillary plexus; a few, however, continue on into the inner medulla, where they feed capillary plexuses at various levels. The inner medullary capillary plexuses perfuse descending and ascending thin limbs of Henle and collecting ducts and are drained by ascending vasa recta that course through the outer medulla exclusively through the vascular bundles.

The venous circulation of the kidney closely follows the course of the arterial system. Thus interlobular and arcuate veins accompany the corresponding arteries and follow them towards the segmental or interlobar vessels. Contrary to previous thought, no significant aglomerular shunt pathways between afferent and efferent arterioles or preglomerular arterial–venous communications exist in the normal kidney.

GLOMERULUS

The glomerulus is a vascular-epithelial organ designed for the ultrafiltration of plasma (Figs. 6–10). The total surface area of the filtering membrane in man approximates one square meter. Each human glomerulus is approximately 200 μm in diameter. As inferred from its embryology and ultrastructure, the glomerulus can be considered to be an invagination of a capillary network into an epithelium lined sac, the Bowman's capsule. The epithelial layer that invests the capillary network (the visceral epithelium) is incorporated into and becomes an intrinsic part of the filtering membrane, whereas the parietal epithelium bounds the Bowman's space, the cavity into which plasma ultrafiltrate first collects.

The anastomosing capillaries of individual glomerular lobules ramify around the mesangium, also called the centrilobular or stalk region of the glomerulus. The mesangium forms a branching, supportive framework for the glomerulus and consists of highly irregular, stellate cells (mesangial cells) embedded in a basement-membrane-like glycoprotein matrix. Mesangial cells contain contractile elements in their cytoplasm and by their contraction are thought to control intraglomerular blood flow and regulate the operation of intraglomerular shunt pathways. The mesangium is also thought to have a "clearing" function. Large macromolecules that might lodge in the glomerular basement membrane find their way into the mesangial matrix and are phagocytosed by the mesangial cells. From the capillary lumen

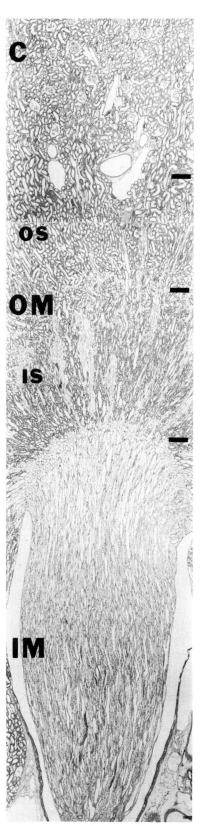

Fig. 2. Low-magnification micrograph of a rat kidney from cortex to inner medulla in transverse section. C, cortex. OM, outer medulla. OS, outer stripe. IS, inner stripe. IM, inner medulla.

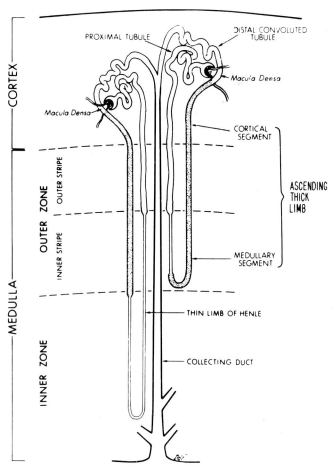

PROXIMAL TUBULE

DISTAL CONVOLUTED TUBULE

Macula Densa

Macula Densa

CORTEX

CORTICAL SEGMENT

ASCENDING THICK LIMB

MEDULLARY SEGMENT

OUTER ZONE

OUTER STRIPE

INNER STRIPE

MEDULLA

INNER ZONE

THIN LIMB OF HENLE

COLLECTING DUCT

Fig. 3. Diagram showing the segmentation of short and long-looped nephrons and zonation of the kidney. The ascending thick limb is also known as the straight part of the distal tubule. [Reprinted from Kidney International with permission—Allen F, Tisher CC: Morphology of the ascending thick limb of Henle. Kidney Int 9:8, 1976.]

to the urinary space, the filtering membrane consists of (1) a thin layer of capillary endothelium, (2) a glomerular basement membrane, and (3) the visceral epithelial cells. The endothelial layer, which is adherent to the lamina rara interna of the glomerular basement membrane (see below), is thin and is pierced by numerous pores or fenestrae, about 700 Å in diameter. An endothelial cell coat, 120 Å thick, covers the cell surface and extends into the fenestrae. The glomerular basement membrane (GBM), is shared between the endothelium and epithelium, is approximately 3200 Å wide in man, and has a central electron-dense layer, the lamina densa, and two peripheral electron-lucent layers, the lamina rara interna and externa. The epithelial cells, or podocytes, exhibit interdigitating foot processes that are embedded in, and adherent to, the lamina rara externa. Adjacent foot processes are separated by 200–300 Å wide filtration slits filled by an epithelial cell coat, which, when examined on the free surfaces of the cells after appropriate staining, measures up to 800 Å in thickness. Filtration slit diaphragms 70 Å thick bridge the narrowest points in the gaps between adjacent foot

processes. The diaphragms are anchored to the plasma membranes of the foot processes; when viewed appropriately they exhibit an orderly subunit structure and multiple repeating rectangular pores, about 40 × 140 Å. Ultrastructural tracer studies have shown that the path taken by molecules filtered across the glomerulus is almost exclusively extracellular, viz., the endothelial fenestrae, the glomerular basement membrane, and the filtration slits including the diaphragms. The GBM is a meshwork of fibrillar material and is chemically a complex glycoprotein consisting of both relatively neutral collagen-like glycopeptides, highly acidic, polyanionic sialoglycopeptides and glycosaminoglycans. It is thought that the acidic moieties are oriented toward the lamina rara externa and interna, in close relationship to the epithelial and endothelial cell coats, both of which also contain negatively charged sialoglycoproteins. The process whereby plasma proteins are hindered from entry into the filtrate is thought to depend not only on steric exclusion from the filter but also on electrostatic interaction with these polyanionic glomerular elements. In addition, podocytes are capable of pinocytosis, a

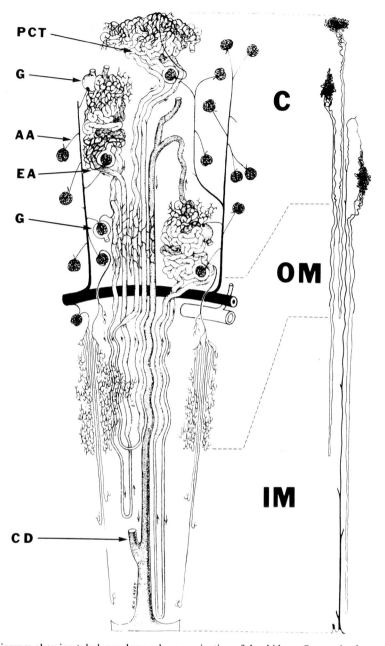

Fig. 4. Diagram showing tubular and vascular organization of dog kidney. One each of a superficial cortical, midcortical, and deep cortical nephron is shown. For simplicity, the venous system has not been included. The vertical scale is compressed on the left and in correct proportion on the right. C, cortex. OM, outer medulla. IM, inner medulla. PCT, proximal convoluted tubule. G, glomerulus. AA, afferent arteriole. EA, efferent arteriole. CD, collecting duct. [Reprinted with permission from Beeuwkes R, Bonventre JV: Tubular organization and vascular tubular relations in the dog kidney. Am J Physiol 229:695, 1975.]

process whereby they imbibe into their cytoplasm any proteins that might leak through the filter; thereby they are thought to "monitor" the process of filtration.

The parietal epithelial cells of the Bowman's capsule are squamous in type, appear to serve only a passive role, and undergo abrupt transition to columnar cells of the first segment of the proximal tubule at the urinary pole of the glomerulus.

PROXIMAL TUBULE

In the human, the proximal tubule (Figs. 11–13) is about 14 mm long. It has two anatomic segments—the tubule first forms several convolutions around the glomerulus of its origin and then takes on a straight course downwards through a cortical medullary ray into the outer stripe of the outer medulla. At the beginning of the inner stripe, it undergoes sudden transition to the

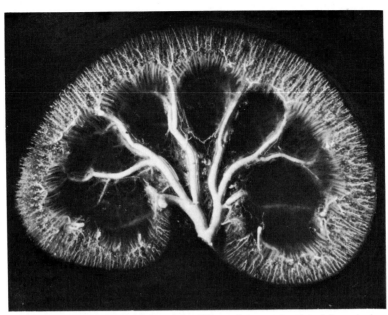

Fig. 5. Photograph of silicone-rubber-injected dog kidney. Segmental or interlobar arteries give rise to arcuate arteries at the corticomedullary junction, which, in turn, give rise to radially oriented interlobular arteries, which go toward the surface of the kidney. [Courtesy of R. Beeuwkes, Department of Physiology, Harvard Medical School.]

descending thin limb of Henle. The following are general features of proximal tubular cells (for cellular subtypes, see below). They possess a greatly expanded luminal plasma membrane, which is thrown into numerous finger-like protrusions or microvilli, visible by light microscopy as a faintly staining brush border. The brush border appears to be the seat of high metabolic activity. Enzyme systems that have been localized to

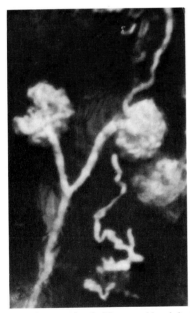

Fig. 6. Photomicrograph of silicone-rubber-injected rat kidney showing interlobular artery, afferent arterioles, two glomeruli, and one efferent arteriole. × 150.

microvilli include disaccharidases, aminopeptidases, 5'-nucleotidase, alkaline phosphatase, and Mg^{2+} activated adenosine triphosphatase (Mg^{2+} ATPase). Between microvilli the plasma membrane is pinched into the cytoplasm in the form of tubules or vesicles that are in continuity with the lumen. The apical cytoplasm also contains a number of free tubulovesicular profiles that are apparently derived from the apical plasma membrane and larger vacuoles formed by the fusion of smaller vesicles. Some of the smaller free vesicles in the apical cytoplasm are thought to be primary lysosomes, derived from the Golgi apparatus, situated deeper within the cell. The apical tubulovesicular system is designed for the function of pinocytosis, i.e., a mechanism by which droplets of fluid in the filtrate are engulfed into the cytoplasm. Proteins that leak through the filter may thus be partially retrieved by the epithelial cells. Following pinocytosis, the vesicles containing imbibed fluid fuse with each other, and with primary lysosomes, eventually forming membrane-bound bodies containing digested residue called secondary lysosomes. Other cytoplasmic organelles include numerous mitochondria, rough and smooth endoplasmic reticulum, and microbodies or peroxisomes. Proximal tubular cells have complex shapes and interdigitate with adjacent cells through primary and secondary processes or ridges that extend from the apical to the basal surfaces of the cells, as well as numerous basal-lateral evaginations that extend from the primary processes. The result is that a capacious, labyrinthine paracellular space is formed toward the lateral and basal aspects of the cells. This space is separated from the tubule lumen by narrow bands of membrane fusion between the

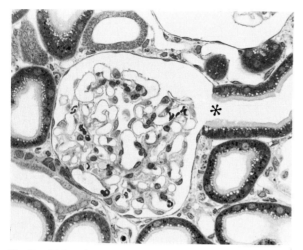

Fig. 7. Light micrograph of rat kidney showing a glomerulus, Bowman's capsule, and transition of the latter to the proximal tubule (asterisk). × 280.

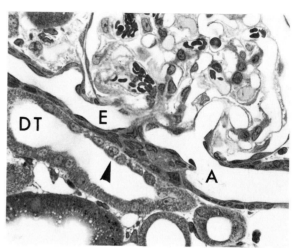

Fig. 8. Light micrograph of rat kidney showing afferent arteriole (A), glomerulus, efferent arteriole (E), distal tubule (DT), and macula densa (arrowhead). In between the two arterioles and macula densa there is a collection of cells, the extraglomerular mesangium or polar cushion. × 450.

plasma membranes of adjacent cells. These shallow intercellular "tight junctions" appear to constitute a low-resistance, "shunt" pathway across the epithelium (i.e., bypassing the transcellular route) and may play a significant role in proximal tubular sodium and water transport. That the junctions can be penetrated by electrolytes has been shown by ultrastructural tracer studies using the lanthanum ion.

By cell type, proximal tubules are divided into three, and in some species four, sequential segments. In the rat, there are three segments, S_1, S_2, S_3. The S_1 segment commences at the glomerulus and terminates

within the proximal convoluted tubule. The S_2 segment is present both in the convoluted portion and the first part of the proximal straight tubule in the medullary ray. S_3 cells are seen only in the straight segment, up to its termination. Differences between S_1, S_2, and S_3 cells are illustrated and outlined in Figs. 12 and 13. Segmentation of the human proximal tubule has not been as well studied.

A sodium pump is thought to be located in the basal-lateral labyrinth of proximal tubular cells. Operation of the pump is by the action of a membrane-bound Na^+ K^+ ATPase and closely situated mitochondria

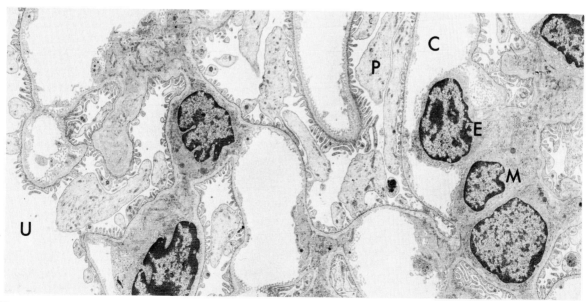

Fig. 9. Electron micrograph of rat glomerulus showing capillaries (C), endothelial cells (E), mesangial cells (M), and visceral epithelial cells or podocytes (P). U, urinary space. × 5200.

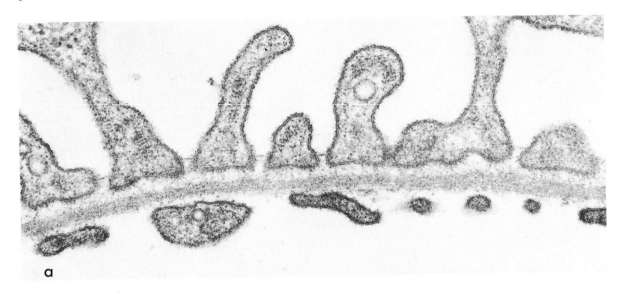

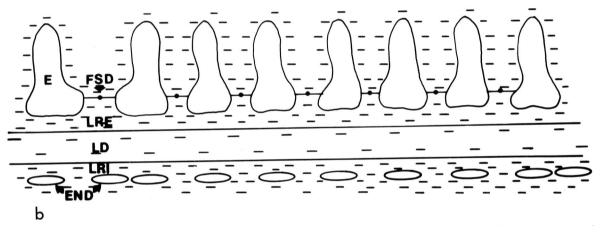

Fig. 10. High-power electron micrograph (a) and diagram (b) of the glomerular capillary wall. From capillary lumen outward toward the urinary space, the capillary wall consists of a fenestrated endothelium (END), the glomerular basement membrane with its three layers, the lamina rara interna (LRI), lamina densa (LD), lamina rara externa (LRE), and the interdigitating foot processes of the epithelium (E). The filtration slits are bridged by filtration slit diaphragms (FSD). The distribution of negatively charged polyanionic elements is indicated in Fig. 10b. Fig. 10a, Original magnification × 73,000.

which supply energy through oxidative phosphorylation. The complexity of the basal-lateral labyrinth decreases progressively along the length of the tubule, and this is associated with a decrease in number and alteration in the configuration of mitochondria. These structural differences are thought to correlate with differences in pump function and modes of sodium transport between the convoluted and straight tubule segments.

THIN LIMBS OF THE LOOP OF HENLE

Human thin limb segments may measure up to 10 mm or more in length. Both descending and ascending thin limbs of Henle are thought not to possess active transport mechanisms but to function as countercurrent exchangers and multipliers by virtue of unique differences in their passive permeability characteristics. In this function, they are aided by their parallel and countercurrent arrangement with respect to each other

and other tubular structures of the renal medulla (ascending thick limbs of Henle, collecting ducts, and vasa recta in the outer medulla; collecting ducts and vasa recta in the inner medulla). The resemblance of medullary structure to model countercurrent multiplier systems (such as industrial heat exchangers) is central to modern concepts of urinary concentration and is illustrated in a cross-sectional view in Fig. 14. The ultrastructural features of thin limb segments do not indicate a high metabolic activity and are consistent with their postulated passive role; unlike other segments of the nephron which exhibit active transport, thin limbs possess flat squamous epithelia with relatively fewer numbers of mitochondria, which are the chief energy source in active transport processes. Distinct differences in epithelial cell shape, the internal structure of plasma membranes, and character of intercellular tight junctions have been found between descending and ascending thin limb segments and between descending segments of short and long loops in the rat. Limited observations suggest that such differences may exist in other species also. However, attempts at the correlation of the structural features of thin limbs with their experimentally demonstrated passive permeability characteristics have been fruitless to date. In view of the complexity of the problem, and the controversey that surrounds structural–functional correlations in this field, a detailed discussion of thin limb ultrastructure is not warranted in this brief review. (For detailed exposition, see Kokko and Tisher.)

THICK ASCENDING LIMB OF HENLE AND DISTAL TUBULE

The thick ascending limb of Henle's loop and distal convoluted tubule (Figs. 12 and 15) have many common features, whereas the macula densa, described in a subsequent section, is composed of cells with a different ultrastructure. As in other segments of the nephron, their ultrastructural features have been well studied in the rat, but many important features appear to be common to most species, including man. In the human kidney, the ascending thick limb is about 9 mm, and the distal convoluted tubule approximately 5 mm long. Ascending thick limbs have a low columnar epithelium. The cell height decreases significantly as the tubule courses through the outer stripe and cortex, but after the macula densa it increases once more to give the cells in the convoluted portion a columnar character. As in the S_1 and S_2 segments of the proximal tubule, distal tubular cells interdigitate with each other through multiple lateral and basal-lateral cytoplasmic processes, causing a great expansion of the paracellular space. Sections of the laterally interdigitating processes appear in electron micrographs as cytoplasmic segments separated by apical cell junctions; the basal plasma mem-

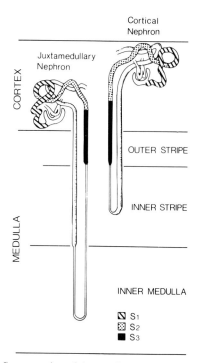

Fig. 11. Segmentation of the proximal tubule in the rat. Three sequential segments S_1, S_2, and S_3 occur in the proximal tubule. S_1 segments occur in the convoluted portions only. S_2 segments extend partially into the straight portions, whereas S_3 segments are present in the proximal straight tubule exclusively.

brane of each segment invaginates deeply upwards, reaching up to two-thirds the height of the cell. The basal-lateral cell processes contain numerous elongated mitochondria oriented perpendicular to the basement membrane. Mitochondria are in close relationship to the plasma membrane and appear to play a crucial role

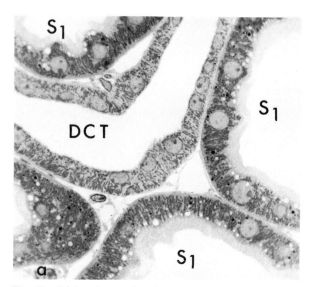
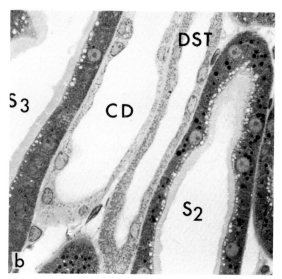

Fig. 12. Light micrographs of tubular structures in the rat renal cortex, (a) (× 670) from the cortex in between the medullary rays and (b) (× 580) from a medullary ray. The proximal tubule segments S_1, S_2, and S_3 all have a brush border, whereas the distal convoluted tubule (DCT), ascending thick limb of Henle or distal straight tubule (DST), and collecting duct (CD) have no brush border.

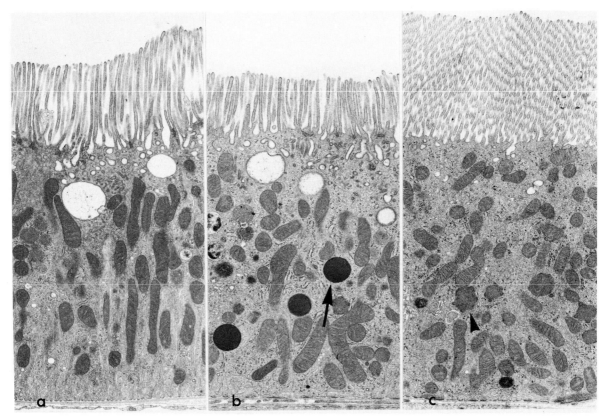

Fig. 13. Electron micrographs of rat proximal tubule segments S_1 (a), S_2 (b), and S_3 (c). All the cells have a brush border, but the microvilli are tallest in S_3, intermediate in S_1, and shortest in S_2. Tubulovesicular profiles and vacuoles in the apical cytoplasm are numerous in S_1 and S_2 and are but few in S_3. Mitochondria are elongated and arranged perpendicular to the basement membrane in S_1; going to S_2 and S_3, mitochondria get shorter and there is progressive disarray in configuration. Secondary lysosomes (arrow) are most numerous in S_2 and microbodies (arrowhead) in S_3. The lateral-basal labyrinth is well developed in S_1, becomes simpler in S_2, and is almost absent in S_3. Original magnification × 8300.

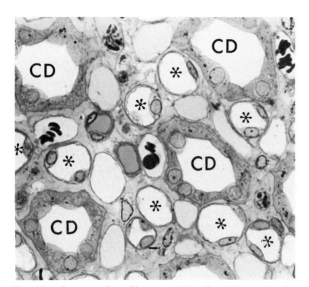

Fig. 14. Cross section of inner medulla of rat kidney showing collecting ducts (CD), thin limbs of Henle (asterisks), vasa recta, and capillaries. The blood vessels contain red blood cells and plasma in their lumina. × 560.

in tubular function by supplying energy to a membrane-associated electrolyte pump. The main enzyme of the pump is a Na^+ K^+ ATPase, which has been selectively localized to the basal-lateral plasma membrane by histochemical and autoradiographic methods.

Cells of the ascending thick limb may be of the rough type (R), with many short, blunt microvilli all over their luminal surface, or of the smooth type (S), with few microvilli except at their lateral cell borders. R cells have more lateral interdigitations (as viewed from the luminal surface) than S cells. Within the inner stripe, S cells outnumber the R cells, but the ratio alters markedly in favor of R cells as the thick limb ascends upwards towards its parent glomerulus; concurrently, the complexity of lateral interdigitations (as viewed from the luminal surface) and density of microvilli also increases. Past the macula densa, the cells appear less complex as viewed from their luminal surface, but they still possess numerous basal-lateral interdigitations. Cells of both segments exhibit numbers of lysosomes, prominent Golgi complexes, and abundant endoplasmic reticulum. The apical cytoplasm contains numerous coated vesicles whose function is not known.

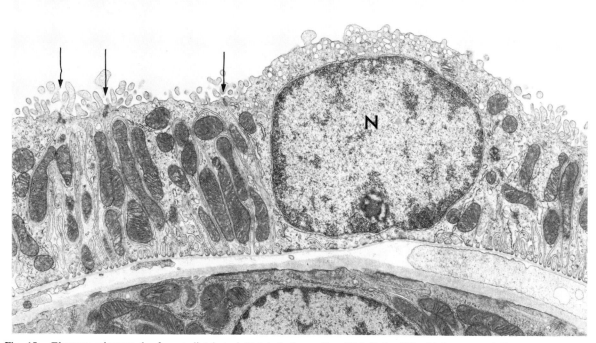

Fig. 15. Electron micrograph of a rat distal straight tubule (ascending thick limb of Henle) from a medullary ray. There are numerous cytoplasmic segments separated by intercellular junctions (arrows) indicative of lateral interdigitation between cells. The basal-lateral labyrinth is well developed, as shown by the numerous basal invaginations of the plasma membrane. Mitochondria are elongated and arranged perpendicular to the basement membrane. Apical cytoplasm has vesicular profiles, and luminal plasma membrane has many short, blunt microvilli. N, nucleus. × 9650.

COLLECTING DUCT

The first portion of the cortical collecting duct (Figs. 16–18) is the initial collecting tubule, which follows the distal tubule and extends up to its first union with another tubule. Sometimes present on the renal surface, this segment has been erroneously considered to be the "late distal tubule" in the past. It is connected by means of an intermediary segment to a descending medullary ray portion of the collecting duct. Following the cortical collecting duct, there is an outer medullary and an inner medullary portion, the latter emptying in the area cribrosa of the papilla as the ducts of Bellini. The human collecting duct measures approximately 20–22 mm long and may measure up to 200 μm in diameter in the inner medulla.

The dominant cell type is the light cell, which exhibits a clear cytoplasm containing small numbers of randomly oriented mitochondria. Other cellular components—the endoplasmic reticulum and Golgi complexes—are also fewer in concentration in the light cells compared to other metabolically active segments of the nephron. As the duct descends, the light cells progressively increase in height and become columnar in Bellini's ducts. The lateral margins of the cells interlock through numerous small processes, and the basal plasma membrane shows numerous small invaginations. Short, blunt microvilli are present on the luminal plasma membrane, as well as a cell coat, or glycocalyx. The intercellular tight junction is well developed and measures 0.3 μm in depth in the rat.

Interposed between the light cells are fewer numbers of a second cell type, the "dark" or intercalated cell. These cells have abundant mitochondria and other organelles and a denser cytoplasmic matrix. Dark cells decrease in frequency along the course of the collecting duct and are virtually absent in the inner medulla. The luminal surfaces of the dark cells are thrown into numerous microvillar processes, longer than in light cells. The number of vesicular profiles observed in the apical cytoplasm is also higher.

The collecting duct appears to have a role in a variety of reabsorptive and secretory functions, but the relative roles played by the light and dark cells are not known. The permeability of the luminal plasma membrane of light cells to water is markedly influenced by vasopressin. It has been demonstrated by autoradiography that isotope-labeled vasopressin binds to the basal surfaces of collecting duct cells. A stimulation of intracellular 3', 5' cyclic adenosine monophosphate production follows and possibly the activation of a protein kinase in the luminal plasma membrane. The final steps of the mechanisms whereby an increase of membrane water permeability is actually achieved is not known, but extrapolation from morphological work done on the toad urinary bladder (an analog of the collecting duct) suggests that there may be a redistri-

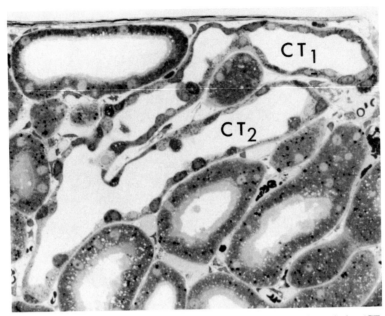

Fig. 16. Light micrograph of rat renal cortex showing two initial collecting tubules (CT₁ and CT₂, derived from two separate nephrons) forming a junction. Both tubules correspond to the so-called "late distal tubules" as usually defined during micropuncture. Note that one of the tubules is just beneath the capsule and thus available for puncture. × 360. [Reprinted with permission from Tisher CC: Anatomy of the kidney, in Brenner BM, Rector FC (eds): The Kidney, vol I. Philadelphia, W.B. Saunders, 1976, p 5.].

bution of particulate subunits in the membrane to form patches or aggregates. These aggregates are presently thought to constitute channels for the increased transfer of water across the membrane provided an osmotic gradient exists. Another morphological expression of increased water flow across the duct may be observed following acute vasopressin administration in animals with water diuresis. Under these conditions, the in-

crease in net flow of water results in temporary swelling of the epithelial cells, increase in number and size of epithelial vacuoles, and the formation of large spaces in the intercellular and basal labyrinth. It has been suggested that the dark, mitochondria-rich cells are involved in acid–base regulatory function, but the evidence appears still inconclusive.

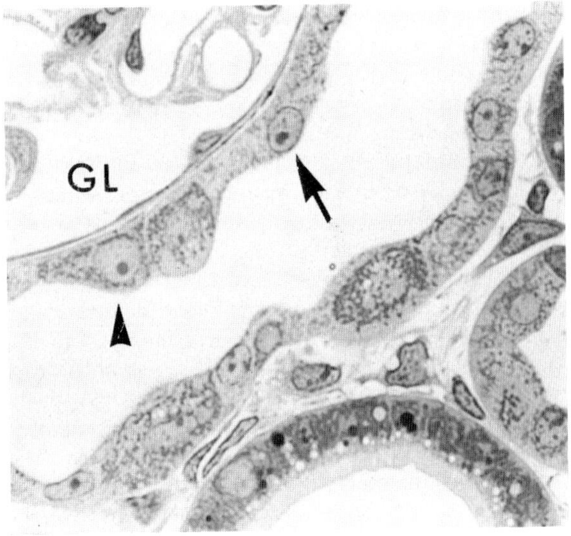

JUXTAGLOMERULAR APPARATUS

The juxtaglomerular apparatus (Figs. 8 and 19) consists of the terminal portion of the afferent arteriole, the efferent arteriole, the macula densa, and the polar cushion or extraglomerular mesangium. The distal tubule returns to the vascular pole of its parent glomerulus, at which region it makes intimate contact with both afferent and efferent arterioles, more extensively so with the latter. Forming the base of a triangular area bounded on two sides by the afferent and efferent arterioles is a specialized plaque-like area of the distal tubule, called the macula densa. Filling the triangular space are irregular branched cells embedded in a basement membrane framework; this polar cushion (polkissen) is apparently an extraglomerular extension of the glomerular mesangium. Situated in the medial tunic of both arterioles are specialized granular myoepithelioid cells; the granules contain a substance immunologically similar to renin, thought to be renin or its precursor. Cells of the polkissen may also contain similar granules, particularly under conditions of increased renin production and storage. The macula densa epithelium differs markedly from the adjacent distal tubular cells. The cells are shorter, and most cellular organelles are situated basally, including the Golgi ap-

Fig. 17. Light micrograph of rat cortical collecting duct showing light cells (arrow) and dark cells (arrowhead). The numerous granules in the cells are mitochondria. GL, glomerulus. × 800.

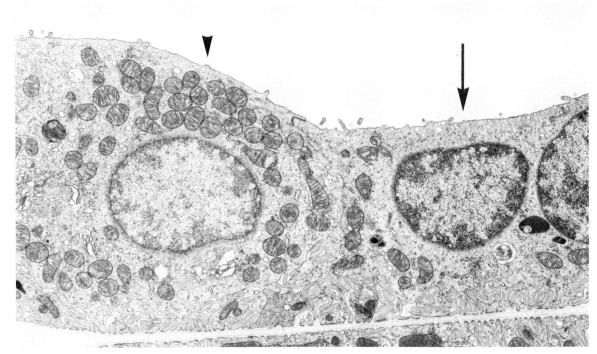

Fig. 18. Electron micrograph of cortical collecting duct from a rat kidney. There is one light cell with few mitochondria (arrow) and one dark cell with numerous mitochondria (arrowhead). × 9600.

paratus. The basal plasma membrane exhibits numerous irregular processes and infoldings. At certain points, the basement membrane of the macula densa is shared by the macula densa cells and the cell processes of the polkissen. Laterally, the epithelium of the macula densa overlies the myoepithelioid cells in the walls of the afferent and efferent arterioles. That the cells of the macula densa are different in character from the surrounding distal tubular epithelium is indicated by marked differences in the histochemical staining properties of the two cell types. The juxtaglomerular apparatus is richly innervated by autonomic nerve endings that make synaptic type of contacts with both granular and agranular cells.

The juxtaglomerular apparatus is the principal source of renin production in the kidney, and it is thought that it is also an important site of conversion of angiotensin decapeptide to the active octapeptide.

INTERSTITIUM

The interstitial space, between the vascular and tubular compartments of the kidney, increases in capacity from the cortex toward the inner medulla. Concurrently, there is an increase in the number of interstitial cells. In the cortex, the interstitial cells are either fibroblasts, which predominate, or a less common cell that has properties similar to that of histiocytes. In the medulla, particularly the inner medulla, there are distinctive interstitial cells of three types. Type I cells, the most common, are rich in lipid inclusions and have numerous cell processes that come in contact with thin limbs of Henle, collecting ducts, and vasa recta. These cells have abundant rough endoplasmic reticulum and

well developed Golgi apparatus in addition to mitochondria, smooth endoplasmic reticulum, and the lipid inclusions. The number of lipid inclusions has been shown to vary predictably in different physiological states. Type II cells are more rounded, have no lipid droplets, and are found in close proximity to type I cells. Type III cells resemble pericytes and are found in the walls of the vasa recta. The lipid inclusions in the type I interstitial cell have been shown to contain significant quantities of triglycerides, long chain fatty acids, and cholesterol. They are particularly rich in the prostaglandin precursor arachidonic acid. The renal medulla is an important source of renal prostaglandins, and the interstitial cells appear to be one site for their production.

INNERVATION OF THE KIDNEY

The kidney is innervated by both cholinergic and adrenergic fibers from the autonomic nervous system. The fibers follow the arteries generally, and nerve endings are present near the smooth muscle cells of the entire arterial tree including afferent and efferent arterioles and the vasa recta up to the inner stripe of the outer medulla. The glomeruli are not innervated, but it is becoming increasingly clear that many tubules are, and that this may have considerable physiological importance.

LYMPHATICS OF THE KIDNEY

A lymphatic circulation has been demonstrated in the renal cortex in most species examined; the existence of lymphatics in the renal medulla is yet to be demonstrated. The cortical lymphatics start as lymphatic capillaries among the tubules and around some glomeruli,

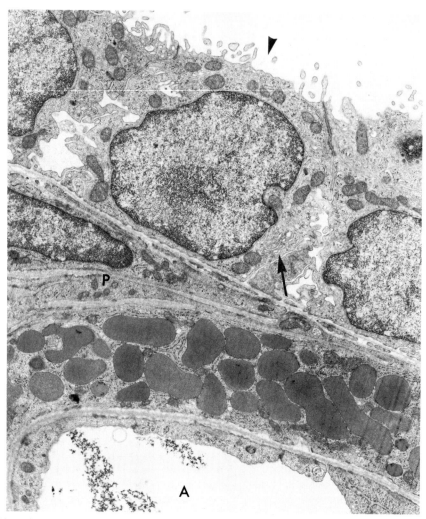

Fig. 19. Electron micrograph of rat juxtaglomerular apparatus showing macula densa epithelium (arrowhead), cells and cytoplasmic processes of the polkissen (P), and afferent arteriole (A). A modified smooth muscle cell in the wall of the arteriole has numerous dense granules, thought to be renin. Note the basal location of the Golgi apparatus (arrow) in the macula densa cell. Original magnification × 10,750.

as well as around the interlobular arteries. They then follow a course that follows the major arteries towards the renal hilus. A lymphatic system is present in the renal capsule and subcapsular space, and this appears to communicate with the cortical lymphatics.

REFERENCES

Allen F, Tisher CC: Morphology of the ascending thick limb of Henle. Kidney Int 9:8, 1976

Barajas L: Innervation of the renal cortex. Fed Proc 37:1192, 1978

Barger AC, Herd JA: Renal vascular anatomy and distribution of blood flow, in Orloff J, Berliner RW (eds): Handbook of Physiology. Section 8, Renal Physiology. Baltimore, Williams & Wilkins, 1973

Beeuwkes R, Bonventre JV: Tubular organization and vascular tubular relations in the dog kidney. Am J Physiol 229:695, 1975

Kokko JP, Tisher CC: Water movement across nephron segments involved with the countercurrent multiplication system. Kidney Int 10:64, 1976

Maunsbach AB: Ultrastructure of the proximal tubule, in Orloff J, Berliner RW (eds): Handbook of Physiology. Section 8, Renal Physiology. Baltimore, Williams & Wilkins, 1973

Osvaldo-Decima L: Ultrastructure of the lower nephron, in Orloff J, Berliner RW (eds): The Handbook of Physiology. Section 8, Renal Physiology. Baltimore, Williams & Wilkins, 1973

Rennke HG, Venkatachalam MA: Structural determinants of glomerular permselectivity. Fed Proc 36:2619, 1977

Tisher CC: Anatomy of the kidney, in Brenner BM, Rector FC (eds): The Kidney, vol I. Philadelphia, W.B. Saunders, 1976

Trump BF, Bulger RE: The morphology of the kidney, in Becker EL (ed): The Structural Basis of Renal Disease. New York, Harper & Row, Hoeber Medical Division, 1968

Normal Renal Function

GLOMERULAR FILTRATION RATE

John D. Conger

Glomerular filtration is the initial step in urine formation. By the filtration process an ultrafiltrate of plasma is formed which is devoid of red blood cells and proteins and in all other respects (allowing for Gibbs-Donnan equilibrium) is quantitatively the same as plasma water. It is this ultrafiltrate which becomes the substrate for tubular modification and the ultimate formed urine.

The actual anatomic barrier within the glomerulus that allows formation of an ultrafiltrate is controversial. This barrier appears to be in part structural and in part electrical with fixed negative charges. The selected negativity repels protein of net negative charge such as albumin which might otherwise pass through the structural barrier.

PHYSIOLOGIC DETERMINANTS OF GLOMERULAR FILTRATION

Glomerular ultrafiltration of plasma water can be visualized as a physical process that is driven by forces of opposite directions and varying magnitudes. The determinant favoring glomerular ultrafiltration is the hydrostatic pressure within glomerular capillaries. The forces which oppose filtration are the hydrostatic pressure within Bowman's space and the oncotic pressure within glomerular capillaries. Equation 1 shows the relationship between these various pressures:

$$P_{UF} = \Delta P - \Delta \Pi \qquad (1)$$

In this equation P_{UF} refers to the net ultrafiltration pressure, ΔP is the difference between the glomerular capillary and Bowman's space pressures, and $\Delta \Pi$ is the difference between the glomerular capillary and the Bowman's space oncotic pressures. Since the protein concentration of the filtrate is negligible, the value of Π for Bowman's space is zero.

In the past few years a great deal of light has been shed upon the actual magnitude of the determinants of glomerular filtration from studies carried out in a mutant strain of Wistar rat (Munich Wistar) with surface glomeruli. Under normal hydropenic conditions, hydrostatic pressures within glomerular capillaries were found to average 45 mm Hg. Bowman's space hydrostatic pressure had a mean value of 10 mm Hg. The initial glomerular oncotic pressure, based on plasma protein concentration, was assumed to be the same as systemic arterial oncotic pressure (approximately 20 mm Hg). Oncotic pressure at the efferent end of glomerular capillaries was determined from the protein concentration in the efferent arteriolar vessels and found to average 35 mm Hg.

The measured values of these determinants of glomerular ultrafiltration indicate that by the efferent end of the glomerulus that, at least in this rat strain, there is filtration equilibrium. Filtration equilibrium means that the hydrostatic pressure driving ultrafiltration equals the glomerular oncotic plus Bowman's space hydrostatic pressures which oppose filtration.

GLOMERULAR ULTRAFILTRATION COEFFICIENT

The finding of filtration equilibrium within the glomerulus not only gave insight into the kinetics of glomerular ultrafiltration but also posed a problem in measuring the coefficient of ultrafiltration for the glomerulus. Since by the efferent end of the glomerulus equilibrium between the forces favoring and opposing filtration had been reached, it was not possible to know at what point along the course of the glomerular capillary that filtration actually ceased; however, it was discovered that by plasma loading Munich Wistar rats, filtration disequilibrium could be imposed. Creating this situation permitted the determination of a minimal estimate of the glomerular ultrafiltration coefficient. The calculated value averaged 4.8 nl/min·mm Hg. It was then possible to determine that the mean net ultrafiltration pressure in the hydropenic state was only 5 mm Hg. When the glomerular plasma flow was varied over a wide range the ultrafiltration coefficient remained relatively constant. It should be pointed out that the ultrafiltration coefficient that is determined by this method does not necessarily represent the actual permeability properties of the capillary wall but rather is a function of the capillary wall permeability and the surface area available for filtration. Using morphologic studies the value of water permeability was calculated as approximately 2520 nl/min·mm Hg·cm². This value is several orders of magnitude higher than that which has been reported for capillaries in other tissues and accounts for the high rate of filtration at relatively low net ultrafiltration pressures.

EFFECTS OF ALTERING THE DETERMINANTS OF GLOMERULAR ULTRAFILTRATION

The finding of filtration equilibrium by the efferent end of the glomerulus has a substantial influence on the importance of various determinants of glomerular ultrafiltration and how each affects its magnitude. The various factors that influence the rate of glomerular ultrafiltration include the transcapillary hydrostatic pressure, the transcapillary oncotic pressure, the rate of glomerular plasma flow, and the ultrafiltration coefficient. Figure 1 shows the predicted effects of varying these four different parameters upon the rate of single nephron filtration. As can be seen in Fig. 1A, where nephron filtration rate is predicted from changes in glomerular plasma flow rate, alteration of this latter parameter has a profound influence on the rate of nephron filtration over the physiologic range of glomerular plasma flow. The linear relationship between glomerular plasma flow and single nephron filtration rate is lost above 100 nl/min of plasma flow because above this level disequilibrium conditions develop, resulting in a decline in the single nephron filtration fraction. The hashed line represents the theoretical linear relationship if single nephron filtration fraction remained at a constant value of 0.33. Varying glomerular plasma flow affects the driving force for ultrafiltration by displacing the point at which filtration equilibrium occurs toward the efferent end of the glomerulus.

Figure 1B shows that changes in the ultrafiltration coefficient would have a significant effect upon the rate of nephron filtration if the former parameter was in a very low range; however, as the ultrafiltration coefficient rises to a value at which filtration equilibrium would occur there is no further increase in nephron ultrafiltration rate despite larger values of the ultrafiltration coefficient. The lack of an effect of increases in the ultrafiltration coefficient on glomerular filtration rate is the result of filtration equilibrium being achieved more readily at higher values of this parameter such that the distance along the capillary over which the net ultrafiltration pressure acts progressively decreases as the ultrafiltration coefficient increases. The calculated value for the rat kidney of 4.8 nl/min·mm Hg is in the flat portion of this relationship, so that major reductions in the ultrafiltration coefficient would have to be encountered in order for this to be a significant determinant of the actual rate of nephron filtration.

The relationship between single nephron glomerular filtration rate and the net hydrostatic pressure across the glomerulus (ΔP) can be seen in Fig. 1C. As filtration is driven by the hydraulic driving pressure, the oncotic pressure within the glomerular capillary progressively increases and blunts the net ultrafiltration pressure increase. Thus an alteration in ΔP has limited effects on changes in nephron filtration rate because of the rise of oncotic pressure and the ultimate achievement of filtration equilibrium.

The relationship between nephron filtration rate and alterations in initial glomerular capillary oncotic pressure is shown in Fig. 1D. In several respects this relationship is very similar to that seen for $\Delta\Pi$. As

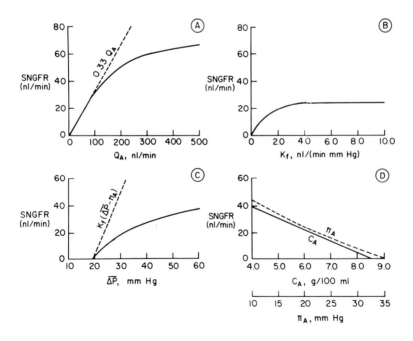

Fig. 1. Effects of varying glomerular plasma flow (Q_A), the ultrafiltration coefficient (K_f), transcapillary hydrostatic (ΔP), and oncotic pressure (Π_A) values on single nephron glomerular filtration rate (SNGFR). [Reprinted with permission from Brenner BM, Rector FC (eds): The Kidney. Philadelphia, W. B. Saunders, 1976, p 257.]

initial glomerular capillary oncotic pressure approaches ΔP there is no net driving force for filtration.

It must be noted that the roles of these various determinants of glomerular ultrafiltration are in large part dependent upon the attainment of filtration equilibrium within the glomerulus. If filtration disequilibrium occurred, then the relative influences of glomerular plasma flow rate and ΔP would be different in terms of the magnitude of their effects on changing nephron filtration rate. In dog studies in which there are indirect estimates of glomerular capillary hydraulic pressure this value has been estimated to be higher than that achieved in the rat and squirrel monkey such that disequilibrium would occur at the efferent end of the glomerulus. Under these conditions theoretical estimates would indicate that alterations in ΔP would have a more profound influence upon nephron filtration rate than alterations in nephron plasma flow.

A final point needs to be made concerning the relationship of glomerular plasma flow to nephron filtration rate. It has been shown with clearance studies that renal vasodilators such as prostaglandins, bradykinin, and acetylcholine increase renal plasma flow without having a major effect on the rate of glomerular filtration. Such a finding would not be compatible with the filtration equilibrium model, in which plasma flow is a primary determinant of nephron filtration rate; however, at least in the rat, it has been shown that these vasodilator substances also reduce the ultrafiltration coefficient of the glomerulus. By their effect on this latter parameter of nephron filtration, there is a blunting of the effect of increased nephron plasma flow to increase glomerular filtration rate.

GLOMERULAR FILTRATION AUTOREGULATION

The manner in which the kidney adjusts intrarenal vascular resistance to maintain relative constancy of renal blood flow and glomerular filtration rate has been examined at the single nephron level in the Munich Wistar rat. As shown in Fig. 2, where renal perfusion pressure was varied between 60 and 115 mm Hg, there was only a small change in single nephron plasma flow and nephron filtration rate when the blood pressure was reduced from the higher value to 80 mm Hg. As can be seen from the middle panel of Fig. 2 there was little change in the hydraulic pressure within the glomerular capillary, and filtration equilibrium seemed to obtain. In order for this constancy of intraglomerular pressure dynamics to be achieved, the changes observed in the third panel occurred. As the renal perfusion pressure

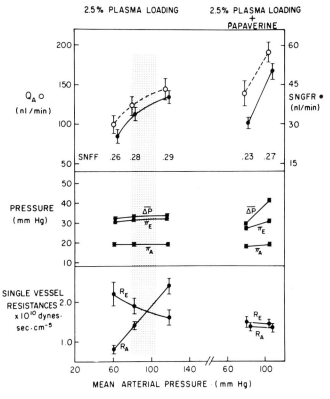

Fig. 2. Effects of graded reductions in renal perfusion pressure on glomerular plasma flow (GPF) and single nephron glomerular filtration rate (SNGFR); glomerular capillary (P_{GC}) and proximal tubular (P_T) hydraulic, efferent (Π_{AA}), and efferent arteriolar (Π_{EA}) oncotic pressures; and afferent (R_A) and efferent arteriolar (R_E) resistances. [Reprinted with permission from Robertson CR, Deen WM, Troy JL, et al: Dynamics of glomerular ultrafiltration in the rat. III. Hemodynamics and autoregulation. Am J Physiol 223:1193, 1972.]

was reduced through the autoregulatory range the was concomitant reduction in afferent arteriolar resistance and increase in efferent arteriolar resistance.

MEASUREMENT OF GLOMERULAR FILTRATION

In order to measure glomerular filtration rate one must have an understanding of the concept of clearance (see the chapter on *Renal Function Tests*). It is the method of measuring renal clearance of a substance that is used to estimate the rate of glomerular filtration. Simply defined, renal clearance means the volume of renal plasma flow from which a particular substance is completely cleared in some finite period of time. Stated mathematically, clearance can be expressed

$$C_x = U_x V / P_x \qquad (2)$$

where C_x represents the clearance of a substance, U_x is the concentration of the substance in the urine, V is the urine flow rate, and P_x is the concentration of the substance in the plasma. Theoretically, the clearance of any substance can be measured by substituting the appropriate values into the above equation; however, if one is interested in using the clearance method to estimate glomerular filtration rate, then the particular substance measured must have some unique properties. This substance must be readily filterable by the glomerulus at its plasma concentration and be neither metabolized nor reabsorbed or secreted by the tubular system. In addition, it must be nontoxic to the kidney such that it does not modify the function that it measures. Since the 1930s the substance found to meet these requirements most ideally has been inulin. The clearance of inulin is independent of its plasma concentration over a wide range, which indicates that it is a freely filterable substance and is neither secreted nor reabsorbed. Using inulin, the average value of glomerular filtration for normal young males is 125 ± 15 ml/min/ 1.73 m² body surface area and that of normal young women averages 110 ± 15 ml/min/1.73 m² body surface area. Filtration tends to be somewhat lower in the newborn and eventually decreases with age.

Because the use of inulin clearance to measure glomerular filtration rate necessitates parenteral infusion of inulin to achieve a steady-state plasma level, this measurement is not convenient for routine clinical use. The clearance of endogenous creatinine has been found to be a useful substitute for inulin clearance and has much greater clinical applicability (see the chapter on *Renal Function Tests*).

REFERENCES

Baylis C, Deen WM, Myers BD, et al: Effects of some vasodilator drugs on transcapillary fluid exchange in renal cortex. Am J Physiol 230:1148, 1976

Brenner BM, Humes HD: Mechanics of glomerular ultrafiltration. N Engl J Med 297:148, 1977

Brenner BM, Rector FC (eds): The Kidney. Philadelphia, W.B. Saunders, 1976, p 257

Chang RLS, Deen WM, Robertson CR, et al: Permselectivity of the glomerular capillary wall. III. Restricted transport of polyanions. Kidney Int 8:212, 1975

Deen WM, Robertson CR, Brenner BM: A model of glomerular ultrafiltration in the rat. Am J Physiol 223:1178, 1972

Farquhar MG: The primary glomerular filtration barrier—Basement membrane or epithelial slits? Kidney 8:197, 1975

Navar LG, Bell PD, White RW, et al: Evaluation of the single nephron glomerular filtration coefficient in the dog. Kidney Int 12:137, 1977

Pitts, RF: Clearance and rate of glomerular filtration, in: Physiology of the Kidney and Body Fluids (ed 2). Chicago, Year Book Medical, 1968, p 62

Robertson CR, Deen WM, Troy JL, et al: Dynamics of glomerular ultrafiltration in the rat. III. Hemodynamics and autoregulation. Am J Physiol 223:1191, 1972

RENAL BLOOD FLOW

Allan E. Nickel and Jay H. Stein

Coincident with the evolutionary development of the mammalian nephron, the renal vascular supply has uniquely evolved to facilitate both filtration and reabsorption of filtrate. Each kidney receives approximately 10 percent of the cardiac output, the highest blood flow per gram of tissue of any major organ excepting the brain. The kidney is both an excretory and a regulatory organ, and the blood flow delivered to each nephron is certainly a controlling factor in both of these types of functions. This chapter focuses on the renal vascular anatomy as it relates to renal function and the physiologic and pharmacologic control of renal blood flow.

RENAL VASCULAR ANATOMY

In man, as in most mammals, the renal artery is usually single but is occasionally double or with an early bifurcation. In either case, once within the hilus the renal vascular tree divides into anterior and posterior divisions. These arteries give rise to several interlobar arteries which further subdivide into arcuate and then interlobular arteries. The interlobular arteries course through the cortex, giving rise to afferent arterioles. Each afferent arteriole gives rise to its own glomerular capillary system. The afferent arterioles are well endowed with smooth muscle and form the major preglomerular resistor. In addition the afferent arteriole contains the special myoepithelial element known as the macula densa in juxtaposition to the distal tubule. This specialized segment in the distal afferent arteriole contains granules and is the site of renin production.

The glomerular capillary system is quite unlike that of other capillaries. Each glomerulus usually contains about 20–40 capillary loops. As with all capillaries, those comprising the glomerular tuft are lined by endothelium, but this endothelium is perforated by large fenestra. The epithelial layer of Bowman's capsule (the first true portion of the metanephric nephron) is uniquely intertwined around these capillary loops. This entire structure is specially designed for a very high permeability to low molecular weight solutes and water, with minimal permeability to larger molecules.

Neither the distribution of glomeruli nor glomerular size are uniform throughout the cortex. After a subcapsular aglomerular area, the density of glomeruli progressively diminishes from outer to inner cortex. Juxtamedullary glomeruli, however, are larger and have higher filtration rates than superficial glomeruli.

The capillary loops from each glomerulus merge to form a single efferent arteriole distinct for each glomerulus. This efferent arteriole variably branches into another capillary system which envelops a group of renal tubules (Fig. 1). Efferent arterioles from the superficial glomeruli tend to supply the capillary network to their own tubular segments, whereas those from deeper glomeruli may supply vessels to distant nephrons in the outer medulla and cortex. In addition, certain of the juxtamedullary glomeruli have efferent arterioles which give rise to the vasa recta that penetrate deep into the medulla to supply the papilla. It is these vessels which are intimately connected with the long loops of Henle and are involved in the countercurrent multiplier system critical to urinary concentration. Whereas total renal blood flow averages approximately 5 ml/min per gram of tissue, papillary flow averages about 0.3 ml/min per gram of papilla. Since the papilla is quite small when compared to the cortical tissue mass, less than 1 percent of the cortical blood flow enters the papilla. Such a low blood flow is critical for the complex urinary concentrating system, just as the very high cortical blood flow is important for initial filtration, reabsorption, and secretion.

The venous drainage of the kidney in general parallels the arterial system, finally ending in a single renal vein which empties into the inferior vena cava.

For many years the presence of a significant anatomical aglomerular pathway or a direct pathway from the afferent arterioles to a postglomerular structure has been debated. Recent data with microspheres have clearly indicated that such pathways do not exist.

AUTOREGULATION OF RENAL BLOOD FLOW

One of the initial and most important observations to be made after techniques to measure renal blood flow were developed was that renal blood flow remained relatively constant over a wide range of perfusion pressures. This phenomenon is termed autoregulation and is illustrated in Fig. 2. This phenomenon varies slightly from species to species, but generally occurs over the range 60–160 mm Hg mean perfusion pressure. In addition to the autoregulation of renal blood flow, glomerular filtration also remains relatively constant over this range. Most investigators believe that autoregulation of GFR is the consequence of the autoregulation of renal blood flow although there are data, which demonstrates dissociation of the two parameters. None-

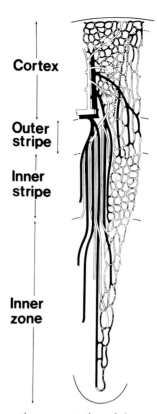

Fig. 1. Schematic representation of the renal vascular network. [Reprinted with permission from Kriz W, Barrett JM, Peter S: The renal vasculature: Anatomic-functional aspects, in Guyton A (series ed): International Review of Physiology. Volume 2: Kidney and Urinary Tract Physiology II; K Thurau (volume ed). Baltimore, University Park Press, 1976, p 3.]

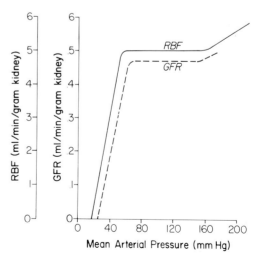

Fig. 2. Phenomenon of autoregulation of renal blood flow and glomerular filtration rate in experimental models.

theless, no clear mechanism for this autoregulation of blood flow has been discovered, and multiple theories have been developed to explain this phenomenon.

The cell separation theory suggested that the progressive change of rheologic properties of flowing blood under pressure was the principal cause of autoregulation. As pressure increased, more axial streaming would occur, leading to a higher functional hematocrit in the interlobular arteries and subsequently greater viscosity and resistance. This increase in resistance would then diminish flow. The converse would occur as perfusion pressure decreased. Direct measurements have been unable to document such changes in hematocrit, however, and autoregulation has been observed when kidneys are perfused with artificial noncellular fluids.

The tissue pressure theory suggests that with changes in perfusion pressure a parallel change in renal interstitial pressure occurs and therefore a rise in renal vascular resistance; however, direct measurements of capillary hydraulic pressure have shown that this pressure remains relatively constant over a wide range of perfusion pressure. There are a number of other experimental findings which have negated this theory.

The myogenic theory of autoregulation is based on Laplace's law of the relationship of wall tension to vessel radius and transmural pressure. As perfusion pressure and hence transmural pressure rises, the wall tension increases and the smooth muscle of the vessel wall constricts to diminish the vessel radius. Hence when perfusion pressure is increased the vessel radius decreases, resistance increases, and flow remains relatively constant. Although no direct observations are contradictory, there are certain theoretical problems with this model.

Most recently the feedback hypothesis has been advocated by Thurau and Schnermann to explain autoregulation. This theory proposes that the delivery of solute to the macula densa controls the release of renin. As sodium chloride delivery into the macula densa increases, more renin is supposedly released, causing an increase in intrarenal angiotension generation and subsequent afferent arteriolar vasoconstriction and diminished blood flow. With a diminished blood flow, a diminished distal tubular delivery would occur, thereby decreasing renin release and completing the cycle. Although there are complicated micropuncture experiments to support this theory, there is also a wide variety of contradictory data. For example, when an increased distal sodium chloride delivery occurs, renal venous and renal lymphatic angiotensin II is diminished, not increased as proposed in this theory. In addition, models using a constant renal angiotensin II infusion still show autoregulation, although it is set at a lower basal level.

No totally acceptable theory to explain autoregulation has emerged, although the myogenic theory has the fewest negative features and most reasonably accounts for this phenomenon.

VASOACTIVE SUBSTANCES AND RENAL BLOOD FLOW

Because of the simplicity of renal blood flow measurement, the renal vasculature has become a prototype for the study of vasoactive substances. Multiple agents, some of pathophysiologic interest and others of pharmocologic interest only, will be discussed in this section. It must be recognized, however, that many of these data are derived from exogenous infusion of vasoactive agents and therefore may have only pharmocologic and not physiologic importance.

Acetylcholine infused into the renal artery of experimental animals at a dose of 1–2 μg/kg/min causes a marked increase in renal blood flow, diuresis, and natriuresis. This effect is mediated by cholinergic renal receptors, since it can be totally blocked by atropine. At large pharmacologic doses or when preceded by guanethidine or phenoxybenzamine, however, acetylcholine becomes a renal vasoconstrictor by an unknown mechanism. Although it is difficult to separate the vasodilatory and natriuretic effects of this agent, it is likely the natriuresis and diuresis is not purely a consequence of the increase in renal cortical blood flow.

Bradykinin is a naturally occurring vasodilatory polypeptide released from an α_2 globulin precursor by the kallikrein enzyme system (see the chapter on *Kinins*). It appears to be the major component of the vasoactive kinins formed in the above manner. Its effects on renal hemodynamics and tubular function are similar to acetylcholine, although the receptor mechanism has not been clarified. Some investigators have suggested that kinins are modulators of renal hemodynamics and sodium excretion. Others have suggested that the effects of the kinins are totally mediated by the release of renal prostaglandins.

Prostaglandins (PG) are long chain unsaturated fatty acid derivatives of arachidonic acid (see the chapter on *Prostaglandins*). The major renal prostaglandins include PGE_2, thromboxanes, $PGF_{2\alpha}$, PGD_2 and PGI_2. It is now clear that the kidney not only excretes these substances but also produces them. Determination of the exact cells responsible for the production of various prostaglandins is likely important and is the focus of much ongoing research. In most mammalian species studied, PGE_2 is quantitatively the major prostaglandin produced in the kidney. Exogenous infusion of this agent has effects similar to acetylcholine and bradykinin, causing renal vasodilatation, natriuresis, and diuresis. Thromboxanes, on the other hand, appear to have a vasoconstrictor effect on the renal vasculature. Although much work is yet to be done, in general renal prostaglandins appear to be locally active hormones whose effects may be variable in different parts of the kidney due to local production and local degradation. Many investigators believe this system is an important physiologic modulator of renal function. Clearly in some pathophysiologic states, inhibition of prostaglandin synthesis is associated with major changes in renal function.

Secretin is a gastrointestinal hormone whose major function is to enhance pancreatic bicarbonate secretion. When infused intrarenally this hormone has been noted to produce marked renal vasodilatation with very minimal change in urinary sodium or water excretion. This observation is of interest because it clearly separates a rise in renal blood flow from sodium and water excretion and implies that the natriuretic and diuretic effect of other renal vasodilators may be mediated by a mechanism other than renal vasodilatation.

Recently the intrarenal infusion of histamine has been shown to increase renal blood flow and induce both a natriuresis and diuresis. Studies using competitive antagonists suggest the presence of both H_1 and H_2 receptors, probably with different effects. The relationship of these findings to renal pathophysiology is yet to be defined.

Isoproterenol, a β adrenergic stimulator, causes renal vasodilation at low doses, an action which is blocked by propranolol. At high doses, however, vasoconstriction occurs, which is partially blocked by the α adrenergic blocking drug phentolamine. Thus there is good evidence for both α and β adrenergic renal vascular receptors.

Norepinephrine and epinephrine, the two major circulating catecholamines, are both renal vasoconstrictors whose effects are dose dependent. These agents may preferentially increase the postglomerular efferent arteriolar resistance and thus increase the ratio of the glomerular filtration rate to the renal plasma flow (filtration faction).

Dopamine is another naturally occurring catecholamine whose major function appears to be predominantly in the central nervous system; however, either through α and β adrenergic or separate dopaminergic receptors, dopamine exerts an effect on vascular smooth muscle. Although essentially a vasoconstrictor in most vascular beds, dopamine vasodilates the renal vasculature through specific dopaminergic receptors. At very high doses α adrenergic receptor stimulation leads to vasoconstriction. Because of its unique properties dopamine has now become a very popular drug for the treatment of noncardiac "shock." Dopamine elevates blood pressure like norepinephrine, but since renal vasodilatation occurs (unless very high doses are used), the complications of progressive renal insufficiency are less common than with norepinephrine.

Angiotensin II is among the most potent renal vasoconstrictors known, but its mechanism of action is unclear. There is evidence for specific renal angiotensin receptors. In almost any state in which circulating levels of renin and angiotensin II are elevated, inhibition of angiotensin II causes a marked fall in blood pressure. Although it would seem that elevated angiotensin II levels would lead to a marked fall in renal blood flow, this vasoconstrictor effect is partially offset by angiotensin II stimulation of vasodilatory renal prostaglandin production. In the basal state when renin and angiotensin II levels are normal or low, blockade of this system has minimal hemodynamic effects. Therefore this system is clearly important in the maintenance of blood pressure in certain states associated with a diminished "effective" volume. The importance of angiotensin II in the normal control of renal blood flow, although vigorously debated, is yet uncertain.

RENAL BLOOD FLOW DISTRIBUTION AND SODIUM EXCRETION

As well as a change in total renal blood flow, the distribution of cortical blood flow and papillary blood flow have been thought to be important in determining the regulation of sodium and water balance. It was once suggested that juxtamedullary nephrons intrinsically had an enhanced capacity to reabsorb sodium. Thus a redistribution of blood flow to these nephrons would seemingly lead to an antinatriuretic state; yet numerous studies utilizing the radioactive microsphere method to measure the distribution of cortical blood flow were not in keeping with that view. Recent micropuncture studies have also shown that the juxtamedullary nephrons reabsorb less sodium than superficial cortical nephrons during extracellular volume expansion. Thus it is possible that any maneuver which redistributes blood toward deep nephrons may enhance sodium excretion. Indeed many vasodilator substances redistribute blood flow in such a manner. On the other hand, other vasodilatory maneuvers which also redistribute blood flow to inner cortical nephrons, including aortic constriction and elevated ureteral pressure, are antinatriuretic states. Most vasoconstrictor substances decrease blood flow uniformly. Hence the distribution of cortical flow would not appear to uniformly correlate with changes in sodium excretion. Changes in papillary flow may, however, play a major role in regulating sodium excretion. Theories have been proposed to explain how a rise in papillary flow with a resultant reduction in papillary tonicity will cause an increase in sodium excretion, yet it should be remembered that water diuresis may increase papillary flow and decrease medullary tonicity without causing a natriuresis.

REFERENCES

Dunn MJ, Hood VL: Prostaglandins and the kidney. Am J Physiol 233 (3):F169–F184, 1977 [or Am J Physiol Renal Fluid Electrolyte Physiol 2 (3):F169, 1977]

Kriz W, Barrett JM, Peter S: The renal vasculature: Anatomic-functional aspects, in Guyton A (series ed): International Review of Physiology. Volume 2: Kidney and Urinary Tract Physiology II; K Thurau (volume ed). Baltimore, University Park Press, 1976, p 3

Stein JH: The renal circulation, in Brenner BM, Rector FC (eds): The Kidney. Philadelphia, W.B. Saunders, 1976

Stein JH, Boonjarern S, Wilson CB, et al: Alterations in intrarenal blood flow distribution; Methods of measurement and relationship to sodium balance. Circ Res Suppl 332:I61, 1973

Stein JH, Lameire NH, Earley LE: Renal hemodynamic factors and the regulation of sodium excretion, in Andreoli TE, Hoffman JF, Fanestil DD (eds): Physiology of Membrane Disorders. New York, Plenum, 1978, p 739

SODIUM TRANSPORT

H. John Reineck and Jay H. Stein

Sodium salts are virtually restricted to the extracellular fluid space (ECF) and comprise the bulk of total solute in this compartment. Because the concentration of sodium is maintained relatively constant by thirst mechanisms and the appropriate release or suppression of antidiuretic hormone, the volume of the ECF is dependent upon the quantity of total body sodium. Maintaining this quantity at a constant level requires that sodium excretion equals sodium intake. Because this latter factor may vary widely, the maintenance of this balance requires a sensitive mechanism for the control of sodium excretion. In mammals, this important responsibility has been assigned to the kidney. This chapter deals with the mechanisms by which this organ carries out this assignment and thus controls the ECF volume.

RENAL REGULATION OF SODIUM EXCRETION

The urinary excretion of sodium is determined by the difference between the rate of sodium filtration by the glomerulus and its rate of reabsorption by the tubule. Theoretically, therefore, urinary sodium excretion can be controlled by altering either of these components.

Glomerular Filtration Rate

In normal man the filtered load of sodium equals approximately 24,000 mEq per day. On a normal diet, the urinary excretion rate is about 1 percent of this amount, 240 mEq per day, indicating that 99 percent is reabsorbed. If the GFR increased by as little as 1 percent and reabsorption remained unchanged, urinary sodium excretion would double. Conversely, small decreases in GFR would be reflected by a relatively large fall in sodium excretion. Therefore it is conceivable that very small and even imperceptible changes in GFR are important in controlling urinary sodium excretion. Several observations make this unlikely, however. First, experimental data clearly demonstrate that an increase in GFR is accompanied by a rise in tubular reabsorption of sodium and that a fall in GFR results in diminished reabsorption. This direct relationship between filtration and reabsorption is termed glomerulotubular balance. Second, if GFR is chronically reduced, either in experimental animals or by disease in man,

the volume of the ECF is controlled as sodium balance is maintained by appropriate adjustments in the rate of tubular reabsorption. Thus even though it is possible that small changes in GFR contribute to the control of urinary sodium excretion, it is clear that the major mechanisms for the control of sodium excretion must reside at the level of the renal tubule.

Tubular Reabsorption

Despite intensive efforts over the past two decades, investigators have been unable to define clearly the factors controlling the rate of tubular sodium reabsorption. Those factors which may be important in determining this rate include aldosterone, the peritubular capillary forces (hydrostatic and colloid osmotic pressures), medullary blood flow, redistribution of renal blood flow or glomerular filtrate, "natriuretic hormone," and sympathetic nerve activity.

Aldosterone. The fact that aldosterone is necessary for the maintenance of normal sodium balance is illustrated by the observation of renal salt wasting in adrenal insufficiency. Since volume depletion stimulates and expansion suppresses aldosterone secretion, it was attractive to credit this hormone with an important regulatory role in controlling urinary sodium excretion and ECF volume. Although the specific site of action of aldosterone is presently controversial, clearance and micropuncture studies have clearly demonstrated the importance of this hormone in the tubular reabsorption of sodium, especially along the distal nephron.

Several observations, however, indicate that aldosterone is not the primary regulator of urinary sodium excretion. First, a variety of studies indicate that the hormone requires at least 30–60 min to exert its effect on sodium transport, presumably because its action requires the induction of an intracellular or membrane-bound protein, yet changes in sodium excretion occur immediately after a wide variety of maneuvers. Second, patients with adrenal insufficiency on a fixed dosage of both mineralocorticoid and cortisone maintain sodium balance despite an inability to regulate secretion of these hormones. Third, the chronic administration of mineralocorticoid causes only a transient period of salt retention after which sodium balance is restored.

This so-called "DOCA escape" phenomenon is illustrated in Fig. 1. A normal 70 kg subject who is ingesting 100 mEq of sodium per day is in the steady state as urinary excretion equals this intake. After mineralocorticoid is administered, a period of sodium and water retention ensues which lasts for 3–5 days. Then, in spite of continued mineralocorticoid administration, a natriuresis occurs and the subject goes back into balance albeit at a higher level of ECF volume.

From these data it would therefore seem clear that factors other than aldosterone secretion must play a role in the regulation of tubular sodium reabsorption. The unequivocal proof of this statement was obtained by de Wardener and his colleagues in a group of classic experiments.

At the time that study was performed (1961), there was still a prevalent view that an unmeasurable increase in GFR and changes in aldosterone secretion might be of major importance in determining the natriuresis which occurs with expansion of the ECF volume. To examine this question, de Wardener decreased the GFR and the filtered load of sodium by reducing the perfusion pressure to the kidneys of dogs with an inflatable balloon placed in the aorta cephalad to the renal artery. In addition, supraphysiologic doses of mineralocorticoid were given prior to and during the experiment. In spite of these maneuvers and a resultant marked fall in GFR, a natriuresis occurred when a large infusion of isotonic saline was given to the animal. Although the natriuresis was certainly greater when the balloon was deflated and the filtered load increased, these studies provided unequivocal evidence that a natriuresis could occur after expansion of the ECF volume independent of GFR and aldosterone. Since that time, a number of laboratories have examined other possible factors which may play a major role in the control of the efferent limb of volume regulation. The main possibilities will be discussed individually.

Peritubular capillary forces. Over a century ago, Ludwig initially proposed that tubular reabsorption was totally a passive phenomenon due to a fall in hydrostatic pressure in the postglomerular capillaries coupled with the concentration of nonfilterable solutes in the capillary circulation. This view was quite intuitive, since Starling's classic description of the forces affecting solute and water movement across the capillary was not to be published until a half century later. But, tubular transport cannot be explained on the basis of the Ludwig hypothesis alone. First, active transport of sodium or its accompanying anion has been demonstrated in virtually every portion of the nephron. Second, the passive reabsorption thesis is not compatible with the ability of the mammalian kidney to both concentrate and dilute the final urine. These two points in particular dissuaded a number of investigators from seriously considering the role of the capillary circulation in the regulation of salt and water balance. Although there is clearly active transport of sodium and/or chloride along the nephron, changes in hydrostatic and/or oncotic pressure in the peritubular capillary circulation may in some manner modify the net reabsorption of electrolytes. In fact, in a recent study it was shown that an effect of oncotic pressure on proximal tubular sodium reabsorption could be demonstrated only in the presence of an intact active transport system. Thus the active transport of sodium and other electrolytes in no way obviates a role for these passive forces in altering the composition of the final urine.

In order to understand more clearly the role of these so-called "physical factors," a few basic comments are warranted. Along the glomerular capillary net ultrafiltration is favored at least in a portion of the glomerulus because of the transcapillary hydrostatic

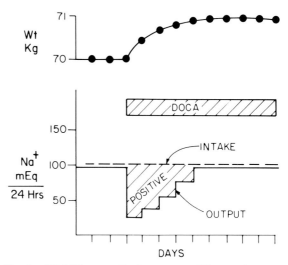

Fig. 1. "DOCA escape" phenomenon. When an individual with constant sodium intake receives mineralocorticoid, a period of positive sodium balance and weight gain occurs. After 3–5 days, however, new steady state ensues with sodium excretion again equal to sodium intake, and no further weight gain occurs.

pressure gradient (ΔP). Because the glomerular capillary is impermeable to protein as filtration occurs, the transcapillary colloid osmotic pressure difference ($\Delta\Pi$) rises until it equals ΔP (see the chapter on *Glomerular Filtration Rate*). The reverse forces are operative in the peritubular capillary. Because of the marked hydrostatic pressure drop from the glomerulus to the peritubular capillary, $\Delta\Pi$ exceeds ΔP and absorption of reabsorbate into the capillary occurs. ΔP is equal to P_C-P_I, where P_C and P_I are the capillary and interstitial hydrostatic pressure, respectively, while $\Delta\Pi$ is equal to $\Pi_C - \Pi_I$, where Π_C and Π_I are the capillary and interstitial colloid osmotic pressures, respectively. Thus the fluid exchanges across the capillary wall at any point can be expressed as

$$J_v = K\,(\Pi_C - \Pi_I) - (P_C - P_I) \qquad (1)$$

where J_v is the net transcapillary fluid flux and K is the effective hydraulic permeability of the capillary wall.

Although it has recently become popular to consider these passive forces totally as a function of the mass balances shown in Equation 1, it must be remembered that the primary regulatory events which alter either ΔP or $\Delta\Pi$ are hemodynamic. For example, increases in renal blood flow caused by various stimuli (e.g., vasodilator agents, extracellular volume expansion, etc.) are usually associated with a fall in filtration fraction (*FF*). As originally derived by Bresler,

$$C_E = \frac{C_A}{1 - FF} \qquad (2)$$

where C_E and C_A are efferent and afferent arteriolar protein concentrations, respectively. Rearranging,

$$FF = 1 - \frac{C_A}{C_E} \qquad (3)$$

From Equation 3 it is clear that at any given C_A a fall in filtration fraction will decrease C_E. In addition, vasodilation will increase P_C because of the fall in resistance at the efferent arteriole. Thus renal vasodilation will decrease C_E and increase P_C, both alterations which would tend to decrease capillary uptake.

Even with this basic understanding of the relationship between capillary uptake and the Starling forces acting across the peritubular capillary, a rather complex mechanism is required to explain how alterations in these parameters may modify urinary sodium excretion. The initial Ludwig hypothesis suggesting a direct osmotic gradient between peritubular capillary and tubular lumen is not seemingly plausible. Recent basic observations, however, have led to the development of a pump_leak model schematically shown in Fig. 2. This model is clearly applicable only to the proximal tubule.

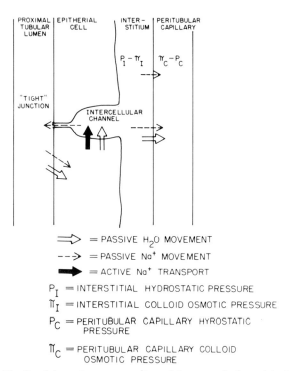

=> = PASSIVE H₂O MOVEMENT

--> = PASSIVE Na⁺ MOVEMENT

⟹ = ACTIVE Na⁺ TRANSPORT

P_I = INTERSTITIAL HYDROSTATIC PRESSURE

π_I = INTERSTITIAL COLLOID OSMOTIC PRESSURE

P_C = PERITUBULAR CAPILLARY HYROSTATIC PRESSURE

π_C = PERITUBULAR CAPILLARY COLLOID OSMOTIC PRESSURE

Fig. 2. Schematic representation of the pump_leak model of proximal tubular sodium reabsorption. Filtered sodium is passively reabsorbed from the tubular lumen into the epithelial cell down a concentration gradient. It is then actively transported into the lateral intercellular channel, which communicates directly with the interstitial space. The uptake of reabsorbate from the interstitium into the peritubular capillary is determined by Starling's forces acting across the capillary wall. If the net force for uptake of reabsorbate into the capillary is decreased, conductive and/or geometric changes in the tight junction_interspace complex may occur which favor increased "back leak" of reabsorbate into the tubular lumen, diminishing net reabsorption.

Electrophysiologic studies have demonstrated that the proximal convoluted tubule possesses typical characteristics of a leaky epithelium. When an electrical current is passed along the proximal convoluted tubule, there is significant shunting across some high-conductance pathway. Virtually all evidence points to the tight junction and/or lateral intercellular space as the site of this shunt pathway. In this model, sodium moves into the cell down a concentration gradient and then is actively transported into the interspace, with water following because of the osmotic gradient created by the sodium transport. In the original formulation of this model, a markedly hypertonic interstitium was predicted, but recent work has suggested that only a small osmotic gradient need be generated to have the system function efficiently. Fluid moves from the intercellular channel into the interstitium by a hydrostatic pressure gradient generated in the channel. The reabsorbate entering the interstitium is then removed at a rate determined by the Starling forces acting across the peritubular capillary. If, in a given setting, the rate of reabsorption exceeds the rate of capillary uptake, interstitial volume will increase. For example, a decrease in capillary oncotic pressure and/or a rise in capillary hydrostatic pressure would decrease the rate of uptake out of the renal interstitium. This alteration in interstitial volume may then lead to a change in the conductance and/or the geometry of the tight junction_intercellular channel complex with a resultant increase in the flux of sodium back into the lumen of the proximal tubule (back leak). The net effect of this particular alteration would be a decrease in net sodium transport in the proximal tubule even though active transport was unchanged. Although a number of the specific aspects of this model are still controversial, the general description would seem to be a reasonable working hypothesis. In any case, from this model one can see how alterations in Starling's forces in the peritubular capillary circulation may modify net sodium transport in the proximal convoluted tubule. Indeed, both clearance and micropuncture studies have confirmed this general relationship between capillary forces and urinary sodium excretion.

Medullary blood flow. In addition to the alterations in net transport in the proximal tubule which may occur by purely passive means, a theory has been formulated to explain how hemodynamic alterations may change sodium transport in the distal nephron. Earley and Friedler proposed that an increase in medullary blood flow as may occur during extracellular volume expansion may depress sodium reabsorption in the ascending limb of Henle's loop as a consequence of the dissipation of the usual hypertonicity of the renal medulla. The theory is as follows: Conditions associated with an increase in medullary blood flow will "wash out" the hypertonic medullary interstitium. This will decrease the abstraction of water out of the descending limb of Henle's loop which normally occurs because of the high medullary tonicity. Thus an increased volume of fluid with the same total content of sodium will be delivered to the water-impermeable ascending limb. If there is a lower limit to the sodium concentration which can be generated along the ascending limb, then more sodium will be delivered to the distal portions of the nephron. Although this hypothesis has not been adequately tested, it does seem to be a reasonable model to explain at least a portion of the natriuresis seen in settings such as extracellular volume expansion.

Redistribution of blood flow and/or filtrate. Alterations in the distribution of renal blood flow have also been suggested to effect urinary sodium excretion. According to this original theory, deep nephrons may have a greater sodium reabsorption capacity than more superficial nephrons, and thus the redistribution of flow to deep nephrons would result in sodium retention. Data to support this hypothesis have been obtained utilizing an inert gas washout technique. A recent review, however, has summarized the current status of this controversial field. With compilation of data from a large number of studies employing the radiolabeled microsphere method, no correlation between the changes in distribution and urinary sodium excretion could be demonstrated. A redistribution of renal blood flow does not necessarily indicate a redistribution of glomerular filtrate. Multiple laboratories have utilized micropuncture methods as well as a technique which determines the nephron uptake of ^{14}C-ferrocyanide (Hanssen technique) to determine the distribution of nephron GFR. The results of these studies are somewhat conflicting, yet it would seem fair to say there is generally no evidence to suggest that a redistribution of glomerular filtrate is consistently noted in a given experimental setting. Therefore it is unlikely that distribution changes in renal blood flow or glomerular filtration are important determinants of urinary sodium excretion.

It should also be recalled that the original hypothesis (the larger juxtamedullary nephrons could reabsorb more sodium) was based strictly on anatomic data. Recently, investigators utilizing the isolated perfused tubule technique have evaluated the transport characteristics of rabbit proximal tubules from superficial and juxtamedullary nephrons. Although fascinating electrophysiologic differences have been noted, the physiologic significance of these findings is unclear. Lastly, it is also worthy of note that recent micropuncture studies have indicated that sodium transport may even be inhibited to a greater extent in juxtamedullary nephrons during Ringer loading. This phenomenon will be discussed in greater detail subsequently.

"Natriuretic hormone." Since the classic studies of de Wardener that demonstrated that factors other than GFR and aldosterone are involved in the control of urinary sodium excretion, a great deal of interest has centered on the identification and isolation of a humoral substance effecting sodium transport; de Wardener himself hypothesized the existence of such a "natriuretic hormone." Many investigators, including de Wardener, have described inhibitors of sodium transport in plasma

or urine of both man and animals after expansion of the ECF volume. In addition, such a substance has been found in the plasma of uremic subjects and postulated to account for the ability of individuals with diminished nephron mass to maintain sodium balance.

In a recent review, Dirks et al. compiled a list of investigators describing the existence of some yet undefined humoral factor which is important in the regulation of sodium excretion. It should be pointed out, however, that attempts to identify chemically this elusive substance have been to date unsuccessful. In addition, recent studies examining the response to ECF volume expansion have clearly demonstrated that exposure of the kidney to the hemodynamic consequences of expansion are necessary for the normal natriuretic response to this maneuver. These findings argue strongly against the existence of a humoral substance of nonrenal origin and in fact cast considerable doubt on the physiologic importance of such a hormone, at least in the response to ECF volume expansion. Thus while the search for a humoral regulator of sodium balance other than aldosterone continues, its very existence as well as its precise role are still uncertain.

Sympathetic activity. Altered adrenergic nervous activity can modify urinary sodium excretion by influencing Starling's forces in the peripheral capillary bed, by affecting the central blood volume and thus the distribution of the ECF, or by changing renal hemodynamics. A more direct effect of the autonomic nerve activity on renal sodium handling has also been demonstrated. Many studies in anesthetized animals have shown that either anatomic or pharmacologic unilateral renal denervation leads to a significant ipsilateral increase in sodium excretion. Conversely, renal nerve stimulation decreases sodium excretion.

The mechanism by which renal nerve activity alters sodium excretion remains controversial. Several authors have demonstrated that an increase in GFR or renal blood flow occurs with renal denervation. Recent studies in the rat and dog, however, describe diminished proximal reabsorption of sodium in the absence of measurable changes in GFR and/or renal blood flow. Further, micropuncture studies indicate that renal hemodynamics are not involved in the diminished proximal sodium reabsorption and postulate that a direct effect on tubular transport may be operative. In this regard, anatomic and histochemical studies have indicated innervation of renal tubules in the rat. Additionally, several in vitro studies have demonstrated that catecholamines directly affect active sodium transport.

It should be noted, however, that several investigators have studied the effect of chronic unilateral denervation in the conscious animal and have found no effect on sodium excretion. Furthermore, renal denervation fails to blunt either the antinatriuretic response to hemorrhage or the natriuretic response to volume expansion in awake dogs. Therefore further studies are needed to better define the role of the renal nerves in the physiologic control of urinary sodium excretion.

SEGMENTAL ANALYSIS
OF SODIUM TRANSPORT

This section evaluates the qualitative and quantitative aspects of sodium transport in the various nephron segments.

Proximal Tubule

The proximal tubule normally reabsorbs 50–75 percent of the filtered load of sodium. Reabsorption along this segment is isosmotic, as evidenced by tubular fluid to plasma osmolar and sodium concentration ratios of unity. That the reabsorption of sodium is at least in part due to active transport has been shown by several well established observations. First, inhibitors of $Na^+ K^+$ ATPase decrease proximal sodium reabsorption by approximately 35 percent. Second, while the exact quantitative value of the early proximal tubular transepithelial potential differential (PD) is controversial, most investigators agree that it is oriented lumen negative. Finally, if a poorly reabsorbable substance such as raffinose or mannitol is placed within the proximal tubular lumen in vivo or in vitro, the ratio of tubular fluid to plasma sodium in the steady state is less than unity. All of these findings are compatible with a transport process which is active in nature. It should be emphasized, however, that passive forces also appear to be involved in the proximal reabsorption of sodium.

Several investigators have demonstrated by both in vivo and in vitro techniques that sodium transport along the proximal convoluted tubule is linked to the active reabsorption of bicarbonate, glucose, and amino acids. According to the theory first proposed by Rector and colleagues, a significant portion of proximal tubular sodium reabsorption is passive following bulk fluid reabsorption but is dependent on active bicarbonate and glucose reabsorption. Subsequently, amino acid transport has also been shown to influence net sodium reabsorption. Recent studies in vivo in the rat and in vitro in the isolated rabbit tubule have described a small but consistent negative PD in the early proximal convoluted tubule which is dependent on glucose and amino acid transport. In the later portion of the proximal tubule, the tubular fluid to plasma chloride ratio exceeds unity, presumably due to the preferential reabsorption of bicarbonate more proximally. This gives rise to the development of a positive PD caused by diffusion of chloride down its concentration gradient in this later portion of the proximal convoluted tubule.

In the straight portion of the proximal tubule (pars recta) sodium reabsorption also occurs. Because this tubular segment is inaccessible to micropuncture, information regarding this portion of the nephron is derived solely from in vitro microperfusion studies of isolated rabbit tubules. When straight proximal tubules from superficial nephrons are perfused with a solution identical to that found at the end of the convoluted tubule, this segment maintains a lumen positive PD and a significant portion of net sodium transport is dependent on this passive chloride gradient. Nonetheless, active sodium reabsorption also occurs, since either

cooling the bath or addition of ouabain to the bath inhibits sodium reabsorption. Recent studies have demonstrated intrinsic differences between straight proximal tubules of superficial and deep nephrons, the former being chloride permselective and the latter more permeable to sodium. The significance of this finding is not clear, however, since net fluid reabsorption did not differ in the pars recta of the two nephron populations.

In addition to affecting net sodium reabsorption, information has accumulated indicating that the proximal straight tubule actively secretes organic solutes. In fact, when exposed to high concentrations of paraaminohippurate, net fluid secretion is observed. Under certain circumstances such secretory activity could alter net sodium and fluid transport in this segment.

While the active transport of organic substances and hydrogen ion secretion may effect sodium reabsorption, passive physical phenomena also appear to play an important role in the regulation of net sodium transport in the proximal tubule. As was discussed previously in detail, the hydrostatic and oncotic pressures in the peritubular circulation are major determinants of net sodium reabsorption in the proximal tubule.

In summary, proximal reabsorption is at least in part due to active transport of sodium. In addition, a portion of sodium reabsorption may be linked to the development of a positive potential difference across the late proximal tubule as well as to bulk flow of reabsorbate. Finally, net sodium reabsorption is further modulated by Starling's forces across the proximal tubule. The relative importance of each of these phenomena is unclear.

Since the advent of micropuncture techniques, many laboratories have documented that ECF volume expansion diminishes both fractional and absolute reabsorption along the proximal convoluted tubule. Conversely, sodium retaining states have been shown to enhance proximal reabsorption. This latter observation has now been demonstrated in a variety of experimental models including diuretic-induced volume depletion, bile duct obstruction, chemically induced hepatic disease, and inferior vena caval ligation. Thus proximal tubular sodium reabsorption appears to respond appropriately to changes in extracellular fluid volume.

Loop of Henle

Current concepts of sodium transport along the loop of Henle are derived largely from in vitro microperfusion studies performed on isolated rabbit tubules. The descending limb of Henle's loop is virtually impermeable to sodium. The thin ascending limb of Henle's loop affects net sodium reabsorption. In vitro studies have provided a model for passive sodium transport in this segment in which net reabsorption is dependent upon the generation of a concentration gradient for sodium between tubular lumen and interstitium. In this regard, in vivo micropuncture studies in the rat demonstrate a sodium concentration gradient from lumen to vasa recta in hydropenic rats, suggesting that passive flux of sodium may indeed occur. The thick ascending segment of Henle's loop has been extensively studied. Several investigators found a lumen positive PD generated by active chloride transport. These findings suggest that sodium reabsorption occurs passively down an electrochemical gradient.

Absolute sodium reabsorption along the loop of Henle of superficial nephrons varies directly with changes in delivery to that segment. The change in fractional reabsorption (i.e., the percentage of delivered sodium reabsorbed) along Henle's loop as a function of delivery is less certain. Nonetheless, there is no evidence that sodium transport in the loop of Henle, at least of superficial nephrons, is inhibited by extracellular volume expansion. It should be cautioned, however, that sodium reabsorption along the loop of Henle of deep nephrons may be affected by changes in ECF volume. Recent studies have demonstrated a greater delivery of sodium to the base of the papillary collecting duct than to the late distal tubule of superficial nephrons (Fig. 3). This finding was interpreted to indicate a greater inhibition of sodium transport in inner cortical nephrons during expansion of the extracellular fluid volume. Further studies localized this greater inhibition of sodium transport to the loop of Henle of these nephrons. Juxtamedullary nephrons have a thin ascending limb in which sodium reabsorption occurs because of a concentration gradient developed by the accumulation of urea in the medullary interstitium. Saline loading markedly decreases the hypertonicity of the medullary interstitium and abolishes this concentration gradient. Thus sodium transport in the thin ascending limb of these nephrons may be markedly decreased during extracellular expansion. In contrast, the loop of Henle of superficial nephrons of the rat is made up only of a thick ascending limb which presumably transports sodium chloride only by an active process which is seemingly not impaired by volume expansion.

Distal Convoluted Tubule

Net sodium reabsorption occurs along the distal convoluted tubule. Electrical measurements indicate a lumen negative PD, the magnitude increasing progressively along the length of the distal convoluted tubule. While the sodium concentration of the tubular fluid varies depending on the model studied, the tubular fluid to plasma sodium concentration gradient is normally less than unity and progressively decreases along the length of the segment. Thus sodium reabsorption occurs against an electrochemical gradient, indicating an active transport process. Unlike the proximal convoluted tubule, which, as discussed above, has a low electrical resistance and high sodium chloride permeability, the electrical resistance is high along the distal convoluted tubule. This property will allow the establishment and maintenance of a high transepithelial sodium concentration gradient.

Micropuncture studies of sodium transport along the distal convoluted tubule during ECF volume expansion demonstrate increased absolute and decreased fractional reabsorption. Furthermore, in vivo microper-

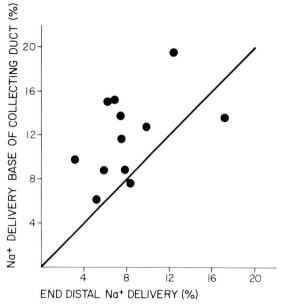

Fig. 3. In 10 of 12 studies sodium delivery to the base of the papillary collecting duct exceeded delivery to the end of distal tubule of superficial nephrons. This finding suggests a greater inhibition of sodium reabsorption in juxtamedullary nephrons in response to ECF volume expansion. [Reprinted with permission from Stein et al: Direct measurement of papillary collecting duct sodium transport in the rat. J Clin Invest 58:767, 1976.]

fusion studies describe a direct correlation between perfusion rate and sodium reabsorption. Saline loading did not qualitatively or quantitatively alter this relationship.

Collecting Duct

Important physiologic differences appear to distinguish the cortical collecting tubule and papillary collecting duct. While some of these differences may be due to the methods utilized and the species under study, it seems appropriate to discuss these two portions of the terminal nephron separately.

Cortical collecting tubule. A large number of in vitro microperfusion studies have demonstrated net sodium reabsorption along this nephron segment. The nature of this sodium transport is not entirely clear, however. Multiple reports indicate that the PD is oriented lumen negative and have found this segment capable of generating and maintaining a sizable sodium concentration gradient. The removal of sodium from the perfusate abolishes this electrical potential, and ouabain inhibits sodium transport and causes transepithelial depolarization. These results suggest that active electrogenic sodium transport occurs along the cortical collecting duct. Recent studies have shown that this negative PD occurs only in the presence of mineralocorticoids, suggesting that mineralocorticoids are necessary for active sodium transport in this nephron segment.

Electrical resistance is high in the cortical collecting tubule compared to the proximal convoluted tubule, and measurements of unidirectional sodium flux indicate that little back leak of sodium occurs. These findings are supported by the morphologic observations that lanthanum permeability across the tight junction of the cortical collecting tubule was quite low. In summary, the cortical collecting tubule is capable of effecting net sodium reabsorption and maintaining a large concentration gradient for sodium. Recent in vitro studies suggest that this phenomenon is mineralocorticoid dependent.

Medullary collecting duct. The ability of this terminal portion of the nephron to reabsorb sodium is now well established. Studies utilizing micropuncture and microcatheterization techniques have demonstrated that the lowest tubular fluid sodium concentrations are achieved and the steepest transepithelial concentration gradients can be maintained along this segment. Recent studies in the hamster describe a significant negative electrical potential which is abolished by the substitution of choline for sodium in the tubular lumen, and the magnitude of this PD varies directly with the sodium concentration of the fluid perfusing the segment. These findings indicate that active electrogenic sodium transport occurs along the terminal collecting duct.

Micropuncture studies comparing end distal delivery and urinary excretion of sodium suggest that fractional reabsorption is depressed by ECF volume expansion. It must be stressed, however, that these studies compared late distal delivery and urinary excretion as an index of sodium reabsorption. Such an extrapolation may be invalid if nephron heterogeneity of sodium reabsorption exists. Indeed, as previously mentioned, there does seem to be a much greater inhibition of sodium transport in more inner cortical nephrons during extracellular volume expansion. Thus this type of comparison is not a valid marker of net collecting duct transport. In fact, several studies using direct micropuncture of the papillary collecting duct have described a marked increase in absolute sodium reabsorption along that segment in response to volume expansion. Therefore at present one would have to conclude that collecting duct sodium transport is not obviously impaired during acute expansion of the extracellular volume. It would seem, however, that the collecting duct must participate in the regulation of sodium balance in chronic steady-state situations.

REFERENCES

de Wardener HE, Mills IH, Claphain WF, et al: Studies on the efferent mechanism of the sodium diuresis which follows the administration of intravenous saline in the dog. Clin Sci 21:249, 1961

Dirks JH, Cirksena WJ, Berliner RW: The effect of saline infusion on sodium reabsorption by the proximal tubule of the dog. J Clin Invest 44:1160, 1965

Dirks JH, Seely J, Levy M: Control of the extracellular fluid volume and the pathophysiology of edema formation, in Brenner BM, Rector FC (eds): The Kidney. Philadelphia, W.B. Saunders, 1976, p 495

Earley LE, Daugharty TM: Sodium metabolism. N Engl J Med 281:72, 1969

Fitzgibbons JP, Geunari FJ, Garfinkel HB, et al: Dependence of saline-induced natriuresis upon exposure of the kidney to the physical effects of extracellular fluid volume expansion. J Clin Invest 54:1428, 1974

Klahr S, Slatopolsky E: Renal regulation of sodium excretion. Arch Intern Med 131:780, 1973

Lameire NH, Lifschitz MD, Stein JH: Heterogeneity of nephron function. Annu Rev Physiol 39:159, 1977

Schrier RW, de Wardener HE: Tubular reabsorption of sodium ion: Influence of factors other than aldosterone and glomerular filtration rate. N Engl J Med 285:1231 and 1292, 1971

Stein JH, Osgood RW, Kunau RT: Direct measurement of papillary collecting duct sodium transport in the rat. J Clin Invest 58:767, 1976

RENAL POTASSIUM TRANSPORT

Robert T. Kunau, Jr.

In the presence of normal renal function, the maintenance of external potassium balance depends almost exclusively upon renal potassium excretion. For example, in the normal adult ingesting 100 mEq of potassium daily, 15 mEq or less is excreted in the stool; the remainder exits via the kidneys. It is now firmly established that renal potassium transport is characterized by both secretion and reabsorption. Much of our current understanding regarding the segmental nature of potassium transport has been derived from micropuncture studies of the rat kidney. Figure 1 illustrates the quantity of potassium as a fraction of the filtered load present at various points along the superficial and juxtamedullary nephrons of the kidney of the normal antidiuretic rat. In the following, the segmental nature of potassium transport in the mammalian nephron which results in the findings observed is reviewed.

PROXIMAL CONVOLUTED TUBULE

Potassium freely traveres the glomerular barrier. Thus the concentration of potassium in the proximal convoluted tubule is the same as, or slightly lower than, the plasma concentration. For the most part, the quantity of potassium reabsorbed in the proximal convoluted tubule is controlled by those factors which govern the amount of glomerular filtrate reabsorbed in this segment. Under antidiuretic conditions, approximately 50 percent of the filtered load of potassium is reabsorbed by the end of the accessible portion of the proximal convoluted tubule. It has recently been shown that under normal circumstances the lumen is electronegative only in the initial one-third of the proximal convoluted tubule but is electropositive in the later two-thirds. It is conceivable that potassium reabsorption in the initial electronegative portion may be active, whereas the positive potential in the the later segments might facilitate reabsorption of potassium by passive means.

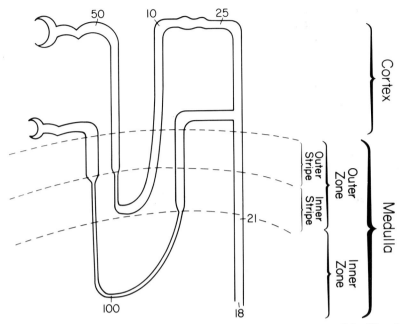

Fig. 1. Numbers indicate the quantity of potassium present as a percentage of the filtered load at the late proximal and early and late distal tubules of the superficial nephron, at the bend of Henle's loop of the juxtamedullary nephron, and at the base and tip of the papillary collecting duct. The values refer to hydropenic conditions in the rat.

PROXIMAL STRAIGHT TUBULE

When isolated segments of the pars recta of the rabbit kidney are bathed in normal rabbit serum under in vitro conditions, net fluid absorption occurs. However, when paraaminohippurate (PAH) is added to the bath, net secretion of potassium, sodium, and water occurs, presumably moving into the lumen through paracellular channels. Therefore in this nephron segment either potassium reabsorption or secretion may be observed.

DESCENDING LOOP OF HENLE

The quantity of potassium present at the bend of Henle's loop of juxtamedullary nephrons may equal or actually exceed that filtered. Recent micropuncture studies in the rat have shown that the amount of potassium present at this site depends upon the concentration of potassium at some point in the collecting system, the potassium presumably moving from the collecting duct into the medullary interstitium and then into the descending limb of Henle's loop. The amount of potassium present at the bend of Henle's loop therefore will depend upon that quantity which escapes reabsorption in more proximal portions of the nephron and that which is added in the descending limb. Since the bend of Henle's loop in superficial nephrons is not accessible to direct study, the amount of potassium at the bend in these nephrons is unknown.

ASCENDING LIMB OF HENLE'S LOOP

The quantity of potassium present at the early distal tubule of superficial nephrons is usually is about 10 percent of that filtered. This indicates that a significant amount of potassium is reabsorbed between the proximal and early distal tubules, presumably in large part in the thick ascending limb. Although the concentration of potassium at the bend of the loop of Henle is considerably higher than plasma, the potassium concentration at the early distal tubule is usually less than one-half that of plasma. Recent in vitro studies have shown that the thick ascending limb of Henle's loop actively transports chloride. As a result, an electropositive potential is developed in the lumen, and a portion of potassium, as well as sodium, reabsorption may occur by passive means.

DISTAL TUBULE

The distal tubule studied on the surface of the rat kidney may consist of several different anatomic and functional components. Thus the nature of potassium transport which is displayed between the early and late distal tubule reflects the net effect of transport processes in this heterogeneous segment. In the rat, reabsorption of potassium occurs here when the animal is ingesting a low potassium diet, whereas when the dietary intake is normal this segment secretes potassium and is a major source of the potassium present in the final urine.

In the early distal tubule, the transepithelial potential difference is oriented with the lumen either slightly positive or modestly negative. At the late distal tubular site, the potassium concentration usually exceeds the plasma concentration by severalfold and the transepithelial potential difference is oriented lumen negative by approximately 50 mV.

The nature of potassium transport in the distal tubule has been envisioned in the following manner. Potassium can move from the peritubular space into the distal tubular cell either by an active component linked to the extrusion of sodium from the cell, a transfer likely related to activity of the ATPase system, or by electrically driven passive movement. Potassium moves from the cells across the luminal border into the tubular lumen at a rate governed by the size of the transport pool of potassium in the cell, the permeability of the luminal membrane to potassium, and the magnitude of the potential difference across the membrane. Although potassium can move passively down an electrochemical gradient from the cell interior into the tubular lumen, the concentration of potassium in the lumen does not reach the level one would expect based upon the magnitude of the transepithelial potential difference. This is felt to be the result of a mechanism in the luminal membrane which actively reabsorbs potassium, thereby lowering the luminal potassium concentration below its equilibrium value. Thus although potassium transfer from cell to lumen in this schema can be considered to occur by passive means, active components of potassium transfer, both in the luminal and peritubular membranes, may play a prominent role in dictating the quantity of potassium found in the urine at this nephron site.

Finally, it should be appreciated that certain aspects of this model may require revision. Recent studies have suggested that potassium may be secreted against an electrochemical gradient in the late distal tubule. In addition, a tight coupling between the transepithelial potential difference and the ratio of the concentrations of potassium in the tubular lumen and in plasma or changes in these parameters has not been uniformly observed.

COLLECTING TUBULE AND DUCT

An assessment of the characteristics of potassium transport along the collecting system has frequently been made from a comparison of the quantity of potassium present at the superficial late distal tubule and in the final urine.

Direct study of the transport characteristics of the cortical collecting tubule can be performed only with the use of in vitro perfusion techniques. When so examined, in contrast to the findings in the distal tubule of the rat, active potassium secretion against an electrochemical gradient has been demonstrated in tubular segments isolated from rabbits maintained on a normal diet. Removal of sodium from the lumen decreases the amount of potassium secreted. This effect of sodium is felt not to be related to a coupled exchange of the two ions but is an interdependence that is more indirect.

Recent in vivo studies have indirectly shown that the cortical collecting tubule may be a significant contributor to urinary potassium excretion. In these experiments, fractional potassium delivery rates to the base of the exposed papilla and to the superficial late distal tubule were compared. Under hydropenic conditions, no net transfer of potassium was observed between late distal and the papillary base, whereas after the acute infusion of Ringer's solution net addition of potassium between late distal and papillary base occurred. This

finding was attributed to enhanced secretion by the cortical collecting tubule. Additional studies indicated that the net addition of potassium between the late distal tubule and the papillary base was not due to a greater contribution from juxtamedullary nephrons.

In vivo micropuncture studies of the terminal collecting duct of normal animals have demonstrated both potassium reabsorption and potassium secretion. Although the character of the potassium secretory process has yet to be defined, the reabsorption observed presumably is an active process as it can proceed against an electrochemical gradient.

FACTORS WHICH ALTER RENAL POTASSIUM TRANSPORT
Sodium

Clearance studies in the dog, performed 20 years ago, demonstrated that an acute reduction of the glomerular filtration rate by approximately 40 percent could reduce both potassium and sodium excretion, yet when agents were used to maintain sodium excretion at near-normal levels despite the reduction in filtration rate, potassium excretion did not fall. Studies such as these prompted the suggestion that potassium secretion in the distal tubule was dependent upon the availability of sodium for a one to one exchange to occur. Micropuncture studies in the mid 1960s directly examined the relationship between sodium reabsorption and potassium secretion in the distal tubule of the rat and observed that the quantity of potassium secreted in the distal tubule to be approximately one-tenth of the quantity of sodium reabsorbed. Since these studies were performed in sodium-deficient rats, the quantity of sodium available at the distal tubule clearly was not rate limiting for one to one exchange with potassium to occur; although potassium excretion was reduced in these rats, this was due to events beyond the late distal tubule. These studies do not exclude the possibility that sodium may have a more indirect effect on potassium transport in the distal tubule, e.g., by influencing the transepithelial potential difference. In addition, it has recently been demonstrated that the infusion of sodium-containing solutions can increase the flow rate of distal tubular fluid (see below) and thereby influence potassium transport. Of these two factors, the influence of sodium on distal tubular flow rate would appear to be more important than the effect of sodium on the transtubular potential difference in affecting distal potassium transport.

Potassium Intake

The renal response to an increase in potassium intake is to accelerate the rate of urinary potassium excretion. This response is in part influenced by the previous level of potassium ingestion, i.e., the kaliuretic response to an acute potassium load being greater in animals that have chronically been fed a high-potassium diet. Chronic high potassium ingestion in the rat increases the quantity of potassium secreted along the superficial distal tubule, whereas in the papillary collecting duct of rats fed a high-potassium diet, as in normal rats, both potassium secretion and reabsorption may be seen. The accelerated distal tubular potassium secretion seen in the potassium-loaded state may be largely due to an increase in the intracellular transport pool of potassium as a result of an increase in the peritubular uptake of potassium, although a chronic increase in potassium intake can result in a more favorable electrical gradient for distal tubular potassium secretion as well. Micropuncture studies suggest that changes in potassium transport in the superficial distal tubule are sufficient to account for the enhanced kaliuresis seen in the potassium loaded animal, yet a supplementary role for the collecting system cannot be excluded. The collecting system may serve to minimize the loss of potassium from the lumen which might occur because of a more favorable gradient of potassium between the lumen and the cell.

Recently, an increase in renal $Na^+ K^+$ ATPase activity has been implicated as playing a role in the kaliuresis associated with chronic potassium loading. Unfortunately, there is not uniform agreement regarding the area of the kidney in which an increase in enzyme activity aids in the ability of the kidney to excrete a potassium load.

In rats maintained on a potassium-deficient diet, potassium reabsorption, rather than secretion, is observed along the distal tubule and the papillary collecting duct.

Mineralocorticoids

It is generally assumed that mineralocorticoids have a profound influence on renal potassium transport by enhancing potassium secretion. The effect of mineralocorticoids on potassium transport takes place in the distal nephron as potassium transport in the proximal nephron is unaffected. Adrenalectomy abolishes the progressive increase in potassium concentration which occurs along the length of the distal tubule in norma rats. This finding may be related to two factors. First aldosterone administration to adrenalectomized rats can increase and thereby normalize the permeability of the luminal membrane of the distal tubule to potassium, an effect not mediated through steroid-induced protein synthesis. Second, chronic but not acute aldosterone administration to adrenalectomized rats results in a restoration of the distal tubular intracellular potassium content. Obviously, both effects of aldosterone would have a favorable influence on distal tubular potassium secretion.

Although mineralocorticoids may increase renal $Na^+ K^+$ stimulated ATPase activity, it is not certain to what extent this is an important aspect of their effect on potassium transport in the distal nephron.

Mineralocorticoids also appear to be capable of exerting an influence on potassium transport in the collecting system. The potential difference measured in an isolated segment of rabbit cortical collecting tubule varies depending upon the mineralocorticoid level of the animal. In tubules from rabbits fed a regular diet, the transepithelial potential difference is oriented lumen positive by approximately 4 mV. After mineralocorticoid stimulation the potential difference was found to be greater than 30 mV, lumen negative. This latter potential could favor either the entrapment of luminal potassium delivered from more proximal sites, or, if a passive element of potassium secretion were present, promote the movement of potassium from cell to lumen.

The kaliuretic effect of mineralocorticoids can be disassociated from their antinatriuretic effect. Nevertheless, when animals are maintained on a diet free of sodium, the kaliuretic response to mineralocorticoid administration can be markedly diminished, if not abolished. There appear to be several reasons for the ability of sodium-free diets to minimize the kaliuretic effect of mineralocorticoids. First, under certain circumstances sodium deficiency may enhance potassium removal from the lumen of the distal tubule. Second, sodium-deficient diets may be associated with a reduction in the flow rate of tubular fluid. Lastly, low concentrations of sodium in the cortical collecting tubule in sodium-deficient states may impair potassium secretion at this site.

Acid–Base Balance

A relationship between urine pH and potassium excretion has been frequently observed. For example, both the infusion of sodium bicarbonate and the administration of a carbonic anhydrase inhibitor render the urine alkaline and enhance potassium excretion. Respiratory and metabolic acidosis can have the opposite effect. Studies of this nature have suggested the possibility that potassium and hydrogen compete for a common secretory site.

Recent data have done much to clarify the effect of acute acid–base variations on renal potassium transport. Figure 2 illustrates the quantity of potassium, expressed as a fraction of the filtered load, present along the distal tubule of the rat under a variety of acute acid–base disturbances. Acute alkalosis of either metabolic or respiratory origin results in a marked increase in potassium secretion along the distal tubule. In contrast, both respiratory and metabolic acidosis result in a diminution of potassium secretion along this segment. The ability of acute acid–base disturbances to alter potassium secretion in the distal tubule is largely related to variations in the chemical gradient of potassium between cell and lumen. For example, acute metabolic alkalosis, induced by sodium bicarbonate infusion, increases the concentration of potassium in the intracellular transport pool by accelerating the active uptake of potassium across the peritubular border. Acidosis presumably has the opposite effect.

In vitro studies in the isolated cortical collecting tubule of the rabbit have shown that the intraluminal pH can have an influence on potassium transport at this site. Lowering of the intraluminal pH of the perfusate from 7.4 to 6.8 decreases potassium secretion by almost 50 percent. The intraluminal pH directly influences potassium transport at this site by altering an active component of potassium secretion.

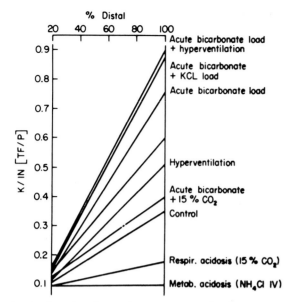

Fig. 2. Quantity of potassium present, as a fraction of filtered load, along distal tubule in various acid–base disturbances. [Reprinted with permission from Malnic G, de Mello-Aires M, Giebisch G: Potassium transport across distal tubular during acid-base disturbances. Am J Physiol 221:1192, 1971.]

Most of the above studies have dealt with acute acid–base disturbances. Under more chronic conditions, the effects of acid–base disturbances on renal potassium transport are more complex and less well understood.

Tubular Fluid and Urine Flow Rate

Recently it was demonstrated that the flow rate of tubular fluid through the distal tubule can be an important modulator of potassium transport at this site. The extent to which distal tubular potassium transport is affected by changes in the flow rate of tubular fluid depends upon the degree to which the net driving forces for cell to lumen potassium movement change as the flow rate varies. If the movement of potassium from cell to tubular lumen increases in proportion to an increase in flow rate, the quantity of potassium present at the late distal tubule will vary directly with the flow rate of tubular fluid. Conversely, should the quantity of potassium which moves from cell to tubular lumen remain constant as the flow rate is increased, the quantity of potassium at the late distal tubule will be unaffected by an increase in flow rate.

Following chronic potassium loading and the infusion of hypertonic solutions, potassium secretion in the distal tubule varies in parallel with changes in flow rate. On the other hand, in rats previously fed a low-potassium diet, the late distal potassium concentration progressively decreases as the flow rate is enhanced and potassium secretion along the length of the distal tubule does not increase as the flow rate is increased.

It was recently suggested that potassium transport in the collecting system may also be influenced by the urinary flow rate. When studied in a number of models in the rat kidney, net reabsorption has been noted along the collecting system during low urinary flow rates, whereas no net transport was apparent at higher flow rates.

REFERENCES

Brenner BM, Berliner RW: The transport of potassium, in Orloff J, Berliner RW (eds): Renal Physiology, Handbook of Physiology, Sect. 8, edited Washington, American Physiological Society, 1973, p 497

Giebisch G: Renal potassium excretion, in Rouiller C, Muller AF (eds): The Kidney, vol 3. New York, Academic Press, 1970, p 329

Grantham JJ: Renal transport and excretion of potassium, in Brenner BM, Rector FC (eds): The Kidney. Philadelphia, W.B. Saunders, 1976, p 299

Malnic G, Klose RM, Giebisch G: Micropuncture study of renal potassium excretion in the rat. Am J Physiol 206:674, 1964

Malnic G, de Mello-Aires M, Giebisch G: Potassium transport across renal distal tubular during acid-base disturbances. Am J Physiol 221:1192, 1971

Wright FS: Sites and mechanisms of potassium transport along the renal tubule. Kidney Int 11:415, 1977

HYDROGEN ION TRANSPORT

Robert T. Kunau, Jr.

Physiologic adjustments in urinary acidification are vital to the preservation of normal acid–base homeostasis. In particular, the regulation of the plasma bicarbonate concentration is for the most part dependent upon the kidney. By reabsorption of all the filtered bicarbonate below a certain threshold level, urinary loss of bicarbonate is avoided. On the other hand, when the plasma bicarbonate concentration is elevated above a threshold level, reabsorption is incomplete and the excess bicarbonate is spilled into the urine. In addition, the kidneys are also responsible for regenerating, and returning to the extracellular fluid, that bicarbonate decomposed by reaction with nonvolatile acids in the extracellular space. The quantity of bicarbonate so regenerated is equivalent to the amount of hydrogen excreted in the urine. Since little free hydrogen is present in the final urine, the quantity of bicarbonate regenerated is equivalent to the hydrogen excreted as titratable acid and ammonium (NH_4^+).

There are data which suggest that hydrogen ion secretion may be the sole means by which bicarbonate is reabsorbed and the urine acidified. As conceived, hydrogen ions produced within the cell are actively transported across the luminal membrane where they react with filtered bicarbonate (Fig. 1a) or with certain salts such as phosphate (A^-) to form titratable acid or with NH_3 to form NH_4^+ (Fig. 1b). In the first instance, filtered bicarbonate is reabsorbed; in the second, bicarbonate is regenerated. Quantitatively, the hydrogen ions utilized for bicarbonate reabsorption greatly exceed the amount which serve to generate new bicarbonate.

Although the effectiveness of the hydrogen secretory mechanism will in large part depend upon the availability of bicarbonate or other buffers within the tubular lumen, the secretory mechanism can be influenced at a number of steps. For example, any factor(s) which would reduce the supply of hydrogen to the pump or affect the membrane permeability to hydrogen ions may have a significant effect on the character of the hydrogen secretory mechanism.

The rate of hydrogen ion secretion is proportional to the chemical gradient against which they must be secreted—i.e., the concentration of buffer in the lumen—and thus is normally highly unsaturated. It is uncertain if the proportionality between hydrogen ion secretion and luminal buffer concentration indicates the presence of secretory pump which varies its rate in response to a pH gradient or a pump–leak system in which a constant pump is opposed by a variable leak of hydrogen ions from the lumen. Also, one system may be present in one segment of the nephron, while the other may be the nature of the hydrogen secretory pump in another.

The hydrogen ions may be produced within the cell by hydration of CO_2, forming carbonic acid (H_2CO_3), which disassociates into hydrogen ions and bicarbonate (Fig. 2a). Alternatively, a redox mechanism may split water into hydrogen and hydroxyl (OH^-) ions with the hydroxyl being neutralized by CO_2 (Fig. 2b). In any case, carbonic anhydrase may serve one of its several functions in the hydrogen secretory process at this step (Fig. 2). In this way, carbonic anhydrase activity would facilitate the delivery of hydrogen ions to the secretory mechanism. In addition, the removal of alkali from the cell, an impairment of which can reduce hydrogen ion secretion, may be diminished by inhibition of carbonic anhydrase. In certain portions of the nephron, luminal carbonic anhydrase may catalyze the dehydration of carbonic acid ($H_2CO_3 \xrightarrow{c.a.} CO_2 + H_2O$) within the lumen, thereby preventing a buildup of carbonic acid and lowering the pH gradient against which hydrogen ions are secreted.

The quantitative importance of carbonic anhydrase in renal hydrogen ion secretion has been a matter of considerable debate. After the systemic administration of an inhibitor of carbonic anhydrase, total renal bicarbonate reabsorption is reduced by approximately 50 percent. Free-flow micropuncture studies of the proximal convoluted tubule have shown that the systemic administration of a carbonic anhydrase inhibitor reduces fractional bicarbonate reabsorption at this site by roughly 30–40 percent. In contrast, recent in vitro studies in the convoluted and straight portions of the proximal tubule and cortical collecting tubule of the rabbit have demonstrated that when an inhibitor of carbonic anhydrase was present in the luminal perfusate, no bicarbonate was reabsorbed. A similar finding has recently been reported from in vivo perfusion studies of the rat proximal convoluted tubule. The reasons for these discrepant findings are not clear; however, until such time that the quantitative role of carbonic anhydrase is clarified, a discussion of the possible means by which hydrogen ion secretion can continue in the absence of this enzyme may properly be postponed.

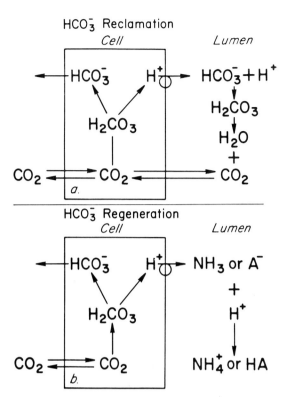

Fig. 1. Hydrogen ion secreted into the tubule lumen may result in reabsorption of the filtered bicarbonate (a) or regeneration of bicarbonate (b).

In the clinical setting, a number of factors would appear to be capable of influencing effective hydrogen ion secretion.

Extracellular fluid (ECF) volume. The state of the degree of expansion of the ECF volume may have

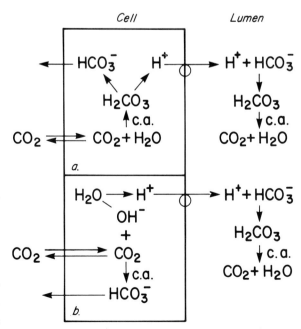

Fig. 2. Possible pathways of intracellular hydrogen ion production.

a profound influence on renal bicarbonate transport. When the plasma bicarbonate concentration is increased in a manner which minimizes the degree of expansion of the ECF volume, the capacity of the renal tubule to reabsorb bicarbonate is enhanced. Conversely, at comparable levels of plasma bicarbonate, expansion of the ECF volume with isotonic fluids results in a decrease in renal bicarbonate reabsorption. This relationship is graphically demonstrated in Fig. 3, in which a theoretical T_m bicarbonate curve is plotted. At lower bicarbonate concentrations, essentially all of the filtered bicarbonate is reabsorbed. At a plasma concentration where bicarbonate is spilling into the urine in the volume expanded state and where reabsorption is incomplete, all of the filtered bicarbonate is reabsorbed in the nonexpanded state. One can readily see that the T_m for bicarbonate or the maximum capacity of the tubule to reabsorb bicarbonate is significantly influenced by the degree of expansion of the extracellular fluid volume.

Micropuncture studies in the rat have shown that at least part of the influence of ECF volume on renal bicarbonate transport is mediated in the proximal tubule. One speculation is that the reduced rate of proximal tubular bicarbonate reabsorption seen during ECF volume expansion is due primarily to an increased back leakage of hydrogen ions.

Carbon dioxide tension (pCO₂). The demonstration of an effect of the arterial pCO_2 on renal hydrogen ion transport has been difficult. Earlier studies which concluded that an acute increase in the arterial pCO_2 raised the bicarbonate T_m were performed without the knowledge of the effect of changes in ECF volume on the T_m phenomena. Acute elevation of the pCO_2 may result in a generalized vasodilatation, a decrease in

effective ECF volume, and thus an enhanced capacity to reabsorb bicarbonate; however, careful studies in which norepinephrine was administered to prevent the vasodilatation have shown a small stimulating effect of pCO_2 on bicarbonate reabsorption.

In the absence of bicarbonate loading, it has not been possible to demonstrate an effect of hypercapnia on bicarbonate reabsorption with micropuncture techniques. After bicarbonate loading, reabsorption of bicarbonate in both the superficial proximal and distal tubules has been shown to increase with an acute elevation in the pCO_2. These findings indicate that the ability of hypercapnia to increase bicarbonate reabsorption depends not only on the increase in hydrogen ion secretion but also on the intraluminal pH and bicarbonate concentration. Under physiologic circumstances, it is possible that renal bicarbonate reabsorption is not significantly enhanced by an elevation in the arterial pCO_2 tension until such time that the intraluminal bicarbonate concentration is spontaneously increased.

Hypocapnia, as expected, has been shown to decrease hydrogen ion secretion in both the proximal and distal tubules. In contrast to hypercapnia, which appears to have a direct effect on hydrogen ion secretion, the effect of hypocapnia may be mediated through the associated increase in pH.

Calcium, phosphorous, and parathyroid hormone (PTH). A number of clinical observations have suggested that PTH may have an inhibitory effect on renal hydrogen ion secretion such that high endogenous levels may induce a metabolic acidosis. For the most part, however, it has been difficult to clearly characterize the effect of PTH on renal hydrogen ion secretion in the experimental animal. In the normal dog, PTH administration reduces renal bicarbonate reabsorption from

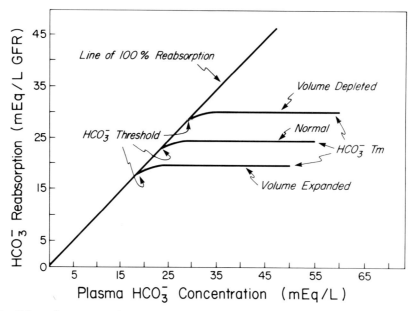

Fig. 3. Schematic representation of the effect of the state of expansion of the extracellular fluid on bicarbonate reabsorption.

around 25 to 23 mM/liter GFR. In the thyroparathyroidectomized animal, the effect is modestly greater, the reduction from 27 to 23 mM/liter GFR. Micropuncture studies, while demonstrating an inhibitory effect of PTH on proximal bicarbonate reabsorption, have not shown an increase in urinary bicarbonate excretion. At present, while it appears that PTH may affect bicarbonate transport, its physiologic role, if any, remains to be fully defined.

Systemic phorphous depletion, induced by the administration of a low-phosphorus diet and aluminum hydroxide gel to bind intestinal phosphorus, results in a modest decrease in the plasma bicarbonate concentration. Bicarbonate titration studies indicate that a decrease in both bicarbonate threshold and T_m are effected by phsophorus depletion. An interaction between the effect of phosphorus depletion and PTH on renal hydrogen ion secretion is possible inasmuch as hyperparathyroid states can induce phosphate depletion. In fact, there is some evidence that sodium phosphate administration can ameliorate the bicarbonaturia observed after the administration of PTH in certain select circumstances.

Acute hypercalcemia, per se, can induce a modest increase in the serum bicarbonate concentration.

Potassium and mineralocorticoids. The metabolic alkalosis which has been assumed to be a common companion of potassium deficiency is in truth a complex and poorly understood disorder. In the rat, the experimental induction of potassium depletion has frequently been accomplished with maneuvers which make an interpretation of the singular effect of potassium deficiency on renal hydrogen ion secretion difficult. In this species, the alkalosis which occurs after mineralocorticoid administration and dietary potassium restriction is corrected when potassium chloride is given to the nephrectomized animal. This finding suggests that the extracellular alkalosis may largely be the consequence of transcellular shifts. On the other hand, an increase in renal hydrogen ion secretion seemingly is essential to the maintenance of the alkalosis, since, if this were not the case, one might anticipate that the "excess" bicarbonate would be excreted in the urine. Nevertheless, it has not been convincingly demonstrated that the renal contribution to the maintenance of the alkalosis is a selective effect of potassium depletion.

In the dog, simple potassium depletion causes a modest metabolic acidosis as a consequence of an impaired ability to maximally acidify the urine. As a result, net acid excretion is diminished. The metabolic acidosis so generated results in an increase in NH_3 production, and, with time, urinary NH_4^+ excretion returns to normal. Of interest is the recent observation that when the potassium-deficiency-induced reduction in mineralocorticoid production is overcome by exogenous aldosterone administration, an acidosis does not develop in the potassium deficient dog. In addition, when infused with sodium bicarbonate, the potassium-deficient dog appears to reabsorb more bicarbonate

than either the normal or acutely potassium loaded dog at any level of ECF volume expansion, a finding which suggests that the capacity of the potassium-deficient dog to reabsorb bicarbonate at elevated levels may be enhanced.

The difference in response between the dog and rat to the potassium-deficient state has not been adequately defined. Conceivably, the magnitude of the contribution of transcellular shifts, variations in mineralocorticoid activity, or the role of other factors such as renal chloride wastage differ in two species.

Mineralocorticoids can induce a metabolic alkalosis when potassium deficiency is permitted to develop during their administration. Under these circumstances, urinary acid excretion and the plasma bicarbonate concentration increase. This response is blocked if the potassium deficiency can be prevented.

Mineralocorticoid deficiency may result in a metabolic acidosis as a consequence of a decrease in the rate of hydrogen ion secretion.

REFERENCES

Crumb CK, Martinez-Maldonado M, Eknoyan G, et al: Effects of volume expansion, purified parathyroid extract and calcium on renal bicarbonate absorption in the dog. J Clin Invest 54:1287, 1974

de Mello-Aires M, Malnic G: Peritubular pH and pCO_2 in renal tubular acidification. Am J Physiol 228:1766–1774, 1975

Giebisch G, Malnic G: Studies on the mechanism of tubular acidification. Physiologist 19:511, 1976

Hulter HN, Ilnicki LP, Harbottle JA, et al: Impaired renal H$^+$ secretion and NH_3 production in mineralocorticoid-deficient glucocorticoid replete dogs. Am J Physiol 232:F-136, 1977

Kurtzman NA: Regulation of renal bicarbonate reabsorption by extracellular volume. J Clin Invest 49:586, 1970

Malnic G, Giebisch G: Mechanism of renal hydrogen ion secretion. Kidney Int 1:280, 1972

Malnic G, Steinmetz PR: Transport processes in urinary acidification. Kidney Int 9:172, 1976

Rector FC Jr: Acidification of the urine, in Orloff J, Berliner RW (eds): Handbook of Physiology, section 8. Washington, D.C., American Physiology Society, p 431, 1973

WATER METABOLISM

Nama Beck

The osmotic concentration of human body fluid is maintained constant within a narrow range, 290±4 mOsm, despite a wide fluctuation of fluid intake. This fine regulatory mechanism is controlled by the thirst–neurohypophyseal–renal feedback system. Both the thirst center and the center of antidiuretic hormone secretion are in the hypothalamus. The two centers are, however, anatomically distinguishable.

THIRST

Drinking is commonly separated into primary and secondary drinking. Primary drinking occurs in response to physiological needs for fluid. Secondary drinking is not induced by an existing need for water, and the mechanisms involved are not clear. The discussion will therefore be limited to primary drinking.

There are two major thirst signals: cellular dehydration and extracellular volume depletion. Cellular dehydration may be induced by water deprivation or administration of hypertonic solutions which do not enter the cells, such as saline. Extracellular volume depletion may be seen after hemorrhage, sodium depletion, vomiting, diarrhea, or sequestration of extracellular fluid by various means.

Thirst–neurophypophyseal–renal responses maintain constant osmolality of body fluids through a feedback system. These responses, however, interact in a complex manner. For example, the drinking response to a given dipsogenic stimulus is attenuated by vasopressin infusion. The kidney also affects the thirst mechanism in a complex manner, in at least three ways. (1) The drinking response to a given dipsogenic stimulus is less in the presence of antidiuresis. (2) Water intake is greater in nephrectomized rats than normal rats in response to a given dipsogenic stimulation. These examples demonstrate fine regulatory feedback mechanisms between thirst and renal responses, since retention of free water and solute excretion through the kidney decrease the amount of water necessary to dilute the osmolality of body fluid. (3) The kidney also influences thirst mechanisms through the renin–angiotensin system.

It has become increasingly clear that the renin–angiotensin system in both the central nervous system and the kidney influences the thirst mechanism. As shown in Fig. 1, the effect of the renin–angiotensin system on the thirst mechanism is complex. The anatomical loci, sensitive to angiotensin-induced drinking, are in the vicinity of the anterior third ventricle in the brain. It has been postulated that the dipsogenic action of angiotensin is induced by vasoconstriction in the periventricular structures. The renin–angiotensin system in cerebrospinal fluid is activated in the central nervous system, and blood-borne angiotensin does not enter the central nervous system. Probably for this reason, angiotensin in the brain is more effective than blood-borne angiotensin to stimulate thirst mechanism. Renal angiotensin, however, may also be involved.

Acetylcholine or carbachol (cholinergic agents) administration induces drinking, and atropine abolishes the dipsogenic effect of these substances, suggesting that cholinergic stimulation induces drinking. The dipsogenic effect of angiotensin is, however, not mediated through cholinergic mechanisms because atropine does not influence the angiotensin-induced dipsogenic response. On the other hand, catecholamines, especially dopamine, interact with the angiotensin response. For example, 6-hydroxydopamine (which destroys catecholaminergic nerve terminals) or haloperidol (which is the antagonist of dopamine) abolish angiotensin-induced drinking without affecting the carbachol-induced thirst mechanism. These results suggest that angiotensin-induced drinking is mediated through the dopaminergic system. Norepinephrine has a more complex series of actions. On the one hand, norepinephrine causes a rapid enhancement of drinking. On the other hand, it attenuates drinking induced by cellular dehydration or carbachol. Norepinephrine, however, does not affect angiotensin-induced drinking.

Clinical Disorders of Thirst

Disorders of thirst can be divided into symptomatic and pathological thirst. Symptomatic thirst includes all cases associated with cellular dehydration or extracellular volume depletion, such as water deprivation, vomiting, diarrhea, diabetes insipidus, sodium depletion, potassium depletion, or hypercalcemia; in these cases, polydipsia is a physiological response to a need for fluid

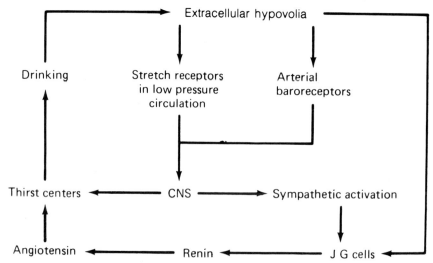

Fig. 1. Possible mechanisms for drinking caused by extracellular dehydration. [Reprinted with permission from Fitzsimons JT: The renin-angiotensin system in the control of drinking, in Martini L, Motta M, Frascini F (eds): Hypothalamus. New York, Academic Press, 1970, p 195.]

repletion. Pathological thirst is present despite normal or overhydration, e.g., brain tumor, trauma or inflammation, compulsive drinking, abnormally high renin–angiotensin, or congestive heart failure. Hypodipsia is usually seen in patients with lesions in the supraopticohypophyseal system.

NEUROHYPOPHYSIS

With the development of immunohistochemical techniques, the mechanisms of vasopressin synthesis and secretion have recently become clear. Vasopressin is synthesized and stored mainly in neurosecretory granules in the magnocellular system in the hypothalamus, particularly in the supraoptic nucleus and the paraventricular nucleus.

Neurophysin is a carrier protein for vasopressin and oxytoxin. It is specific for vasopressin and oxytocin, and it does not bind other hormones. Neurophysin is a large protein, approximately 10,000 daltons molecular weight; and it is also synthesized and stored in the magnocellular system. Vasopressin is loosely bound to this carrier protein, forming the Van Dyke protein. There are two immunologically distinct neurophysins: neurophysin I and neurophysin II. Oxytocin is bound to neurophysin I and vasopressin to neurophysin II. Accordingly, estrogen stimulates release of the neuro-

physin I–oxytocin complex, and nicotine stimulates release of the neurophysin II–vasopressin complex.

Oxytocin and vasopressin are closely related in chemical structure, anatomical site of synthesis, and secretory mechanism. These two hormones and their specific neurophysins are distinguishable, however, and can be found in separate perikarya in the supraoptic and the paraventricular nuclei.

Vasopressin is loosely bound to neurophysin II, and this complex is secreted by exocytosis. There are three major secretory pathways (Fig. 2): The major pathway is the supraoptic–hypophyseal tract to the posterior lobe of the pituitary. Two other minor pathways lead to the external zone of the median eminence for secretion into the hypophyseal portal capillaries to the third ventricle for secretion into cerebrospinal fluid. The second pathway, the external zone of the median eminence, is augmented in the absence of adrenocortical steroids. The physiological role of the local release of vasopressin in cerebrospinal fluid is not clear.

Vasopressin and neurophysin are stored in granules and transported along the beaded axonal pathways. Transport of the hormone can be evaluated by injecting ^{35}S-cysteine into the sites of vasopressin synthesis and measuring the appearance of ^{35}S in the posterior lobe of

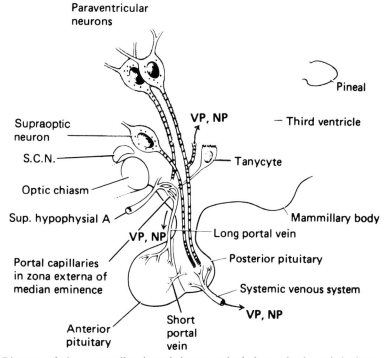

Fig. 2. Diagram of the mammalian hypothalamus and pituitary gland, sagital view, depicting pathways secreting vasopressin (VP) and neurophysin (NP). The hormone and carrier protein are formed in magnocellular perikarya in the supraoptic and paraventricular nuclei, transported in granules along their axons and secreted at three sites: (a) posterior pituitary gland (systemic circulation), (b) zona externa of the median eminence (hypophysial portal circulation), and (c) third ventricle (cerebrospinal fluid). Parvicellular neurons in the suprachiasmatic nucleus (SCN) in rat and mouse also contain VP and NP. [Reprinted from Kidney International with permission — Zimmerman EA, Robinson AG: Hypothalamic neurons secreting vasopressin and neurophysin. Kidney Int 10:14, 1976.]

the pituitary. Most of the injected ^{35}S-cysteine appears in the posterior lobe after 2–3 hours.

Factors Influencing ADH Secretion

There are many factors influencing vasopressin secretion. The osmoregulatory mechanism is the major factor modulating vasopressin secretion. There are, however, many other nonosmolar regulatory mechanisms.

Osmoregulatory mechanisms. Robertson et al. developed a sensitive radioimmunoassay for vasopressin, and the results of their work show that the threshold of plasma osmolality for the osmoregulatory mechanism is 280 mOsm. The sensitivity of the osmoregulatory mechanism is impressive—the plasma vasopressin concentration rises 0.34 pg/ml of plasma for the increment of plasma osmolality of 1 mOsm (Fig. 3).

The antidiuretic response of the kidney to vasopressin is even more sensitive (Fig. 4). For an increment of 1 pg vasopressin/ml plasma, the increase of urine osmolality is approximately 250 mOsm. In other words, for a rise of plasma osmolality of 1 mOsm the increase in plasma vasopressin concentraion is 0.34 pg/ml, and the increase in the final urine osmolality is approximately 100 mOsm, which is a 100-fold gain.

It is noteworthy that when plasma osmolality rises

to 294 mOsm, healthy subjects experience thirst in addition to a rise in plasma vasopressin. These mechanisms provide double protective measures for water deprivation. In this way, the osmolality of body fluid is maintained constant within a narrow range.

In considering the relationship between plasma osmolality and plasma vasopressin, the magnitude of the hormonal response to a given stimulus is dependent upon the rate of change as well as the absolute level of plasma osmolality. The basis for this rate-dependent mechanism is not known.

Nonosmoregulatory factors influencing ADH release. Baroreceptor and volume receptor. Baroreceptor and volume-receptor responses also influence ADH release. A change in perfusion pressure is detected by baroreceptors located in the carotid sinus and the aortic arch, and a change in blood volume is detected by stretch receptors located in the cardiac atrium. There are many other humoral and nonhumoral factors which influence ADH secretion independent of plasma osmolality. Nonosmolar factors augment ADH secretion commonly through stimulation of baro- or volume receptors. These receptors are probably not as sensitive as the osmoreceptor. The stimulation of the baro- or volume receptor is, however, more potent. For example, in the event of acute hemorrhage, stimulation by baro- and/or volume-receptor mechanisms augment ADH secretion often at the expense of plasma osmolality and result in an abnormally low plasma osmolality.

Catecholamines. There have been extensive studies regarding the effect of catecholamines on the urinary concentrating mechanism. Alpha adrenergic stimulation induces diuresis, while beta adrenergic stimulation causes antidiuresis. The diuretic effect of alpha adrenergic stimulation is mediated through an inhibition of secretory mechanisms for ADH release in the brain and also via a direct effect on water excretion in the kidney, such as an alteration of renal hemodynamics and/or cellular action of ADH.

The antidiuretic mechanism of beta adrenergic stimulation has been more extensively investigated. Beta adrenergic stimulation increases ADH release through stimulation of the extracranial baroreceptor. Possible effects of catecholamines in the cerebrospinal fluid on ADH release are, however, not clear. Although evidence is not conclusive, beta adrenergic stimulation appears to also alter renal water excretion independent of the ADH release mechanism.

Thyroid hormone. Patients with hypothyroidism are unable to properly excrete a water load. There are three possible mechanisms to account for the impaired water excretion in hypothyroidism—inappropriate secretion of ADH, impairment of metabolic inactivation of ADH, or an abnormal increase in renal response to ADH. None of these possibilities, however, has been confirmed.

Adrenal corticoids. Adrenal insufficiency is also commonly associated with an impairment of water excretion. It appears that both glucocorticoids and

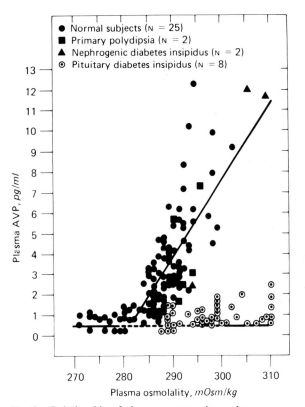

Fig. 3. Relationship of plasma vasopressin to plasma osmolality in healthy adults and patients with different types of polyuria. [Reprinted with permission from Robertson GL, Mahr EA, Arthur S, et al: Development and clinical application of a new method for the radioimmunoassay of arginine vasopressin in human plasma. J Clin Invest 52:2346, 1973.]

mineral corticoids stimulate ADH secretion in the presence of low plasma osmolality through the stimulation of baroreceptor mechanisms. The mechanisms involved in stimulation of baroreceptors are different between the two hormones, however. These hormones may also influence water excretion through other mechanisms, such as alteration of Na^+ reabsorption and the countercurrent mechanism.

Renin–angiotensin. The effect of the renin–angiotensin system on renal water excretion is conflicting. In certain experimental models, infusion of angiotensin II increases plasma ADH level. In other models, infusion of angiotensin II induces diuresis. The mechanism of ADH release induced by the renin–angiotensin system is not clear. The results of in vitro studies indicate a direct stimulatory effect of angiotensin on the ADH secretory mechanism. The physiological significance of these results is not clear.

Prostaglandin E. Prostaglandin E is produced mainly in the kidney; however, it is a ubiquitous hormone, and it elicits multiple physiological effects, among which is the attenuation of the antidiuretic effect of ADH in the kidney through both an alteration of the countercurrent mechanism induced by an increase in medullary blood flow and a decrease in the sensitivity of ADH to increase water permeability in the collecting duct at the step of cyclic AMP generation. There is also information suggesting an increase in ADH secretion through the stimulation of the baroreceptor or through direct effects of prostaglandin E on ADH release mechanisms in the central nervous system.

Drugs. Drugs can also influence water metabolism through an alteration of either the ADH secretory mechanism or the renal response to ADH.

Oxytocin has less antidiuretic effect than vasopressin. A large dose of oxytocin may, however, induce a significant antidiuresis and water intoxication.

Nicotine stimulates ADH secretion through multiple mechanisms. It increases ADH release through the stimulation of the baroreceptor mechanism. Direct administration of nicotine into the third ventricle or the subarachnoid space also causes antidiuresis.

Chlorpropamide induces antidiuresis possibly through multiple mechanisms. Chlorpropamide may stimulate ADH secretion as well as augment the antidiuretic response of the kidney to ADH.

Clofibrate induces antidiuresis in patients with diabetes insipidus. The antidiuresis is thought to be due to augmentation of ADH secretion.

Morphine induces antidiuresis through the stimulation of ADH secretion. Chronic administration of morphine, however, diminishes the antidiuretic response of the kidney to ADH and induces diuresis in rats.

Tricylic compounds also induce antidiuresis through the stimulation of ADH release. Water intoxication after the use of tricyclics has been reported.

Vincristine and cyclophosphamide also induce antidiuresis through an increase in ADH release. The

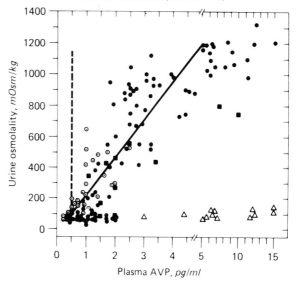

Fig. 4. Relationship of urine osmolality to plasma vasopressin in healthy adults and patients with different types of polyuria. [Reprinted with permission from Robertson GL, Mahr EA, Arthur S, et al: Development and clinical application of a new method for the radioimmunoassay of arginine vasopressin in human plasma. J Clin Invest 52:2346, 1973.]

effect of these drugs on ADH release is important, since fluid intake is commonly encouraged in patients on chemotherapy in order to prevent the precipitation of uric acid stones.

Ethanol, dilantin, and oxilorphan suppress ADH release and induce water diuresis.

REFERENCES

Fitzsimons JT: Physiological basis of thirst. Kidney Int 10:3, 1976

Fitzsimons JT: The renin-angiotensin system in the control of drinking, in Martini L, Motta M, Frascini F (eds): Hypothalamus. New York, Academic Press, 1970, p 195

Fitzsimons JT: Thirst. Physiol Rev 52:468, 1972

Robertson GL, Mahr EA, Arthur S, et al: Development and clinical application of a new method for the radioimmunoassay of arginine vasopressin in human plasma. J Clin Invest 52:2346, 1973

Robertson GL, Shelton RL, Athar S: The osmoregulation of vasopressin. Kidney Int 10:25, 1976

Robinson AG, Frantz AG: Radioimmunoassay of posterior pituitary peptides: A review. Metabolism 22:1047, 1973

Schrier RW, Berl T: Non-osmolar factors affecting renal water excretion. N Engl J Med 292:81, 141, 1975

Verney EG: The antidiuretic hormone and the factors which determine its release. Proc R Soc Lond (Biol) 135:25, 1947

Zimmerman EA, Robinson AG: Hypothalamic neurons secreting vasopressin and neurophysin. Kidney Int 10:14, 1976

ORGANIC ANION SECRETION AND URATE HANDLING BY THE KIDNEY

Meyer D. Lifschitz

ORGANIC ACID SECRETORY PATHWAY

In the early days of renal physiology, there was some controversy concerning the possibility that urine was formed by filtration versus the possibility that it might be formed via secretion. Marshall and his co-workers were able to perform definitive experiments indicating tubular secretion of certain organic anions. Although it is now recognized that urine is formed by both filtration and by reabsorption and secretion, the original experiments by Marshall still stand as the first clear demonstration of the organic acid secretory pathway. Although a large number of weak organic acid compounds (Table 1) can be actively transported by this pathway, paraaminohippuric acid (PAH) is used as the prototype because it is both the most thoroughly studied and one of the substances most effectively transported by this pathway.

The most direct evidence for tubular secretion of a substance in clearance observations occurs when the clearance of the test substance is greater than the clearance of inulin. Since inulin is felt to be a marker of glomerular filtration rate, when the clearance of the substance of interest is greater than the clearance of inulin, it is safe to conclude that it must be added to the urine by some mechanism in addition to filtration—i.e., secretion. From a practical point of view, this approach has been formalized in the expression of a clearance ratio: the clearance of the test substance divided by the clearance of inulin. The clearance ratio of PAH is frequently between 2 and 4 in most mammalian species. In fact, PAH is so effectively removed from the plasma entering the kidney that the extraction of PAH in one passage of the kidney is frequently greater than 80 percent. Thus it has become common to use PAH clearance as an approximation of renal plasma flow. On those occasions when it is important to obtain a more accurate measurement of renal plasma flow, the extraction of PAH can be directly determined by comparing

Table 1

Some Classes of Organic Compounds Transported by Organic Acid Secretion

Classes	Examples
Carboxylic acids	
Oxyacetic acid	Phenoxyacetate, ethacrynic acid
Amino acid	3,5-diiodo-L-tyrosine
Benzoate	Salicylate
Hippurate	Paraaminohippurate
Glucuronide	Salicylglucuronide
Heterocyclic	Penicillin, diodrast
Dicarboxylic acids	Oxalate
Phenols	2,4-dinitrophenol
Sulfonic acids	Phenol red
Sulfonamides	Acetazolamide

renal vein PAH concentration with peripheral vein PAH concentration and calculating true renal plasma flow by the Fick principle.

PAH secretion, and presumably most organic acid secretion, occurs mainly in the proximal tubule. PAH secretion can occur in both the proximal convoluted tubule and in the proximal straight tubule, but recent studies suggest that the proximal straight tubule is much more effective in this regard. Present observations suggest that the process whereby tubular secretion occurs involves active transport of organic acids from the peritubular side into the tubular cell. The concentration of PAH within proximal straight tubules has been shown to be 20–50 times greater than the concentration on the peritubular side of the cell. Thus a large concentration gradient exists for PAH to move from the tubular cell into the tubular lumen, and it is presently felt that this downhill transport is passive. On the other hand, active accumulation within the cell is an energy requiring process and can be inhibited by cold, ouabain, and inhibitors of energy production such as dinitrophenol. In isolated preparations of pars recta, PAH can be transported into the lumen at such a rate that salt and water follow and fluid then accumulates within the lumen of the pars recta, leading to net fluid secretion; however, there is little evidence to suggest that this phenomenon is quantitatively important in terms of whole kidney function or in clinical conditions.

Transport, at the organic acid secretory site, can be competed for by a number of different organic acids. Figure 1 demonstrates the typical response when PAH is added in increasing amounts to the plasma of a normal man. Although the amount filtered and excreted continues to rise with increasing plasma concentrations, the amount secreted reaches a plateau. This plateau is referred to as a tubular maximum and for PAH is referred to as the tubular maximum for PAH. When an additional organic acid such as phenol red is added at the same time, the tubular maximum for PAH is lowered, presumably because portions of the organic acid secretory sites are transporting phenol red rather than PAH. There may well be more than one class of organic acid transport sites in the proximal tubule. Although the major class of sites appears to have a relatively high affinity for PAH transport, other classes of organic acid transport sites may have variable affinities for different classes of organic acids.

In evaluating the renal excretion of a particular substance, a number of factors come into play. The first consideration is whether the substance is freely filterable at the glomerulus. Although PAH is not protein bound, a number of other organic acids may be bound to protein to some extent and thus be relatively unavailable for filtration. As discussed above, the potential for tubular secretion for organic acids (and to some extent along separate pathways for organic bases) exists within the proximal tubule. In addition, there are reabsorptive sites for certain organic anions along some segments of the nephron. PAH has very limited reabsorption, particularly when compared to some other organic acids.

Organic acid secretion not only plays a role in facilitating the excretion of a number of organic acids produced within the body, such as hippurate and benzoate, but also is responsible for the excretion of a number of drugs. One of the best examples is that of penicillin, which has a high affinity for the organic acid secretory pathway and is cleared by the kidney at a rate similar to PAH. At a time when penicillin was quite expensive, it seemed important to try to reduce the renal clearance and excretion of penicillin. To effect this, probenecid, another drug with a high affinity for the organic acid secretory pathway, was developed. Probenecid is not only secreted by the organic acid secretory pathway, but is subsequently reabsorbed further down the nephron. Thus probenecid is excreted at a relatively slow rate but markedly retards the rate of excretion of penicillin and thus reduces penicillin clearance. Although this is no longer a critical clinical issue, it does point out the fact that when two drugs, both of which are transported by the organic acid secretory pathway, are administered to the same patient, they may affect each other's rate of excretion.

RENAL HANDLING OF URATE

Because of the association of hyperuricemia with gout and several other diseases, a number of studies have been directed at elucidating the mechanism whereby the body excretes urate. Although both the kidney and intestine can be sites for urate excretion, under normal conditions the kidney is quantitatively the most important excretory organ.

There is still considerable controversy concerning urate handling by the kidney. Figure 2 is a schematic drawing representing our present state of knowledge. Uric acid, which is almost completely ionized at the normal pH of blood, is not presently felt to be bound to any quantitative extent to plasma proteins. Thus urate is freely filterable at the glomerulus. In addition, there is both secretion and reabsorption of urate. The greatest transport in both directions occurs in the proximal convoluted and, to some extent, in the straight portion of the proximal tubule. Distal convoluted tubules appear to be generally impermeable to urate, although there may be some very limited degree of reabsorption in quite distal segments of the nephron. In proximal convoluted tubules, reabsorption and secretion of urate occur at similar sites. Where studied, urate secretion appears to be similar to secretion of other organic acids in that the pars recta or straight portion of the proximal tubule has a greater secretory potential than the pars convoluta. The dynamics of urate reabsorption are less well understood but can be altered by a number of drugs. In addition, certain organic acids, in particular, lactate, beta hydroxybutarate, and acetoacetic acid acutely decrease excretion and clearance of urate, probably by inhibiting urate secretion.

Studies in man are, for obvious reasons, usually the result of clearance studies in which drug manipu-

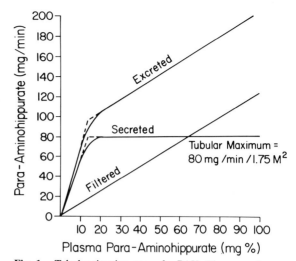

Fig. 1. Tubular titration curve for PAH. The curve for secretion is the difference between those for excretion and filtration. Note the rapid rise in PAH secretion until the tubular maximum is reached.

lations are performed. On the basis of such information, it is presently felt that there are at least two reabsorptive sites for urate along the nephron (Fig. 2), one quite early and one somewhat more distal, beyond the usual secretory site within the nephron. A number of drugs affect renal transport of urate in a quantitatively important manner. Table 2 lists a number of drugs that either increase or decrease the rate of renal excretion of urate. As will be noted, certain drugs may alter urate excretion in either direction depending on the dosage utilized.

Aspirin is perhaps the best example of a drug which at low doses decreases urate excretion and at high doses increases the excretion of the organic acid. In addition, a number of diuretics affect the renal handling of urate, including a relatively recent diuretic, tricrynafen, which markedly increases the rate of uric acid excretion. From an experimental point of view, pyrazinamide is commonly used to inhibit urate secretion

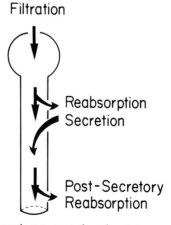

Fig. 2. Schematic representation of urate transport along the nephron. Urate is filtered at the glomerulus. There are reabsorptive sites both before and after the site of secretion.

Table 2
Some Drugs Which Alter Urate Excretion

Increase	Decrease
Probenecid	Pyrazinamide
Sulfinpyrazone	Aspirin in low dose
Ticrynafen	Thiazide diuretics
Acetylsalicylic acid in high dosage	Ethambutol
Phenylbutazone in high dosage	Nicotinic acid
Halofenate	
Radiocontrast media (diatrizoate, etc.)	
Orotic acid	
Ascorbic acid	
Glyceryl guaiacolate	
Acetoheximide	
Glycine	

and probenecid to inhibit urate reabsorption. Although these drugs, in general, seem to be reasonably selective, it should be kept in mind that both drugs can have the opposite effects in certain species. Still, the model as shown in Fig. 2 is based, in large part, on results of changes in urate excretion following the administration of pyrazinamide and probenecid in man.

REFERENCES

Diamond HJ, Paolino JS: Evidence for a post-secretory reabsorptive site for uric acid in man. J Clin Invest 52:1491, 1973

Grantham JJ, Qualizza PB, Irwin RL: Net fluid secretion in proximal straight renal tubules in vitro: Role of PAH. Am J Physiol 226:191, 1974

Marshall EK Jr, Vickers JL: The mechanism of the elimination of phenolsulphone-phthalein by the kidney—A proof of secretion by the convoluted tubule. Bull Johns Hopkins Hosp 34:1, 1923

Steele TH: Urate excretion in man, normal and gouty, in Kelley WM, Weiner IM (eds): Handbook of Experimental Pharmacology. New York, Springer, 1978, p 257

Tune RM, Burg MB, Patlak CS: Characteristics of p-aminohippurate transport in proximal renal tubules. Am J Physiol 217:1057, 1969

Weiner IM: Transport of weak acids and bases, in Orloff J, Berliner RW (eds): Handbook of Physiology. Section 8, Renal Physiology. Baltimore, Williams & Wilkens, 1973, p 521

Weiner IM, Mudge GH: Renal tubular mechanisms for excretion of organic acids and bases. Am J Med 36:743, 1964

GLUCOSE

Meyer D. Lifschitz

The kidney plays a key role in glucose handling by the body because large amounts of glucose are filtered and reabsorbed by the kidney each day and because the kidney can serve as an important site for both glucose synthesis and glucose metabolism. This chapter reviews the normal handling of glucose by the kidney and certain disease states associated with glycosuria.

TUBULAR TRANSPORT

Glucose is freely filterable at the glomerulus and normally is not detectable in voided urine. Thus the renal tubule has the ability to reabsorb all, or virtually all, filtered glucose. The great majority of filtered glucose is reabsorbed in the proximal tubule, which is to say over 95 percent of glucose filtered at the glomerulus is reabsorbed by the end of the proximal tubule. In addition there appears to be some limited capacity for glucose reabsorption in more distal nephron sites, perhaps between the late distal tubule and the final urine. Glucose reabsorption is an active process requiring energy, and there appears to be a relationship between glucose reabsorption and the reabsorption of other electrolytes. In particular, sodium reabsorption and glucose reabsorption appear in part to be linked such that the rate of sodium reabsorption from the proximal tubule will be increased when glucose is present in the tubule lumen. Tubular glucose reabsorption can be inhibited by a compound called phlorizin (Phloretin-B-glucoside). The best evidence would suggest phlorizin acts as a competitive inhibitor of glucose transport by competing with glucose for binding to a carrier which is involved in the reabsorption of glucose. In addition to glucose reabsorption there is a finite but quite small potential for glucose secretion into the tubular lumen. This phenomena is not presently felt to be quantitatively important.

T_m for Glucose

The concept of a tubular maximum (T_m) originally derived from studies of glucose handling by the kidney (Fig. 1). A number of investigators have found, in various species, that as one raises the amount of glucose in the blood, and thus the filtered amount of glucose, almost no glucose appears in the urine until some theoretical level referred to as the T_m for glucose is achieved, after which the rate of glucose excretion in the urine will increase with the rate of increase in filtered glucose. Although theoretically there is a specific filtered load of glucose after which glycosuria begins and after which the increase in urine glucose reflects increase in filtered glucose, there is usually some gradual increase in glycosuria as one approaches the T_m for glucose; this absence of a sharp appearance of glycosuria is referred to as splay. The exact explanation for splay in glucose titration curves is not clear but may be related to either differences in the filtered load of glucose per nephron or perhaps differences in glucose reabsorptive potential per nephron.

RENAL GLUCOSE METABOLISM

Glucose can be used by both kidney cortex and medulla as a source of energy. While the energy metabolism of the cortex is quite complex and may depend on other fuels for substrate as well as glucose, the renal medulla derives the largest fraction of its energy supply from glucose metabolism. Much of this may be relatively anaerobic, since the partial pressure of oxygen in the deeper regions of the kidney is quite low. In addition to glucose serving as a substrate for energy metabolism in the kidney, glucose can also be synthesized de novo by the kidney cortex. In fact, under certain conditions renal gluconeogenesis may be the largest single source for glucose synthesis in the body.

Renal Glycosuria

Although glucose is not normally present in the urine, a number of clinical conditions exist in which renal glycosuria is present and at times can be clinically important. Glucose can be detected in the urine by a relatively nonspecific reaction with either tablets or tape that will also detect other reducing substances, or it can be detected by the much more specific glucose oxidase reaction. The presence of glucose in the urine can be explained on the basis of two major phenomena, (1) increase in filtered load of glucose which exceeds the tubule maximum for glucose reabsorption or (2) decrease in tubular glucose reabsorption per se. The most common clinical condition leading to renal glycosuria is that which occurs when the filtered load of glucose is markedly increased by an elevation of the plasma glucose concentration. Hyperglycemia occurs commonly in diabetes mellitus, and one of the most readily detectable signs of diabetes mellitus is glycosuria in association with hyperglycemia. A number of other, usually transient, conditions can be associated with hyperglycemia and glycosuria. As a rule of thumb most normal people will not excrete glucose in their urine until the plasma glucose concentration is greater than 200 mg/100 ml.

Idiopathic Glycosuria

In addition to glycosuria occurring due to an elevation of plasma glucose concentration and thus the filtered load of glucose, there is a group of clinical conditions in which renal glycosuria occurs even though the filtered load of glucose can be normal. From a physiological point of view, perhaps the most clearcut condition is one in which the tubule's ability to reabsorb glucose is impaired although the tubule's ability to reabsorb other substances is apparently normal. This condition is frequently familial and is characterized simply by a lower T_m for glucose than normal. It usually is not associated with other functional abnormalities and does not regularly lead to renal dysfunction other than that of glucose reabsorption.

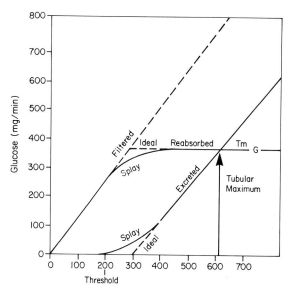

Fig. 1. Schematic representation of the relationship among filtered, reabsorbed, and excreted glucose. Filtered glucose is a linear function of plasma glucose. In this figure, up to a plasma glucose concentration of 200 mg/dl all filtered glucose is reabsorbed and thus none is excreted. Once plasma glucose exceeds 400 mg/dl the tubular maximum for glucose reabsorption (T_{mG}) is reached and no further increment in glucose excretion occurs. Thus as plasma (and filtered) glucose increase further there is a linear increase in glucose excretion.

Fanconi's Syndrome

An abnormality of glucose reabsorption can occur in association with other abnormalities of reabsorption in the proximal tubule. When there is a defect in reabsorption of glucose, phosphate, bicarbonate, and calcium the clinical condition is usually referred to as Fanconi's syndrome (see the chapter on *Transport Disorders*). A number of clinical disease states, including immunologically mediated tubular disease, tyrosinemia, and hereditary fructose intolerance, to name a few, are associated with renal glycosuria. In addition, this condition can be familial. Certain of the diseases which lead to Fanconi's syndrome can be treated; if they are brought under control the renal glycosuria will disappear.

Abnormal Splay

Beyond these two groups of categories there are also individuals who have an abnormal splay to their glucose titration curve such that the threshold for glucose appearance in the urine occurs at a lower level of plasma glucose than in normal people even though the total capacity for glucose reabsorption may well be normal. This latter condition also appears quite benign clinically and does not have a progressive renal abnormality associated with it. All of the above-discussed conditions occur in individuals with normal or near-normal glomerular filtration rate. In addition, recent studies have addressed the question of renal glucose reabsorption in moderate renal failure. It appears that in this condition—although the T_m for glucose may not be markedly altered—there is a greater degree of splay such that small amounts of renal glycosuria will occur at lower than normal plasma levels but that the total amount of glucose reabsorbed as plasma glucose rises will be close to normal.

REFERENCES

Knight T, Sansom S, Weinman EJ: Renal tubular absorption of D-glucose, 3-O-methyl-D-glucose, and 2-deoxy-D-glucose. Am J Physiol 233:F274, 1977

Mudge GH, Berndt WO, Valtin H: Tubular transport of urea, glucose, phosphate, uric acid, sulfate and thiosulfate, in Orloff J, Berliner RW (eds): Handbook of Physiology. Section 8, Renal Physiology. Baltimore, Williams & Wilkins, 1973, p 587

Wen S: Micropuncture studies of glucose transport in the dog: Mechanism of renal glycosuria. Am J Physiol 231:468, 1976

CALCIUM TRANSPORT

Nama Beck

In man, the plasma calcium concentration is approximately 2.5 mM, 47.5 percent (1.18 mM) of which is in ionized form; 46.0 percent (1.14 mM) is bound to protein, mainly albumin, and approximately 0.08 mM is in the form of a Ca–phosphate or Ca–citrate complex. The Ca–phosphate or Ca–citrate complex is filterable through the glomerulus but is not as readily reabsorable at the tubules as ionized Ca^{24}. Under ordinary conditions, the fractional excretion of Ca^{24} is only 0.5–1.0 percent, indicating that the kidney is an important organ to conserve and regulate Ca^{24} balance.

SITE OF Ca^{2+} REABSORPTION IN THE NEPHRON

In the nephron, the sites of tubular reabsorption of Ca^{2+} are similar to those of Na^+. Approximately 50–55 percent of the filtered load of Ca^{2+} is reabsorbed in the proximal tubule, 20–30 percent in the loop of Henle, 10–15 percent in the distal convoluted tubule, and 2–8 percent in the collecting duct. In the proximal tubule, Ca^{2+} reabsorption is closely associated with that of Na^+, and many factors affecting tubular reabsorption of Na^+ also affect Ca^{2+} reabsorption in a parallel fashion. In the distal nephron, Ca^{2+} reabsorption is, however, dissociated from Na^+ reabsorption under certain conditions. In this and the succeeding two chapters, the factors affecting the renal handling of Ca, phosphorus, and magnesium will be outlined.

Common features of the renal handling of Pi (plasma inorganic phosphorus), Ca^{2+}, and Mg^{2+} include the following: (1) The major stores of Pi, Ca^{2+}, and Mg^{2+} are in bone; the kidney, however, regulates the balance of these substances; (2) The major fractional tubular reabsorption of Pi, Ca^{2+}, and Mg^{2+} are in the proximal tubule (50–80 percent); (3) The final urinary excretion of Pi, Ca^{2+}, and Mg^{2+} are regulated by the distal nephron; (4) An increase in the glomerular filtration rate may increase the filtered loads of Pi, Ca^{2+}, and Mg^{2+}, but these increases do not increase the final urinary excretion of these substances, i.e., glomerulotubular balance; (5) Saline infusion inhibits the proximal tubular reabsorption of Pi, Ca^{2+}, and Mg^{2+} and increases the final urinary excretion of these substances; (6) Vitamin D has no direct effect on renal tubular reabsorption of Pi, Ca^{2+}, and Mg^{2+}; (7) PTH inhibits the proximal tubular reabsorption of Pi, Ca^{2+}, and Mg^{2+}, but the effects of PTH on the distal tubular reabsorption of Pi, Ca^{2+}, and Mg^{2+} are different; (8) Diuretics, such as furosemide or thiazide, inhibit the tubular reabsorption and increase the urinary excretion of Pi, Ca^{2+}, and Mg^{2+}. Table 1 details important differences in the renal handling of these ions.

FACTORS INFLUENCING URINARY Ca^{2+} EXCRETION

Glomerular filtration rate. An increase in the GFR increases the filtered load of Ca^{2+} and tubular Ca^{2+} reabsorption, i.e., glomerulotubular balance. Therefore the final urinary Ca^{2+} excretion is usually not altered.

Renal hemodynamics. Vasodilatation by acetylcholine or bradykinin, or an increase in perfusion pressure by angiotensin II, increases urinary Ca^{2+} excretion by mechanisms not clearly defined.

Parathyroid hormone. PTH is the major hormone affecting urinary Ca^{2+} excretion, both directly and indirectly. In contrast to the inhibition of tubular reabsorption of Pi in both the proximal and distal tubules, PTH has dual effects on Ca^{2+} reabsorption. In the proximal tubule, PTH inhibits Ca^{2+} reabsorption as well as Pi and Na^+. In contrast, PTH augments Ca^{2+} reabsorption in the distal nephron. In general, the final urinary Ca^{2+} excretion is regulated by the distal nephron, and PTH elicits an anticalciuric effect. The exact locus of the distal action of PTH and the biochemical mechanism involved are not clear.

Vitamin D and thyrocalcitonin. Vitamin D and calcitonin are important hormones for Ca^{2+} homeostasis; however, neither vitamin D nor calcitonin appears to have a conclusive direct effect on renal tubular reabsorption of Ca^{2+}.

Phosphorus. In Pi depletion, urinary Ca^{2+} excretion is increased. The hypercalciuric mechanism is independent of PTH or plasma Pi. Systemic infusion of Pi, but not intrarenal infusion, reverses hypercalciuria; hypercalciuria persists in isolated perfused kidney obtained from a Pi-depleted rat, suggesting that an extrarenal mechanism resets the tubular reabsorptive capacity for Ca^{2+}.

Plasma Ca^{2+}. An increase in the plasma Ca^{2+} concentration inhibits the distal tubular reabsorption of Ca^{2+} and increases the final urinary Ca^{2+} excretion. The distal tubular effect probably occurs through dual mechanisms—a direct effect of hypercalcemia and the inhibition of PTH release by hypercalcemia.

Magnesium. Mg^{2+} infusion increases urinary excretion of Ca^{2+} and Na^+ through a direct effect on distal tubular Ca^{2+} reabsorption and also through the inhibition of PTH release.

Sodium excretion. Saline infusion increases Ca^{2+}

Table 1
Different Features of Renal Handlings of Pi, Ca^{2+}, and Mg^{2+}

	Pi	Ca^{2+}	Mg^{2+}
↓ plasma Pi or ↓ dietary Pi	↓UV	↑UV	↑UV
↑ plasma Pi	↓ plasma Ca^{2+}		
	↑PTH		
	↑UV	↓UV	
↓ plasma Ca^{2+}	↑PTH		
	↑UV	↓UV	
↑ plasma Ca^{2+}	↓PTH		
	↓UV	↑UV	↑UV
↑ plasma Mg^{2+}	↓UV	↑UV	↑UV
↑ PTH	↑UV	↓UV	↓UV
Metabolic acidosis		↓PTH effects	
	↓UV	↑UV	
Metabolic alkalosis	↑PTH		
	↑UV		
Glucocorticoids		↑GI absorption	
		↑UV	

↑UV, an increase in urinary excretion; ↓UV, a decrease in urinary excretion; ↑PTH, an increase in PTH secretion; and ↓PTH, a decrease in PTH secretion.

excretion. This is probably caused by the inhibition of tubular reabsorption of Ca^{2+} in both proximal and distal nephron segments.

Diuretics. Ethacrynic acid and furosemide, acting mainly in the ascending limb of Henle's loop, inhibit the distal tubular reabsorption of Ca^{2+} and induce hypercalciuria. The effect of thiazide on Ca^{2+} excretion is complex. An acute administration of thiazide elicits variable effects. Chronic administration of a thiazide, however, decreases urinary Ca^{2+} excretion. There are two possible explanations for the hypocalciuria after chronic thiazide administration. The first sequence of events is that thiazides induce natriuresis, decrease extracellular fluid volume, increase the proximal tubular reabsorption of Ca^{2+} as well as Na^+, decrease the delivery of Ca^{2+} to the distal nephron, and decrease urinary Ca^{2+} excretion. Second, it has been suggested that thiazides potentiate the anticalciuric effect of PTH.

Glucocorticoids. Glucocorticoids inhibit Ca^{2+} absorption from the intestine. An acute administration of the hormone, however, does not elicit any direct effect on the renal handling of Ca^{2+}. Chronic administration, on the other hand, induces hypercalciuria. Chronic glucocorticoid administration increases bone resorption, plasma Ca^{2+} concentration, the filtered load of Ca^{2+}, and the delivery of Ca^{2+} to the distal nephron.

Acid–base balance. Urinary Ca^{2+} excretion is usually increased in metabolic acidosis. Acidosis probably has a direct inhibitory effect on the tubular reabsorption of Ca^{2+}. Also, metabolic acidosis appears to suppress PTH release and inhibits the anticalciuric effect of PTH in the kidney. The effect of metabolic alkalosis and respiratory acidosis or alkalosis on urinary Ca^{2+} excretion is not clear.

REFERENCES

Goldberg M, Agus ZS, Goldfarb S: Renal handling of phosphate, calcium, magnesium, in Brenner BM, Rector FC Jr (eds): The Kidney. Philadelphia, W.B. Saunders, 1976, p 344

Massry SG, Friedler RM, Coburn JW: Excretion of phosphate and calcium. Physiology of their renal handling and relation to clinical medicine. Arch Intern Med 131:828, 1973

Sutton RAL, Dirks JH: Renal handling of calcium. Fed Proc 37:2112, 1978

Walser M: Divalent cations: Physicochemical state in glomerular filtrate and urine and renal excretion, in Orloff J, Berliner RW (eds): Handbook of Physiology. Section 8, Renal physiology. Baltimore, Williams & Wilkins, 1973

PHOSPHORUS TRANSPORT

Nama Beck

Plasma inorganic phosphorus (Pi) concentration is 1.14 mM (3.5 mg/dl) in man. Pi is, however, the major intracellular anion, and a large amount of Pi is stored in bone. Furthermore, phosphorus is present in the human body in many different chemical forms, and they are continuously exchanged. Therefore plasma Pi concentration may not reflect Pi kinetics in the body. In the complex system of Pi kinetics, the kidney is the major organ regulating the Pi balance.

SITES OF Pi REABSORPTION IN THE NEPHRON

Approximately 70–80 percent of the Pi filtered at the glomerulus is reabsorbed in the proximal tubule. The amount of Pi reabsorbed in the distal nephron is obviously small, but distal Pi reabsorption plays an important role in the fine homeostatic regulation of the final urinary Pi excretion. There is little evidence to indicate Pi reabsorption along the ascending limb of Henle's loop. The evidence for tubular secretion of Pi in the mammalian kidney is not conclusive.

FACTORS AFFECTING URINARY
Pi EXCRETION

There are many factors that can alter tubular Pi reabsorption. These factors may, however, have different effects at the different sites of the nephron. The final urinary excretion of Pi depends on the combination of effects on the proximal tubule and the distal nephron and the maximal tubular reabsorptive capacity (T_m) for Pi at these sites along the nephron. These various factors regulating Pi reabsorption along the nephron include the following:

Glomerular filtration rate. A modest increase in the GFR would increase the filtered load of Pi and would substantially increase urinary Pi excretion if tubular Pi reabsorption remains unchanged. The T_m for Pi, however, rises with an increase in GFR, i.e., glomerulotubular balance for Pi, and the final Pi excretion does not rise substantially.

Plasma Pi concentration. A rise in plasma Pi concentration would induce the following chain reaction: a decrease in the plasma concentration of ionized Ca^{2+}, stimulation of parathyroid hormone (PTH) release, an inhibition of tubular Pi reabsorption, and an increase in urinary Pi excretion. The effect of plasma Pi concentration on the final urinary Pi excretion is variable, however, depending upon the basal state of plasma Pi.

Parathyroid hormone. PTH is the major hormone affecting tubular Pi reabsorption in the kidney. PTH inhibits tubular Pi reabsorption both at the early proximal tubule and in the distal nephron. The biochemical mechanisms of the phosphaturic effect of PTH are as follows: The hormone binds to its specific receptor, located at the serosal side of the tubule, and activates adenyl cyclase bound in the serosal plasma membrane. This leads to an increased cyclic AMP generation by converting ATP to cyclic AMP. An increased cyclic AMP generation then results in activation of protein-kinase and consequent induction of subsequent reactions of as yet unknown nature which inhibit tubular Pi reabsorption.

Vitamin D. The kidney is the major organ activating 25(OH)-cholecalciferol to 1,25(OH)$_2$-cholecalciferol. Information concerning the direct effect of vitamin D on renal tubular Pi reabsorption is inconclusive. This hormone may, however, affect urinary Pi excretion through indirect mechanisms. An increase in vitamin D activation would cause a rise in both Ca^{2+} absorption from the intestine and Ca^{2+} mobilization from bone, which would suppress PTH release, augment tubular Pi reabsorption, and decrease the final urinary Pi excretion.

Calcium. The evidence for the direct effect of Ca^{2+} on renal tubular Pi reabsorption is inconclusive Ca^{2+}, however, alters urinary Pi excretion through complex indirect mechanisms. An increase in plasma ionized Ca^{2+} concentration suppresses PTH release, increases tubular Pi reabsorption at both proximal and distal tubules, and decreases the final urinary Pi excretion. Second, an increase in intracellular Ca^{2+} inhibits

the phosphaturic effect of PTH. Third, an acute Ca^{2+} infusion into the renal artery decreases urinary Pi excretion. This decrease is probably due to a decrease in renal blood flow, GFR, and the filtered load of Pi. In chronic hypoparathyroid patients, chronic Ca^{2+} infusion, however, increases urinary Pi excretion. The mechanism of this increase is not clear.

Magnesium. An increase in dietary Mg^{2+} decreases urinary Pi excretion, and Mg^{2+} deprivation increases Pi excretion. The mechanisms involved are not clear.

Sodium excretion. Saline infusion induces a substantial increase in urinary Pi excretion as well as sodium excretion. There are at least two different mechanisms involved. Saline infusion inhibits Pi reabsorption as well as sodium reabsorption in the proximal tubule. Second, a decrease in plasma Ca^{2+} concentration due to hemodilution would stimulate PTH release, inhibit tubular Pi reabsorption, and increase the final urinary Pi excretion.

Diuretics. There are at least three mechanisms involved in phosphaturia induced by diuretics. First, inhibition of sodium reabsorption in the proximal tubule would also inhibit Pi reabsorption. Second, diuretics which inhibit carbonic anhydrase activity in the kidney (e.g., acetazolmalide, furosemide, or thiazide derivatives) would inhibit HCO_3^- reabsorption in the proximal tubule and increase the ratio of HPO_4^{2-}/HPO_4^-. HPO_4^{2-} is less reabsorbable than HPO_4^-. Third, the diuretics with calciuric effect (e.g., ethacrynic acid or turosemide) would decrease plasma Ca^{2+} concentration, stimulate PTH release, inhibit tubular Pi reabsorption, and increase Pi excretion.

Acid–base balance. The direct effect of changes in pH or the plasma HCO_3^- concentration on renal handling of Pi is difficult to assess. The administration of $NaHCO_3$ increases urinary Pi excretion, but there is more than one mechanism involved. The Na^+ administration along with HCO_3^- would suppress Na^+ reabsorption in the proximal tubule, which would also suppress Pi reabsorption. Second, an acute metabolic alkalosis would decrease the plasma concentration of the ionized Ca^{2+}, which would then stimulate PTH release and increase Pi excretion. Third, alkalosis would increase the ratio of HPO_4^{2-}/HPO_4^-. HPO_4^{2-} is less permeable than HPO_4^- across the tubular cell membrane. Fourth, metabolic alkalosis may potentiate the phosphaturic effect of PTH in the kidney, possibly through an augmentation of PTH-dependent cyclic AMP generation in the kidney.

Glucose and insulin. Hyperglycemia probably increases urinary Pi excretion by decreasing the T_m for Pi. Glucose may compete with Pi for tubular reabsorption in the proximal tubule. On the other hand, insulin increases Pi reabsorption in the proximal tubules and decreases urinary Pi excretion independent of glucose.

REFERENCES

Goldberg M, Agus ZS, Goldfarb S: Renal handling of phosphate, calcium and magnesium, in Brenner BM, Rector

FC Jr (eds): The Kidney. Philadelphia, W.B. Saunders, 1976, p 344

Knox FG, Osswald H, Marchand GR, et al: Phosphate transport along the nephron. Am J Physiol 2:F261, 1977

Popovtzer MM, Mehandru S, Saghafi D, et al: Interactions between PTH, vitamin D metabolites, and other factors in tubular reabsorption of phosphate, in Massry SG, Ritz E, Rapado A (eds): Homeostasis of Phosphate and Other Minerals. Plenum, New York, 1978, p 11

Massry SG, Friedler RM, Coburn JW: Excretion of phosphate and calcium. Physiology of their renal handling and relation to clinical medicine. Arch Intern Med 131:828, 1973

MAGNESIUM TRANSPORT

Nama Beck

Studies on magnesium (Mg^{2+}) are limited, and information regarding the renal handling of Mg^{2+} are not clear. Plasma Mg^{2+} concentration varies from 0.62 to 1.10 mM, and the cause of this variation is not clearly understood. Approximately 0.53 mM (55 percent) of plasma Mg^{2+} is in an ionized form, 0.30 mM (32 percent) is bound to plasma protein, and 0.03 mM (3 percent) is in a Mg-phosphate complex. Bone contains huge stores of Mg^{2+} as well as Ca^{2+} and Pi (plasma inorganic phosphorus), and approximately 50 percent of the total body Mg^{2+} is in bone. Hypomagnesemia is not uncommon in a variety of clinical disorders. Hypermagnesemia is rarely seen, however, since the kidney has the capacity to excrete a large amount of Mg^{2+}.

SITES OF Mg^{2+} REABSORPTION IN THE NEPHRON

Renal handling of Mg^{2+} is similar to that of Ca^{2+}. Both Ca^{2+} and Mg^{2+} are reabsorbed at common sites by similar mechanisms. In dogs, approximately 60 percent of the filtered Mg^{2+} is reabsorbed in the proximal tubule. The major fraction of the Mg^{2+} delivered to the distal nephron is reabsorbed probably in the loop of Henle and early distal tubule. The final fractional excretion of Mg^{2+} in urine is only 4 percent under ordinary conditions. Mg^{2+} reabsorption along the collecting duct is probably negligible, and there are no conclusive data to suggest Mg^{2+} secretion.

Glomerular filtration rate. An increase in GFR increases the filtered load of Mg^{2+}, as well as the T_m for Mg^{2+}, but these increases do not augment the final urinary Mg^{2+} excretion, i.e., glomerulotubular balance for Mg^{2+}.

Hemodynamics. Vasodilatation and an increase in perfusion pressure increase urinary excretion of Mg^{2+} as well as Ca^{2+}.

Parathyroid hormone. The effect of PTH on urinary Mg^{2+} excretion is biphasic. In the early phase, PTH augments tubular Mg^{2+} reabsorption and decreases urinary Mg^{2+} excretion. These findings are similar to the effect of PTH on Ca^{2+} excretion. In the later phase, PTH elicits a different effect by increasing plasma Ca^{2+} concentration and augmenting urinary Mg^{2+} excretion.

Vitamin D and calcitonin. The effect of these hormones on renal handling of Mg^{2+} is not clear, and the results of studies are not conclusive.

Plasma Ca^{2+}. Acute Ca^{2+} infusion inhibits Mg^{2+} reabsorption in both proximal and distal tubules and increases urinary Mg^{2+} excretion. This finding is similar to the effect of hypercalcemia on urinary Ca^{2+} excretion. The inhibitory effect of hypercalcemia on tubular Mg^{2+} reabsorption is independent of PTH, the GFR, and Na^+ excretion, and the increase of Mg^{2+} clearance in hypercalcemia parallels the increase of Ca^{2+} clearance.

Dietary Mg^{2+}. Dietary deprivation of Mg^{2+} decreases urinary Mg^{2+} excretion as well as Ca^{2+} and Na^+ excretion. Mg^{2+} deprivation, however, increases urinary K^+ excretion through an unknown mechanism.

Sodium. Saline infusion increases urinary Mg^{2+} excretion probably by the inhibition of both proximal and distal tubular reabsorption of Mg^{2+}.

Diuretics. Ethacrynic acid, furosemide, and mercurial diuretics act mainly in the distal nephron and increase urinary Mg^{2+} excretion through a mechanism similar to that for Ca^{2+}. Thiazides increase urinary Mg^{2+} excretion, unlike their anticalciuric effects. The mechanism involved is not clear.

Glucocorticoid. This hormone does not elicit any acute effect on tubular reabsorption of Mg^{2+}. Chronic administration, however, induces magnesiuria through mechanisms similar to those for hypercalciuria: increased bone resorption increases Mg^{2+} mobilization, plasma Mg^{2+}, and the filtered load of Mg^{2+}. Hypercalcemia from bone resorption suppresses PTH release and decreases PTH-dependent tubular reabsorption of Mg^{2+} as well as Ca^{2+}.

Acid–base balance. Acute metabolic acidosis directly inhibits tubular reabsorption of Mg^{2+} and increases urinary Mg^{2+} excretion through a mechanism similar to that for Ca^{2+} excretion. In chronic metabolic acidosis, urinary Mg^{2+}, however, is not altered. The mechanism of renal adaptation to chronic metabolic acidosis is not clear.

REFERENCES

De Rouffignac C, Morel F, Moss N, et al: Micropuncture study of water and electrolyte movements along the loop of Henle in Psammomys with special references to magnesium, calcium and phosphorus. Pflugers Arch 344:309, 1973

Dirks JH, Quamme GH: Renal handling of magnesium, in Massry SG, Ritz E, Rapado A (eds): Homeostasis of Phosphate and Other Minerals. Plenum, New York, 1978, p 51

Goldberg M, Agus ZS, Goldfarb S: Renal handling of phosphate, calcium, and magnesium, in Brenner BM, Rector FC Jr (eds): The Kidney. Philadelphia, W.B. Saunders, 1976, p 344

Walser M: Divalent cations: Physiochemical state in glomerular filtrate and urine and renal excretion, in Orloff J, Berliner RW (eds): Handbook of Physiology. Section 8, Renal Physiology Baltimore, Williams & Wilkins, 1973

Hormonal Action on Renal Function

RENIN–ANGIOTENSIN SYSTEM

Meyer D. Lifschitz

Since the discovery by Tigerstedt and Bergman in 1898 of a pressor substance in saline extracts of the kidney, a large body of information has accumulated concerning the physiological and pathophysiological role of the renin–angiotensin system in health and disease. This chapter reviews the components of the renin–angiotensin system and discusses the role that activation of the renin–angiotensin system is presently felt to play in normal physiology.

The important features of the renin–angiotensin system, as presently understood, are depicted in Fig.1. A high molecular weight polypeptide, referred to as renin substrate, is synthesized in the liver and released into the circulation. Circulating renin substrate, sometimes referred to as angiotensinogen, is cleaved by a proteolytic hormone called renin, which is released from the kidney, liberating a ten amino acid peptide called angiotensin I. Angiotensin I by itself is relatively inactive, but a series of converting enzymes which exist in lung and other tissues (including kidney) convert it to an eight amino acid chain called angiotensin II. Angiotensin II is a potent vasoconstricting agent and in addition stimulates aldosterone synthesis in the adrenal gland. It may also have direct effects on renal tubular sodium reabsorption as well. Angiotensin II can further be cleaved by angiotensinase to angiotensin III, a seven amino acid peptide which can also stimulate aldosterone production and may have a relatively selective renal vasoconstricting potential as well. Even smaller peptide products of angiotensin, six amino acids or less, are not presently felt to have important physiological roles.

RENIN SUBSTRATE

Renin substrate, or angiotensinogen, is the protein substrate from which renin enzymatically cleaves angiotensin I. Most evidence indicates that angiotensinogen in the circulation is produced by the liver. Although the exact structure of human angiotensinogen has yet to be described, its molecular weight has been approximated to be between 66,000 and 110,000 daltons, and at present it is felt to be a glycoprotein. The concentration of angiotensinogen in plasma can be increased by the administration of adrenocorticosteroids, estrogens, and angiotensin II and by nephrectomy. Under most physiological circumstances glucocorticoids and angiotensin II are probably the most important physiological regulators, but estrogens are presumably responsible for the increase in plasma angiotensinogen which occurs during pregnancy. Although at one time it was felt that low levels of angiotensinogen might be responsible for the lower level of blood pressure in certain patients with cirrhosis of the liver, present findings do not support this conclusion.

RENIN

Renin is a glycoprotein and a very specific carboxyl protease that cleaves the leucine-10–leucine-11 bond in renin substrate to release angiotensin I. Renin has an apparent molecular weight of 37,000–43,000 daltons. More recent studies would suggest that there are larger forms of renin or prorenin which may be synthesized and stored in the kidney, and some other organs, and these forms of renin may be activated by alterations in pH or temperature. The number and variety of structures of either prorenin or big renin are still at issue. Renin or its precursor is synthesized and stored in specialized cells located along the afferent arteriole of glomeruli. These cells are referred to as juxtaglomerular cells or as Goormaghtigh cells, and they can be shown to stain for renin with an antibody directed against renin. Renin can be released from these cells into the general circulation of the kidney, where it can act upon renin substrate either within the kidney itself or in the generalized circulation. In addition, some renal renin is released into the interstitial fluid of the kidney and leaves the kidney via the renal lymph. Additionally, a small amount of renin can be found in the urine.

Anatomically the juxtaglomerular cells are in close proximity to a specialized region of the distal tubule referred to as the macula densa. This combination of juxtaglomerular cells and macula densa is commonly referred to as the juxtaglomerular apparatus. The mechanism whereby alterations in either the afferent arteriole or in the macula densa effect renin release will be discussed subsequently.

CONVERTING ENZYME

The action of renin on substrate yields antiotensin I, a relatively inactive ten amino acid peptide. It is activated to angiotensin II by converting enzyme. Converting enzyme exists in large concentration in the lung. While at one time most converting enzyme activity was

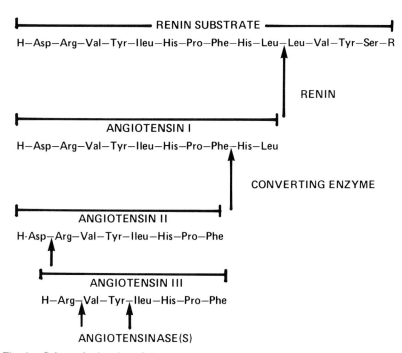

Fig. 1. Schematic drawing of the major components of the renin–angiotensin system.

felt to be present only in lung, there is now evidence for converting enzyme activity in the kidney, in other organs, and possibly in peripheral plasma as well. Although the presence of converting enzyme has been known for some time, the enzyme has assumed greater clinical significance since the description of drugs which are relatively specific converting enzyme inhibitors. One of the best known of these is a nonapeptide orginally isolated from the venum of the snake Bothrops jaracaca. This nonapeptide has been isolated and its structure determined. It has subsequently been synthesized and given the number SQ20881. A number of clinical studies have used this substance to inhibit angiotensin II conversion from angiotensin I. In addition, since converting enzyme is also involved in the inactivation of bradykinin, administration of SQ20881 also augments the level of bradykinin. More recently, a single amino acid form of proline with several side branch substitutions has been shown to also be a potent inhibitor of converting enzyme. This agent, referred to as SQ14225, is presently undergoing clinical studies, some of which will be referred to subsequently.

ANGIOTENSINS

Angiotensin I, the primary product of renin's action on substrate, is a ten amino acid chain, as shown in Fig. 1, and is relatively inactive physiologically. It is converted to the eight amino acid chain referred to as angiotensin II, which is the most potent vasoconstricting agent, on a molar basis, yet described and which in addition is a potent stimulator of aldosterone production in the adrenal cortex. Angiotensin II is further degraded by a series of enzymes referred to as angiotensinases. No enzyme to date has been identified which uses angiotensin II as its specific substrate. One of the

smaller products of angiotensin II des-aspartyl angiotensin II is referred to as angiotensin III. This seven amino acid polypeptide is potent at stimulating aldosterone production in the adrenal cortex, similar to angiotensin II, and is relatively ineffective as a vasoconstricting agent, with the possible exception of the renal vasculature. Data to date would suggest that angiotensin III may be a relatively selective renal vasoconstricting substance.

CONTROL OF RENIN RELEASE

A number of factors have been demonstrated to affect the rate of release of renin from the kidney. Although there is some controversy as to which factor or factors are primary, all of the following would appear to play an important role at least in certain settings: (1) the baroreceptor system, presumably functioning at the level of the afferent arteriole, (2) the macula densa of the distal tubule sensing delivery or load of sodium or chloride, (3) the sympathetic nervous system, (4) potassium concentration, and (5) circulating levels of angiotensin II and possibly antidiuretic hormone (ADH).

In 1959 Tobian et al. suggested that a baroreceptor or stretch receptor was located in the region of the afferent arteriole and functioned to regulate the rate of renin release. Subsequent studies by a number of other groups have gathered data to support this theory. As presently put forth the baroreceptor theory for the control of renin release would suggest that a preglomerular pressure or stretch receptor, perhaps in the afferent arteriole itself, can sense pressure or stretch within the renal arterial system and that as perfusion pressure diminishes renin release increases and as perfusion pressure increases renin release diminishes.

Because of the close proximity of the macula densa cells of the distal tubule to the juxtaglomerular cells of the afferent arteriole a number of workers have performed studies and gathered data to suggest that some function of load, delivery, or transport in this region of the distal tubule would affect renin release from the juxtaglomerular cells. Although this area is still quite controversial, the majority of the data at present would suggest than an increase in the amount or concentration of either sodium or chloride delivered to or transported across the macula densa would appear to play a role in inhibiting renin release.

In addition to the baroreceptor and macula densa theory, present evidence also suggests a role for the sympathetic nervous system in stimulating renin release from the kidney. Stimulation of the renal nerves has been shown to directly stimulate renin release, and anatomical studies have shown that branches of the sympathetic nervous system lead directly to the afferent arteriole. In addition, stimulation of certain regions of the central nervous system appears to be able to augment renin release by transmitting signals down the sympathetic nervous system directly to the kidney or perhaps also by augmenting circulating levels of catecholamines. A beta receptor at the level of the kidney appears to play a role in augmenting renin release. This latter observation has been used clinically, since the administration of the beta blocker propranolol commonly leads to suppression of renin release and can thus be used as a pharmacological tool to alter circulating levels of renin.

Potassium loading and hyperkalemia tend to decrease plasma renin activity and renin release, whereas potassium depletion tends to stimulate renin release. Whether these are direct effects of potassium on the juxtaglomerular apparatus or whether alterations in potassium function through some more complicated system, perhaps affecting the rate of sodium or chloride transport, is presently unclear.

Angiotensin II, the potent vasoconstrictor product of renin's action on substrate, can directly inhibit renin release from the juxtaglomerular cells. On the basis of a number of studies in which these observations have been found it has been suggested that there is, in fact, a short feedback loop in which the product of the renin–angiotensin system, angiotensin II, inhibits release of renin from the kidney.

Vasopressin also appears to have a negative influence on renin release. The exact balance among all of these factors in clinical and pathophysiological conditions on the control of renal renin release is still under investigation.

ROLE OF THE RENIN–ANGIOTENSIN SYSTEM IN NORMAL PHYSIOLOGY

Until quite recently, most information concerning the role of the renin–angiotensin system in clinical and pathophysiological states was derived from measurements of either plasma renin activity or plasma renin concentration. Angiotensin II and its precursor, angiotensin I, have been quite difficult to measure in normal plasma because of their relatively low concentrations. Thus until recently the role of the renin–angiotensin system had been inferred simply on the basis of measuring alterations in plasma renin activity or concentration. In the past few years the use of the competitive antagonist of angiotensin II, saralasin, and the converting enzyme inhibitors SQ20881 and SQ14225 have, for the first time, offered direct evidence for the role of the renin–angiotensin system in a number of clinical conditions. Because saralasin is not only a competitive antagonist but also has some agonistic activity of its own, results with this agent would tend to underestimate the role of the renin–angiotensin system. Conversely, since converting enzyme is involved not only in activating the conversion of angiotensin I to angiotensin II but also in inactivating bradykinin, an effect seen with converting enzyme inhibition might exaggerate or overestimate the role of the renin–angiotensin system because bradykinin and angiotensin tend to antagonize each other. The results to be described are a synthesis of studies in which plasma renin activity has been measured and both a competitive angiotensin II antagonist such as saralasin and a converting enzyme inhibitor have been used.

There is little question that the renin–angiotensin system can, at times, play an important role in regulating mean arterial pressure. For many years it has been known that a low sodium intake is a potent stimulus for increasing plasma renin activity, and recent studies have demonstrated that normal individuals on a low sodium intake utilize the renin–angiotensin system to maintain normal levels of blood pressure. In addition to systemic vascular resistance being regulated by angiotensin II, there is also a growing body of literature to suggest that renal vascular resistance per se, in normal individuals, can be regulated by the renin–angiotensin system. To date no studies have been performed which directly demonstrate alterations in glomerular filtration rate under similar conditions in normal man.

Aldosterone, a mineralocorticoid produced by the adrenal cortex, is regulated, at least to some extent, by circulating levels of angiotensin. Although there is no question that acute alterations in angiotensin are paralleled by similar changes in aldosterone, there are now recent studies to suggest that chronic elevations of angiotensin II do not necessarily lead to chronic elevation in aldosterone levels. Since angiotensin II can both stimulate aldosterone secretion and decrease renal plasma flow, both factors which would be expected to diminish the rate of renal sodium excretion, it is not surprising that a number of studies have demonstrated that angiotensin II tends to lead to a decrease in sodium excretion. Recent studies have also suggested that there may be a direct effect of angiotensin II on renal tubular sodium transport independent of these other two factors. Whether or not angiotensin, or the renin–angiotensin system itself, does play an important role in the overall regulation of sodium balance is still somewhat unclear.

A number of studies have described a renin–angiotensin system within the central nervous system, but its exact role in physiology is presently unclear.

In addition to the above-described direct effects of the renin–angiotensin system, there is now a growing body of evidence to suggest that angiotensin can interact with other hormonal systems, particularly the catecholamine system and the prostaglandins, and it may well be that in the next few years additional studies will demonstrate that interactions between the renin–angiotensin–catecholamine and renin–angiotensin–prostaglandin systems play important roles in normal physiology.

REFERENCES

Renin-angiotensin system and sodium metabolism, Blair-West Jr: in Thurau K (ed): Kidney and Urinary Tract Physiology II, vol II Baltimore, University Park Press, 1976, p 95

Mechanisms regulating renin release. Davis JO, Freeman RH: Physiol Rev 56:1, 1976

The angiotensin I converting enzyme. Erdos EG: Fed Proc 36:1760, 1977

Freeman RH, Davis JO, Lohmeier TE, et al: Des-asp-l-angiotensin II: Mediator of the renin-angiotensin system? Fed Proc 36:1766, 1977

Peach MJ: Renin-angiotensin system: Biochemistry and mechanism of action, Physiol Rev 57:313, 1977

Peach MJ, Vaughan ED: Sar¹-Ala⁸-angiotensin II Kidney Int 15 [Suppl 9], 1979

The renin-angiotensin system. Reid IA, Morris BJ, Ganong WF, Annu, Rev Physiol 40:1377, 1978

Sambhi MP:Renin substrate reaction. Circ Res [Suppl II] 41:1, 1977

ALDOSTERONE

Michael J. Hanley

Aldosterone is the secretory product of the zona glomerulosa of the adrenal cortex. Since this adrenal corticosteriod stimulates active transepithelial sodium transport at physiologic concentrations, it can be classified as a mineralocorticoid. Aldosterone is produced only in the zona glomerulosa of the adrenal, since this is the only zone containing the mitochondrial enzymes necessary for the formation of the 18-aldehyde group, the final step in its biosynthesis. Aldosterone accounts for less than 0.25 percent of the total adrenal steroid output, circulates in very low concentrations (10^{-9}–10^{-10} M), and is rapidly cleared by the liver.

A large body of literature demonstrates beyond doubt that the regulation of aldosterone secretion is much more complex than the feedback relationship between ACTH and cortisol. Controversy concerning the regulation of aldosterone secretion is engenered by the complexity of the control system. The four major recognized influences on aldosterone secretion are (1) the renin–angiotensin system, (2) ACTH, (3) potassium balance, and (4) sodium balance. While changes in the rate of aldosterone removal may significantly influence its plasma level, it appears that aldosterone is for the most part regulated by changes in secretion rather than clearance rate.

REGULATION OF ALDOSTERONE SECRETION
Renin–Angiotensin System

Release of the enzyme renin from the kidney results in a biologic cascade of events (see the preceding chapter). Renin acts on a plasma–2–globulin to release the decapeptide angiotensin I, which is rapidly converted into the octapeptide angiotensin II in the pulmonary circulation. Angiotensin II is a potent vasoconstrictor and a specific stimulus for adrenal aldosterone production. The COOH-terminal heptapeptide fragment of angiotensin II also appears to possess an equipotent stimulatory action on aldosterone secretion, but the exact physiologic role for this agonist is not settled at this time. The rate-limiting production of renal renin in the above cascade appears to be mediated directly by a real or sensed whole body salt (NaCl) deficit. While in the past the renin–angiotensin system may have been promoted as the prime regulator of aldosterone production, this position is now thought to be too rigid.

ACTH

It is at present difficult to define the precise role of ACTH in aldosterone regulation, but it is important to note that ACTH may have a number of significant interactions with other known stimuli. The role of ACTH in the control of aldosterone secretion has generally been accepted as only permissive, subservient to the renin–angiotensin system and potassium, since in many studies pharmacologic doses of ACTH have been required to increase aldosterone secretion. Recent data from several laboratories, however, suggest that aldosterone may be stimulated by quantities of ACTH likely to be secreted by normal man without sodium restriction. In these studies neither plasma antiotensin II nor serum potassium were altered, which suggests that these potent mediators of aldosterone secretion were not involved in the observed aldosterone response and that ACTH acted directly on the adrenal zona glomerulosa. Current data thus imply that physiologic levels of ACTH may play a role in regulating the circadian secretion of aldosterone but do not exercise trophic control of the adrenal glomerulosa cells to other stimuli.

Potassium

Potassium has a potent influence on aldosterone production. Evidence for the effect of potassium is derived from three types of studies: (1) alteration of potassium intake, (2) alteration of potassium concentration in the adrenal blood supply, and (3) in vitro studies of isolated adrenal cells. In total, these studies indicate that increments of serum potassium of as little as 0.2 mEq/liter can significantly increase plasma aldosterone. The mechanism whereby potassium regulates aldosterone secretion remains unclear at this time. Blood levels of potassium and intracellular potassium stores have both been supported as the mediator of its effect.

Sodium

In contrast to changes in potassium concentration, all studies to date indicate that aldosterone production is influenced only by large changes (10–20 mEq/liter) in sodium concentration. Reduction in the plasma sodium concentration increases aldosterone secretion and increases in plasma sodium concentration decrease aldosterone release from the adrenal gland. Studies indicate that multiple steps in the aldosterone biosynthetic pathway are stimulated by sodium depletion.

ALDOSTERONE–TARGET CELL INTERACTION

Like all steroid hormones, aldosterone enters the target cell (probably by diffusion) and binds to specific cytoplasmic receptors. This steroid–protein complex undergoes some alteration and migrates to the cell nucleus, where it binds to the chromatin, initiating RNA transcription and protein synthesis. In terms of this model the latent period in aldosterone action (60–90 min) is the time necessary for the synthesis of the presumed sodium transport protein. Actinomycin D, an inhibitor of transcription, abolishes the effect of aldosterone on sodium transport but has no effect on potassium excretion. This strongly suggests that the kaliuretic and antinatriuretic effects of the hormone are mediated by entirely different mechanisms. At least three types of aldosterone–protein complexes have been identified in the cytosol of the rat kidney. Type I sites have a high affinity for aldosterone and deoxycorticosterone and a low affinity for corticosterone and dexamethasone. Type II sites have a high affinity for dexamethasone, corticosterone, and aldosterone in decreasing order. Type III sites have a high affinity for corticosterone, with much lower affinities for other steroids. Type I sites are believed to be mineralocorticoid receptors and types II and III glucocorticoid receptors. Aldosterone in pharmacologic concentrations will occupy all these sites and thus demonstrate glucocorticoid activity.

PHYSIOLOGIC RESPONSE TO ALDOSTERONE
Effect on Sodium, Potassium, and
Acid Excretion

Sodium. In a normal subject receiving a normal diet the daily administration of mineralocortocoid causes a decrease in sodium excretion until a total of 300/500 mmoles of sodium is retained but without apparent edema. At this point, sodium excretion again equals intake and the subject again comes into balance. The speed with which escape occurs depends on how quickly the excess sodium is accumulated and therefore on sodium intake and the dose of mineralocorticoid. The generally accepted hypothesis for this escape phenomenon is that the extracellular volume expansion

results in increased sodium delivery out of the proximal tubule which overcomes the increase in sodium reabsorption stimulated in the distal nephron by the excess hormone. When aldosterone is selectively injected into a single renal artery one observes a fall in sodium excretion (beginning at 30 min) with no change in GFR, which implies a direct tubular effect of the hormone. It is now generally held that early data implicating a proximal nephron site of action of aldosterone were due to secondary, nonmineralocorticoid effects of the hormone. Recent data demonstrate that the hormone acts principally on the distal nephron. Distal tubular micropuncture data demonstrate that adrenalectomized rats have a reduced capacity to lower intraluminal sodium concentration and that this functional impairment can be corrected by the administration of a relatively small dose of aldosterone. Microperfusion studies in the rabbit suggest that the target tissue for aldosterone is not the distal tubule but the collecting tubule. These findings were reconciled by morphologic studies in the rat which demonstrated that distal tubule micropuncture studies in this species often examine an epithelium characteristic of the collecting tubule.

Potassium. The exogenous administration of a mineralocorticoid to a normal subject on a normal diet (100 mmoles K^+ per day) results almost immediately in an increased potassium excretion. Unlike sodium excretion, which readily adjusts to intake, potassium excretion is unrelenting and potassium loss continues until severe potassium deficiency results. Potassium loss will not occur if sodium intake is restricted. Under normal circumstances, the major fraction of urinary potassium is secreted by the distal nephron, and aldosterone's effect on urinary potassium excretion is thought to be localized to this portion of the nephron. Micropuncture data indicates that potassium concentration increases along the length of the distal tubule. This potassium concentration rise is abolished in adrenalectomized animals and restored by the administration of aldosterone.

Acid excretion. Observations in humans and animals suggest that mineralocorticiods play a role in acid/base balance. Mineralocorticoid administration results in increased urinary hydrogen ion excretion culminating in a moderate metabolic alkalosis. Initially the urine becomes acidic with increasing titratable acid and ammonium ion. Eventually the urine again becomes alkaline with hydrogen ion excretion being equal to production, but the metabolic alkalosis is maintained. a low-sodium or high-potassium diet can prevent the alkalosis.

Mechanism of Aldosterone Action

Subcellular. As previously discussed, the initial event in aldosterone action is receptor binding, leading to the transcription of an effector protein in the target cells. How the induced proteins stimulate sodium transport is not clear. Three modes of action for the transport proteins have been proposed: (1) the pump theory maintains that aldosterone increases the number or

activity of contraluminal membrane sodium pumps, (2) the permease theory maintains that aldosterone facilitates entry of sodium into the cell across the mucosal or luminal membrane providing more substrate for the sodium pump, and (3) the energy theory maintains that aldosterone is able to increase the supply of energy for the operation of the sodium pump. Experimental measurements of sodium transport pools, epithelial resistance, and high-energy phosphate pools have not been able to conclusively implicate any single mechanism of aldosterone action and all may be operational.

Cellular. Although the reciprocal relationship between sodium reabsorption and potassium secretion in response to aldosterone is well known, the stoichiometric nature of this relation is not completely understood. Over the past several years a working model has evolved principally because of the work of Giebisch and Malnic. Initial whole animal studies lead to the conjecture that aldosterone acted by stimulating sodium reabsorption and—coupled to this—increased sodium reabsorption was an increased potassium or hydrogen ion secretion depending on the intracellular availabilities of these two species. While this model was simple and appeared to adequately explain the whole animal data, it failed to adequately explain two micropuncture observations: (1) the amount of sodium reabsorbed by the distal nephron is ten times the amount of potassium secreted by this segment, and (2) distal hydrogen ion and potassium secretion could be both augmented simultaneously (during metabolic alkalosis). Recent measurements of the potential profile along the distal nephron together with transepithelial concentration profiles and intercellular ion activities has allowed a more complete description of aldosterone action. Details of the model outlined below could easily change as more

measurements of various parameters are made. Whether a species is designated as actively or passively transported depends on the measured concentration and potential profiles. The current concepts regarding the aldosterone sensitive cell are embodies in Fig. 1. The two critical observations included in this model are (1) a transepithelial PD which is dependent on the luminal sodium concentration and (2) an intercellular potassium concentration of 50 mmoles/liter as determined by K^+-specific microelectrodes.

The sequence of events can be described as follows: (1) Aldosterone enters the cell and acts to increase sodium transport out of the cell across the peritubular membrane by direct action on the sodium pump located on the blood side of the cell (Fig. 1) and on luminal membrance sodium permeability. Because the transepithelial potential is a function of the luminal sodium concentration this pump is envisioned as electrogenic or without a one to one coupling with potassium entry into the cell (shown schematically in Fig. 1 by the smaller K^+ component entering the cell). A component of passive potassium entry from the blood into the cell is also shown in Fig. 1. The aldosterone-sensitive sodium pump on the peritubular membrane lowers the intracellular sodium concentration (60 mEq/liter) so that passive sodium entry into the cell occurs across the luminal membrane (sodium moves down an electrochemical gradient from lumen into the cell due to the potential drop across the luminal membrane). The action of the sodium pump on the peritubular membrane thus brings about sodium reabsorption from the tubular lumen. (2) As shown, potassium is delivered into the aldosterone-sensitive cell from the blood both passively and via an active transport process. Under the influence of aldosterone, potassium then moves into the tubular

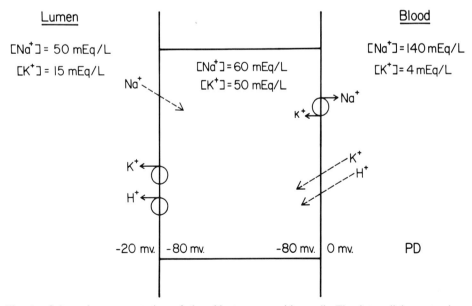

Fig. 1. Schematic representation of the aldosterone-sensitive cell. The intercellular potassium concentration is that determined by direct puncture with a potassium-sensitive electrode. Dotted arrows represent passive ion movement and $\overrightarrow{O}$ denotes presumed specific active transport systems.

lumen. Given the concentration and potential profiles shown, this step requires active potassium transport from cell to lumen as shown in Fig. 1. (3) There is a paucity of data on aldosterone-dependent hydrogen ion transfer. The available information seems to indicate that the critical factor in tubular fluid acidification is the size of a mobile intracellular hydrogen ion pool. Some data suggest that distal cell hydrogen ion activity is low giving rise to passive H^+ entry into the cell across the peritubular membrane but necessitating an active H^+ extrusion process across the luminal membrane. In isolated cortical collecting tubule studies luminal acidification does not require sodium; therefore this process is shown as not being coupled with sodium entry. This model is only tentative and subject to change as new techniques are devised to measure critical parameters. Note especially that there are little data regarding anion transport in the aldosterone sensitive segment. Given the nature of this epithelium it would not be surprising to find transcellular chloride and bicarbonate transport either as independent events or directly coupled to sodium transport.

REFERENCES

Giebisch G: Renal Potassium Excretion, in Rouiller C, Miller AF (eds): The Kidney vol 3. New York, Academic Press, 1971, p 329

Giebish G: Some reflections on the mechanism of renal tubular potassium transport. Yale J Biol Med 48:315, 1975

Ludens J, Fanestil D: The mechanism of aldosterone function. Pharmacol Ther 2:371, 1976

Parllard M: Effects of aldosterone on renal handling of sodium, potassium and hydrogen ions. Adv Nephrol 7:83, 1977

PARATHYROID HORMONE

Nama Beck

Parathyroid hormone (PTH) functions to maintain the concentration of ionized calcium (Ca^{2+}) in the extracellular fluid within a narrow desired range. In PTH metabolism, the kidney plays an important role: (1) Ca is the principal factor known to regulate PTH synthesis and secretion from parathyroid glands, and the kidney modulates Ca^{2+} balance; (2) the kidney is a major target organ of PTH, and the kidney modulates Ca and Pi (plasma inorganic phosphorus) metabolism and vitamin D activation in response to PTH; and (3) the kidney catabolizes and inactivates PTH.

PTH BIOSYNTHESIS AND SECRETION

The amount of PTH secretion is determined by three factors: biosynthesis of PTH, degradation of PTH in parathyroid glands, and secretion of hormone from these glands.

PTH is a single-chain polypeptide of 84 amino acids. In parathyroid glands, larger PTH precursors (pre-pro-PTH and pro-PTH) are biosynthetized, and these larger precursors are cleaved to PTH. The cleavage steps are probably regulated events and serve as control mechanisms(s) which vary in response to extracellular Ca^{2+}.

In addition, beta adrenergic receptors are linked to the cyclic AMP system in parathyroid glands and may modulate PTH secretion.

EFFECTS OF PTH ON THE KIDNEY

There are two major organs known to be target organs for PTH: bone and kidney. In addition, PTH indirectly increases Ca absorption from the intestine by enhancing 1α-hydroxylation of 25(OH)-D_3 in the kidney. The liver also has PTH receptors and a PTH-dependent adenylate cyclase, implicating a possible role for PTH in the liver. The physiological role of PTH in the liver is not known, however.

In the kidney, PTH has multiple physiological effects: (1) PTH increases tubular Ca reabsorption in the distal nephron; (2) PTH inhibits tubular Pi reabsorption in both the proximal and distal enphron; (3) PTH activates vitamin D by 1α-hydroxylation of 25(OH)-D_3 to 1,25(OH)$_2$-D_3; and (4) the kidney catabolizes and inactivates PTH. In subjects with chronic renal failure, renal degradation of PTH is decreased. The decreased PTH degradation may contribute in part to the increase in immunoassayable PTH in chronic renal failure. The physiological importance of PTH degradation in the kidney under basal condition, however, is not presently clear.

Ca reabsorptive and phosphaturic effects of PTH on the kidney are mediated through the cyclic AMP system. This involves binding of PTH to its specific receptors in renal tubular cells, activation of adenylate cyclase, activation of cAMP-dependent protein kinase, and subsequent biochemical reactions as yet not delineated.

PTH receptors and PTH-sensitive adenylate cyclase have recently been identified in the glomerulus, and the glomerular ultrafiltration coefficient (K_f) is decreased by PTH. In contrast, the single-nephron glomerular filtration rate is increased in thyroparathyroidectomized animals and PTH injection reverses this change, suggesting that PTH may have a physiological effect on glomerular dynamics.

REFERENCES

Abe M, Sherwood LM: Regulation of parathyroid hormone secretion by adenylate cyclase. Biochem Biophys Res Commun 48:396, 1972

Arnaud CD: Calcium homeostasis: Regulatory elements and their integration. Fed Proc 37:2557, 1978

Habener JF, Potts JT Jr: Biosynthesis of parathyroid hormone. N Engl J Med 299:580, 1978

Hayer GP Hurst JG: Sigmoidal relationship between parathryroid hormone secretion rate and plasma calcium concentration in calves. Endocrinology 102:1036, 1978

ANTIDIURETIC HORMONE

Larry D. Barnes

Antidiuretic hormone (ADH) increases the reabsorption of water in the kidney by increasing the water permeability of the distal nephron. The physiologic consequences are a decrease in plasma osmolality, a decrease in urine volume, and an increase in urine osmolality. Although ADH can cause constriction of the vascular system (hence the basis for its synonym, vasopressin), the plasma concentration of ADH required to exert a pressor effect is two orders of magnitude greater than the concentration required for the antidiuretic effect. The physiologic and biochemical aspects of the antidiuretic effect of ADH in the mammalian kidney are discussed.

PHYSIOLOGIC ASPECTS

ADH is a nonapeptide hormone synthesized in the supraoptic and paraventricular nuclei of the hypothalamus. The hormone is axonally transported in secretory granules to the posterior pituitary, where it is stored prior to release. ADH is associated with neurophysin, a carrier protein, during the transport to and storage in the posterior pituitary. Plasma hyperosmolality is the main stimulus for release of ADH. An increase in plasma osmolality above 280–285 mOsm/kg, caused by dehydration or addition of hypertonic solutions, stimulates osmoreceptors located in the internal carotid arteries and the hypothalamus to trigger the secretion of ADH in man. Stimulation of baroreceptors by a 10–15 percent reduction of vascular volume or by a 5 percent decrease in blood pressure also increases the release of ADH.

Osmoregulation and baroregulation of ADH release may be either agonistic or antagonistic. For example, the effects of hyperosmolality and hypervolemia on the release of ADH tend to negate each other, while hyperosmolality and hypovolemia complement each other as stimuli. The renin-angiotensin system and adrenocortical hormones have been proposed as participating in the release of ADH, but data are equivocal. Cold temperature and emesis are also stimuli for the release of ADH.

The normal plasma concentration of ADH in hydrated man is approximately $1–5 \times 10^{-12} M$ (1–5 pg/ml) as measured by radioimmunoassay. Several studies have demonstrated a positive correlation between the plasma osmolality and the plasma concentration of ADH with plasma levels of ADH progressively increasing above a plasma osmolality of 285 mOsm/kg. Patients with primary polydipsia or nephrogenic diabetes insipidus have a plasma ADH concentration similar to that in normal subjects for a particular plasma osmolality. Patients with hypothalamic diabetes insipidus or inappropriate secretion of ADH have markedly decreased (less than 1 pg/mg) and increased (up to 100 pg/mg) levels of circulating ADH, respectively. The half-time of removal of ADH from the circulatory system has been estimated as 8–24 min in man. ADH is removed by glomerular filtration and proteolysis in the liver and kidney.

ADH is transported by the circulatory system to the mammalian kidney, where it passes from the peritubular vessels into the renal interstitium. It subsequently binds to specific receptors on the basal and lateral membranes of epithelial cells of the nephron for initiation of its physiologic function. Perfusion of ADH into the lumen of isolated segments of collecting tubules does not elicit a physiologic response. ADH acts on collecting tubules of renal cortex, medulla, and papilla to increase the permeability of the luminal membrane to water (Fig. 1). Data suggest that ADH may also act on a specific portion of the distal convoluted tubule in some mammalian species but not in others. ADH has not been demonstrated to affect the water permeability of segments of the nephron proximal to the juxtaglomerular apparatus.

Studies of the physiologic function of ADH in amphibian skin and bladder complement and support results obtained in the mammalian kidney. ADH increases both the water and urea permeability of frog skin and toad urinary bladder. The hormone has no effect on active sodium transport in the collecting tubules of mammalian nephrons, but it stimulates sodium transport in amphibian skin and bladder.

BIOCHEMICAL ASPECTS

The initial steps in the biochemical mechanism of action of ADH have been determined; however, the terminal steps in the biochemical mechanism remain unknown, even though some components have been identified.

The physiologic response to ADH is initiated by the synthesis of cyclic AMP. Several experimental approaches have clearly established cyclic AMP as the intracellular mediator. Reversible binding of ADH to specific receptors on the basal and lateral membranes of target cells causes stimulation of a membrane bound adenylate cyclase. ADH-sensitive adenylate cyclase is present in medullary thick ascending limb, distal convoluted tubule, and collecting tubules of the cortex and medulla as measured on isolated segments of nephrons from rabbits. The greatest stimulation of adenylate cyclase by ADH occurs in the collecting tubules. The significance of ADH-sensitive adenylate cyclase in the thick ascending limb is unknown because no effect of ADH on the water permeability of this portion of the nephron has been detected. The apparent binding constant of ADH to its receptor is approximately equal to the concentration of ADH which half-maximally stimulates adenylate cyclase, and the degree of stimulation is proportional to the number of receptor sites bound with the hormone.

Stimulation of adenylate cyclase by ADH increases the intracellular levels of cyclic AMP by three to ten times depending upon experimental conditions such as the presence of inhibitors of cyclic AMP phosphodies-

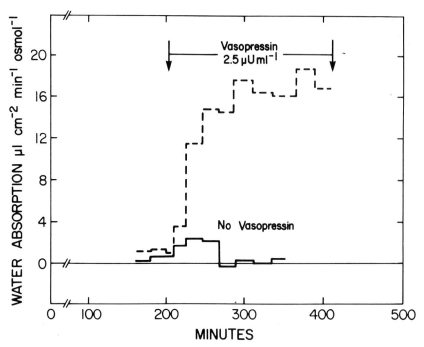

Fig. 1. Permeability to water of collecting tubules in the steady state preceding and after administration of vasopressin. Results from two tubules are depicted. [Reprinted with permission from Grantham JJ, Orloff J: Effect of prostaglandin E on the permeability response of the isolated collecting tubule to vasopressin, adenosine 3,′5′-monophosphate and theophylline. J Clin Invest 47:1154, 1968.]

terase. Although the activity of phosphodiesterase is not affected by ADH, catabolism of cyclic AMP by this enzyme and modulation of its activity by different drugs may alter the physiologic response to ADH. Cyclic AMP and analogs such as dibutyryl cyclic AMP and 8-p-chlorophenylthio cyclic AMP mimic the effect of ADH by increasing the water permeability in isolated, perfused cortical collecting tubules.

Several substances can affect the action of ADH at the level of cyclic AMP metabolism. Calcium decreases the synthesis of cyclic AMP by inhibiting both the binding of ADH to its receptor and adenylate cyclase activity. The physiologic significance is unknown because the concentrations of calcium used in the in vitro experiments exceed the physiologic levels of unbound calcium. Prostaglandin E_1 (PGE_1) decreases the water permeability response to ADH in isolated, perfused collecting tubules by inhibiting the stimulation of adenylate cyclase; however, PGE_1 stimulates the basal activity of adenylate cyclase in the absence of hormone. It has been proposed that in intact renal medulla, where prostaglandins are synthesized in interstitial cells, prostaglandins may serve in a feedback mechanism to modulate the response to ADH. Although such a feedback mechanism has not been conclusively demonstrated, renal prostaglandins are probably local modulators of ADH action. Adrenal steroids such as aldosterone appear to enhance the water permeability response to ADH in toad bladder by inhibiting phosphodiesterase. Although adrenalectomized rats have a lower maximal

response to ADH, the role of adrenal steroids on ADH action in mammalian kidneys is unknown. Adrenergic agents may either inhibit (α adrenergic substances) or potentiate (β adrenergic substances) the hydroosmotic effect of ADH in the toad bladder, but corresponding roles of such agents in mammalian kidneys have not been elucidated. Data suggest that adrenergic agents affect the release of ADH rather than the cellular mechanism in mammals.

The biochemical mechanism of ADH action subsequent to the generation of cyclic AMP is unknown, but at least two components have been identified: cAMP-dependent protein kinase and microtubules.

One hypothesis for the mechanism of ADH in the kidney is that cyclic AMP stimulates a protein kinase, which catalyzes the phosphorylation of specific protein(s) in the luminal membrane of collecting tubules. Such phosphorylation would induce an increase in the water permeability of the membrane. Subsequent dephosphorylation of the membrane proteins, catalyzed by a protein phosphatase, would return the membrane to a relatively water impermeable state. Only certain aspects of this hypothesis are supported by experimental data. A cAMP-dependent protein kinase is present in the cytosol of renal medullary cells, and the enzyme catalyzes the in vitro phosphorylation of a plasma membrane preparation. A membrane preparation which contains a cAMP-dependent protein kinase has also been isolated from bovine renal papilla. This protein kinase catalyzes the phosphorylation of its own membrane preparation. A

protein phosphatase which catalyzes the dephosphory-lation of ^{32}P-labeled membrane preparations in vitro is present in the cytosol of renal medullary cells. Studies with tissue slices of renal medulla demonstrate that the cytosolic protein kinase is activated in situ by elevated intracellular levels of cyclic AMP in response to stimulation by ADH. The degree of activation is a function of the levels of cyclic AMP and the concentration of ADH. Although the components necessary for phosphorylation and dephosphorylation of membrane proteins are present and activation of protein kinase does occur in intact cells, the correlation between phosphorylation of specific proteins and increased water permeability of the luminal membrane is lacking.

Taylor and co-workers first demonstrated that microtubules have a role in the action of ADH. Alkaloids, such as colchicine, vinblastine, and podophyllotoxin, which disrupt the structure of microtubules inhibit the antidiuretic effect of both ADH and cyclic AMP in toad bladder. The alkaloids also block ADH-induced antidiuresis in both conscious and anesthetized rats but do not affect renal hemodynamics or the excretion of solutes. Colchicine and vinblastine do not inhibit the activities of enzymes associated with the mechanism of action of ADH. Thus microtubules are probably re-

quired in steps after the generation of cyclic AMP, but how microtubules are involved is unknown. Microtubules may serve as a cytoskeleton for the localization and translocation of components between the basal-lateral membranes, where ADH receptors are located, and the luminal membrane, where the change in water permeability occurs. Microtubules may have a more active role such as interacting with the luminal membrane and affecting the water permeability. This hypothesis is supported by the finding that colchicine inhibits the rearrangement of intramembranal granules induced by ADH in toad bladder. Interestingly, microtubules are closely associated with protein kinase during isolation. In addition tubulin, the subunit of microtubules, and microtubule-associated proteins can be phosphorylated by protein kinase; however, a possible relationship between the participation of protein kinase and microtubules in the action of ADH has not been established.

The biochemical basis of the change in water permeability of the luminal membrane is unknown. Experimental data have been mustered to support the hypothesis that ADH increases the pore size of aqueous channels in the membrane, thereby increasing bulk water flow. But data also support the hypothesis that

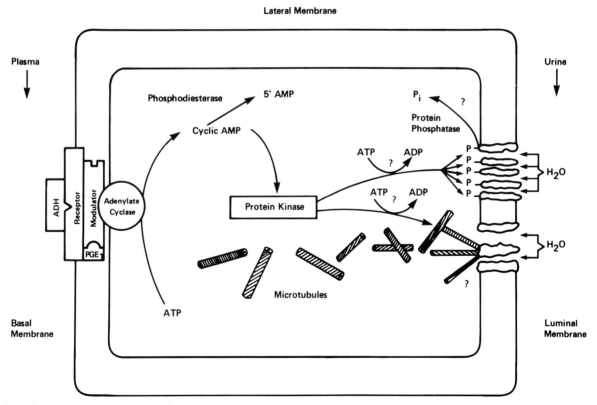

Fig. 2. Schematic illustration of a current hypothetical mechanism of antidiuretic hormone in mammalian kidney. A representative ADH-sensitive adenylate cyclase unit with its receptor, modulator, and catalytic components is depicted on the basal membrane. Protein kinase, after activation by cyclic AMP, may catalyze the phosphorylation of membrane proteins or microtubules, which could increase the water permeability of the luminal membrane. The illustration of pores in the luminal membrane does not imply the actual physicochemical means of water movement. Microtubules may be located in the cytosol and/or interact with the luminal membrane. Question marks indicate hypothetical steps.

water movement occurs by diffusion and that ADH increases the area and number of membrane sites for such diffusion. Conceivably, an effect of microtubules on membrane components and/or conversion of hydrophobic to hydrophilic areas of the membrane by phosphorylation would be compatible with either hypothesis. A schematic diagram of a current hypothesis of the biochemical mechanism of ADH in the mammalian kidney is shown in Fig. 2.

REFERENCES

Andreoli TE, Schafer JA: Mass transport across cell membranes: The effect of antidiuretic hormone on water and solute flows in epithelia. Annu Rev Physiol 39:451, 1976

Dousa TP, Barnes LD, Kim JK: The role of the cyclic AMP-dependent protein phosphorylations and microtubules in the cellular action of vasopressin mammalian kidney, in Moses AM, Share L (eds): Neurohypophysis. Basel, S. Karger, 1977, p 220

Grantham JJ: Action of antidiuretic hormone in the mammalian kidney, in Thurau K (ed): Kidney and Urinary Tract Physiology. Baltimore, University Park Press, 1974, p 247

Grantham JJ, Orloff J: Effect of prostaglandin E on the permeability response of the isolated collecting tubule to vasopressin, adenosine 3,'5'-monophosphate and theophylline. J Clin Invest 47:1154, 1968

Handler JS, Orloff J: The mechanism of action of antidiuretic hormone, in Orloff J, Berliner RW (eds): Handbook of Physiology. Section 8, Renal Physiology. Baltimore, Waverly Press, Inc., 1973, p 791

Hays RM, Levine SD: Vasopressin. Am J Physiol 6:307, 1974

Robertson GL: The regulation of vasopressin function in health and disease, in Greep RO (ed): Recent Progress in Hormone Research, vol 33. New York, Academic Press, 1977, p 333

Strewler GM, Orloff J: Role of cyclic nucleotides in the transport of water and electrolytes, in Greengard P, Robinson GA (eds): Advances in Cyclic Nucleotide Research, vol 8. New York, Raven Press, 1977, p 311

Taylor A: Role of microtubules and microfilaments in the action of vasopressin, in Andreoli TE, Grantham JJ, Rector FD (eds): Disturbances in Body Fluid Osmolality. Baltimore, Waverly Press, 1977, p 97

KININS

Meyer D. Lifschitz

The kinins are a series of biologically active polypeptide hormones. At present three major kinins are recognized: bradykinin, a nonapeptide; kallidin, a decapeptide (lysyl-bradykinin); and an undecapeptide, methionyllysylbradykinin. The kinins are released from a specific plasma alpha 2 globulin (kininogen) by a peptidase referred to as kallikrein (or sometimes referred to as kinin-forming enzymes, kininogenases, or kininogens). Kallikrein is widely distributed and can be found in plasma and circulating granulocytes as well as in a number of glands and organs. The kallikrein in plasma may well be different from the kallikrein in different organ systems.

Because the kinins are very potent vasodilators and because they are relatively short-lived in plasma the kallikrein–kinin system has been proposed as a regulator of both local organ and systemic vascular resistance. The renal kallikrein system has been proposed as a local hormonal system involved in the regulation of renal blood flow, renal sodium excretion, and renal water excretion. Until recently the measurement of kallikrein and kinin concentration has been difficult, so that it is only in the past few years that any quantitative data have been available concerning their production by various organ systems. The kidney makes kallikrein and in part excretes it into the urine. It would appear that urinary kallikrein derives from a region of the kidney beyond the proximal tubule. Isotopic studies suggest that urinary kallikrein does not derive from plasma. Kinins are also present in the urine, do not represent plasma kinin, and also appear to be derived from a portion of the tubule beyond the proximal nephron.

Although kallikrein and kinin activity in the urine reflects renal production, it is not yet clear whether these urinary measurements, in fact, do realistically reflect renal kinin production and activity. Further studies will be required to address this issue. The best evidence to date to suggest an intrarenal role for the kinins is found in studies in which bradykinin or other kinins have been administered into the renal artery of animals. When this is done there is a marked and rapid increase in renal blood flow. In addition to the increase in renal blood flow there is a concomitant increase in sodium excretion, urine volume, and free water clearance. Additional studies have demonstrated a decrease in medullary osmolality and an increase in papillary plasma flow. Bradykinin is also a potent stimulus to renal prostaglandin E production, and some authors have suggested that certain of the effects of bradykinin administration are mediated by renal prostaglandin synthesis. When the administration of intrarenal bradykinin is discontinued there is a prompt return of renal blood flow, urine flow, sodium excretion, and osmolality to previous control values.

Because of the potent effects of bradykinin in experimental animals a role for the kallikrein–kinin system in the regulation of renal function has been proposed. Evidence to support this contention to date has been quite limited. Aldosterone appears to be an important regulator of renal kallikrein excretion. In patients with primary aldosteronism there is an elevation of renal kallikrein excretion, and the administration of spironolactone decreases the rate of kallikrein excretion. In addition, studies in normal man have demonstrated an inverse relationship between the change in sodium intake and excretion and renal kallikrein excretion.

It has been suggested that a deficiency of the kallikrein–kinin system might play a role in certain forms of both experimental and human hypertension. While some preliminary data have been gathered to support this contention, additional studies clearly will be necessary before a definitive role for the kallikrein–kinin system in the regulation of either systemic or renal hemodynamics can be accepted. Recent studies have demonstrated alterations in the kallikrein–kinin system in patients with Bartter's Syndrome and after furosemide administration, but it is not yet clear what role these factors play in the alteration of renal hemodynamics and electrolyte excretion.

REFERENCES

Abe K, Irokawa N, Yasujima M, et al: The kallikrein–kinin system and prostaglandins in the kidney: Their relation to furosemide-induced diuresis and to the renin-angiotensin-aldosterone system in man. Circ Res 43:254, 1978

McGiff JP (Chairman): Kinins, renal function and blood pressure regulation. Fed Proc 35:172, 1976

Pisano JF, Austen KF (eds): Chemistry and Biology of the Kallikrein–Kinin System in Health and Disease. Washington, D.C., DHEW Publications Publication No. (NIH) 76:791, 1976

Vinci JM, Gill JR Jr, Bowden RE, et al: The kallikrein–kinin system in Bartter's syndrome and its response to prostaglandin synthetase inhibition. J Clin Invest 61:1671, 1978

PROSTAGLANDINS

Meyer D. Lifschitz

The prostaglandins are a series of fatty acids which are derived from the metabolism of arachidonic acid. The presently recognized structures and their sequence of synthesis are depicted schematically in Fig. 1. Arachidonic acid is a structural lipid which is bound to plasma membranes. The first step in the initiation of prostaglandin (PG) synthesis is the activation of phospholipase A_2, which cleaves arachidonic acid from the membrane. Next a series of enzymes synthesize PGG_2 and PGH_2, cyclic endoperoxides, which are quite unstable chemically and exist for only a very short period of time. From the cyclic endoperoxides three major pathways then exist. The first is to the classical prostaglandins PGE_2, $PGF_{2\alpha}$, and PGD_2. The other two major pathways involve the synthesis of relatively recently described structures PGI_2 (PGX, prostacyclin) and thromboxane A_2.

ANATOMICAL LOCATION WITHIN THE KIDNEY

The classical prostaglandins PGE and PGF are made in large part in the medulla and papilla of the kidney. In fact, the renal medulla is one of the richest sources for prostaglandin production in the body. Recent evidence would suggest that PGD is also synthesized within the medulla of the kidney. There is also some potential for synthesis of the classical prostaglandins in the cortex, but this is quantitatively much less than that which occurs in the medulla. In contrast, PGI_2 appears to be made in large part in the cortex, and only a modest amount of PGI_2 synthesis has been identified in the deeper regions of the kidney. It may be that PGI_2 synthesis is located specifically in glomeruli and perhaps within the vascular endothelium. This would seem reasonable because many blood vessels in the body have been shown to have PGI_2 synthetase. Thromboxane synthesis exists within the kidney but has not been localized to a specific region.

RENAL TRANSPORT

Since the classical prostaglandins are fatty acids, it is not surprising that data exists which demonstrate that PGE_2 and $PGF_{2\alpha}$ can be secreted into the tubular lumen by the organic acid secretory pathway. In addition, there is limited evidence from microinjection studies to suggest that some amount of PGE_2 may be reabsorbed from the tubular lumen perhaps in the loop of Henle; however, since the kidney has such a relatively large potential for prostaglandin synthesis, urinary prostaglandins presently are felt to reflect renal prostaglandin synthesis rather than the amount of prostaglandins delivered to the kidney by the blood stream.

PROSTAGLANDIN SYNTHETASE INHIBITORS

Because it has been quite difficult to measure the various prostaglandins much of the present information concerning the effect of prostaglandins in physiological and pathophysiological conditions derives from studies in which drugs which alter prostaglandin synthesis have been used. The first enzyme in prostaglandin synthesis, phospholipase A_2, can be partially blocked by cortisol, aldosterone, and mepacrine. The cyclooxygenase step can be blocked by a number of nonsteroidal antiinflammatory agents, including aspirin, indomethacin, and naproxin. Although at present there are no specific inhibitors of the classical prostaglandin synthetase pathway beyond PGH_2 or of PGI_2 synthesis, imidazole appears to be a relatively specific inhibitor of thromboxane A_2 synthesis.

PHYSIOLOGY OF THE RENAL PROSTAGLANDINS

Prostaglandins are synthesized at the level of the cell, and at least for the classical prostaglandins it is felt that they act mainly within the region where they are synthesized. Anatomical and enzymatic evidence exists for prostaglandin synthetase both within the renal interstitial cells and the collecting ducts. There may well be prostaglandin synthetase in other anatomical structures in the kidney as well. Because the classical prostaglandins, in particular PGE_2, are rapidly inactivated in one passage through the lung, it is presently felt that PGE_2 plays its role upon the kidney by local production and action. This same generalization does

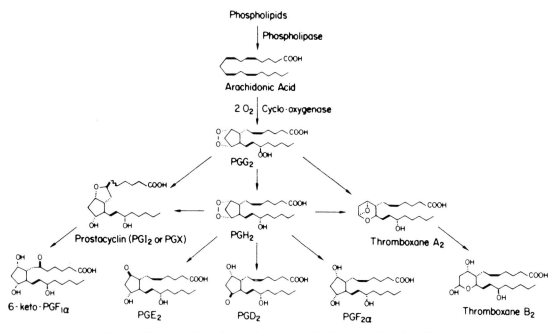

Fig. 1. Sequence of synthesis of prostaglandins from arachidonic acid.

not hold as well for PGI_2 because PGI_2 is not very well extracted or inactivated by the lungs and thus may be released by the kidney and perhaps other anatomical sites and can act as a circulating hormone on the systemic circulation. The exact systemic or renal regulatory role of thromboxane A_2 is still unclear.

At this point, there are major considerations for the role that prostaglandins may play in the regulation of renal function: (1) prostaglandins may regulate renal hemodynamics, (2) they may be involved in the regulation of sodium excretion, (3) they may be involved in renal water excretion, and (4) they may play a role in modulating the renin–angiotensin system.

RENAL BLOOD FLOW

The classical prostaglandins PGE_2 and PGD_2 both are potent renal vasodilating agents, and PGI_2 also vasodilates the kidney, while thromboxane A_2 is a potent renal vasoconstricting agent. While the administration of the inhibitors of prostaglandin synthesis does not markedly effect renal blood flow in awake studies, there is usually a fall in blood flow in the anesthetized animal, suggesting that endogenous prostaglandin release may play a role in the maintenance of blood flow in this latter setting; however, recent evidence would suggest that the administration of the thromboxane synthetase inhibitor imidazole is associated with an increase in renal blood flow, suggesting that the kidney of anesthetized animals may make thromboxane A_2 as well. It may be that rather than playing a primary role in controlling renal blood flow

the renal prostaglandins modulate renal blood flow by attenuating the response of the kidney to vasoconstricting agents such as angiotensin II and norepinephrine.

SODIUM EXCRETION

Considerable controversy exists at present as to the role that the renal prostaglandins may play in altering renal sodium excretion. Acute experiments have demonstrated that the intrarenal administration of PGE_2, PGD_2, or PGI_2 leads to both an increase in renal blood flow and renal sodium excretion; however, since the effect of intraarterial administration may be quite different from the physiological effect of local prostaglandin production, interpretation of these experiments is not simple. In studies in which inhibitors of prostaglandin synthesis have been administered some investigators find an increase and others find a decrease in sodium excretion. There is also similar controversy over whether or not changes in the rate of production of the classical prostaglandins exists in conditions in which chronic alterations in sodium balance are achieved. Recent studies have demonstrated an increase in PGE_2 during the administration of the loop diuretics, furosemide and ethacrynic acid; however, there is no direct evidence to suggest that the increased prostaglandin production induced by certain diuretics necessarily is an important determinant of the diuretic action of these agents.

RENAL WATER EXCRETION

Studies both in vitro and in vivo have demonstrated that PGE_2 has the ability to antagonize the hydroosmotic effect of antidiuretic hormone. This phenomenon has been observed in the isolated cortical collecting tubule, in the isolated toad bladder, and in clearance studies in both dogs and rats. On the basis of such findings it has been suggested that renal PGE_2 may play a role in modulating the hydroosmotic effect of vasopressin on the collecting system. This suggestion is supported by observations in which the administration of an inhibitor of prostaglandin synthesis such as indomethacin or meclofenamate enhances the renal response to a fixed amount of antidiuretic hormone administration. Although $PGF_{2\alpha}$ does not have the ability to antagonize antidiuretic hormone, studies have not been performed to date to determine whether PGI_2 or other prostaglandins may also modulate the concentrating mechanism.

RENIN–ANGIOTENSIN SYSTEM

On the basis of several lines of evidence it has been suggested that the prostaglandins play an intimate role in modulating the level of activity of the renin–angiotensin system. Angiotensin II is a potent stimulus for renal prostaglandin production, since angiotensin II stimulates phospholipase A_2 activity. Although in vivo studies with PGE_2 given into the renal artery have demonstrated an increase in plasma renin activity, PGE_2 does not appear to stimulate renin release in vitro, while PGI_2 does. Nonsteroidal antiinflammatory agents that inhibit cyclooxygenase and subsequent prostaglandin synthesis also lower the level of plasma renin activity in most experimental situations. Thus most evidence to date would suggest a parallel change between the level of prostaglandin synthesis and the level of activity of the renin–angiotensin system; however, recent studies have also demonstrated that at least under unique situations one can disassociate the level of the renin–antiotensin system from the level of renal prostaglandin synthesis. Further studies will obviously be necessary to clarify the potential role of the renal prostaglandins in the regulation of renal function.

REFERENCES

Anderson RJ, Berl T, McDonald KM, et al: Prostaglandins: Effects on blood pressure, renal blood flow, sodium and water excretion. Kidney Int 56:420, 1976

Dunn MJ, Hood VL: Prostaglandins and the kidney. Am J Physiol 233:F169, 1977

Frolich JC, Wilson TW, Sweetman BJ, et al: Urinary prostaglandins: Identification and origin. J Clin Invest 55:763, 1975

Lee, JB, Patak RV, Mookerjee BK: Renal prostaglandins and the regulation of blood pressure and sodium and water homeostasis. Am J Med 60:798, 1976

Lee JR (ed): The Renal Prostaglandins, vol. 1. St. Albans, Vt., Eden Press, 1977

McGiff JC, Itskovitz MD: Prostaglandins and the kidney. Circ Res 33:479, 1973

Zins GR: Renal prostaglandins. Am J Med 58:14, 1975

VITAMIN D
Nama Beck

Vitamin D is a sterol hormone and serves as a major physiological regulator of calcium (Ca) and phosphorus (Pi—plasma inorganic phosphorus) metabolism. In both vitamin D biosynthesis and the mechanism of action of vitamin D on Ca and Pi metabolism the kidney plays a pivotal role. The mechanism(s) of action of vitamin D is complex. Vitamin D affects at least three major organs (the intestine and bone as well as the kidney) and functions in concert with parathyroid hormone (PTH). All of these factors are closely interrelated in the physiological effects of vitamin D and therefore must be considered together to obtain a clear understanding of the physiological role of vitamin D.

VITAMIN D SYNTHESIS

Man's supply of vitamin D derives from both dietary intake and conversion in the skin of 7-dehydrocholesterol to vitamin D_3 by the ultraviolet rays of the sun. Vitamin D_3 (cholecalciferol) is metabolized to 25-hydroxycholecalciferol, $25(OH)-D_3$, mainly in the liver. $25(OH)-D_3$ has modest biological activity on G-d Ca absorption. Further, 25-hydroxylation of vitamin D_3 in the liver microsomal fraction is not a regulated step. For example, the plasma concentration of $25(OH)-D_3$ may rise as much as 30-fold simply by increasing the intake of vitamin D. Thus, $25(OH)-D_3$ is probably a metabolic intermediate of vitamin D.

$25(OH)-D_3$ is metabolized to 1α, 25-dihydroxycholecalciferol, $1,25(OH)_2-D_3$, in the kidney. This produce is extremely potent in facilitating Ca absorption in the intestin, and its mode of onset is rapid compared to other vitamin D products. Thus $1,25(OH)_2-D_3$ is felt to be the major active form of vitamin D; however, the possibility that $1,25(OH)_2-D_3$ may be further metabolized to yield products with biological activity in target organs cannot be excluded. The 1α-hydroxylation of vitamin D occurs exclusively in the mitochondria of the renal cortex, and this step is tightly regulated. The primary effect of $1,25(OH)_2-D_3$ is on Ca and Pi metabolism. In addition, Ca and Pi directly and indirectly influence 1α-hydroxylation of $25(OH)_2-D_3$. Thus $1,25(OH)_2-D_3$ appears to be under "feedback control." The step of 1α-hydroxylation in the kidney is, however, not a simple feedback-regulated reaction. The biochemical mechanism of action of $1,25(OH)_2-D_3$ involves binding to its specific receptor in cell cytosol, activation of selected genes, and the biosynthesis of new messenger RNA (mRNA) which then codes for proteins capable of changing cellular functions.

FACTORS REGULATING 1α-HYDROXYLATION OF VITAMIN D

The following factors are known to modulate 1α-hydroxylation of vitamin D in the kidney:

Parathyroid hormone. PTH stimulates 1α-hydroxylation of vitamin D in the kidney. The stimulatory effect of PTH is mediated by two processes: (1) PTH has a direct stimulatory effect on $1,25(OH)_2$-D_3 production in the kidney. For example, a simple injection of PTH enhances $1,25(OH)_2$-D_3 production. (2) Another effect of PTH on 1α-hydroxylation of vitamin D is an indirect stimulatory mechanism—PTH increases urinary Pi excretion and decreases plasma Pi. Hypophosphatemia, then, stimulates $1,25(OH)_2$-D_3 production in the kidney.

Calcium. Lowering of dietary Ca intake increases $1,25(OH)_2$-D_3 production in the kidney; however, the effect of Ca is an indirect mechanism rather than a direct stimulatory effect. Hypocalcemia requires intact parathyroid glands to elicit its stimulatory effect on 1α-hydroxylation of vitamin D, and parathyroidectomy eliminates the increase in $1,25(OH)_2$-D_3 in response to dietary Ca deprivation. Thus the effect on Ca on 1α-hydroxylation is felt to involve the following chain of events: a decrease in dietary Ca intake lowers plasma Ca, hypocalcemia stimulates PTH secretion, and the increased enhances $1,25(OH)_2$-D_3 production in the kidney.

Phosphorus. Dietary Pi deprivation or hypophosphatemia stimulates and hyperphosphatemia inhibits $1,25(OH)_2$-D_3 production in the kidney. In contrast to Ca, Pi has direct effect on 1α-hydroxylase in the kidney, and Pi-mediated 1α-hydroxylation does not require PTH.

$1,25(OH)_2$-D_3. In vitamin D deficiency, there is a marked increase in the renal 1α-hydroxylase enzyme.

In contrast, administration of physiological doses of vitamin D_3, $1\alpha(OH)$-D_3 or $1,25)OH)_2$-D_3 causes a virtual disappearance of this enzyme from the kidney. During this suppression of 1α-hydroxylase activity induced by vitamin D metabolites, 24-hydroxylase activity is stimulated in the kidney. Thus the regulation of enzyme activities between 1α-hydroxylase and 24-hydroxylase has an inverse relationship. $1,25(OH)_2$-D_3 may also influence the 1α-hydroxylase activity through an indirect mechanism. $1,25(OH)_2$-D_3 may suppress PTH secretion, leading to a removal of the stimulatory effect of PTH on 1α-hydroxylation. Thus $1,25(OH)_2$-D_3 limits its own production via dual mechanisms.

Calcitonin. Calcitonin leads to stimulation of 1α-hydroxylation of vitamin D in the kidney through an indirect effect on 1α-hydroxylation. The calcitonin-mediated 1α-hydroxylation involves a chain of events: hypocalcemia, an increase in PTH secretion, and the activation of 1α-hydroxylase by PTH.

Prolactin. The need for calcium is increased in women during lactation, and vitamin D is a hormone regulating Ca and Pi metabolism. Thus it is conceivable that vitamin D metabolism might be altered during lactation. Indeed, an injection of prolactin activates 1α-hydroxylase activity in the kidney and increases $1,25(OH)_2$-D_3 production; and circulating $1,25(OH)_2$-D_3 is elevated in lactating rats, implying that prolactin may have physiological effect on 1α-hydroxylation of vitamin D.

Estrogen. In pregnancy, Ca metabolism is also

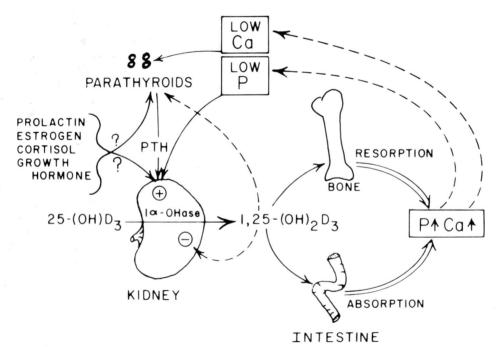

Fig. 1. Regulation of $1,25(OH)_2$-D_3 biosynthesis. Solid arrows indicate a positive effect, and dashed arrows refer to negative feedback. [Reprinted by permission from Haussler MR, McCain TA: Basic and clinical concepts related to vitamin D metabolism and action. N Engl J Med 297:974, 1977.]

altered, and it is expected that changes in vitamin D activity may contribute to the alteration of Ca metabolism in pregnancy. An injection of estrogen stimulates 1α-hydroxylase activity in the kidney, and plasma $1,25(OH)_2$-D_3 is elevated in pregnancy. Thus estrogen is felt to influence vitamin D activation under physiological conditions.

Glucocorticoids. The effect of vitamin D on Ca transport in the intestine is antagonized by glucocorticoids. On the other hand, cortisol has been shown to augment $1,25(OH)_2$-D_3 formation. Since cortisol has been shown to enhance PTH secretion, the effect of cortisol on vitamin D activation may be mediated through PTH.

In the kidney, vitamin D may be hydroxylated at the 24-position and may produce $24,25(OH)_2$-D_3 or $1,24,25(OH)_3$-D_3; however, the physiological role of these vitamin D metabolites is not clear.

In summary, $1,25(OH)_2$-D_3 is a hormone regulating Ca and Pi metabolism. Activation of vitamin D to $1,25(OH)_2$-D_3 in the kidney is tightly regulated by Pi and PTH and indirectly by Ca. Low Pi directly stimulates 1α-hydroxylation, whereas the low Ca^{2+} signal feeds through the parathyroid glands, with PTH being the mediator of the signal to 1α-hydroxylation. Once $1,25(OH)_2$-D_3 production is enhanced, the hormone acts on the intestine and bone. In the intestine, $1,25(OH)_2$-D_3 enhances absorption of both Ca and Pi. In bone, $1,25(OH)_2$-D_3 also augments mobilization of Ca and Pi. Thus plasma concentrations of both Ca and Pi rise by

an enhancement of $1,25(OH)_2$-D_3 production in the kidney. This activation of vitamin D corrects the original hypophosphatemia and/or hypocalcemia.

In addition, $1,25(OH_2$-D_3 governs its own synthesis through multiple mechanisms. An increase in plasma Pi directly suppresses PTH secretion, which in turn removes the stimulatory effect of PTH on 1α-hydroxylation. Thus the mobilization of calcium and phosphorus from bone and intestine as a result of $1,25(OH)_2$-D_3 activation closes the feedback loop regulating 1α-hydroxylase activity.

A possible direct effect of $1,25(OH)_2$-D_3 on the renal handling of Ca and Pi has been postulated. At the present time, however, data are inconclusive about indicating a direct effect of $1,25(OH)_2$-D_3 on Ca or Pi metabolism in the kidney. On the other hand, changes in Ca and Pi metabolism as a result of $1,25(OH)_2$-D_3 activation may indirectly alter renal handling of Ca and Pi and also PTH secretion.

REFERENCES

DeLuca HF: Vitamin D metabolism. Clin Endocrinol 7 Suppl:1S, 1977

Haussler MR, McCain TA: Basic and clinical concepts related to vitamin D metabolism and action. N Engl J Med 297:974, 1977

Holick MF, Clark MB: The photobiogenesis and metabolism of vitamin D. Fed Proc 37:2567, 1978

Methods of Diagnosing Renal Disease

URINALYSIS

Michael J. Sweeney and Marvin Forland

The important role which the kidneys play in homeostatic control of body fluid composition and volume requires their daily perfusion by quantities of blood equal to many times total body fluid volume. Urine is the major endproduct resulting from renal processing of these large volumes of perfusate. Hence appropriate analyses of urine often can provide valuable insights into homeostatic or pathologic events effecting body fluids. Moreover, unlike organ systems such as the heart and lungs, the general physical examination often reveals little or no information regarding the functional status or anatomic integrity of the kidneys and lower urinary tract. Therefore clinical evaluation of the upper and lower urinary tract generally requires further use of a variety of diagnostic studies. In the above contexts, "routine" urinalysis is one of the oldest and simplest but still most useful and informative of diagnostic tests.

This chapter describes urine collection procedures as well as the physical, chemical, and microscopic methodologies employed for "routine" examination of urine and discusses interpretation of the results of "routine" urinalyses.

"ROUTINE" URINALYSIS
Tests Performed

At the present time, "routine" urinalysis in office, clinic, and hospital settings generally consists of the following series of urine studies: (1) color and appearance, (2) specific gravity, (3) pH, (4) semiquantitative measurement of concentrations of protein, glucose, ketoacids, and heme-containing materials (erythrocytes, hemoglobin, myoglobin), (5) under some circumstances semiquantitative measurement of bilirubin and urobilinogen concentrations, and (6) microscopic examination of the urine sediment for the presence of erythrocytes, leukocytes, epithelial cells, various types of renal tubular casts, crystals, bacteria, and miscellaneous materials such as spermatozoa, mucuous threads, and fat droplets.

Because changes in pH and degeneration of cells and casts can occur with standing, particularly at room temperature, routine urinalyses should be performed within 1 hour after urine collection. If such is not possible, the specimen should be refrigerated until shortly before urinalysis is done.

Collection of Urine Specimens

Bladder urine is the ideal specimen for analysis, but except in special circumstances practical considerations preclude use of catheterization or needle puncture for obtaining such specimens. Thus routine urinalyses usually are done on voided specimens, the most satisfactory type of which is the so-called midstream urine. The procedure for obtaining the latter type of specimen from cooperative children and adults is as follows: (1) the specimen is collected in a clean glass or disposable plastic container; (2) males in a standing position and females seated with vulva spread initiate voiding into the toilets; (3) approximately halfway through voiding, and without interrupting urination, the container is positioned to "catch" several ounces of urine, after which the remainder of the urine is voided into the toilet. If bacteriologic studies also are desired, the midstream technique is employed along with a sterile container and initial cleansing of the external genitalia with a mild antiseptic solution. Use of the midstream technique is particularly important in females because it avoids vaginal reflux of urine and consequent contamination of the specimen with leukocytes, epithelial cells, and bacteria normally present in the vagina.

Because they cannot or will not void on demand, collection of urine specimens from infants and young children or from uncooperative or comatose patients can present difficulties. Careful catheterization may be necessary in comatose or uncooperative patients. The commonest technique used for obtaining specimens from infants and young children is to attach a specially designed plastic bag around the child's external genitalia and simply wait until the child voids into the bag. Some of the problems encountered with this technique include leakage, contamination with stool, and, in females, contamination of the urine with vaginal secretions and microorganisms. If the routine urinalysis is to be coupled with bacteriolgic studies of the urine, either a suprapubic needle aspiration of the bladder or careful urethral catheterization may be necessary in these young patients.

Timing of Urine Collection and Patient Dietary and Hydration Status

Most routine urinalyses are performed on random specimens collected without particular regard to the patient's hydration status or time of most recent food intake. Such specimens are satisfactory for most purposes; however, with some patients the type of information desired by the physician requires particular attention to the above variables, as illustrated by the following examples: (1) evaluation of renal concentrating or diluting capabilities, which requires appropriate manipulation of patient hydration status; (2) avoidance of the "alkaline tide" which can follow a meal, when simple evaluation of renal ability to form an acid urine is desired; (3) demonstration of orthostatic proteinuria, which requires collection of two urine specimens, one after the patient has been recumbent for several hours and the other after the patients has been up and active for several hours (see the chapter on Proteinuria); and (4) detection of postprandial glycosuria in a patient with diabetes mellitus.

Performance and Interpretation of Routine Urinalysis

Today, many of the older, more cumbersome methods for performing various components of routine urinalyses have been replaced by use of a variety of chemically impregnated reagent strips and tablets (Table 1). The chemical reactions between urine and the strips or tablets produce color changes which by use of appropriate charts permit semi-quantitative evaluation of the urinary constituents under study. Because many of these color changes are time dependent, test results should be read at the intervals given in the manufacturer's instructions.

The remainder of this section will be devoted to discussion of the performance and interpretation of the individual tests making up a routine urinalysis.

Urine Color and Appearance

Normal urine is clear and, depending on urine concentration, varies in color from light yellow (dilute urine) to dark brown (concentrated urine). A cloudy urine may indicate presence of large numbers of cells or crystals. The solubility of phosphates and urates is

Table 1

Chemically Impregnated Reagent Strips and Tablets Currently Available for Routine Urinalysis

Test	Reagent Strip	Reagent Tablet	Comment
pH	pH range 5–9	—	Nitrazine indicator papers cover pH range 4–8; precise pH measurement requires pH meter
Protein	Indicates approx. concentrations per decaliter: 5–20 mg (trace), 30 mg (1+), 100 mg (2+), 300 mg (3+), and 1000 mg (4+)	—	Highly alkaline urine may give false positives; many nephrologists prefer to use the sulfasalicylic acid turbidometric method
Glucose	Specific for glucose with lower range of sensitivity about 100 mg/dl; positive test results are light (1+), medium (2+), dark (3+)	Not specific for glucose; lower range of sensitivity about 200 mg/dl; positive test results range from trace (250 mg/dl) through 4+ (2000 mg/dl)	Strips use glucose oxidase; high urinary concentrations of ascorbic acid may cause false negative with strips; tablets detect glucose, lactose, galactose, fructose, pentose, gluconates, and ascorbic acid
Ketoacids	Positive results are small (1+), moderate (2+), and large (3+)	Positive results are small, moderate, large	Strips and tablets react with acetoacetic acid, are relatively insensitive to acetone, and do not react with beta hydroxybutyric acid
Blood	Positive results are small (1+), moderate (2+), and large (3+)	—	Reaction extremely sensitive to small quantities of heme; does not distinguish among erythrocytes, free hemoglobin, and free myoglobin; much less sensitive to intact erythrocytes; cannot be used to semiquantitate degree of hematuria
Bilirubin	Positive results are small (1+), moderate (2+), and large (3+)	Positive results not graded, but bilirubin concentration proportional to speed and intensity of color reaction	Strips are relatively insensitive and may give false negatives at low urine bilirubin concentrations; tablets quite sensitive and will detect bilirubin concentrations as low as 0.1 mg/dl urine
Urobilinogen	Positive results are read as 0.1, 1, 4, 8, and 12 Ehrlich units per dl urine	—	Concentrations of 0.1 and 1 considered normal; strongly alkaline urines show higher values and strongly acid urines lower values; porphobilinogen and p-aminosalicylic acid in urine give falsely high values

less at lower temperatures, and crystals may precipitate out in large quantities in refrigerated urines. Generally, these crystals will go back into solution with the simple warming of urine to room temperature. Infections of the lower urinary tract, prostate, and urethra, as well as vaginal reflux of urine, may be associated with presence of visible mucous strands in the urine.

A large number of exogenous and endogenous substances and pigments can lead to an abnormal urine color. Occasionally the abnormal color may represent an important clue to a particular disease process. A partial listing of abnormal urine colors and their causes includes the following:

1. Brown: bilirubin (to olive green on standing), blood, hemoglobin, myoglobin, homogentistic acid (to black on standing), quinine, cascara, phenacetin
2. Purple: porphyrin (on standing)
3. Black: melanoma
4. Yellow: Atabrine, riboflavin
5. Orange: Pyridium, Azulfidine
6. Red: phenytoin, phenolphthalein, vegetable dyes, beets, fresh blood, free hemoglobin
7. Green-blue: methylene blue, indigo blue, biliverdin

Urine Specific Gravity and Osmolality

Actual evaluation of kidney concentrating and diluting capacities requires measurement of urine osmolalities in the presence of water deprivation or a water load, respectively; however, in the absence of abnormal quantities of "heavy" molecules, which elevate specific gravity while producing little increase in osmolality, such as glucose, mannitol, radioopaque dye used for intravenous urograms, etc., urinary specific gravity can be used as an indirect measure of kidney concentrating and diluting capabilities. The normal range of urine specific gravity is about 1.003–1.030, corresponding to urine osmolalities of about 40 mOsm/kg water to slightly above 1000 mOsm/kg water. Random urine samples usually have specific gravities ranging from 1.005 to 1.020 and osmolalities ranging from about 100–600 mOsm/kg water.

Urine specific gravity reflects the weight of 1 cc of urine, a mixture of water and solute, compared to the weight of 1 cc of pure water. Osmolality reflects the total solute particle population per kg of urine water. Urine specific gravity can be measured with either a urinometer or a refractometer. The urinometer consists of a glass cylinder for holding the urine specimen and a hydrometer which is marked to indicate specific gravity (SG) values ranging from 1.000 to 1.060 at 0.001 intervals. The instrument is calibrated so that pure water has a SG of 1.000 at 20°C; for clinical purposes, correction of urine SG measurements for temperature is not necessary. Depending on the size of the hydrometer, 10–60 ml of urine are placed in the cylinder. The hydrometer is floated in the urine, and the specific gravity is read at the point where the urine meniscus crosses the hydrometer stem. Estimation of specific gravity with an appropriately calibrated refractometer depends on the close correlation between urinary specific gravity and refractive index. The refractometer is more expensive then the urinometer, but it has the advantage of requiring only a drop or so of urine. Urine osmolality generally is estimated by use of an instrument which measures the freezing point of the urine, an osmometer, and it depends upon the fact that 1 Osm (1000 mOsm) of solute per kilogram of water depresses the freezing point 1.83°C. The instruments are designed to provide a readout of osmolality rather than freezing point temperature.

Inability to produce urine specific gravities or osmolalities much above the minimum values with water deprivation occurs in diseases which produce diabetes insipidus or diabetes-insipidus-like syndromes. Renal failure, from whatever the cause, impairs both concentrating and diluting abilities, with eventual development of relative "fixation" of urine specific gravity and osmolality independent of patient hydration status— that is, urine specific gravities of 1.010± 0.003 and urine osmolalities of about 300± 100 mOsm/kg water. Other clinical settings with relative fixation of urine specific gravity and osmolality include acute tubular necrosis, chronic diuretic therapy, and osmotic diuresis. When renal disease is associated with heavy proteinuria, urine specific gravities often will be above 1.030 while osmolalities are similar to, or are only modestly greater than, serum osmolality. Another relatively common example of this dichotomy is seen with the heavy glycosuria of uncontrolled diabetes mellitus; specific gravities as high as 1.050 may occur when urine osmolalities are about 300. "Rules of thumb" for correcting urine specific gravities for presence of glucose or protein are as follows: reduce measured specific gravity by 0.004 units for each g/dl concentration of glucose and by 0.003 units for each g/dl concentration of protein.

Urine pH

The normal kidney can generate a urine pH ranging from about 4.5 to slightly greater than 8, corresponding to free hydrogen ion concentrations ranging from about 0.03 to 0.00001 mEq/liter. The pH of most freshly voided, random urine specimens is around 6, on the acid side of a neutral pH of 7. The pH of specimens left standing at room temperature tends to rise with time because of conversion of urea to ammonia by microorganisms growing in the urine and because of loss of carbon dioxide into the atmosphere. Therefore specimens which cannot be studied immediately should be refrigerated in capped containers whose volume is about the same as that of the urine specimen.

As shown in Table 1, the commonest method for measuring urine pH is colorimetric and makes use of paper strips which are chemically impregnated with pH-sensitive indicator dyes. Generally, these strips also are used for performing other components of the routine urinalysis and thus are impregnated with a number of chemical reagents at separate points along their surface.

The color and pH spectra of the strips are indicated on the label of the container in which they are purchased. While one pH unit is the increment shown on the color chart, the color changes usually permit estimation of 0.5 pH units. If a more precise measurement is desired, a pH meter must be used.

As a simple generalization, the pH of a particular urine specimen reflects the acid or base excretory load imposed on the kidney at the time of production of the specimen; however, when interpreting the significance of urine pH, the following points must be kept in mind: (1) catabolism of the usual diet generates a metabolic hydrogen ion load of about 30–50 mEq/m^2/day, essentially 100 percent of which is excreted by the kidney in a buffered form, either as titratable acidity or as ammonium ion; (2) as previously stated, even at the most acid urine pH the free hydrogen ion concentration in urine is minuscule; (3) an acid urine pH reflects the ratio of the concentrations of the base and acid components of the buffers making up titratable acidity, and thus demonstration of an acid urine pH does not provide information about the overall functional status of the kidney (ability to form an acid urine often is retained in far advanced renal disease) or about the quantities of metabolic hydrogen ion excreted either as titratable acidity or ammonium ion (measurement of both of these are research laboratory procedures); (4) while systemic acidosis usually is associated with a low urine pH, detection of a very acid urine does not necessarily indicate systemic acidosis; (5) when the urine pH is less than 6.1, the pK_1 of the bicarbonate ion/carbonic acid buffer pair, the urine contains little bicarbonate ion; (6) conversely, when the pH of essentially sterile, freshly voided urine is about 6.1, bicarbonate will be present in amounts which are directly related to the pH value (actual quantitation of the amount is a research laboratory procedure); (7) systemic alkalosis usually is accompanied by an alkaline urine, but the reverse is not necessarily true—alkaline urine may result from a postprandial "alkaline tide," from an alkaline diet, or from therapeutic use of the carbonic anhydrase inhibitor acetazolamide.

Some clinical situations in which urine pH may provide an important diagnostic clue include (1) the persistence of a very acid urine and absence of an alkaline tide seen in some patients who develop uric acid stones; (2) the acid urine seen in some patients with metabolic alkalosis and a severe total body potassium deficit; (3) the combination of a systemic hyperchloremic metabolic acidosis coupled with inability to generate a urine pH less than about 6, features which characterize the distal variety of renal tubular acidosis; (4) the combination of a systemic, hyperchloremic metabolic acidosis with formation of an acid urine when serum bicarbonate concentrations are below 17–18 mEq/liter but formation of an alkaline urine when the latter concentrations are exceeded, features which characterize the proximal variety of renal tubular acidosis; and (5) the persistently alkaline urine associated with urinary tract infection with microorganisms which split urea to form ammonia.

Proteinuria

(See the chapter on *Proteinuria* for discussion of pathophysiology and etiology of proteinuria.) As indicated in Table 1, detection of proteinuria in routine urinalyses usually is achieved with either colorimetric or tubidimetric methods. These tests provide semiquantitative information regarding protein concentration in the particular urine specimen under study; the minimum concentrations they will detect are about 5–10 mg/dl.

In healthy individuals, the daily volume of urine usually is large enough to prevent rise in concentration of the normally excreted quantities of urine protein to levels exceeding the minimal sensitivity of the tests. The test results generally reflect 24-hour urine protein excretory rates, but they are not substitutes for the latter measurements.

The most commonly used colorimetric tests employ a chemically impregnated reagent strip (the dipstick). The method depends on the ability of protein to change the color of a pH indicator dye in the absence of any change in pH. The indicator dye–pH-buffer combination used in these strips is tetrabromphenyl blue dye and pH 3 citrate buffer. At pH 3 the dye is yellow in the absence of protein; it changes to green and then to blue with increasing protein concentrations. Color changes are rather subtle and must be carefully compared to the color chart on the label of the reagent strip container. Positive results range from trace, representing protein concentrations of 5–20 mg/dl, through 4+, representing protein concentrations above 1000 mg/dl. The indicator dye is considerably more sensitive to albumin than to globulins, and thus the reagent strip may not detect hemoglobin, Bence Jones protein, or the globulins associated with so-called tubular proteinuria. It also will not detect Tamm-Horsfall mucoprotein. Because the indicator dye turns blue at pH above 3 highly alkaline urines may cause false positive results by overcoming the citrate buffer impregnated in the strip.

The sulfosalicylic acid (SSA) turbidimetric method is preferred by many nephrologists because test results are less subtle than the color changes occurring with reagent strips. The SSA method depends upon the fact that protein in solution precipitates in the presence of an acid. Thus addition of SSA to urine containing detectable concentrations of protein will produce turbidity which varies directly with protein concentration. Commonly used SSA concentrations are 3 percent and 20 percent. When 3 percent SSA is employed, about 0.5 ml of solution is thoroughly mixed with 0.5 ml of urine, and when 20 percent SSA is used, two or three drops of solution are mixed with 3–5 ml of urine. Development of turbidity usually indicates elevated urine protein concentrations and is reported on the scale of 0-4+ as shown in Table 2.

False positive results with the SSA method may occur with urines which are cloudy or which contain x-

Table 2
SSA Turbidimetric Method

Report	Protein Concentration (mg/dl)	Appearance
0	5	Clear
Trace	5–10	Slight turbidity
1+	15–30	Definite turbidity
2+	40–100	White cloud—no ppt
3+	150–300	White cloud—ppt present
4+	600–2000	Flocculant ppt

ray contrast media, metabolites of tolbutamide, or large amounts of penicillin. False negative results can occur with highly buffered alkaline urines.

Glucosuria and Other Reducing Substances in the Urine

As shown in Table 1, two colorimetric tests—a reagent strip and a reagent tablet—are in common use for detection of abnormal glucosuria. The reagent strip is specific for glucose and will detect concentrations greater than 100 mg/dl. The reagent tablet will detect glucose concentrations greater than 200 mg/dl, but it also gives positive results with fructose, galactose, lactose, pentose, glucuronates, and ascorbic acid. Thus a positive tablet test does not necessarily signify glucosuria unless the strip test also is positive. On the other hand, a positive tablet test, in the absence of a positive strip test, is good evidence that reducing substances other than glucose are present in the urine, a distinction which sometimes can be of considerable clinical importance, as in the lactosuria commonly seen during pregnancy and in some rare inherited diseases such as galactosemia.

The specificity of the reagent strip is based on the use of glucose oxidase and an indicator dye. When the strip is dipped into a urine containing detectable concentrations of glucose, a complex set of chemical reactions occur which result in enzymatic degradation of the glucose and production of a color change in the dye (red to deep lavender) that is roughly proportional to the glucose concentration. The reaction and consequent color change are time dependent, and the color should be compared with the chart on the strip container at the recommended time interval. False positive reactions are rare but can occur because of contamination of the urine with strong oxidizers such as peroxides or hypochlorite. False negative reactions can occur in the presence of high concentrations of ascorbic acid, a strong reducing agent.

The reagent table (Clinitest) is a modern-day adaptation of the long-used Benedict's test. Benedict's reagent consists of copper sulfate dissolved in an alkaline solution. When glucose, or one of the other substances previously listed, is added to the blue colored Benedict's solution and the mixture is heated, cuprous ions are reduced to cupric ions, and a color change occurs, ranging from green to orange, which is propor-

tional to the concentration of reducing substances in the mixture. The reagent tablet is a solid mixure of copper sulfate, sodium hydroxide, sodium carbonate, and citric acid. The test is performed by dropping a tablet into a test tube and adding five drops of urine and ten drops of water. The reaction between the fluid and the tablet releases heat and carbon dioxide and causes the solution to boil. Approximately 15 sec after boiling has stopped, the tube is shaken and the solution color is matched with the accompanying color chart. The color change is read from negative to 4+ and corresponds to the following glucose concentrations shown in Table 3.

As stated above, false positive tests for glucose will occur if urine contains any of a variety of other reducing substances. False negative reactions do not occur unless the tablets have deteriorated because of prolonged exposure to the atmosphere during storage. Because the tablets contain a strong alkali (sodium hydroxide) they are corrosive and can produce severe lye-type burns if ingested. Hence they should be stored out of reach of children.

Diabetes mellitus is the most common disease associated with glucosuria. In this disease, the so-called renal tubular threshold for glucose is normal (or even elevated in some patients), but higher than threshold blood sugar concentrations (about 180–200 mg/dl) result in delivery of more glucose in the glomerular filtrate than can be handled by proximal tubular glucose reabsorption sites. A similar mechanism accounts for the transient glucosuria frequently noted in nondiabetic patients receiving intravenous glucose solutions. A lower than normal tubular threshold can result in detectable glucosuria in the presence of normal blood sugar concentrations in a number of renal diseases, including hereditary renal glucosuria, Fanconi's syndrome, acquired and hereditary glomerulonephritides, and exposure to a variety of nephrotoxins.

Ketonuria

By definition, ketonuria refers to elevated urinary concentrations of beta hydroxybutyric acid, acetoacetic acid, and acetone. Independent of the absolute urinary concentrations of these three ketone bodies, beta hydroxybutyric acid generally makes up about 78 percent of those present, acetoacetic acid 20 percent, and acetone 2 percent. This relatively constant distribution of urinary ketone bodies is most fortunate because the most frequently employed tests for demonstrating ketonuria do not detect beta hydroxybutyric acid, and are about tenfold more sensitive for acetoacetic acid than for acetone. Thus for the most part acetoacetic acid is the ketone body actually detected by these methods. As with glucose, reagent strip and reagent tablet methods (Table 1) are in common use and represent modern day adaptations of the colorimetric test first described by Rothera in 1908, the development of a pink to purple color in proportion to urinary ketone concentrations when a mixture of ammonium sulfate and sodium nitroprusside is introduced into the urine and the urine is then overlayed with ammonium hydroxide.

The modern day reagent strip test usually is one of several on multipurpose strips. The test area is impregnated with nitroprusside, glycine (as the nitrogen source), and a strongly alkaline buffer. When the strip is dipped in urine containing acetoacetic acid, a purple color develps, the intensity of which is roughly proportional to the urinary concentration of ketone bodies. Because color development is time dependent, the color change must be compared with the chart on the strip container at the suggested time interval. Test results are read as negative, 1+, 2+, or 3+, with positive results translated as indicating small, moderate, and large urinary concentrations of ketone bodies, respectively.

The reagent tablets (Acetest) are white and consist of a mixture of sodium nitroprusside, aminoacetic acid (as the nitrogen source), an alkaline buffer, and lactose. In addition to detection of ketonuria, the tablets can be used to demonstrate ketonemia. A negative result is indicated when the tablet color does not change. Positive results reflect development of an increasingly intense purple color, which is graded as 1+, 2+, 3+, representing small, moderate, and large ketone body concentrations, respectively.

Ketonuria and ketonemia occur when body energy needs require utilization of fatty acids in amounts and at rates which exceed the body's capacity to metabolize them to carbon dioxide and water. Clinical settings in which such may occur include (1) dietary fat intake greatly in excess of that for carbonhydrate, e.g., ketogenic diets, (2) markedly decreased total caloric and carbohydrate intakes, as in acute starvation, acute illnesses, etc., and (3) impaired carbohydrate metabolism, as in diabetes mellitus and certain glycogen storage diseases. Ketonuria without evidence of systemic acidosis indicates that body fluid acid–base homeostatic mechanisms and renal hydrogen ion excretory rates are able to keep up with the acid loads imposed by metabolic formation of excess ketone bodies. When ketonemia occurs, ketonuria becomes more severe, and a metabolic acidosis develops whose severity often is proportional to the degree of ketonemia. The life threatening severe metabolic acidosis associated with uncontrolled, insulin deficient diabetes mellitus is the classical clinical example of ketoacidosis.

Table 3
Reagent Tablet Test

Reading	Glucose Concentration (g/dl)
Negative	<0.20
Trace	0.25
1+	0.50
2+	0.75
3+	1.00
4+	2.00

Heme Pigmenturia

Heme pigmenturia can result from (1) hematuria, (2) intravascular hemolysis with delivery of free hemoglobin into the urine via the glomerular filtrate, or (3) muscle injury with delivery of free myoglobin into the urine via the glomerular filtrate. Hematuria is by far the most common cause of heme pigmenturia.

A colorimetric test for detection of elevated urinary concentrations of heme pigments is incorporated in most of the multipurpose reagent strips. The test area is chemically impregnated with orthotolidine and a buffered organic peroxidase. Presence of a heme pigment in the urine catalyzes the reaction between the peroxidase and orthotolidine to produce a blue color, the intensity of which is roughly proportional to the free heme concentration in the urine. As with other time-dependent colorimetric tests, after dipping of the strip in the urine the color change must be compared with the chart on the strip container at the recommended time interval. Positive test results are graded as 1+, 2+, and 3+, representing small, moderate, and large heme concentrations, respectively. False positive and false negative reactions are not common. The former may occur if the urine is contaminated with strong oxidizing agents such as hypochlorite or microbial peroxidases in urines with high bacterial counts. False negatives may occur in the presence of high urinary concentrations of ascorbic acid because the reducing activity of the latter can interfere with peroxidase.

For the most part, the pigmenturia detected with hematuria probably represents free hemoglobin derived from hemolysis of small numbers of erythrocytes after their arrival in the urine. The lower limit of sensitivity of the strip test is a heme concentration of about 30 μg/dl, equivalent to the heme content of a red cell concentration of about 10/mm^3; that is, the reagent strip test is much more sensitive for free hemoglobin than it is for hemoglobin contained in intact erythrocytes. Consequently, the test cannot be used to quantitate the magnitude of hematuria, and demonstration of erythrocyturia by microscopic examination of the urine sediment is mandatory before equating a positive result with hematuria. Finally, the reagent strip test does not distinguish between hemoglobinuria secondary to intravascular hemolysis and myoglobinuria caused by muscle injury. Therefore if such is desired acrylamide gel electrophoresis or immunodiffusion techniques provide the most definitive differentiation.

Bilirubinuria

The only form of bilirubin appearing in the urine is that previously conjugated in the liver with glucuronic acid. In health, urinary concentrations of bilirubin are less than 0.02 mg/dl. Obstruction of the biliary ducts and hepatocellular disease are the major causes of abnormal bilirubinuria.

Bilirubin imparts a brown color to the urine, but not until concentrations considerably above normal are reached. Bilirubin also produces a yellow foam on shaking, but only at concentrations greater than 2 mg/dl. Thus neither of these tests will detect relatively low but still abnormal urinary bilirubin concentrations. The most commonly used methods (Table 1) for detecting abnormal bilirubinuria are colorimetric and employ either a reagent strip or a reagent tablet (Ictotest). the reagent tablet is quite sensitive and will detect bilirbun glucuronide concentrations on the order of 0.05–0.1 mg/dl. The reagent strip is convenient for general screening purposes, but the tablet is preferred for detection of hepatitis in its earlier phases. Both tests are more sensitive to bilirubin glucuronide than to free bilirubin. The importance of this fact is that on standing, and particularly if simultaneously exposed to light, the glucuronide may undergo hydrolysis. Further, the bilirubin may undergo oxidation to biliverdin, which is not detectable by either test. Hence both tests should be performed on freshly voided urine.

The reagent strip test area is impregnated with stabilized, diazotized 2,4-dichloroanaline, which reacts ·with bilirubin to form a tan to brown colored azobilirubin compound. The strip is dipped into urine in the usual manner. Color changes with a positive urine are quite subtle and time dependent, and they must be carefully compared with the chart on the strip container at the recommended time interval. Positive results are read as 1+, 2+, and 3+, representing small, moderate, and large urinary bilirubin concentrations.

The reagent tablets consist of a mixture of p-nitrobenzenediazonium, p-toluenesulfonate, sulfosalicylic acid, and boric acid. A positive result is indicated by development of a blue or purple color around the tablet. The urinary bilirubin concentration is proportional to the speed and intensity of the color reaction, but such is not specifically graded as are the strips. A negative result consists of development of no blue or purple color within 30 sec.

False positive reactions with either the strip or tablet may occur if the urine contains large amounts of phenothiazine metabolites. Pyridium-like drugs will give a red color, and this may cause false negative results because the red color may obscure a slightly positive bilirubin test.

Urobilinogenuria

Urinary excretion of urobilinogen in normal individuals is on the order of 1–4 mg/24 hours. Excretion rates vary during the 24 hours and reach maximum values in midafternoon. The semiquantitative tests most commonly employed to detect urinary urobilinogen are colorimetric, and they make use of Ehrlich's reagent in an acid medium. The tests are not specific for urobilinogen but also detect other chromogens, including porphobilinogen, excreted by patients with acute porphyria, and the drug paraaminosalicylic acid. Hence results usually are expressed as Ehrlich units/dl of urine. Normal individuals excrete less than 1 Ehrlich unit per 2 hours during the time of maximum excretion (midafternoon), and urine concentrations usually do not exceed 1 Ehrlich unit/dl.

As indicated in Table 1, a reagent strip test is available for semiquantitative measurement of urinary concentrations of chromogens which react with Ehrlich's reagent. The test area on the strip is impregnated with paradimethylaminobenzaldehyde and an acid buffer. Ehrlich's reagent consists of a mixture of the former and hydrochloric acid. The ideal urine specimen to study is one collected over a 2-hour midafternoon period. The reagent strip is dipped in the urine in the usual maner, and color changes are compared to those on the strip container chart at the time interval directed by the manufacturer. Very low concentrations or absence of urobilinogen from the urine cannot be detected by the strip. If the clinical setting suggests the need to distinguish between urobilinogen and porphobilinogen, more elaborate chemical analyses are required.

Urobilinogen is formed in the gut as a result of microbial action on bilirubin glucuronide excreted into the duodenum via the biliary tract. In turn, bilirubin is a major endproduct of hemoglobin catabolism. About half of the urobilinogen formed in the intestine is excreted in the feces either as colorless urobilinogen or as its brown-colored oxidation product, urobilin. The half is reabsorbed into the portal circulation and, except for a small quantity which escapes into the systemic circulation and is excreted in the urine, is reexcreted by the liver into the intestine. Urinary excretion of greater than normal quantities of urobilinogen occurs (1) in diseases which cause increased rates of hemoglobin catabolism and thus increased rates of hepatic formation and excretion of bilirubin glucuronide, particularly hemolytic anemias, and (2) in diseases which impair hepatic excretion of urobilinogen, hepatocellular diseases. Conversely, abnormally low or absent urinary excretion of urobilinogen occurs (1) in diseases producing biliary tract obstruction and (2) in clinical settings which require use of antibiotics that reduce the intestinal population of bacteria capable of converting bilirubin to urobilinogen. Thus as illustrated in Table 4 simultaneously obtained tests for bilirubinuria and urobilinogenuria can be helpful in diagnosing and/or monitoring patients with hemolytic anemias, hepatocellular disease, and biliary obstructive disease.

MICROSCOPIC EXAMINATION OF URINE SEDIMENT

General

The urine sediment has been described as an "exfoliative biopsy" of the upper and lower urinary tract. The variety of elements which may be present in the

Table 4
Simultaneous Bilirubin and Urobilinogen Tests

	Normal	Hemolytic Anemias	Hepatocellular Disease	Biliary Obstruction
Urine bilirubin	Absent	Absent	Increased	Increased
Urobilinogen	Normal	Increased	Increased	Low

urine sediment is shown in Table 5. In comparison to the chemical portions of a routine urinalysis, proficient performance of the microscopic examination of the urine sediment requires considerable practice. The most suitable specimen for study is a freshly voided, concentrated first morning urine collected with the midstream technique; however, practical considerations often result in sediment examination of "random" urines collected at a time convenient for the patient and the laboratory. Because of the tendency for bacterial growth to occur and for casts to disintegrate and red cells to lyse when urine stands at room temperature, particularly if the urine is alkaline, refrigerator storage of the specimen is indicated when prompt examination is not possible.

Preparation of Urine Sediment for Study

Although procedures used by most laboratories are similar, universally accepted standards for preparation of urine sediments for study have not been established. Such can lead to confusion among physicians and laboratories regarding the boundary line between normal and abnormal. The techniques most commonly recommended in the literature are as follows:

1. Warm refrigerated specimens to room temperature. Amorphous urates present in acid urines tend to precipitate with cold storage but go back into solution with warming. Amorphous phosphates in alkaline urines tend to precipitate with cold storage and indeed even at room temperature; they will go back into solution if the specimen is acidified with a few drops of acetic acid, but care must be taken because red cells will lyse if too much acid is added.

2. After shaking the specimen to disperse formed elements which settled out with standing, place 10–15 ml of urine in a conical tube and centrifuge at 2000 rpm for 5 min. If total volume is less than 10–15 ml, centrifuge the entire speciman. If specimen contains large amounts of formed elements, as with gross hematuria or severe pyuria, a shorter centrifugation time may be indicated because centrifugation for 5 min may result in a sediment pellet which cannot be resuspended.

3. Following centrifugation, quickly invert the tube once and pour the supernatant urine off; stand the tube upright for a few seconds to allow urine on walls to cover sediment, and then shake gently to resuspend the sediment in the remaining fluid.

4. Place a drop of the suspension on a *clean* slide, top with a *clean* coverslip, and study while still wet.

5. Using a standard microscope and subdued light, study at least ten low-power (LPF) and ten high-power fields (HPF) and report the various sediment elements seen as follows: average number of leukocytes and erythrocytes per high-power field; average number of each type of cast per low-power field; bacteria as occasional (1+), few (2+), many (3+), or a great many (4+) per high-power field; and epithelial cells, crystals, amorphous material, oil droplets, mucous threads, spermatozoa, and the like as occasional (1+), few (2+), many (3+), or a great many (4+) per low-power field.

EVALUATION OF RESULTS OF SEDIMENT STUDY
General

In health, the sediment obtained after 5 min centrifugation of a randomly collected, freshly voided, clean, midstream urine specimen often contains no more than an occasional cell of any type, no casts, a

Table 5
Elements Which May Be Present in Urine Sediment

Cells	Casts	"Normal" Crystals and Amorphous Material	"Abnormal" Crystals	Other
1. Erythrocytes	1. Hyaline	Acid urine	Acid urine	1. Bacteria
2. Leukocytes	2. Red blood cell	1. Uric acid	1. Cystine	2. Yeast
3. Glitter (Schilling)	3. White blood cell	2. Sodium urate	2. Leucine	3. Protozoa
4. Epithelial	4. Fatty	3. Amorphous urates	3. Tyrosine	4. Parasites
Squamous	5. Granular	4. Calcium oxalate	4. Sulfonamide	5. Spermatozoa
Transitional	Coarse	Alkaline urine		6. Mucous threads
Tubular	Fine	1. Ammonium biurate		7. Oil droplets
Oval Fat Bodies	6. Renal failure	2. Calcium carbonate		8. Fecal, vaginal or
Tumor	Waxy	3. Calcium phosphate		perineal
	Broad	4. Triple phosphates		contaminants
	7. Pseudocasts	(ammonium–magnesium–		
	Crystals	calcium)		
	Amorphous	5. Amorphous phosphates		

few crystals, and a scattering of amorphous material. As a generalization, the most important pathophysiologic ''messages'' imparted by an abnormal urine sediment relate to increased numbers of one or more of the types of cells and/or casts listed in Table 5. Thus presence of ''normal'' crystals (Table 5) generally is of no clinical significance except in relatively unique circumstances which will be discussed in more detail below. Similarly, many of the items listed in the ''Other'' column in Table 5 are of no pathologic significance or become so only when vaginal, perineal, or fecal contamination has not occurred during collection of urine. Finally, the disease states or clinical settings in which the ''abnormal'' crystals listed in Table 5 are found are quite rare, but their detection may provide a clue to the patient's problem.

Cells

Erythrocytes. Semiquantitative studies of urinary erythrocyte excretion rates indicate normal individuals excrete 30,000–50,000 RBCs/m²/hour, equivalent to 1–2 million RBCs per 24 hours. In normal individuals, the sediment from a centrifuged, properly collected, random urine contains 0–2 RBCs/HPF, while highly concentrated urines may contain as many as 4 RBC/HPF. Values greater than 4 RBC/HPF, particularly if persistent, are abnormal.

Erythrocytes in urine have a pale to slightly greenish tinge, and depending on urine osmolarity may have shapes varying from the biconcave discs to swollen, shrunken, or crenated cells. Formed elements which may resemble erythrocytes include oil droplets, yeast cells, amorphous urates in an acid urine, and degenerated epithelial cells.

Abnormal erythrocyturia can vary from microscopic to gross hematuria and is a relatively nonspecific diagnostic sign because it can occur in a wide variety of diseases. Because of the diversity of etiologies, investigation into the cause of hematuria in individual patients will vary in nature and extent dependent on the overall clinical situation.

Nucleated cells. Polymorphonuclear leukocytes (''pus'' cells) and a variety of epithelial cells (Table 5) make up the nucleated cell populations found in the urine sediment. Not infrequently, these cell populations are lumped together under the heading ''white blood cells.'' Semiquantitative studies indicate that the upper limit of normal for leukocyte excretion is 2 million per 24 hours and that the upper limit of normal for total white cell excretion is 4 million per 24 hours. The sediment of centrifuged, randomly collected, midstream urine specimens from normal males contains 0–2 leukocytes per high-power field, and that from females contains 0–5 leukocytes per high-power field. Similar values obtain for epithelial cells. The larger cell numbers in females reflect the difficulty in completely preventing urine contamination with vaginal secretions.

Most leukocytes are neutrophils and are about 1.5 times the size of erythrocytes. They are relatively easy to identify because of the lobulated shape of their nuclei (Fig. 1). A unique type of leukocyte is the so-called ''glitter'' or Schilling cell. This leukocyte is larger than usual and appears pale blue with Sternheimer-Malbin stain, and its granules show Brownian movement. At one time these cells were considered pathognomonic for pyelonephritis; however, subsequently they were found to be the result of a hypotonic medium, and their frequent observation in patients with pyelonephritis reflects the urinary concentrating defect often seen in this disease.

If external contamination can be ruled out, the presence of more than 2 leukocytes per high-power field in the male and more than 5 per high-power field

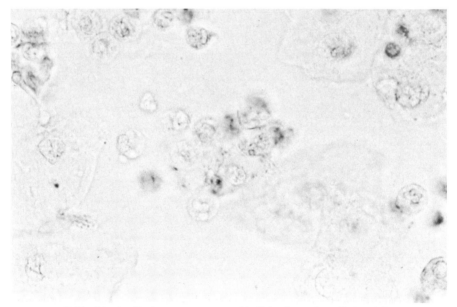

Fig. 1.   White blood cells, large, squamous epithelial cells, and motile bacteria. × 400.

in the female suggests the presence of an inflammatory process somewhere in the upper or lower urinary tract. Such may or may not be infectious in origin, and consideration must be given to results of the chemical portion of the urinalysis as well as the presence or absence of red cells and casts in the sediment. Thus sterile pyruia frequently accompanies the hematuria and/or cylinduria seen in various types of acute and chronic glomerulonephritis and noninfectious interstitial nephritis. Nonpyrogenic infections such as tuberculous pyelonephritis can produce an apparently sterile pyuria and will not be detected unless special efforts are made to culture the organisms from the urine. If the midstream collection technique is not used, pyuria without bacteriuria may be seen in males with nonspecific prostatitis or urethritis. Presence of more than 30–40 leukocytes per high-power field, particularly if some of the cells are in clumps or are associated with leukocyte casts, suggests an active infection and indicates need for quantitative bacteriologic studies of the urine. Thus as with erythrocyturia selection of further diagnostic studies to evaluate pyuria will vary in accordance with the overall clinical situation.

Squamous epithelial cells are large and flat and contain a single small nucleus (Fig. 1). These cells are of no pathologic significance and generally represent contaminants derived from the vulva or vagina and sometimes from the urethra. Transitional (also known as bladder) epithelial cells are intermediate in size between leukocytes and squamous cells, have a single moderate-sized round nucleus, usually are seen singly but occasionally occur in clumps, and can vary in shape from flat to cuboidal to columnar. They are derived

from the bladder and sometimes the renal pelvis, and most often simply represent normal desquamation. Occasionally, however, they represent exfoliative lesions of neoplastic orgin. Renal tubular epithelial cells are round, slightly larger than leukocytes, and each contain a single large nucleus. They can be confused with degenerating leukocytes. They usually occur singly or in groups of two or three, and, like transitional cells, are thought to represent desquamation. Occasionally, large numbers may be seen with diseases causing tubular degeneration. A special type of renal tubular cell is the oval fat body (Fig. 2). These are degenerated, swollen, fat-filled tubular cells which may appear dark in subdued light but refractile in bright light. The refractile material is made up of cholesterol esters which, under polarized light, shine brightly and have the shape of a Maltese cross. The presence of oval fat bodies in the urine indicates heavy proteinuria and the nephrotic syndrome or a disease capable of producing the nephrotic syndrome.

Casts. Casts are cylindrical masses of agglutinated material which represent a mold of a tubular lumen (Fig. 3). Because of their shape, a term frequently used to indicate the presence of casts in the urine is cylinduria. Casts usually are formed in the distal convoluted or collecting tubules. As shown in Table 5, several different varieties may be found in the urine sediment. Semiquantitative studies indicate normal individuals may excrete up to 10,000 casts per 24 hours. This is a small number in comparision to normal red and white cell excretion rates, and frequently scanning of the entire sediment reveals no or, at the most, one or two casts.

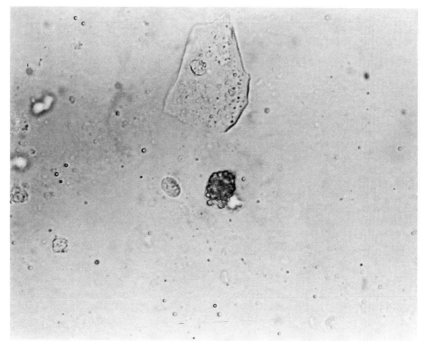

Fig. 2. Lipid-laden oval fat body above faintly outlined hyaline cast. Squamous epithelial cell at top of field. × 250.

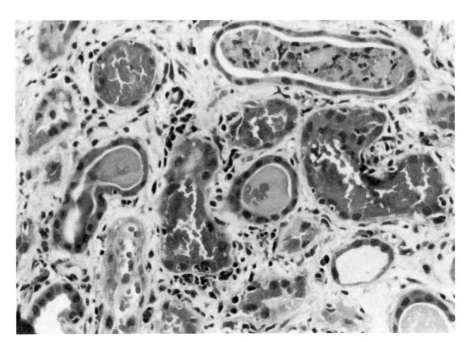

Fig. 3. Interstitium and tubules from patient with acute glomerulonephritis demonstrating cast formation. In situ precipitation of proteinaceous and cellular material is evident within many tubules. H & E. × 250.

The matrix for most casts is believed to be the Tamm-Horsfall mucoprotein, which is secreted by the distal nephron. This protein is produced in increased amounts in many renal parenchymal diseases and appears to be least soluble in slow-moving acidic tubular fluid. Disintegration of casts in an alkaline urine may be related to the latter solubility characteristics of the mucoprotein. When the mucoprotein precipitates, immunoglobulins, albumin, cells, cellular debris, and pigments also present in the tubular fluid become incorporated in the casts.

Hyaline casts are colorless, homogeneous, and transparent (Fig. 4). They consist of a mixture of Tamm-Horsfall mucoprotein and varying amounts of albumin

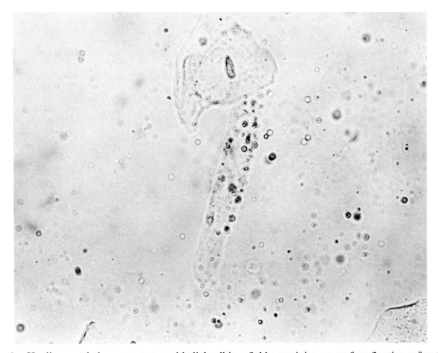

Fig. 4. Hyaline cast below squamous epithelial cell in a field containing many free-floating refractile lipid droplets. × 250.

and immunoglobulins. They are best seen with subdued light, and they usually have rounded or "squared" ends which help to distinguish them from mucous threads. They occur in large numbers in renal parenchymal diseases characterized by slow urine flow, acid pH and heavy proteinuria, as in the nephrotic syndrome. Their excretion often is increased with febrile illnesses, congestive heart failure, and physical exercise.

Red blood cell casts are hyaline casts which contain erythrocytes in their matrix or attached to their surface (Fig. 5). The hemoglobin in the cells imparts an orange-red color to the casts. Individual red blood cells may be distinct, or they may be difficult to identify if large numbers have been incorporated in the matrix and/or have undergone degeneration. The latter type of casts frequently are termed blood or hemoglobin casts. Red blood cell casts are pathognomonic of renal parenchymal disease, particularly that in which an active glomerulitis is present, although they may be seen in acute tubular necrosis.

White blood cell casts are hyaline casts which contain leukocytes or renal tubular cells. As with red blood cell casts, individual leukocytes or tubular epithelial cells may or may not be easy to identify, and thus distinguishing between casts filled with degenerating leukocytes and with degenerating epithelial cells may be difficult. Moreover, some casts may contain a mixture of red cells, leukocytes, and tubular cells. Leukocyte casts are indicative of a renal parenchymal inflammatory process which may or may not be due to bacterial infection. The diagnosis of pyelonephritis requires more evidence than the simple presence of leukocyte casts. Casts containing renal tubular cells can occur in any renal parenchymal disease associated with tubular degeneration and hence are relatively nonspecific.

Fatty casts are hyaline casts which contain highly refractile fat globules, termed oval fat bodies or neutral fats. Like free oval fat bodies, those incorporated in fatty casts contain cholesterol esters and will show the typical Maltese cross when studied by polarized light (Fig. 6). The neutral fats probably are derived from degenerating tubular cells incorporated in the casts, and such fat droplets will stain bright orange with Sudan III. Fatty casts have the same significance as oval fat bodies and are most commonly seen in patients with heavy proteinuria who have either an overt nephrotic syndrome or a disease capable of producing a nephrotic syndrome.

Granular casts are hyaline casts in which debris from degenerated cells has become incorporated. Depending on the size of the granules, these casts are further subdivided into coarsely and finely granular varieties (Figs. 7 and 8). Presence of granular casts in the urine sediment usually is indicative of significant renal parenchymal damage.

Renal failure casts typically are broader than other types of casts and often have a waxy appearance. Presumably, they are formed in the dilated, thin-walled tubules characteristic of chronic renal failure of any cause. Urine flow through the tubules is markedly diminished and slow, and the residence time of cellular casts formed in them is prolonged. Thus once such casts finally are excreted into the urine, they are broad in dimension and may have a homogeneous waxy appearance because of complete degeneration of any

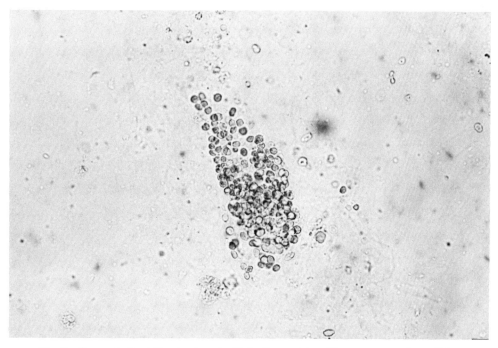

Fig. 5. Segment of red blood cell cast with hyaline matrix evident at upper pole. × 400.

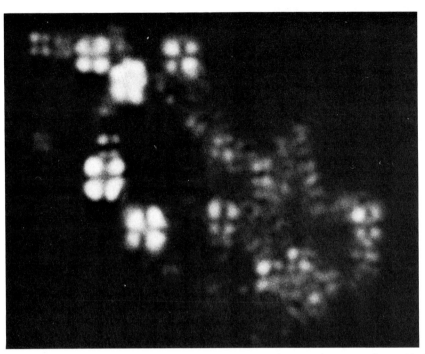

Fig. 6. Doubly refractile fat droplets in a lipid-laden granular cast from a patient with focal glomerular sclerosis and nephrotic syndrome. Oil immersion, polarized light. × 1000.

cellular material which originally was incorporated in them.

Pseudocast is the term applied to conglomeration of crystals or amorphous materials such as urates or phosphates in a form that resembles cellular or granular casts.

Crystals

Many types of crystals can be found in the urine sediment. As a general rule, presence of crystals designated in Table 5 as "normal" is of little or no clinical importance. An exception to the rule is calculous disease of the urinary tract, wherein the type(s) of crys-

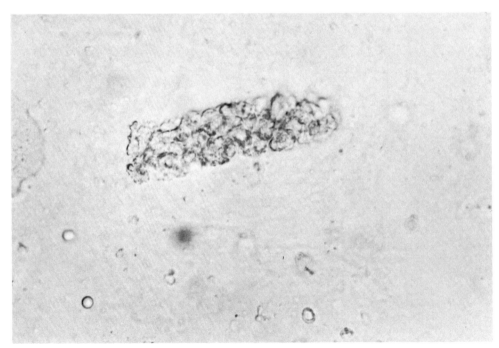

Fig. 7. Coarsely granular cast; cellular elements are still evident. × 400.

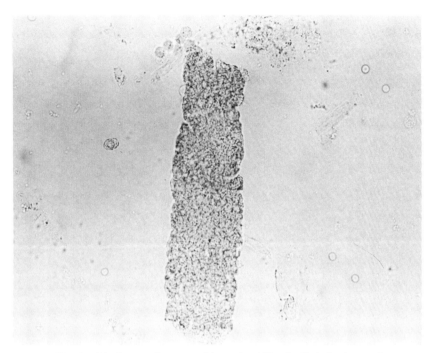

Fig. 8. Finely granular cast; white and red blood cells in background.

tal(s) found in the sediment may provide a diagnostic clue regarding stone chemical composition. Conversely, detection of the crystals designated in Table 5 as "abnormal" virtually always has diagnostic and/or pathologic significance. As also indicated in Table 5, urine pH is an important determinant for the type of crystals found in any particular urine specimen. Since the hydrogen ion load derived from the usual diet results in an acid urine, an alkaline urine with its characteristic crystalluria may or may not have clinical significance. For example, an alkaline urine in an otherwise healthy individual may reflect an alkaline ash diet or the normal postprandial alkaline tide; however, probably the most common cause for an alkaline urine in such individuals is postvoiding proliferation of urea-splitting organisms. Thus as with other components of the urine sediment evaluation of crystalluria should be performed on freshly voided urine specimens. On the other hand, a persistently alkaline urine pH in the freshly voided urine of an individual ingesting the usual diet and not receiving medications which alkalinize the urine is of concern. This may indicate presence of distal renal tubular acidosis or urinary tract infection with urea-splitting organisms which place the patient at risk for development of calculi whose chemical composition is similar to that of the "normal" crystals found in an alkaline urine.

"Normal" crystals found in an acid urine. *Uric acid crystals* usually are yellow-brown in color and rhombic or hexagonal in shape. Sometimes they may appear as sheaves or as prismatic rosettes. While patients with uric acid disorders or uric acid stones may have increased urinary concentrations of uric acid and its salts, presence of uric acid or urate crystals in the sediment does not imply increased urinary concentrations.

Sodium urate crystals are colorless or have a yellowish hue, and they appear as prisms or needles arranged in fan or sheave-like clusters.

Amorphous urates are yellow-brown granules about one-tenth the size of red cells. They tend to occur in conglomerations which sometimes can be mistaken for granular casts, pseudocasts. For the most part, they are composed of sodium urate.

Calcium oxalate crystals are colorless and are mostly envelope or dumbbell shaped. They also can be seen in neutral or slightly alkaline urines. Calcium oxalate is one of the most common constituents of renal stones, but presence of such crystals in the urine does not imply stone disease. They may be present in relatively large numbers in the sediments of patients with one of the hereditary or acquired oxaloses, such as ethylene glycol intoxication.

"Normal" crystals found in an alkaline urine. *Ammonium biurate crystals* are yellow, spherical bodies usually with long spicules and are likened in appearance to thorn apples. When they occur within spicules, they may be confused with yeast spores or red cells. They may be present in large numbers in normal urines which have become alkaline with standing.

Calcium carbonate crystals are colorless granules which can appear singly or in masses and often have a dumbbell shape. Calcium carbonate frequently is present in small amounts in renal calculi.

Calcium phosphate crystals generally are colorless and can take the forms of relatively large, irregular plates or of stellate prisms. As with triple and amorphous phosphate crystals (see below) they may be present in relatively large numbers in urines which have become alkaline on standing or in urines which are alkaline at the time of voiding because of urinary tract infection with urea-splitting organisms.

Ammonium–magnesium–calcium phosphate (triple phosphate) crystals are colorless and have the form of "coffin lids" or feathery leaves. Triple phosphates are frequently found in renal calculi.

Amorphous phosphates are relatively colorless small granules composed mostly of calcium phosphate. Like amorphous urates, they tend to conglomerate, and they occasionally may form pseudocasts.

"Abnormal" crystals found in an acid urine. Cystine crystals are colorless, highly refractile, rather thick hexagonal plates whose appearance has been likened to benzene rings. Their presence in the urine sediment suggests the patient has one of the hereditary cystinurias; the homozygous variety may be associated with urinary tract cystine calculi.

Leucine and tyrosine crystals may be seen in the urine sediment of patients with acute liver necrosis of any cause. Leucine crystals are highly refractile yellow or brown spheres with delicate radial or concentric striations. Tyrosine crystals are colorless, fine needles and usually are grouped in clusters or sheaves.

Sulfonamide crystals can assume a great variety of forms depending on the parent compound. Many of the sulfonamides employed a number of years ago, such as sulfonilamide and sulfapyridine, were relatively insoluble in acid urines, and their crystals sometimes led to renal damage following their deposit in renal tubules. Hence their appearance in the urine suggested the patient was at risk for such crystal deposition. The newer sulfonamides, such as sulfisoxazole, are much more soluble in acid urines and have not been associated with renal crystal deposition problems.

MISCELLANEOUS OTHER CONSTITUENTS OF THE URINE SEDIMENT

As shown in Table 5, the urine sediment also may contain a variety of items other than those described above, including several types of living organisms, spermatozoa, oil droplets, mucous threads, and materials derived from fecal, vaginal, or perineal contamination of the urine. The main problem caused by many of these materials is that they may obscure important findings or may be mistaken for components of the urine sediment which have real diagnostic or pathologic significance. In many instances, these materials come from outside the urinary tract, and the difficulties they cause can be eliminated by examination of freshly voided urines collected by the midstream method.

Bacteria, Yeast, Protozoa, Parasites, etc.

The probability of significant bacteriuria (colony count greater than 10^5 per ml) is high when microscopic examination of a properly collected midstream speci-

men reveals any bacteria in an uncentrifuged urine or more than 20 bacteria per high-power field in a centrifuged urine. Since enteric organisms are the most common cause of urinary tract infections, these bacteria usually are rod shaped and will be gram-negative on staining. Ziehl-Neelsen stains of the centrifuged urine sediment may reveal acid-fast bacilli, but definitive identification of tubercle bacilli requires culture because smegma contains nonpathogenic acid-fast organisms.

Candida (yeast) infections of the urinary tract do occur, often in patients with diabetes mellitus, but most frequently detection of these cells in the urine sediment reflects contamination from the external genitalia or perineal areas or from the air in improperly stored specimens. If yeast cells are found in the sediment of freshly catheterized or voided midstream urines, the probability of a *Candida* urinary tract infection is significant. Yeast cells may be confused with erythrocytes, but budding frequently is seen and helps to distinguish them from red cells.

With the exception of *Schistosoma hematobium* ova in patients with schistosomiasis, detection of parasites, parasitic ova, or cysts in the sediment almost always reflects fecal or vaginal contamination of the urine. Trichomonads from either the vagina or rectum are the most common parasites found in the sediment. In a rare patient, cysts or various pathogenic and nonpathogenic entamoeba species may be seen in the sediment as fecal contaminants.

Spermatozoa, Oil Droplets, Mucous Threads, and Other Contaminants and Artifacts

Spermatozoa often are present in the urine of men following ejaculation or nocturnal emissions. Occasionally, they may be seen as vaginal contaminants in the urine of females following coitus. Presence of mucous threads in the urine may represent external contamination, but they also may reflect inflammatory disease involving the lower urinary tract. Occasionally, mucous threads can be confused with hyaline casts, but the long, narrow, wavy, shred-like form of the threads helps to distinguish between the two. Oil or ointment droplets may contaminate the urine and can be confused with red cells, oval fat bodies, or yeast cells. The structureless nature and varying size of the droplets often helps to distinguish them from cells.

A variety of other contaminants and artifacts may be found in the sediment, including cotton threads, hair, starch granules, wood and wool fibers, and partially digested meat fibers. Most of the time these can be recognized as contaminants, but occasionally they may be confused with the cells or casts.

REFERENCES

Ames Company: Modern Urinalysis, a Guide to the Diagnosis of Urinary Tract Diseases and Metabolic Disorders. Elkhart, Miles Laboratories, 1974

Free AH, Free HM: Urinalysis in Clinical Laboratory Practice. Cleveland, CRC Press, 1975.

Kark RM, Lawrence JR, Pollak VE, et al: A Primer of Urinalysis (ed 2). New York, Harper & Row, Hoeber Medical Division, 1964

Kurtzman NA, Rogers PW: A Handbook of Urinalysis and Urinary Sediment. Springfield, Ill., Charles C. Thomas, 1974

Lippman RW: Urine and the Urinary Sediment (ed 2). Springfield, Ill., Charles C. Thomas, 1957

Spencer ES, Pedersen I: Hand Atlas of the Urinary Sediment (ed 2). Baltimore, University Park Press, 1976

RENAL FUNCTION TESTS

Edward A. Alexander

Clinical tests measuring renal function are a part of the regular evaluation of all patients. These tests provide an estimate of filtration rate and tubular function, and as such provide valuable information for the physician. They are, however, rarely helpful in the diagnosis of a specific renal disease with the exception of some tubular disorders. This discussion is primarily concerned with those tests which are available for the routine examination of blood and urine.

GLOMERULAR FILTRATION RATE (GFR)

Exact measurement of the GFR can be made by the use of inulin, a substance which is freely filtered at the glomerulus and is neither reabsorbed nor secreted by the renal tubule. In the case of such a marker, the amount of the substance excreted in the urine per unit time must equal the amount filtered at the glomerulus in that time. The amount in the urine per minute is the urine volume per minute (V) times the concentration of the substance in the urine (U). The amount filtered per minute is the GFR per minute times the plasma concentration of the material (P); that is, GFR $\times P$ (the amount filtered) $= UV$ (the amount excreted). If GFR $\times P = UV$, GFR $= UV/P$. The term UV/P is defined as the "clearance" of the material. Hence the clearance of inulin provides an exact measure of the GFR. Note that the clearance of inulin is independent of the rate of urine flow (V). If V increases, U falls, but UV remains constant, since it always equals GFR $\times P$; however, determination of the inulin clearance requires intravenous infusion of inulin and is not a convenient routine clinical technique.

The urinary excretion of a number of substances normally present in human plasma has been studied in an attempt to find one which, like inulin, is freely filtered by the glomerulus and not handled by the tubules. No such substance has been discovered. Therefore no exact clinical measure of the GFR is available. The renal excretory mechanism for creatinine, however, is sufficently close to that of inulin to make the creatinine clearance the most satisfactory clinical method for measuring GFR. The creatinine clearance is usually somewhat higher than the inulin clearance, since 15–20 percent of the creatinine in urine is added by tubular secretion.

While it is necessary to measure the clearance of creatinine to determine the absolute magnitude of the GFR, changes in GFR can be inferred from changes in the plasma level of creatinine. Plasma creatinine represents a balance between production by metabolism and excretion by the kidney. The rate of production of creatinine is quite steady, since it is related only to the muscle mass of the individual and is the endproduct of muscle creatine metabolism. In the steady state, what is produced must be excreted (UV). Since production $= UV$ and GFR $\times P = UV$, production must equal GFR $\times P$ in the steady state. If production is constant, GFR $\times P$ will be constant. Therefore GFR and P are inversely related over their entire range. If the GFR is halved, plasma creatinine must double. Conversely, if we find that the plasma creatinine has doubled, we can infer that the GFR has fallen 50 percent.

If changes in plasma creatinine accurately indicate inverse changes in GFR, why is it necessary to measure the clearance of creatinine? For a given patient, a plasma level of 1.2 mg/dl may reflect a normal GFR or may represent a 50 percent reduction in GFR (if the plasma concentration has risen from 0.6 to 1.2). To obtain an absolute measure of filtration, one must relate the plasma creatinine (P) to the production of creatinine [shown previously to equal excretion (UV)]. This relation of UV to P, UV/P, is the clearance of creatinine. It is therefore important to get an initial creatinine clearance in order to have a baseline value. Subsequently, changes in the plasma creatinine concentration will suffice as an index of the change in GFR.

While it is well accepted that the best clinical test for estimation of GFR is the endogenous creatinine clearance (C_{cr}), there are many pitfalls in the use of this parameter. It has been clearly demonstrated that while males excrete about 20–25 mg/kg and females 15–20 mg/kg body weight, individual variation in carefully collected daily urine creatinine excretion may vary by 20–50 percent of the mean excretion. Hence any one 24 hour collection may be in error by a considerable amount even when carefully collected. Since daily plasma creatinine varies no more than 10 percent, it is likely, as has been suggested from simultaneous inulin clearance measurements, that there is considerable day-to-day variation in GFR. This fact must be recognized, and hence clinical decisions should not be formalized until several measurements of creatinine clearance have been obtained. While most clinicians utilize a 24 hour urine collection in measuring C_{cr}, studies indicating much shorter urine collections (even 1 hour) yield similar results if accurately timed. Several methods of estimating C_{cr} utilizing the plasma concentration and variables such as age, body weight, body length, and sex have been suggested, but their use has not received widespread acceptance.

It is particularly important that clinicians be aware of the data demonstrating a steady reduction in C_{cr} with increasing age. This is reflected not by an increase in plasma creatinine concentration but by a reduction in daily creatinine excretion so that by about the ninth decade creatinine excretion is reduced 50 percent. It is likely that this represents a reduction in muscle mass in the elderly.

In summary, as long as it is appreciated that C_{cr} is an estimate of GFR and that multiple measurements over several days are necessary for accurately predicting renal function, the test is clinically valuable. Having established the relationship between C_{cr} and the plasma concentration or when significant renal failure exists, renal function may be evaluated by plasma creatinine alone. In fact, recently it has been suggested that there is a linear relationship between the reciprocal of plasma creatinine and time and that an analysis of this relationship gives an estimate of the progression of the disease in any individual patient.

The blood urea nitrogen concentration (BUN) has also been used to estimate renal function. In view of the ready availability of plasma creatinine concentration, use of the BUN does not seem appropriate. While creatinine varies only in relationship to renal function and muscle mass, urea is the major endproduct of nitrogen metabolism. BUN varies with alterations in nitrogen load including protein intake, rate of catabolism, and absorption of blood from the GI tract and also with urine flow. In addition, disproportionately elevated BUN/creatinine ratios may be helpful in suggesting a diagnosis of prerenal azotemia or urinary tract obstruction.

Other substances utilized for measuring GFR include radioisotopes of sodium iothalamate, sodium diatrizoate, EDTA, vitamin B_{12}, and other compounds (see the chapter on *Radionuclide Evaluation of Renal Disorders*). None has gained wide acceptance in the regular evaluation of renal function. In addition to the routine complete urine collection technique for estimating GFR, other methods have been utilized which do not require urine collection. These include the single injection and constant infusion techniques. In the single injection technique GFR is calculated from blood samples alone assuming that the decrease in blood concentration is proportional to the renal clearance of the substance. The constant infusion method has been suggested particularly for children. This method is based upon the fact that the rate of infusion must equal the rate of urinary excretion of a glomerular marker once a steady state has been achieved. Intravenous infusion is necessary for about 3 hours, however, to be certain of constant plasma levels. Again, these methods have not achieved the popularity in routine clinical work of the endogenous creatinine clearance.

RENAL PLASMA FLOW (RPF)

There is no simple technique for the quantitative measurement of renal plasma flow which is useful for routine clinical evaluation. RPF has been estimated in patients with the clearance of *p*-aminohippurate (PAH), Diodrast, or other such markers which are almost completely extracted by the kidney during one circulation. These tests necessitate the performance of careful clearance techniques, including constant intravenous infusion, timed urine collections, and blood sampling. RPF is calculated by an equation based on the Fick principle, where RPF equals the amount excreted in the urine divided by the arterial plasma concentration minus the renal vein concentration. Since the peripheral venous concentration is virtually identical to the arterial concentration, venous samples are adequate. Furthermore, since the amount of the marker present in the renal vein is quite small, measurement of the renal vein concentration is rarely performed, and the equation then is reduced to the simple clearance formula RPF = UV/Px. Other specialized methods which have been utilized in man for the measurement of total and intrarenal blood flow distribution include the inert gas washout technique and the measurement of the transit time of radio labeled erythrocytes or plasma bound indicators. As noted above, none of these methods is applicable for routine clinical use. In practice, qualitative or semiquantitative estimates of renal perfusion are obtained by use of radiologic contrast media or radionuclide scanning (see the chapter on *Radionuclide Evaluation of Renal Disorders*). These methods provide a very rough gauge of differences between the two kidneys rather than a determination of absolute renal perfusion.

CONCENTRATION AND DILUTION

The most simple and regularly performed test of tubular function is the measurement of the renal concentrating ability. This test, however, is quite nonspecific and it depends not only on tubular integrity but on several other factors, including the patient's prior fluid intake, the ability to synthesize and secrete ADH, solute excretion, GFR, renal plasma flow, and urea production and excretion. Furthermore, many commonly prescribed medications interfere with both concentrating and diluting ability. In spite of these limitations, some measurement of urine concentration is a part of every urinalysis.

Measurement of urine specific gravity has been most commonly performed utilizing a simple hydrometer. This method may be challenged on at least two grounds: (1), the test does not measure precisely what the physician wants to know, and (2), the test itself is often inaccurately performed without sufficient attention to calibration of the instrument. Refractometry is a technically superior method of estimating urine specific gravity, is equally simple, and can be performed with only a drop of urine; however, when an osmometer is available, the preferred measurement of urine concentration or dilution is the urine osmolality. Osmolality is a measure of the number of solute particles per unit of solvent, while the specific gravity is a measure of the number and nature of the particles in solution. Thus large particles such as glucose, radiologic contrast media, or plasma volume expanders raise the specific gravity proportionately more than the identical number of small molecules such as urea. In clinical practice maximum urinary concentration is tested by measuring the urine concentration reached after some arbitrary period of dehydration, usually 18–24 hours, during which time the patient ingests no fluids. Normal concentrating ability after this period of dehydration will raise urine osmolality to over 900 mOsm/kg. To avoid prolonged dehydration, however, 5 units of pitressin tannate in oil may be injected and urine concentration measured after a period of at least 6 hours. If only specific gravity testing is available, a value over 1.023 probably indicates normal concentrating ability. It should be appreciated that the inability to maximally concentrate urine is a nonspecific finding and does not aid in specific disease diagnosis. The diseases which impair concentration are varied, and the mechanisms of concentrating defects are multifactorial. Investigation of the patient with an abnormality in concentrating ability manifested by polyuria is discussed in the chapter on *Polyuria*.

Evaluation of urinary diluting capacity provides even more limited information. Examination of diluting capacity is important in the evaluation of a patient thought to have some disorder related to excess water reabsorption. When plasma osmolality is reduced more than 1–2 percent below normal, urine osmolality should be reduced below 100 mOsm/kg or to a specific gravity of less than 1.005. Values above these suggest the abnormal presence of ADH, an ADH-like material, or an abnormality in filtration or reabsorption of solute.

URINE ACIDIFICATION

The kidney plays a major role in the maintenance of acid–base balance by the reabsorption of bicarbonate and the net secretion of hydrogen ion. The diagnosis of either typical proximal or distal renal tubular acidosis (RTA) is relatively simple, and testing for these abnormalities is easily accomplished in most clinical situations. Diagnosis of incomplete or hybrid forms of renal tubular acidosis may require more sophisticated testing than that described below.

When an inappropriately elevated urine pH is noted in the presence of metabolic acidosis, the diagnosis of some tubular defect in acid excretion or bicarbonate reabsorption should be considered. If a random urine pH measurement is greater than 5.5 and simultaneous blood pH is less than 7.35, this is presumptive evidence for the diagnosis of an acidification defect. In less clear situations or to more fully define the abnormality in acidification, several tests are available which may be easily performed.

The administration of ammonium chloride (0.1 g/kg) should lower urine pH to less than 5.5 after 2 hours providing that adequate absorption produces a reduction in blood pH to at least 7.35. Because ammonium chloride may not be adequately absorbed and because it is contraindicated in patients with liver disease, calcium chloride may be substituted (2 mEq/kg). Metabolic acidosis occurs because of the production of calcium carbonate in the small bowel and hence the loss of bicarbonate into the gastrointestinal tract. Reduction of urine pH below 5.5 indicates normal distal secretion of hydrogen and rules out the distal form of RTA.

In proximal RTA a failure to adequately reabsorb bicarbonate in the proximal tubule leads to bicarbonate wasting and metabolic acidosis. These patients are able to adequately acidify their urine (pH < 5.5) only when serum bicarbonate concentration is markedly reduced, usually to less than 15 mEq/liter. Hence the diagnosis of this defect is dependent upon the demonstration of a normally acid urine at reduced plasma bicarbonate levels, while at plasma bicarbonate levels greater than 15 mEq/liter bicarbonaturia occurs and urine pH is abnormally elevated in the presence of systemic acidosis.

It is not possible to test properly urinary pH in patients with urinary infection and persistently alkaline urine because the organisms may split urea to ammonia.

Recently the measurement of urinary pCO_2 has been proposed as a simple method for the assessment of urinary acidification in the distal nephron. This test is based upon the following theory: The secretion of hydrogen ion into a tubular fluid of high bicarbonate concentration will form carbonic acid. In the absence of carbonic anhydrase and when urine flow is high, the dehydration of carbonic acid is minimal. Exactly these conditions occur along the lumen of the distal nephron during an alkaline diuresis. Carbonic acid is formed as hydrogen ion is secreted. This nondehydrated carbonic acid is then delivered out of the kidney. Subsequent dehydration of carbonic acid in the bladder results in the formation of urinary CO_2. Measurement of the urine pCO_2 then reflects distal hydrogen ion secretion. The test is simple to perform, since it requires only an oral sodium bicarbonate load to achieve maximal urine alkalinity and then the measurement of urinary pCO_2. In this setting, urinary pCO_2 should exceed the plasma pCO_2 by at least 20 mm Hg.

ANION GAP (AG)

While the anion gap (AG) may not be thought of initially as a test of renal function, with this parameter important information concerning the patient's acid–base status can be rapidly obtained. The sum of all serum cations must be equal to the sum of all anions to maintain electroneutrality. Sodium, chloride, and bicarbonate are routinely determined in most patients, and these constituents make up most of the ionic composition of the serum. The difference between the concentration of sodium and the sum of the chloride and bicarbonate concentrations constitute what is called the AG. In normal individuals AG equals sodium (142) − chloride (105) + bicarbonate (25). Usually potassium is not included, since the concentration is relatively small and quite constant. The normal AG = 12 mEq/liter ± 2 SD. Consistent AG measurements which exceed ± 5 mEq/liter from this range probably are of clinical importance. It should be emphasized that the calculation of the AG is clearly one of convenience, utilizing those commonly measured cations and anions which constitute most of the ionic activity of serum. The normal AG is composed of anions present but not routinely measured such as phosphate, sulfate, organic acids, and anionic proteins.

The AG is most useful in diagnosing metabolic acidosis. The common causes of an increased AG include increases in endogenous anions whose excretion is decreased or whose production is increased. These include phosphate, sulfate, lactate, and ketone acids. Exogenously ingested anions producing an increased AG include salicylate, formate, and antibiotics such as carbenicillin. Some anions incompletely identified include those accumulating after the ingestion of methanol, ethylene glycol, and paraldehyde.

A decreased or "negative" AG is usually a laboratory error but may be a clue to the presence of an abnormal anion such as bromide. Most clinical laboratories utilize a colorimetric method to measure serum halides which does not distinguish between chloride and bromide. For any given concentration of halide, bromide produces a more intense color than chloride. Since the test is based on the color intensity being proportional to the concentration of halide, the laboratory will report a spuriously evelated chloride value producing a reduced or "negative" AG. Another cause of a reduced or negative AG is the presence in the serum of an abnormal cationic protein (for example, in patients with multiple myeloma).

URINARY ELECTROLYTES

Since the advent of wide availability of automated tests for the determination of sodium and potassium, measurement of urinary electrolytes has become a very common clinical practice. The usefulness of these tests is limited, however, and they infrequently supply information which helps in the diagnosis or management of the patient. The major determinants of urine electrolyte concentration are dietary electrolyte and water intake. In view of the widespread use of diuretics, results often reflect only the drug's action and provide no information with regard to disease states.

Urinary sodium concentration may be helpful in the evaluation of the oliguric or volume depleted patient. If an oliguric patient has a urinary sodium concentration below 10 mEq/liter, it is unlikely that he or she has acute tubular necrosis and more likely that the patient is volume depleted. In contrast, a urine sodium concentration above 50 mEq/liter in an oliguric patient is compatible with the presence of acute tubular necrosis.

As noted above, the kidney strikingly lowers urine sodium concentration during volume depletion. Hence the finding of an elevated urine sodium in a volume depleted patient suggests renal sodium wasting. This may occur because of renal insufficiency, adrenal insufficiency, or the administration of diuretics. Renal salt wasting may also be found during the recovery phase of acute tubular necrosis, after renal transplantation, and after the relief of urinary tract obstruction.

Measurement of urinary sodium may also be useful in the assessment of plasma renin determinations and in the diagnosis of surreptitious diuretic ingestion.

Urinary potassium levels are helpful only in determining the site of potassium loss in patients with hypokalemia. Urine concentrations of less than 10 mEq/ liter in the hypokalemic patient almost certainly point to the gastrointestinal tract as the site of potassium loss. Values greater than 10–15 mEq/liter suggest renal potassium wasting. This most commonly occurs in patients ingesting diuretics or in patients with mineralocorticoid excess, either endogenous or exogenous.

REFERENCES

Arruda JAL, Kurtzman NA: Metabolic acidosis and alkalosis. Clin Nephrol 7:201, 1977

Bennett WM, Porter GA: Endogenous creatinine clearance as a clinical measure of glomerular filtration rate. Br Med J 4:84, 1971

Brochner-Mortensen J, Rodbro P: Selection of routine method for determination of glomerular filtration rate in adult patients. Scand J Clin Lab Invest 36:35, 1976

Cockcroft DW, Gault MH: Prediction of creatinine clearance from serum creatinine. Nephron 16:31, 1976

Emmett M, Narins RG: Clinical use of the anion gap. Medicine (Baltimore) 56:38, 1977

Harrington JT, Cohen JJ: Measurement of urinary electrolytes—Indications and limitations. N Engl J Med 293:1241, 1975

Kassirer JP: Clinical evaluation of kidney function—Glomerular function. N Engl J Med 285:385, 1971

Levinsky NG, Levy M: Clearance techniques, in: Handbook of Physiology. Section 8, Renal Physiology. Baltimore, Williams & Wilkens, 1973

Rowe JW, Andres R, Tobin JD, et al: Age-adjusted standards for creatinine clearance. Ann Intern Med 84:567, 1976

Wolfe AV, Pillay VKG: Renal concentration tests. Am J Med 46:837, 1969

RENAL RADIOGRAPHY

J. Daniel Johnson and Howard M. Radwin

The urinary tract, more than any other organ system, is accessible to radiologic evaluation. Used in combination with other diagnostic modalities, a well planned radiographic workup will yield an accurate diagnosis for which specific therapy can be instituted in most clinical situations.

While the discussion that follows concentrates on renal abnormalities, it should be emphasized that lower tract evaluation is essential in most cases. A retrograde urethrogram or cystogram may quickly explain an obscure hematuria or recurrent infection. The radiographic examination of the kidneys is discussed in terms of technique, indications, pathophysiology, and complications, but specific findings with specific diseases are not exhaustively listed or pictured.

PLAIN FILM OF THE ABDOMEN

The plain film of the abdomen is often considered merely the preliminary part of intravenous pyelography, but a great deal of valuable information may be learned from its careful examination. Patient position is critical; one must visualize the abdomen from the diaphragm to the symphysis pubis to adequately evaluate the urinary tract. Upper pole renal and adrenal masses may be obscured by improper positioning. Small ureteral calculi near the ureterovesical junction, bladder stones, and calculous prostatitis will be overlooked if the position of the patient is improper. Wide separation of the pubis symphysis is a constant radiographic sign of exstrophy of the bladder (Fig. 1).

Proper technique is essential in evaluating soft tissue structures such as masses, psoas muscle margins, and renal size and shape. Bones may appear deceptively sclerotic with underpenetration; faintly radioopaque stones such as cystine or matrix may be overlooked completely in overpenetrated films.

Orderly interpretation of plain abdominal films should proceed systematically, with noting of specific findings on each film. The bones should be examined carefully for lytic or blastic lesions, and the degree of demineralization or sclerosis should be evaluated. Frac-tures of the pelvis and ribs and compression fractures of the spine should be noted. Excretory urography is indicated with fractures of the 10th, 11th, or 12th ribs or any lumbar transverse process even in the absence of hematuria. Evaluation of the urethra is essential with a pelvic fracture. Pathologic fractures caused by metastatic disease or Pott's disease of the spine may warrant further evaluation of the urinary tract. Congenital anomalies such as spina bifida or sacral defects may be critical clues to the correct diagnosis.

Opacifications of all types should be noted (Fig. 2). Renal, ureteral, vesical, or prostatic calculi are of obvious importance. Vascular calcifications may be critical as well, suggesting aortic or renal artery aneurysms. Linear hypogastric artery calcifications are seen typically in diabetics. Calcified seminal vesicles are also frequently encountered in diabetics or patients with genital tuberculosis. Nephrocalcinosis may be seen in numerous pathologic conditions, including renal tubular acidosis (nephrocalcinosis is present in 38 percent), medullary sponge kidney, and renal tuberculosis. Calcifications in renal masses deserve special mention. While cystic masses with thin "eggshell" calcification in their rims are usually benign, up to 20 percent will contain carcinoma if studied histologically. If the cal-

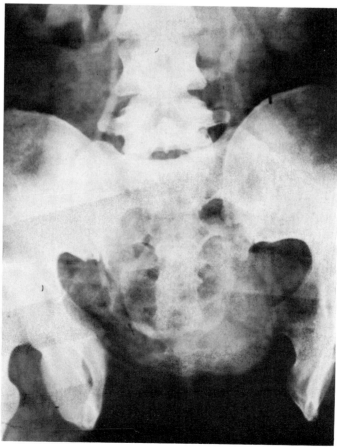

Fig. 1. Plain film of the abdomen demonstrating absent pubis bone in a patient with exstrophy of the urinary bladder.

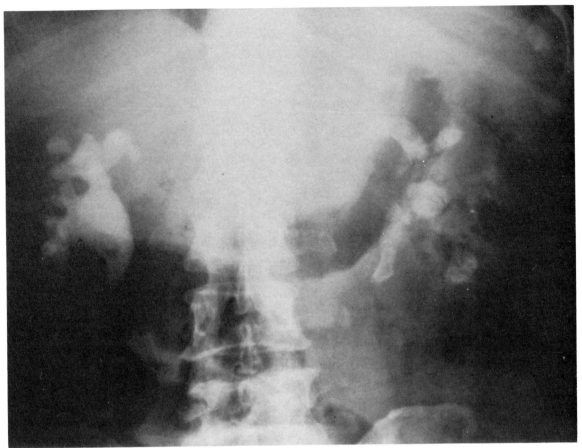

Fig. 2. Staghorn calculi as illustrated here are commonly associated with urinary infection by urea splitting organisms. Exact definition of the stones may require tomography without contrast.

cium is located centrally or in combination with peripheral rim deposits, renal cell carcinoma will be found in 87 percent (Fig. 3). These facts should emphasize the need for thorough evaluation and aggressive therapy of those patients with calcified renal masses.

Renal size, contour, and evidence of soft tissue masses should be carefully noted. While the pathologist may quote statistical limits of normal renal dimensions, one can more practically estimate normal renal size by comparison to a constant anatomic feature on the films. The vertebral bodies are convenient to use. Ninety-seven percent of normal kidneys fall within the range of the distance from the top margin of L1 to the bottom of L3, including disc spaces, as the lower limit of normal and from L1 to the inferior margin of L4 as the upper limit of normal. Small kidneys suggest vascular insufficiency, chronic infection, hypertensive nephrosclerosis, or chronic glomerulonephritis. Modestly enlarged kidneys can be noted in diabetics, and they also may be seen with acute pyelonephritis or renal vein thrombosis. Very large kidneys should alert one to polycystic disease, tumor, or hydronephrosis. Evidence of soft tissue masses in the abdomen, including a distended bladder, should be noted. Intraperitoneal

inflammation, retroperitoneal masses, or blood will often obscure the psoas muscle margins.

The bowel gas pattern may reflect retroperitoneal pathology. Ileus is commonly associated with renal colic and is seen focally near an abscess in the retroperitoneum. The "colon cutoff" gas pattern may be seen in inflammatory conditions of the kidney. The urinary tract itself may be noted to contain gas when an enterovesical fistula or infection with gas-forming organisms is present. Perinephric abscess may be revealed by gas bubbles around the kidney whose outline is otherwise indistinct.

INTRAVENOUS PYELOGRAM

Visualization of the kidneys by systematically administered contrast medium was first noted in 1923, when Roundtree observed pyelograms in luetic patients receiving potassium iodide therapy. The first successful visualization of the kidneys by an intravenously administered contrast agent, Uroselectan, was reported in 1929 by Moses Swick. The history of intravenous pyelography from that point until the mid-1950s may be summarized as a search for a nontoxic iodinated agent which is rapidly cleared and concentrated selectively by the kidney and which does not alter renal function.

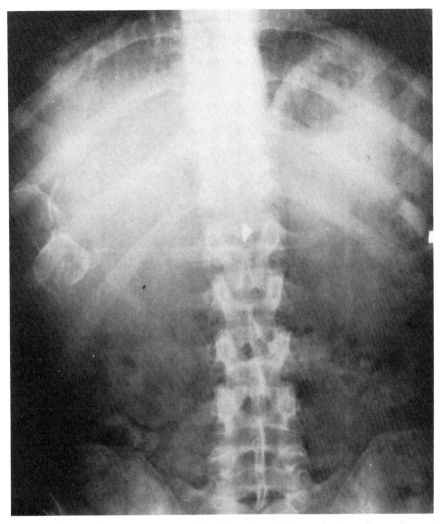

Fig. 3. Calcified renal masses are commonly malignant, as in the renal cell carcinoma demonstrated here.

CONTRAST PATHOPHYSIOLOGY

Currently used agents are triiodinated substituted benzoic acid derivatives which are primarily excreted by the kidney. The agent is cleared by glomerular filtration. Inadequate clearance will occur if the glomerular filtration rate is altered by various factors, ranging from hypoperfusion to glomerulonephritis. There is direct correlation between the filtered load and the urinary content of contrast material. Even with renal insufficiency of an advanced degree, adequate contrast concentrations in the urine may be maintained by altering the dose (up to 2 cc/kg of body weight) to increase plasma concentration, which is translated directly into filtered load. By this same reasoning, bolus injection, with its higher peak plasma concentration, should yield a greater filtered load than a slower infusion of contrast, thus placing a maximal number of iodide molecules in the tubular urine.

After filtration, the contrast is subject to the normal concentrating effects of the tubules. The integrity of the tubule is essential for optimal pyelography. Attempts to manipulate tubular function with dehydration or exogenous pitressin probably do not improve visualization more than the use of large doses of contrast and may act to the detriment of the patients' renal function. The impairment of tubular concentration coupled with decreased glomerular filtration is responsible for the poor-density pyelogram obtained in the patient with renal insufficiency.

There is little advantage and much potential for harm in the routine use of a vigorous bowel preparation with enemas, purgatives, and intentional dehydration prior to pyelography. Citrate of magnesia prior to the urogram usually gives an adequate abdominal preparation with a minimum of obscuring bowel gas. Dehydration exaggerates the toxicity of contrast and should be avoided. If adequate detail is obscured, judicious use of tomography will more safely allow visualization of renal detail. In patients at increased risk to suffer toxic side effects from iodinated contrast, hydration should be assured with intravenous fluids prior to initiating the urogram.

Dehydrated patients are not the only group with increased risk of renal toxicity from the contrast medium. Patients with renal insufficiency may demonstrate a decrease in creatinine clearance and elevation of serum creatinine following intravenous pyelography. Patients with multiple myeloma, especially if dehydrated, are thought to be susceptible to acute renal failure after exposure to iodinated contrast material. Acute renal failure following urography has been reported in diabetic patients as well as patients with hyperuricemia. In addition to hydration, prophylactic alkalinization and low-dose aspirin administration may decrease the uricosuric activity of contrast media. When multiple radiologic procedures are required in a diagnostic evaluation, they should be adequately spaced to avoid dehydration by multiple bowel preparations. In high-risk patients renal function should be checked after x-ray procedures of any kind using iodinated contrast, including angiography, oral cholecystography, or intravenous cholangiography.

TECHNIQUE

After a suitable plain film of the abdomen is reviewed, adult patients are routinely injected with 100 cc of contrast material using an indwelling intravenous catheter or scalp vein injection set which should be left indwelling until the termination of the procedure. This will provide rapid vascular access should a contrast reaction occur. This complication will be discussed later.

Exposures are made routinely at 30 sec, 5 min, and 10 min following the injection of contrast. Right posterior oblique and left posterior oblique films are next made. The 30 sec nephrogram film will allow the best visualization of the renal outlines as well as assessment of the equality and promptness of renal function. Viewed in combination, the remaining four films should reveal every part of the urinary tract.

After the patient urinates, a postvoid film should be obtained. Prior to beginning the study, the patient should empty his bladder, since a full bladder may cause a spurious diagnosis of hydronephrosis. This is more commonly a problem in children, whose upper tracts seem more sensitive to the increased hydrostatic pressure created by the distended bladder.

Rather than a timed sequence of films, some prefer to obtain a film following abdominal compression, which increases upper tract filling, and a release film. Filling of otherwise incompletely seen anterior calyces may be accomplished with a prone film. If delayed excretion of contrast due to ureteral obstruction is detected, delayed films should be obtained until the exact site of obstruction is visualized (Fig. 4). In this regard, it is essential that the patient void prior to each delayed exposure so that a site of obstruction in the distal ureter is not obscured by a bladder full of contrast material. If the patient cannot empty his bladder, a catheter should be employed. When the contralateral unobstructed kidney is no longer visible, after excretion of all the contrast material, a repeat injection of contrast material will allow the study to be continued until the site of obstruction is determined. Spontaneous extravasation in the region of the renal sinus is occasionally seen on a urogram in the presence of obstruction by a ureteral calculus. While this appears alarming, no specific therapy is usually required. When the contrast-material-induced diuresis slows or the obstruction is relieved, the extravasation will cease.

Excellent excretory urograms are not obtained by rigidly following a routine. The most profitable examinations will be obtained if each film in the study is scrupulously monitored and those maneuvers necessary to visualize the entire urinary tract in the degree of detail necessary for a diagnosis are performed.

NEPHROTOMOGRAPHY

Use of nephrotomography was first described in 1954 by Evans and associates who obtained exposures 15–18 sec after injection to visualize the aorta and arterial flush in the kidney. The study has become an integral part of the evaluation of renal masses since 1964, when Schenecker popularized nephrotomography with contrast material infusion in an effort to differentiate solid and cystic masses. Tomographic diagnosis of benign simple cyst may be made only if all the specific criteria are met on the study. These criteria include (1) a uniformly radiolucent mass on all tomograms with no opacification by contrast; (2) a paper-thin cyst wall must be present as well as a smooth margin adjacent to the renal substance; (3) the margin must extend outside the renal substance; and (4) the margin of the renal substance and the mass should form a "beak" sign (Fig. 5).

Diagnosis of many cystic masses which meet the above criteria as well as the "benign criteria" obtained with other soft tissue techniques such as ultrasonography and computer assisted tomography may be safely resolved by the use of cyst puncture with fluid analysis and renal cystography. This approach will minimize the morbidity of higher-risk diagnostic approaches such as angiography and surgical exploration in carefully selected patients. It should be stressed that all criteria of a benign cyst must be strictly met or surgical exploration is indicated in most patients.

Routine use of nephrotomography as part of every urogram has recently been employed with detection of a significant number of renal masses which otherwise would have been overlooked. At the Mayo Clinic, use of three routine tomographic cuts on all urograms resulted in the diagnosis of 28 percent more renal masses than would have been identified on the simple intravenous pyelogram. In a recent prospective study, 29 percent of 109 masses detected by excretory urography were demonstrated only on the routine tomographic films.

Use of tomography during the arterial phase and

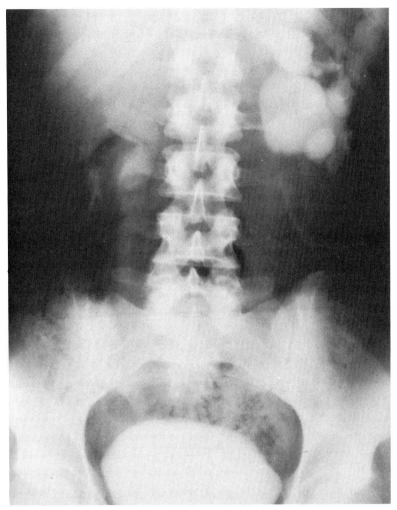

Fig. 4. Stenosis of the ureteropelvic junction caused by aberrant vessels or an intrinsic defect will result in hydronephrosis, demonstrated on this 1-hour delayed film from an IVP.

venous phase of the urogram was studied in 200 renal masses which were subsequently explored. The tomograms used in this manner were found to be 82 percent accurate in diagnosing tumors and 85 percent accurate in diagnosing benign cysts.

UROGRAPHY IN UREMIC PATIENTS

Nephrotomography obtained after injecting a high dose bolus of contrast material first suggested by Schwartz and associates in 1963, will often supplant the need for instrumentation and retrograde pyelography in the azotemic patient. At Cook County Hospital, 38 patients with acute and chronic renal failure of various etiologies were studied with nephrotomograms exposed after injection of 2 cc of contrast material per kilogram body weight. Nephrograms were seen in all patients, and adequate visualization of collecting system was made in 29 of the 38. There is no upper limit creatinine level which eliminates the reasonable chance of obtaining a valuable urogram performed in this manner.

Evaluation of the uremic patient with pyelography may be improved if the study is performed immediately following a vigorous hemodialysis. In a study of eight uremic patients with no visualization of the collecting system prior to dialysis, six adequate pyelograms were obtained after dialysis. Increased sodium and water reabsorption coupled with decreased osmotic diuresis with lower BUN level is a proposed mechanism for the increased concentration of contrast material which improves visualization. The value of this technique when compared to high-dose bolus injection and nephrotomography as previously described is questionable.

Plain tomograms of the kidneys without injection of contrast are also an important adjunct in the evaluation of renal calculi. Many small calyceal stones which are obscured on plain films can be detected by the use of tomography. This study is particularly useful for kidneys containing staghorn calculi or in those with stones associated with chronic infection by urea-splitting organisms in which matrix material is obscured on routine x-rays.

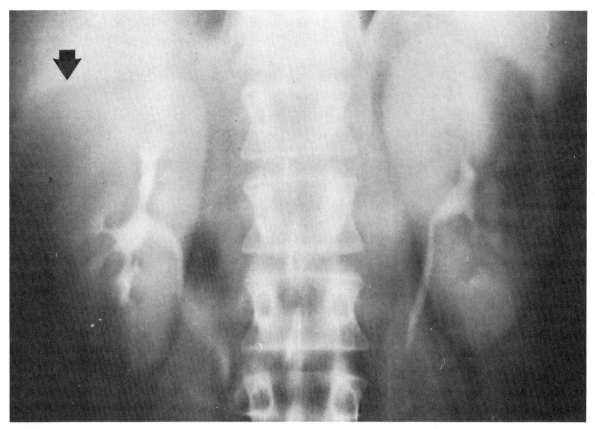

Fig. 5. Benign renal cysts should extend beyond the renal margin and appear relatively radiolucent. The adjacent renal parenchyma should form a "beak sign," pictured in this nephrotomogram.

UROGRAPHY IN PREGNANT PATIENTS

The use of excretory urography in pregnancy should be limited to specific indications in selected patients. One should not, however, hesitate to perform the study if the patient's condition demands it. Ureteral calculus complicating pregnancy is the most common acute painful condition requiring hospitalization. Its specific diagnosis requires urographic confirmation, particularly in differentiating obstructive from nonobstructive pyelonephritis. In this regard, the scout film should not be eliminated from the study in an attempt to minimize radiation. Since each exposure delivers about 0.2 roentgens to fetal and maternal gonads, a three exposure protocol of scout, 20 min, and 60 min films will result in only 0.6 roentgens and will usually be diagnostic. This will allow increased time to visualize collecting systems obstructed by the physiologic hydronephrosis of pregnancy, yet allow definition of an offending ureteral calculus. While asymptomatic or minimally symptomatic infections or hypertension occurring during pregnancy do not demand immediate urography, the integrity of the urinary tract should be assured 6 weeks after delivery by intravenous pyelography.

UROGRAPHY IN THE NEWBORN

The excretory urogram may be useful in evaluation of the neonate. If the contrast is administered slowly over 90 sec to a nondehydrated infant and a relatively high dose of contrast (3–5 cc/kg) is used, the pyelogram is almost always useful and safe. The risks of a closely monitored study are minimal, although excessive radiation should be avoided. There is no upper limit of serum creatinine or BUN above which pyelography should not be attempted. Patients should be selected carefully, and pyelography in the neonate should never be considered routine.

Multiple conditions require urographic evaluation in the neonate, since renal anomalies are frequently associated. All children with multiple anomalies, malformed ears, one umbilical artery, imperforate anus, bladder exstrophy, ambiguous genitalia, or prune belly syndrome should have an intravenous pyelogram due to the high incidence of urinary tract malformations associated. Ascites in the newborn is most commonly associated with obstructive uropathy (usually posterior urethral valves), and excretory urograms may confirm the diagnosis. Spontaneous pneumothorax is often associated with an increased incidence of renal anomalies. All children with sepsis of obscure origins, unexplained anemia, or failure to thrive deserve pyelographic evaluation.

UROGRAPHY IN HYPERTENSIVE PATIENTS

The rapid sequence pyelogram has been used as a screening test to diagnose renovascular hypertension. Exposures are obtained at 30 sec and 1, 2, 3, and 5 min. The relative quantity of blood flow can be judged by the appearance of contrast in each kidney as well as comparison of renal size. In the presence of significant renal artery stenosis, due to either atherosclerosis or fibrous dysplasia, there will be delayed appearance of contrast in the affected kidney in 83 percent of patients with proved renovascular hypertension due to diminished blood flow. With slowed transit time through the renal tubules, there will be increased sodium and water reabsorption resulting in a prolonged, intense nephrogram. The affected kidney will frequently be smaller. A positive study demands angiography and renal vein renin determination if the patient is a candidate for surgical correction of hypertension.

Because of the frequency of repairable lesions found in these age groups, it has been suggested that all patients with the onset of significant diastolic hypertension before age 35 or after age 55 years should be screened with a rapid sequence pyelogram. A sudden increase in hypertension or refractoriness to pharmacologic control may occur in patients who have renal artery lesions whose correction will cure or improve their hypertension and which may be initially detected by a rapid sequence urogram. Angiography and renal vein renin determinations can often be reserved for those patients in whom a renal etiology is suggested by pyelography. A negative rapid sequence pyelogram does not necessarily eliminate the need for further angiographic examination, however, since multiple significant lesions on both sides or intrarenal branch artery lesions may be associated with a deceptively normal urogram. A positive study likewise is not an infallible prognosticator of curability, since 81 percent of surgical failures in a large cooperative study had a positive rapid sequence urogram.

INTERPRETATION OF THE UROGRAM
Renal Position and Shape

After injection of contrast material the position and axis of the kidneys should be examined. A vertical axis rather than the normal oblique axis parallel to the psoas muscle margin is suggestive of an upper pole renal or adrenal mass lesion or a horseshoe kidney, which will usually lie lower than normal and demonstrate malrotation. In the pediatric age group the position of the kidney is important in differentiating Wilms' tumor, which will generally deform the kidney, from neuroblastoma, which will displace the kidney. While the left kidney is usually higher than the right, this is not invariable. Anomalies of position and malrotation are associated with pathologic abnormalities but may have no significance.

Irregularities in the renal outlines should be noted, since these may represent significant mass lesions or pathologic changes such as segmental hypertrophy adjacent to a pyelonephritic scar. Fetal lobulation is the most common cause of an irregular renal contour. This may be differentiated from pyelonephritic scarring. The indentations between fetal lobulations tend to be located between calyceal systems, while pyelonephritic scars will be adjacent to a calyx which is usually blunted due to papillary atrophy. The overlying cortex will be thin.

Collecting System

Careful evaluation of the collecting system should be made, especially when the patient has hematuria. All filling defects must be pursued as if they were malignant tumors. Transitional cell carcinoma accounts for 85 percent of renal pelvis tumors. Squamous cell carcinoma is usually associated with stones, chronic inflammation, or transitional cell carcinoma of the pelvis.

Other changes suggesting chronic interstitial inflammatory disease such as chronic pyelonephritis will be the widening and foreshortening of the infundibulae. Tuberculosis is the exception to this and generally causes infundibular stenosis. Peripelvic cyst, peripelvic lipomatosis, and polycystic disease typically cause stretching and elongation of the calyces without significant obstruction.

There are benign conditions causing intrapelvic filling defects. Uric acid stones comprise 4 percent of all renal stones and are associated with invariably acid urine. While stones are usually smooth, matrix stones, usually occurring in the presence of Proteus infection, will appear irregular. Clot from trauma, anticoagulant therapy, or tumor will also appear irregular but should change or disappear in a short time when repeat examination is made. Infections and inflammatory processes may create filling defects. Papillary necrosis will show a typical "target" deformity of the affected calyx as well as debris of the sloughed papilla which passes down the ureter. Fungus balls created by Candida infection will cause irregular filling defects, and ureteropyelitis cystica will cause multifocal, smooth defects. Peripelvic cysts, renal artery aneurysms, renal sinus lipomatosis, intrahilar vascular branches, and renal cell carcinoma may cause an extrinsic deformity of the pelvis. Gas bubbles due to enterovesical fistulae, gas-forming infection, or air introduced during retrograde pyelography are occasionally seen in the renal pelvis.

The thickness of the renal cortex is normally the same throughout the kidney when measured from calyx to the overlying renal margin. Decreased cortical thickness when measured this way suggests cortical atrophy secondary to infection or segmental infarction. Increased thickness signals a space-occupying mass lesion even though a normal reniform shape may be maintained. Hypernephroma, a nonfunctioning duplicated segment, and the excluded calyx of tuberculosis are often responsible for this finding. While simple cysts often displace the calyces, they present the appearance of undrained renal substance less frequently. Retrograde pyelography may be required occasionally in the normal kidney to fill out the collecting system adequately.

In the presence of obstruction and hydronephrosis, there is always some delay in the appearance of collecting system opacification. A large extrarenal pelvis which requires longer than usual to fill out completely— simply on the basis of volume—may masquerade as a hydronephrotic pelvis with a ureteropelvic junction obstruction. The calyces will usually aid in the correct interpretation, since they will be the first portion of the collecting system to dilate in the presence of a urodynamically significant obstructive lesion. The diagnosis of ureteropelvic junction obstruction may also be revealed by the use of a diuretic after the injection of the contrast to exaggerate the functional obstruction. Careful patient monitoring may reveal reproduction of the pain in the flank which caused the patient to seek medical attention. If coexistent disease such as infection has deformed the calyces, renal pelvic pressure determination with constant infusion may be required to make the differentiation.

Ureters and Bladder

The course and caliber of the ureters should be noted. Small inconsistent deviations in their course, caused by peristaltic waves, are often seen. Major deviations in the ureteral course are found on the right with a retrocaval ureter or on either side in the presence of malignant disease in the retroperitoneal nodes. Retroperitoneal fibrosis characteristically draws the middle third of the ureter to the midline with straightening and significant obstruction. Previous abdominoperineal resection also typically causes deviation of the pelvic ureters toward the midline without functional disturbance. Distal ureteral stenosis may occasionally be seen as a result of a congenital abnormality, but a more common etiology in the adult patient is urinary tuberculosis. Elevation of the ureterovesical junction with the characteristic "hooking" of the distal ureter is a consistent sign of prostatic enlargement. In the patient suffering penetrating trauma, extravasation from the ureter may be seen occasionally, but its absence does not rule out ureteral injury.

Filling defects previously described in the renal pelvis can also occur in the ureter with roughly the same differential diagnosis. Segmental filling defects which are persistent, especially in the pediatric or young adult patient, may indicate an obstructed, redundant duplicated ureter from a nonfunctioning renal segment causing extrinsic compression as it crosses the more normal ureter. Lateral deviation of the ureter above the iliac vessels and medial deviation below is also characteristic of an unseen duplication with obstruction. While not diagnostic, dilatation of the pelvic ureter, especially on a postvoiding film, suggests vesicoureteral reflux, which may be confirmed with cystography. The distal ureter may demonstrate a ureterocele with its typical "cobra head" configuration and a surrounding halo of relative radiolucency. These lesions may be obstructive and may contain stones. Stones lodged in the distal ureter may simulate a ureterocele with periureteral edema forming the halo. This is termed a pseudoureterocele.

The bladder is often difficult to evaluate on excretory films. Rarely is it completely filled, and this leads to errors in interpretation of irregularities and filling defects. Persistent filling defects and larger diverticula can be seen and these demand cystoscopic evaluation. A postvoid film if properly performed may eliminate the need for instrumentation of the lower urinary tract

for direct measurement of the residual volume. A voiding film may be of diagnostic value, since it will reveal lesions such as posterior urethral valves, bladder neck obstruction, and congenital strictures which might otherwise be obscured by diagnostic techniques requiring urethral instrumentation. Neurogenic bladders may assume a characteristic pine cone shape or appear smooth when distended and may empty poorly. Cystoscopic, neurologic, and urodynamic evaluation are required for an accurate and specific diagnosis. Elevation of the bladder base by an enlarged median lobe of the prostate may be noted, but its significance is important only when considered in context. Extravasation in the victim of blunt or penetrating trauma should be confirmed with cystography. Pelvic hematoma and bladder displacement in the patient suffering pelvic fracture may indicate an injury to the epimembranous urethra which should be demonstrated by retrograde urethrography.

RETROGRADE PYELOGRAPHY

Although its employment has diminished in recent years with concurrent improvements in intravenous pyelography and nephrotomography, the retrograde pyelogram remains an essential diagnostic tool for the urinary tract evaluation. Performance of this study is accompanied by cystoscopy and allows collection of urine samples for cytology, differential cultures, and differential renal function. The therapeutic potential of passing a catheter beyond an obstructing lesion or stone may occasionally be a life-saving maneuver.

The particular techniques involved in obtaining retrograde pyeloureterograms are not germane to this discussion, but multiple views and drainage films are often helpful. Retrograde pyelography is indicated when more detail or finer definition of those parts of the collecting system not completely visualized on excretory urography is desired (Fig. 6). Examples would be the study of the nonfunctioning kidney, the collecting system incompletely filled on excretory urography when tumor is suspected, and the visualization of the ureter distal to an obstructing lesion. One should employ retrograde pyelography only when indicated in carefully selected patients, but fear of complications should never cause avoidance of the study when it is necessary. The renal pelvis can be filled with air intentionally on occasion to delineate soft tissue or faintly radiopaque filling defects such as matrix stones.

While there is always the risk of introducing infection into the upper tracts by retrograde pyelography, this is an uncommon occurrence if gentle technique and proper catheter selection are employed. In the presence of obstruction, elective retrogrades should be reserved until one is ready to provide definitive drainage immediately thereafter in the event infection is introduced. The addition of 500 mg neomycin to each liter of contrast material has been helpful in preventing the injection of infected material into the upper tracts or into the systemic circulation. Ureteral instrumentation always results in some degree of reactive edema at the ureterovesical junction. When larger catheters are used,

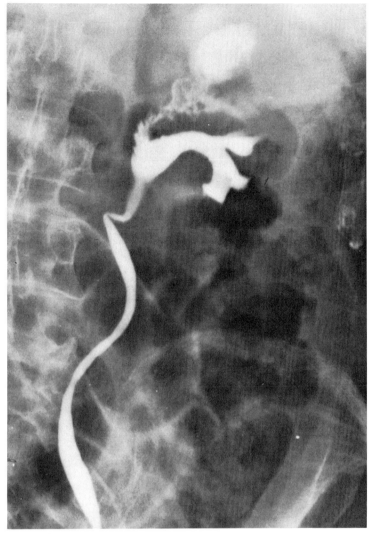

Fig. 6. Filling defect demonstrated on this retrograde pyelogram is typical of transitional cell carcinoma of the renal pelvis.

as in the collection of split renal function studies or passage of a stone basket, this may produce colic and hydronephrosis. These problems are usually transient. Traumatic instrumentation with resultant perforation or extravasation may be devastating and should be treated promptly. Unless specifically indicated, bilateral instrumentation during one endoscopy should be avoided.

Backflow

Pyelorenal backflow during retrograde pyelography is a phenomenon of questionable significance. Four general types have been identified, all of which may represent variations of the same process. If this is true, the common factor appears to be increased pressure in the renal sinus with the pattern depending on the degree and rapidity of the pressure elevation. Pyelosinus backflow is most common and may be seen spontaneously in patients passing ureteral calculi. The mechanism involves a small tear in the urothelium of the renal fornices with leakage into the renal sinus. Occasionally,

enough contrast material to cause a urogram in the opposite kidney will extravasate. Rarely when retrograde pyelography is performed because of a history of adverse reaction to intravenous contrast material, a similar reaction may ensue by this mechanism. Once it has entered the renal sinus, the contrast material enters the lymphatic circulation rapidly. The lymphatics may be visualized as a series of parallel lines approaching the renal hilum, and this is termed pyelolymphatic backflow.

Pyelotubular backflow is diagnosed when contrast material refluxes into the renal papilla. The reason this less common form of backflow is seen is unclear, but its significance is a matter of concern in the patient with vesicoureteral reflux. It is felt by some that reflux into the collecting tubules and the interstitial tissues may lead to interstitial nephritis. This mechanism has been implicated in the etiology of endstage renal disease. Patients with endstage renal failure, no history of infection, and gross vesicoureteral reflux may have succumbed to a disease process similar to this. Future investigations will hopefully resolve the significance of this entity.

Direct reflux into the renal veins is the least common form of backflow. High intraluminal pressure is required in the normal kidney, but in the diseased kidney this form of backflow may be seen at lower pressures. Backflow into necrotic tumor is rarely seen, and it appears to be a grave sign.

ANTEGRADE PYELOGRAPHY

In many clinical settings, percutaneous antegrade pyelography may be preferable to retrograde pyelography. The risk of infection from urethral instrumentation is eliminated, and temporary drainage may be achieved by placing an indwelling percutaneous nephrostomy. Selective renal function studies and pressure determinations may be performed when needed. The procedure may be guided by fluoroscopic visualization of the targeted kidney or by sonographic localization. The

most common indication for this procedure is high-grade ureteral obstruction at any level. Selective catheterization of the ureter with ureteral stenting from above has been reported in the treatment of uretero-cutaneous fistula. The equipment required should be available in any angiography suite, and local anesthesia is usually adequate except in the neonatal or pediatric age groups. Failure to establish adequate drainage occurs in up to 12 percent of large published series. Complications have been minimal (4 percent), and no deaths have been reported.

RENAL CYST PUNCTURE

Using similar techniques, cystic renal masses may be explored radiographically and defined by percutaneous cyst puncture and cystography (Fig. 7). The cyst should meet criteria of a benign lesion on other studies such as tomography, ultrasonography, and CT scan prior to puncture. While seeding of a tumor in the needle tract is rare, it has been reported.

With fluoroscopic or sonographic guidance, the

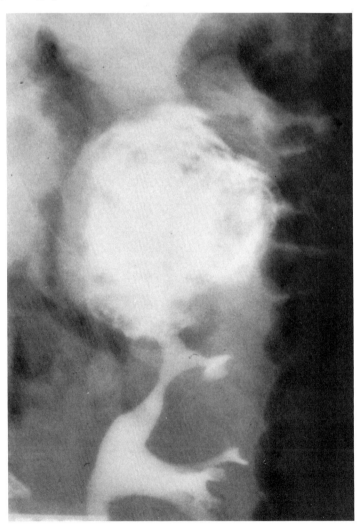

Fig. 7. Percutaneous cyst puncture with instillation of contrast material should reveal a smooth-walled cavity filled with clear fluid to be considered benign. An irregular margin, as illustrated here, is suspicious for neoplasm.

cyst is punctured under local anesthesia. After the fluid is aspirated, the cyst cavity is refilled with contrast material or an equal volume of air and contrast material. X-ray exposures are obtained with the patient in multiple positions until all margins of the cavity are visualized. Aseptic technique is of paramount importance, since injection of infected material into a closed space will result in abscess formation.

The fluid collected is analyzed for LDH enzymes, fat, and cytology. Fluid in the benign cyst should be clear and straw colored. The renal cystogram should demonstrate a smooth-walled cavity without septae or compartmentalization. Careful attention to the cyst wall adjacent to the renal substance should be given, since irregularities here may reveal tumor.

Use of a sclerosing contrast agent such as pantopaque has been recommended because it causes destruction of the cyst cavity. This is of debatable therapeutic value, since the cyst does no real harm and since if the contrast agent is extravasated during injection an intense perinephric inflammatory response is initiated with significant patient morbidity.

If all criteria for benign disease are not fulfilled by the cyst puncture, films, and fluid analysis, angiography usually follows. If all criteria are met, the accuracy of cyst puncture has been reported to be approximately 97 percent.

ANGIOGRAPHY

Since 1929, when dosSantos performed the first translumbar aortogram, angiographic evaluation of the kidneys has become an indispensable diagnostic tool. Seldinger's description of the percutaneous use of directable catheters to obtain selective renal arteriograms, coupled with the introduction of better contrast media and high-speed film changers in the mid 1950s, ushered in the modern era of arteriography.

Normal Angiogram

Familiarity with the normal renal arteriogram is essential to recognize abnormal findings. The two main divisions of the arterial circulation should be recognized, although some variability may normally exist. Multiple main renal arteries may be noted in 25 percent of normal kidneys. Peripheral arborization of the arteries should be orderly and conform to the anatomy of the normal kidney.

The normal angiogram can be divided into three phases, the first being the arterial phase. During the first 2 sec following contrast injection, the arteries will be identified out to the end arteries. Each segmental vessel should be identified and should appear normal. The nephrogram phase lasts 15–20 sec and is characterized by intense parenchymal opacification by contrast material initially in the arterioles and glomeruli, then in the tubular lumen. Since collateral arterial supply in the peripheral parenchyma is minimal, portions of the kidney without direct end artery supply will not be opacified. The venous phase is difficult to visualize initially, obscured by the intense nephrogram. This phase begins about 5 sec after the contrast material

is injected and lasts about 5 sec additional. Early venous visualization suggests abnormal shunting secondary to an arteriovenous fistula or a tumor.

It is usually possible to visualize the main renal vein on late films; failure to do so, when renal carcinoma has been diagnosed, demands vena cavography to rule out obstruction by tumor thrombus. Vena cavography or renal venography may also be diagnostic in the clinical setting of renal vein thrombosis. Renal venograms may be used to differentiate the atrophic kidney from renal agenesis.

Abnormal Angiograms

Renal masses. Many disease entities have characteristic angiographic appearance, but the technique has been employed most frequently and successfully to evaluate renal masses. Early reports claimed 95–99 percent accuracy in the arteriographic diagnosis of renal cell carcinoma. More recent studies with histologic confirmation of the diagnosis have shown an accuracy rate of 86–92 percent in the evaluation of renal mass lesions. The most common masses to be misdiagnosed are angiomyolipoma, tuberculosis of the kidney, chronic inflammatory conditions such as xanthogranulomatous pyelonephritis, and avascular renal cell carcinomas. Typical renal cell carcinoma is characterized by disorganized hypervascularity with early venous filling and puddling of the contrast material in the mass (Fig. 8). Parasitization of blood supply from capsular vessels by smaller tumors and from adjacent organs by larger tumors is common, as is obstruction of the renal vein by tumor thrombus.

Hypertension. Hypertension is another disease which can be evaluated by arteriography when indicated. The main advantages of the arteriogram in hypertension are (1) an excellent anatomic definition of renal arterial lesions, (2) demonstration of other vascular lesions such as atherosclerosis in the opposite renal artery, the abdominal aorta, pelvic vessels, splenic vessels, and carotid arteries, and (3) excellent visualization of the renal cortex which might be poorly seen on excretory urography when there is a severe stenosis of the renal artery.

The arteriogram is not a good predictor of curability even when a lesion is identified, nor is every lesion functionally significant. Because the most common stenosing renal artery lesion, atherosclerotic plaque, occurs in the proximal one-third of the renal artery, careful evaluation of this portion of the artery and the renal artery ostium is required. This is best accomplished by injection of contrast material into the aorta adjacent to the renal artery ostium which is best viewed with the patient in the oblique position. If no main renal artery lesion is seen, selective angiography is used to examine the peripheral intrarenal circulation for segmental stenotic lesions. In the presence of an atherosclerotic plaque, selective catheterization of the main renal artery carries increased risk.

Fibrous lesions and their significance. Renal artery stenosis caused by fibrous dysplasia can usually be

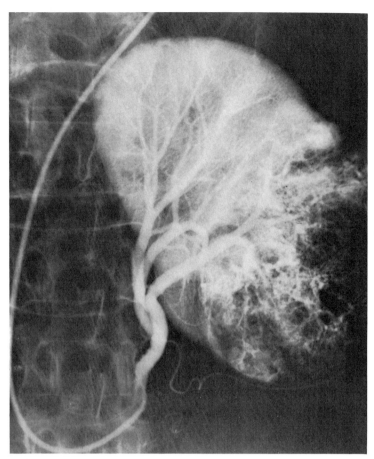

Fig. 8. Angiographic appearance of renal cell carcinoma, typified by increased vascularity arranged in a haphazard fashion with "puddling" of contrast material in neovascular spaces. Neoplastic AV shunts are often identified.

characterized by angiography. The angiographic appearance of the lesion also aids in the determination of the prognosis and directs the therapy. Intimal fibroplasia occurs typically in the proximal one-third of the renal artery. It forms a short, high-grade stenosis, tends to progress and dissect, and should be repaired. This is the most common form of renal artery stenosis in children. True fibromuscular hyperplasia, the rarest fibrous lesion, is radiographically indistinguishable from intimal fibroplasia. Because of its progressive nature, revascularization of the kidney with this arterial lesion is recommended. Medial fibroplasia tends to form a series of multiple stenoses separated by aneurysms in the distal two-thirds of the artery (Fig. 9). The lesions are often multifocal, involve intrarenal vessels, and are generally associated with mild, controllable hypertension in middle-aged women. This lesion is not progressive. Subadventitial or perimedial fibroplasia also forms a series of stenoses and aneurysms, but this lesion is recognizable because the aneurysms are always smaller in diameter than the caliber of the normal renal artery. The lesion is associated with severe hypertension in young women and tends to dissect and thrombose.

Repair or nephrectomy is indicated in most of these patients.

Trauma. Blunt renal trauma is frequently evaluated by angiography. If the patient's vital signs are stable, all kidneys presumably injured by blunt trauma which are nonfunctioning, which show significant defects in the renal outline, or which show extensive extravasation should be evaluated angiographically. Renal arterial injury should be demonstrated or disproved. Major intrarenal arterial injuries can be defined, and this will allow precise planning of reparative surgery or transcatheter embolization. Penetrating injuries less commonly lend themselves to arteriographic evaluation because of the need for immediate exploration. Percutaneous needle biopsies are occasionally complicated acutely by hemorrhage and on a delayed basis by arteriovenous fistula or false aneurysm formation. These lesions can be defined angiographically and occasionally treated by selective embolization.

Miscellaneous indications. The investigation of persistent hematuria occasionally includes arteriography. Occult vascular tumors are often suspected, but other abnormal vascular lesions may be found. Prepa-

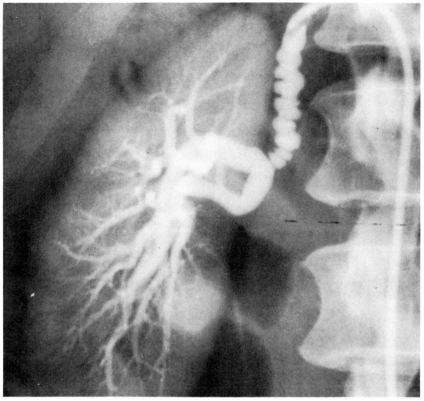

Fig. 9. Medial fibroplasia, the most common of the stenosing fibrous lesions of the renal artery. It is diagnosed by the angiographic appearance of multiple areas of stenosis interposed with aneurysmal dilatations.

ration for major renal surgery, especially on a previously operated kidney or anomalous kidneys such as the horseshoe kidney, is often aided by exact angiographic definition of the renal circulation. In the renal transplant patient, angiography will demonstrate the integrity of renal arterial anastomosis, and the characteristic appearance of acute rejection with "pruning" of the end arteries may be diagnostic. Other inflammatory lesions have characteristic findings on the angiogram, such as the peripheral microaneurysms of polyarteritis nodosa. Patients with acute unexplained renal insufficiency are often most precisely and efficiently diagnosed with an arteriogram. The severely hydronephrotic kidney which is poorly defined by excretory urography can be visualized. The study may reveal splaying of the arterial branches and the quantity of functioning cortex.

Special modifying techniques can be employed by the angiographer to improve the diagnostic accuracy of the study. Since tumor vessels have no muscle, they are unresponsive to the vasoconstricting action of epinephrine or angiotensin. Injection of one of these agents prior to injection of the contrast material will result in generalized vasoconstriction throughout the kidney, leaving the unconstricted tumor vessels more obvious. Subtraction films can further emphasize abnormal vas-

cular patterns by eliminating or at least deemphasizing other elements such as bowel gas, overlying ribs, and the normal renal shadows. Magnification techniques are now available which allow resolution down to 100 μm, making evaluation of vessels on the magnitude of glomeruli (200 μm) possible. This may allow specific diagnosis in certain parenchymal diseases such as hypertensive nephrosclerosis.

In experienced hands, arteriographic complications are uncommon. Minor hematoma or vasospasm occurs in less than 5 percent of patients, and serious life- or limb-threatening vascular complications occur in 0.5 percent. The serious complications include thrombosis, hemorrhage, dissection, embolization, and false aneurysms or AV fistula formation.

Contrast injected directly into the renal circulation has exaggerated toxicity as compared with that associated with intravenous administration. These problems are generally transient and with adequate patient hydration are rarely clinically significant. Anaphylactoid contrast reaction may occur but is less commonly associated with angiograms than with intravenous administration of the contrast material. A catheter introduced into the renal artery may also cause problems. Atheromata may be dislodged and embolized. Intimal abrasion may lead to renal artery thrombosis or dissection. Careful use of small catheters which are not left indwelling in the renal artery longer than necessary will minimize these problems.

CONTRAST REACTIONS

Contrast reactions may be divided into two major types—(1) chemoreceptor responses such as hot flushing, chills, nausea, dizziness, and bitter taste, and (2) serious reactions such as urticaria, angioedema, bronchospasm, laryngospasm, and cardiovascular collapse.

In large retrospective studies, the incidence of life-threatening reactions was 0.09 percent, with one death in 30,000–40,000 patients. Dermal reactions occurred in 1.56 percent. A large prospective series showed the incidence to be two times greater when reactions were sought with anticipation, and deaths occurred once every 10,000 injections. Serious reactions are more common in middle-aged adults and are distinctly rare in children and the elderly.

Patients who claim allergy of any type are known to suffer an increased incidence of contrast reactions. Reactions may occur without prior exposure, and there is no potentiation of the reaction with repeat exposures, making classic anaphylaxis a poor model. Prior reaction does appear to increase the incidence of repeat reactions up to 35 percent, but most authorities feel that a previous reaction is not a contraindication to a necessary repeat urogram. A repeat serious reaction has never been reported, and no deaths have been reported in such patients.

There are data to support some type of immunologic mechanism, but inconsistencies cast doubt. There is no evidence that antibodies or antigen–antibody complexes are involved in the reaction. The reaction is similar to a histamine release reaction, and animal models have demonstrated histamine release associated with contrast injection, but not necessarily with an adverse reaction. It is probable that some of the reactions are due to histamine release from mast cells or basophiles. Direct activation of complement factor C3 may also be involved in a manner demonstrated with other drugs. Although the triiodobenzoic acid salts are too small to be antigenic, there is evidence that contrast does increase IgE synthesis in rabbits, and lymphocyte transformation to organic iodides suggests a cell-mediated response. The inflammatory pathways and mechanisms may vary among different patients.

Pretreatment with an antihistamine, such as Benadryl, decreases nausea and anxiety but does not alter the incidence of serious anaphylactoid reactions. High doses of corticosteroids as a pretreatment have not been shown to be beneficial in a significantly large series, although the recurrent reaction rate was reduced to about 10 percent in a small series. There is no relationship between the dose of contrast or the rate of injection and serious reactions, although a rapid injection seems to intensify the chemoreceptor responses. A test dose by any route of administration does not correlate with subsequent mild or serious reactions or deaths and may cause a lethal reaction itself. Anxiety

is commonly associated with contrast reactions and may explain the increased incidence in repeat reactors in the absence of a solid immunologic explanation.

Urticaria, flushing, or nausea usually requires no therapy, and Benadryl is adequate for treating angioedema. Benadryl may also be beneficial in serious reactions by blocking unbound histamine, but epinephrine and aminophylline are the main therapeutic agents for laryngeal edema and bronchospasm. The therapy for cardiovascular collapse should be suggested by the pulse rate. Bradycardia signals a vagal stimulatory mechanism, most likely anxiety related. Atropine should correct the bradycardia and subsequently the hypotension. When tachycardia is detected, the patient will respond as a victim of anaphylaxis. Capillary dilatation will render the patient relatively hypovolemic, and successful therapy will center on volume expansion, epinephrine, and pressor agents such as dopamine. Corticosteroids have no acute effect but may contribute to maintenance of patient microcirculation and stabilization of lysosomal membranes following the hypotension.

The radiographs may offer a clue to an impending or progressing contrast reaction by showing a delayed intense nephrogram due to slowed intrarenal transit. If possible, one should continue to obtain exposures during and after the resuscitation, since an opportunity to examine the patient's urinary tract may not occur again.

ULTRASOUND

Although not a radiographic technique, ultrasonography of renal tissue is another recently developed diagnostic technique which is used most often in conjunction with the radiologic evaluation of the kidneys. The study is obtained by scanning the kidneys with high-frequency sound waves emitted by a transducer applied to the skin. As the sound waves penetrate tissues of different acoustic impedance, an acoustic interface is encountered and the sound waves are reflected. These echoes are displayed on an oscilloscope. Homogeneous structures with no acoustic interfaces such as fluid are anechoic. Complex tissues with blood vessels, fat, and connective tissues tend to have multiple interfaces, producing a complex pattern of internal echoes. These properties have allowed ultrasound to gain wide acceptance as a means of differentiating solid masses from simple cysts.

Ultrasonographic equipment used clinically is undergoing a rapid evolution and is currently in its third generation. Originally described by Goldberg and Pollack in 1971 as a means of defining renal masses, A-mode ultrasound was used. It reveals received echoes by a deflection from a baseline signal. B-mode ultrasound, rather than giving a pattern of linear deflections, records each echo as a point in the scanning area resulting in the generation of an image. The most recent development, gray scale ultrasound, presents point signals of variable intensity depending on the strength of the echo. This results in much better resolution image due to the variable intensity of the gray tones, which allows improved definition of the mass. Although the technique is not without fault, as technology and experience have progressed, the accuracy of sonography used in conjunction with other radiographic techniques has made it clinically useful.

There are significant sources of error with which the clinician should be familiar to improve his use of sonographic data. Masses which are perfectly homogeneous may be solid and anechoic. Transitional cell carcinomas with this property have been reported. Necrotic tumors may appear cystic. Resolution is generally limited to 2.5 cm. Smaller masses cannot be reliably evaluated, and small tumors in the lining of simple cysts may not be evaluable. Multiple or contiguous cysts will demonstrate a complex pattern of echoes. Left upper pole renal masses are often difficult to study because of the superimposed positions of the spleen, lung, and kidney, all of which are obscured by overlying ribs.

Sonography is a poor means of screening for renal masses not previously detected by urography. Its prime value appears to be characterization of known masses. A sonographically benign cyst should meet three criteria: (1) the interior should be echo-free at low and high gain, (2) the margins should be smooth and sharply defined, and (3) there should be amplification of the echoes on the posterior wall of the cyst.

Ultrasonography has been successfully used with multiple renal abnormalities in addition to kidney masses. Congenital anomalies can be diagnosed, including obstructed duplicated segments, multicystic kidneys, and congenital ureteropelvic junction obstruction. Perinephric abscess and intrarenal carbuncles can be seen. Hydronephrosis of any etiology may be diagnosed, and often the obstructed ureter can be identified with the site of obstruction defined. Ultrasound has been used in pregnancy for localization of fetus and placenta. The intrauterine diagnosis of congenital hydronephrosis caused by posterior urethral valves has recently been reported. Intraoperative A-mode and B-mode ultrasound, using equipment applied directly to the renal surface, has been used to localize obscure intrarenal calculi as an aid for their removal.

When compared with nephrotomography and computer assisted tomography, ultrasound is the best technique for the diagnosis of polycystic disease of the kidneys and liver. It has been found to be the most accurate means of localizing the kidneys for percutaneous biopsy when compared to radioisotopic renal scan, excretory urography, and fluoroscopy. Because their superficial position allows excellent imaging, renal allografts can be biopsied percutaneously safely by ultrasonic guidance with retrieval of diagnostic tissue in over 90 percent of patients. In addition to characterizing masses, sonography can be used to measure lesions and guide the needle for cyst puncture or antegrade pyelography and percutaneous nephrostomy. Hepatic tissue can best be differentiated from the right renal upper pole by gray scale ultrasonography. If the

ribs obscure an upper pole renal mass, an anterior scanning approach can be utilized by changing the gain of the ultrasonic signal and scanning through the liver tissue.

Specific advantages of ultrasonography should be noted. No ionizing radiation is required; thus it can be safely used in pregnancy, or when radiation exposure limitations are desired but multiple exams are needed. When no renal function is observed on excretory urography, sonography can with no risk to the patient quickly differentiate the obstructed hydronephrotic kidney from a nonfunctioning kidney due to vascular insufficiency or intrinsic renal disease. Minimal patient cooperation is needed, and prolonged cessation of respiration is not required. Finally, the capital investment required for ultrasonographic equipment is about 10 percent of that for computer assisted tomography.

COMPUTER ASSISTED TOMOGRAPHY (CAT)

Since Hounsfield's description in 1973, computer assisted tomography (CAT) has vaulted into prominent clinical use. Over 95 percent accuracy in the diagnostic characterization of renal masses has been claimed for the noninvasive CAT scan. The kidneys may be visualized especially well with CAT because they are surrounded by relatively radiolucent fat. The distribution of fat throughout the retroperitoneum allows identification of vascular and lymphatic structures as well. The absence of fat between the right upper renal pole, the adrenal, and the liver make definition in this region less sharp.

The mechanism of CAT is complex and the technology sophisticated. An x-ray source emits a fan-shaped beam in either an axial or linear orientation. The scan lasts 3–20 sec and produces a 1.3 cm tomogram. The source then rotates 10° and the scan is repeated, until 180° of rotation is completed. Rather than being collected on film, the x-ray beam is received by photomultiplier tubes which intensify the images and feed them into a computer. When all scans are received, the computer reconstructs them into an image which can be photographed. Additionally, the computer can calculate the relative radiodensities of each image, and this gives an objective criterion for determining the solid or cystic nature of homogeneous masses. The photographs are of high quality with excellent contrast and resolution, and they may be enhanced by use of contrast media to emphasize the kidneys.

The bones cause no significant impediment to the CAT scanner, whose x-rays penetrate them and can demonstrate metastasis within them. Fat can be demonstrated in angiomyolipoma to help differentiate it from renal cell carcinoma. Retroperitoneal lymphadenopathy can be readily demonstrated, but the differentiation of metastatic from inflammatory nodes is not possible. Vascular pathology such as renal artery or aortic aneurysms and renal vein thrombosis may be pictured and diagnosed. Adrenal masses are most accurately visualized with the CAT scanner.

The CAT scan allows high enough resolution to

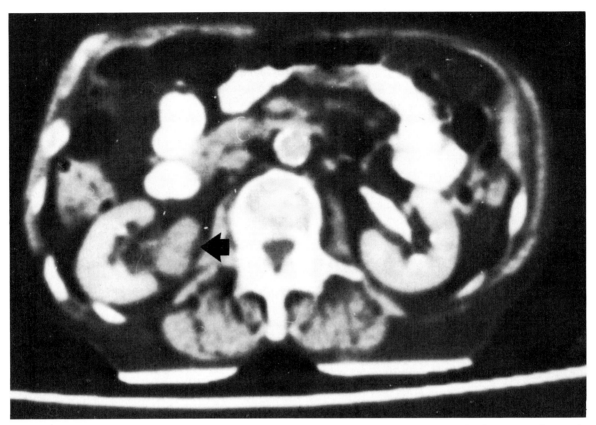

Fig. 10. Squamous cell carcinoma metastatic to the kidney was not clearly defined by angiography, but its extrarenal extension medial to the kidney is demonstrated by the CAT scan (arrow).

visualize masses of less than 2 cm. The extent of disease is also well demonstrated, and invasion of neighboring structures by malignant disease may be seen (Fig. 10). Renal masses may be characterized by their structure (solid, cystic, loculated, septate) and density. The differentiation of filling defects seen in the collecting system on intravenous or retrograde pyelography can often be accomplished with computed tomography. Uric acid stones, for instance, are radiolucent on routine x-rays but appear very dense on the CAT scan as compared with the lesser "tissue density" of tumor.

Some patient cooperation is required for high-quality CAT scans, since a good image requires the subject to hold his breath for 3–5 sec for each scan. The radiation exposure is about 4–8 rads per study, and the risk inherent with iodinated contrast administration is present if contrast enhancement is used. The accuracy of the examination is diminished in the cachectic patient or in children due to absence of retroperitoneal fat, which limits the sharpness of the structures of interest. The accuracy is also decreased by internal foreign bodies such as nasogastric tubes, surgical clips, or barium.

In most centers, the CAT scan has not yet replaced more dangerous invasive diagnostic techniques used to characterize renal masses such as angiography, but it has instead assumed the role of an adjuvant study. This technique, however, has extraordinary potential as a noninvasive diagnostic tool. As the technology improves and experience increases clinical confidence in the data obtained, the CAT scanner may replace more hazardous techniques with no loss and possible improvement of diagnostic accuracy.

REFERENCES

Daniel WW, Hartman GW, Witten DM, et al: Calcified renal masses—A review of ten years' experience at the Mayo Clinic. Radiology 103:503, 1972

Green LF, Segura JW, Hattery RR, et al: Routine use of tomography in excretory urography. J Urol 110:714, 1973

Mamdani BH, Melita PK, Makurkar SD, et al: High dose bolus urography, a superior technique in advanced renal failure. JAMA 234:1054, 1975

Rieble RA, McCarron JP, Kayam E, et al: Computed tomography in urologic patients. Preliminary assessment. Urology 10:529, 1977

Rosenfield AT, Taylor KJW: Gray scale nephrosonography. Current status. J Urol 117:2, 1977

Siegle RL, Lieberman P: Review of untoward reactions to iodinated contrast material. J Urol 119:581, 1978

Stewart BH, Dustan HP, Kiser WS, et al: Correlation of angiography and natural history in evaluation of patients with renovascular hypertension. J Urol 104:231, 1970

Swick M: The discovery of intravenous urography: Historical and developmental aspects of the urographic media. Bull NY Acad Med 42:128, 1966

RADIONUCLIDE EVALUATION OF RENAL DISORDERS

Martin L. Nusynowitz

Recent advances in imaging equipment and radiopharmaceutical development assure the continued application of nuclear medicine technics to the study of urinary tract disorders, since these methods are noninvasive, are relatively inexpensive, are associated with low radiation dosage, and possess the ability to generate rapid sequential images which permit dynamic studies of pathology and pathophysiology.

IMAGING EQUIPMENT AND RADIOPHARMACEUTICALS

Current scintigraphic technics employ relatively high resolution gamma cameras to which are coupled digital data image processing devices, essentially digital computers with electronic components and programming capabilities allowing for acquisition, storage, processing, and display of sequential images in digital format. The digital data thus acquired may be used to provide accurate and precise quantitative indices of renal function. These devices allow the specific delineation of the kidneys and other portions of the urinary tract with exclusion of radioactive "noise" from surrounding structures, such as great vessels. Previously used probe detectors suffered from the inability to separate information originating from the area of interest from that of surrounding sources. Simultaneous visualization of both kidneys and collecting systems is possible, thus providing data for bilateral comparison of function.

Compounds of technetium-99m are ideally suited for imaging applications, since the 140 keV photon emitted matches peak camera efficiency, and the short half-life (6 hours) and lack of particulate emission allow employment of millicurie amounts while radiation dose is kept at acceptable levels. Technetium-99m stannous diethylenetriamine pentaacetic acid (Tc-99m SnDTPA) is handled exclusively by glomerular filtration and is administered in doses of 10–15 mCi to adults. The total radiation dose to the kidney is approximately 1 rad, compared to doses of approximately 1 rad *per film* to both skin and gonads in conventional radiographic procedures. A bolus injection followed by rapid sequential imaging allows delineation of renal perfusion; subsequent timed sequential images permit visualization of the radiopharmaceutical as it passes through the renal parenchyma, calyces, pelves, ureters, and bladder. Tc-99m iron ascorbate DTPA complex is partially handled by glomerular filtration but also localizes in the renal parenchyma. Instead of clearing the parenchymal

tissue completely, a significant proportion remains while lower portions of the urinary tract are visualized. As a result, the renal radiation dose is higher (5 rads) than with technetium-99m SnDTPA but is still at very acceptable levels. Tc-99m dimercaptosuccinic acid (Tc-99m DMSA) localizes, by virtue of the organic mercury contained, to the tubules of the renal cortex. Its concentration in the cortex allows for high-resolution cortical images; the collecting system and lower urinary tract are not seen. The usual 5 mCi adult dose results in 7 rads to the kidney. The gonadal dose from these radiopharmaceuticals seldom exceeds 300 mrad in normal adults of either sex, and bladder doses are no more than 5 rads.

Iodine-labeled compounds are also in wide use, particularly when studying renal function, since these compounds are very pure radiochemically, containing insignificant amounts of the free iodine label. I-131 orthoiodohippurate (OIH) is an analog of PAH and is used primarily for effective renal plasma flow determinations and renography. It may also be used for generating renal images, and doses limited to 400 μCi deliver only approximately 400 mrads to the kidney. The entire urinary tract is visualized, but because of the lower photon yield and higher photon energy compared to Tc-99m compounds image quality is not as good. I-125 iothalamate is handled solely by glomerular filtration and is used for determination of glomerular filtration rate, employing doses of less than 50 μCi. Radiation doses are insignificant.

RADIOPHARMACEUTICAL CLEARANCE TECHNIQUES

Radiopharmaceuticals may be used in determining clearances by standard infusion techniques with measurement of the radioactivity in plasma and urine, but the disadvantages of bladder catheterization, accurate urine collection, constant intravenous infusion, and repeated plasma samplings remain. Single injection clearance techniques, on the other hand, are particularly suitable for use with radiopharmaceuticals, and the hazards and inconveniences of the constant infusion methods are obviated, while precision, accuracy, and ease of measurement, as compared to the more cumbersome chemical methods, are maintained. Furthermore, urine collection is not required, and in patients with low urine outputs the associated inaccuracies are avoided.

Although a variety of methods of performing single injection renal clearance measurements has been described, the most widely applied is based upon the two-compartment model; the principle of this method was described by Sapirstein. This model assumes that an injected tracer cleared by the kidney is distributed in only two major compartments, an excellent approximation, since contributions by other compartments are miniscule. Following a single injection of radiotracer, a series of timed plasma samples are obtained and counted for concentration of radioactivity. A curve plotting time versus logarithmic concentration of radioactivity is drawn (Fig. 1), and the disappearance half-time (T_A) and concentration at zero time (A) of the slowly disappearing component is obtained by back extrapolation of the straight portion of the curve. The subtraction of the concentrations of this slow component from the plasma concentrations at corresponding times produces the concentrations of the fast component of disappearance. These are plotted as log concentration versus time. The disappearance half-time (T_B) and the zero time concentration (B) of the fast component are determined, and the clearance is given by

$$\text{Clearance (ml/min)} = \frac{0.693I}{A(T_A) + B(T_B)}$$

where I is the amount injected (counts/min or cpm), A the zero time concentration of the slow component

(cpm/ml), B the zero time concentration of the fast component (cpm/ml), T_A the disappearance half-time of the slow component (min), and T_B the disappearance half time of the fast component (min).

This procedure may be simplified even further by external counting of a blood pool (cerebral, for example) to monitor the blood disappearance of tracer; this curve is calibrated by only two timed plasma samples. A one-compartment model of clearance has also been applied to the analysis. While data reduction is simpler than that of the two-compartment model, clearances are generally overestimated and accuracy suffers.

Depending on the radiopharmaceutical used, one may apply single injection clearance methods to determine either glomerular filtration rate or effective renal plasma flow.

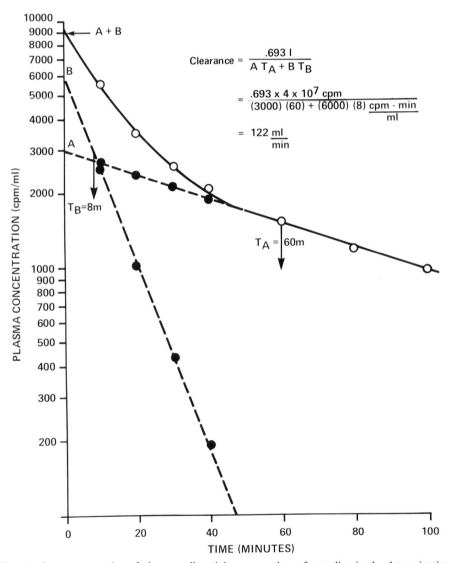

Fig. 1. Log concentration of plasma radioactivity versus time of sampling in the determination of renal clearance by the two-compartment model. The method of curve analysis is demonstrated.

GLOMERULAR FILTRATION RATE (GFR)

Radiolabeled inulin has not generally been used for measurement of glomerular filtration rate because labeling with ^{14}C necessitates the use of inconvenient beta counting methods and labeling with other radioisotopes results in compounds which are either unstable or unlike native inulin. A number of substances with renal handling properties similar to inulin have been developed, and I-125 iothalamate appears to possess the requisite attributes. The renal clearances obtained agree closely with those of standard inulin clearances. Since iothalamate clearance occurs rather slowly, sampling must be obtained as late as 2–3 hours after injection in order to accurately delineate the slow component. Correlation with standard inulin clearances is excellent, with a coefficient r of greater than 90 percent.

EFFECTIVE RENAL PLASMA FLOW

The two-compartment single injection technic has been applied to the measurement of effective renal plasma flow using I-131 orthoiodohippurate, a substitute for the classically employed PAH. Like PAH, OIH is cleared, in large measure, by a single passage through the kidney by tubular secretion. Neither PAH nor OIH is perfectly extracted in a single pass, but the extraction ratio for PAH is higher than that of OIH. If differences in extraction ratio are taken into account, the renal plasma flows, as obtained for both compounds, are identical. Uncorrected clearance values of hippuran are slightly lower than those of PAH. Nevertheless, the correlation with standard PAH clearances is excellent.

DIFFERENTIAL RENAL FUNCTION

Two special methods have been used in the determination of differential renal blood flow. Indicator dilution methods are invasive, necessitating catheterization of and injections into the renal artery and sampling from the renal vein. No adequate separation of cortical from medullary flow has been described by this technique. The radioactive inert gas washout method involves the use of a highly diffusible gas, such as xenon-133 or krypton-85. Renal artery catheterization is necessary, and a bolus of the gas in solution is rapidly injected. Rapid diffusion of the gas establishes almost immediate equilibrium between tissue and blood, and the renal washout curve is monitored by external counting. This curve has three or four components, each of which is isolated from the total washout curve by the above-described curve peeling technic. The flow rate of each component in milliliters per minute per gram of renal tissue (F) is related to the slope (k) of that component by the equation $F = k\rho$, where ρ is the gas partition coefficient between tissue and blood. It is generally agreed that the first component represents cortical blood flow. Anatomical correspondence of subsequent components has never been proved. The mean renal blood flow may also be calculated from this technique.

Qualitative estimates of comparative renal blood flow may be ascertained by the bolus injection of Tc-99m labeled radiopharmaceuticals. Rapid sequential images allow the comparison of relative perfusion of the two kidneys. Small differences in intensity may normally be seen due to differences in kidney position. Good estimates of the quality of renal perfusion may be obtained by this method (see Renal Transplantation Evaluation, below). Various measurements of activity and appearance times in time–activity histograms generated over kidney regions have been used to give a semiquantitative assessment of renal perfusion.

Another noninvasive method of estimating differential renal plasma flow is based on the notion that the slope of the second segment of the renogram curve (Fig. 2), as obtained from counting over each kidney following the injection of I-131 OIH, is proportional to the blood flow to that kidney, since the extraction ability of the renal tubular cell is large relative to the quantity of tracer used and blood flow is the limiting factor. Thus if the effective renal plasma flow is determined, the differential renal plasma flow may be calculated by comparison of the slopes of the extraction phase of the individual renograms; however, the method is only approximate, since distortion of the slope occurs with reduction of renal function exceeding 50 percent, by low urine flow rates, and by dilatation of the calyces. Similar methods have employed the integration of renal activity accumulated during the extraction phase and comparison of results from each kidney. The limitations are identical to those of the extraction phase slope method. A stop flow technique employing ureteral compression, by external pneumatic bands, has the ability to provide quantitative differential information relative to renal blood flow.

A detailed review of these methods may be found in Freeman and Blaufox.

RADIOISOTOPE RENOGRAPHY

For many years, the probe radiorenogram has been used as a test of differential renal function. This test results in a time–activity curve for each kidney which represents the vector sum of the physiologic processes involved in the extraction and excretion of I-131 OIH by renal tissue (Fig. 2). As a result, the curve is complex and not easily amenable to analysis; nevertheless, valuable clinical information has been obtained. As stated, the majority of iodohippurate is removed by the proximal tubular cells of the cortical glomeruli in a single pass, and the concentration of material does not exceed the maximum transport capability of the tubular cells, except with severe cellular damage. Hence the net amount in the kidney is equal to that amount of material extracted from the blood less that amount excreted into the urinary tract. The radiorenogram records changes in the net amount as a function of time.

Radiorenography has found clinical utility in a number of circumstances—(1) screening for the presence or absence of renal disease, with particular application to renovascular hypertension; (2) sequential

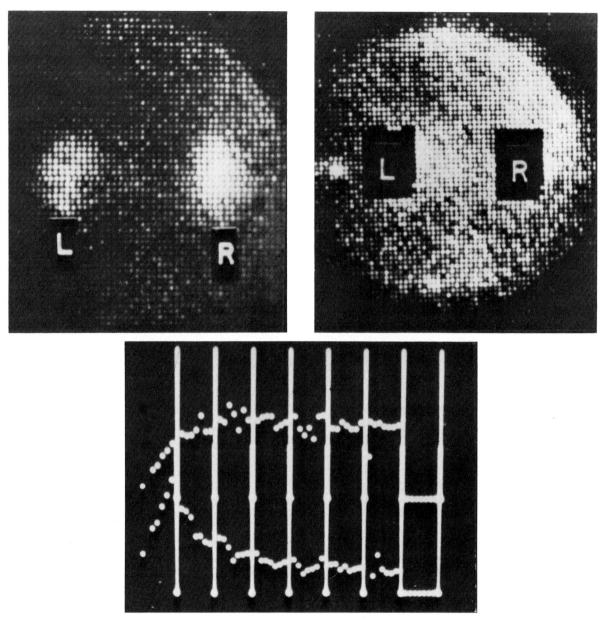

Fig. 2. I-131 iodohippurate radiorenography generated from sequential renal images in a patient with left-sided renovascular hypertension. Upper left, computer display of kidneys; upper right, areas of interest analyzed in renogram, below. The almost vertical initial phase is vascular in origin; the subsequent section, rising to the peak, is due to renal radiopharmaceutical extraction; the decreasing portion is the "excretory" phase. Note the lower slope of the second phase in the upper (left renal) curve. Each point represents 30 sec.

studies for the progression of renal disease; (3) evaluation and followup of patients with ureteral obstruction, especially after pelvic surgery or in cases of pelvic carcinoma; (4) evaluation of renal function and obstructive uropathy in pregnancy; and (5) evaluation of patients with known sensitivity to contrast media. Because of the complexities of the curve, only estimates of renal function can be ascertained, and since no anatomical information is obtained, the site of pathophysiology is difficult to evaluate.

Simple probe radiorenography has in large meas-

ures been replaced by sequential renal imaging and analysis of the digitized images. In fact, rather elaborate analyses have been performed which have shown a very good correlation with constant infusion PAH clearances and split ureteral function studies, and anatomical information is simultaneously obtained.

Radioisotopic techniques may also be employed to determine residual urine volume without the necessity for catheterization. Iodohippurate is injected and sufficient time is allowed for excretion so that the overwhelming proportion of material is in the bladder.

Counts are made over the bladder with either a camera–computer combination or with simple external probe before and immediately after the patient voids. The voided volume is measured; from these data, a calculation of residual volume may be made.

RENAL IMAGING TECHNIQUES

In general, renal imaging techniques suffer in comparison to radiologic techniques in representing renal morphology primarily because image resolution of conventional radiography is several orders of magnitude better. Nevertheless, a number of situations exist where because of the constraints upon the use of radiopaque contrast material or because of extremely poor renal function renal imaging has an important adjunctive role in providing morphologic information.

The indications for renal imaging include (1) radiocontrast media sensitivity, (2) diminished renal function precluding excretory urography, (3) assessment of renal function (in conjunction with quantitative analytical methods), (4) evaluation of patients for specific renal conditions, such as renovascular hypertension, cyst, abscess, trauma, pyelonephritis, and obstructive uropathy, and (5) renal transplant evaluation.

Radiopaque Contrast Media Sensitivity

Conventional excretory urography employs gram amounts of intravenously injected organic iodide, which may result in severe and even fatal hypersensitivity reactions. Thus excretory urography is precluded in patients with iodine hypersensitivity. The location, shape, size, and function of the kidneys and the presence of space-occupying lesions can be ascertained with radiopharmaceutical technics. The Tc-99m radiopharmaceuticals do not result in adverse reactions in patients with iodine sensitivity; even iodine-labeled compounds such as orthoiodohippurate may be used almost with impunity, since the quantity of iodine administered in a 200–400 μCi dose is minute, on the order of approximately 10^{-3} μg.

Diminished Renal Function Precluding Excretory Urography

In those circumstances where renal insufficiency has proceeded to the point where concentration of radiopaque contrast materials in the urinary tract is inadequate for visualization, radioisotopic methods are usually successful in demonstrating the kidneys and the lower urinary tract. Localization of the kidneys for renal biopsy in cases of renal failure is an excellent example of the application of these techniques.

Assessment of Renal Function

As previously discussed, sequential renal imaging analysis of areas of interest, either visually or more elegantly with quantitative techniques, can provide estimates not only of overall renal function but also comparative function of one kidney with the other and regional abnormalities within each kidney.

Specific Applications in Renal Disease

Renovascular hypertension. Iodohippurate renography has been extensively used to screen for renovascular hypertension. Depending on the specific methods employed and the analytic criteria utilized, performance parameters are variable, but test sensitivity of 85 percent and specificity of 90 percent are representative. These figures are somewhat better than those of intravenous pyelography in screening for renovascular hypertension, and a combination of both procedures identifies the vast majority of patients having renovascular lesions. Those patients having an abnormality on the screening studies would be selected for the more definitive angiographic procedures. In recent years, however, it has been appreciated that not all hypertensive patients with renal artery lesions have renovascular hypertension. The diagnosis depends on radioassay techniques, such as determination of bilateral renal vein renin activity. Furthermore, not all agree that renovascular hypertension should necessarily be treated surgically, and many believe that there is no compelling reason for precise diagnosis when response to drug therapy is adequate. The cost-effectiveness of such screening has been extensively studied by McNeal et al. Nevertheless, there is still a role for renography in case finding and localization, especially in selected populations.

Renal trauma. The use of radionuclide studies in the evaluation of renal trauma has certain advantages over excretory urography, which usually performs poorly in identifying extent and location of injury. The advantages include (1) no necessity for patient preparation, (2) noninterference by gas and feces, (3) adequate images even with poor renal function, and (4) low radiation doses allowing repeated evaluation. Contusion and the effects of small vessel occlusion result in mild to moderate decreases in activity on the affected side; main renal artery occlusion or pedicle rupture, on the other hand, produces nonvisualization, a very important distinction. Contusion abnormalities return to normal after several weeks. Renal infarction, on the other hand, results in persistent abnormalities, and the clinician should follow the patient closely for possible renal hypertension in these circumstances. Renal rupture results in distinct bands of absent activity across the kidney image. With major degrees of renal trauma, such as capsular rupture and perirenal hemorrhage or major segmental occlusion, renal scintigraphy is as sensitive as angiography.

Space-occupying lesions. The value of scintigraphic evaluation of space-occupying lesions is limited, since excretory urography, angiography, and ultrasonography produce excellent results. Peripheral cortical lesions may be seen better on scintigraphy, since excretory urography is best when there are deformities of the collecting system by the lesion. The combination of perfusion studies and static imaging may help differentiate an avascular cyst from a vascular tumor.

Obstructive uropathy. Scintigraphy may provide ancillary information about the function of the obstructed kidney, particularly when nonvisualization with excretory urography occurs. Thus an estimate of functional renal mass might provide important information

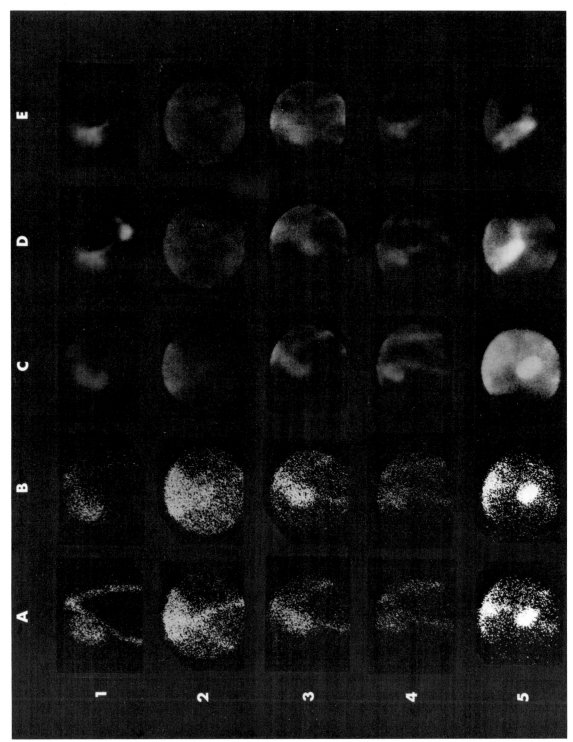

Fig. 3. Tc-99m iron ascorbate DTPA renal images after renal transplantation. A and B, 2 sec flow images obtained seconds after appearance of the radiopharmaceutical bolus in the abdominal aorta. C, static image obtained 1 min after injection. D and E, obtained after 10 and 20 min. Case 1, normal transplant study. Case 2, acute rejection reaction. Case 3, acute tubular necrosis. Case 4, ureteral obstruction. Case 5, ureteral leak. See Table 1.

Table 1
Complications of Renal Transplantation and Results of Scintigraphy

	Complication	Vascular Phase	Parenchymal Phase	Excretory Phase	Bladder Phase
Prerenal	Renal artery occlusion	Absent	Absent	Absent	Absent
Renal	Hyperacute rejection	Absent	Absent	Absent	Absent
	Acute rejection	Normal to decreased	Normal to decreased	Normal to decreased	Present
	Chronic rejection	Decreased to absent	Decreased to absent	Decreased to absent	Decreased to absent
Postrenal	Ureteral obstruction —complete	Normal	Normal	Increased	Absent
	Ureteral obstruction —partial	Normal	Normal	Normal	Delayed
	Ureteral leakage	Normal	Normal	Normal	Decreased to absent; ectopic accumulations

as to whether nephrectomy or simple relief of obstruction is indicated. In pregnancy, the low radiation dose associated with the small amount of radiopharmaceutical employed with probe renography makes this the screening procedure of choice in determining the presence of obstruction, the degree of impairment of renal function resulting from obstruction, and the course of the pathologic process.

Cystography. In children especially, scintigraphy, because of its low radiation dose, provides an excellent method for following the course of a variety of urinary tract disorders. For example, the extent and course of vesicoureteral reflux may be conveniently evaluated. Sequential gamma camera images are obtained prior to, during, and following voiding, and information on bladder volume, residual bladder volume, and reflux volume is obtainable with the application of quantitative techniques.

Renal Transplantation Evaluation

Radiopharmaceutical techniques are excellent in the evaluation of the status of a transplanted kidney. The complications of renal transplantation are varied and frequent and are enumerated in Table 1; differentiation of these complications can usually be made by scintigraphy.

Conventional methods of evaluation of transplanted kidneys have a number of disadvantages. Excretory urography is of limited value with poor renal function because visualization of the transplanted kidney is poor; renal angiography and biopsy are invasive and may result in bleeding or infection; standard clearance techniques require catheterization and measureable urine output. In contrast, the radioisotopic methods are atraumatic, without side effects, reproducible, and repeatable.

Renal function in the transplanted kidney has been evaluated by both quantitative function studies and by imaging, with the latter having the widest application. One commonly employed method involves the intravenous injection of a 10–15 mCi bolus of technetium-99m iron ascorbate DTPA. Rapid sequential images are made of vascular perfusion in the transplanted kidney, followed by sequential images at timed intervals so that both renal parenchymal function and the renal drainage system may be evaluated. The study normally takes approximately 30 min to complete.

Four phases may be visualized—(1) vascular perfusion, (2) renal parenchymal function, (3) pyeloureteral transport (excretory phase), and (4) bladder function. Insight into the specific abnormalities present may be better appreciated by studies performed at intervals after the transplant surgery.

Normally functioning transplanted kidneys show prompt visualization of the aortic bifurcation and common iliac arteries within seconds after injection, followed by rapidly increasing radioactivity in the renal parenchyma (Fig. 3). Within a few minutes, visualization of the pelvis occurs, followed by passage of the material into the ureter and bladder. During the study, the intensity of radiopharmaceutical in the collecting system increases while background activity decreases. Bladder function may be appreciated by obtaining views immediately before and after the patient voids. In renal artery occlusion and renal cortical necrosis, all four phases are absent, since the radiopharmaceutical is not delivered to the kidney. It is difficult to distinguish this from the hyperacute rejection reaction, since the rapid destruction of parenchymal renal vasculature also results in nondelivery of the radiopharmaceutical. Acute and chronic rejection reactions are characterized by diminution in the vascular, parenchymal, and excretory phases to varying degrees, depending on the severity and duration of the rejection reaction (Fig. 3). The bladder phase is present but occurs late and with a diminished rate of radioactivity accumulation. In the endstages of rejection reaction, all phases are absent.

In contrast, the renal parenchyma is primarily involved in acute tubular necrosis and the vessels are spared. Thus early scintiphotos show a normal vascular phase, but later views show diminished parenchymal concentration, and excretory and bladder phases are absent (Fig. 3). The background activity increases with time as the radiopharmaceutical diffuses into the extravascular spaces instead of being cleared by the kidney.

The postrenal complications of transplantation may be due to ureteral obstruction or to urinary extravasation. In complete obstruction, the vascular and parenchymal phases are normal or nearly so, but pelvic and ureteral activity is increased proximal to the obstruction. Bladder activity is absent. In partial obstruction, all phases are normal except for the bladder phase, which shows delayed appearance of radioactivity. With urinary extravasation, all phases are normal but for the bladder phase, which is decreased or absent. The persistent ectopic accumulation of activity persists even after the patient voids (Fig. 3).

As an alternative to the use of Tc-99m DTPA, a combination of Tc-99m pertechnetate and I-131 OIH may be employed. The former is used for evaluation of the vascular phase, whereas the OIH, secreted by the tubule, is used for the parenchymal, excretory, and bladder phases. Both methods generally give equivalent information.

Attempts have been made to develop more specific indicators of transplant rejection, and labeled fibrinogen, Tc-99m sulfur colloid, and Ga-67 citrate accumulation have been reported to localize in rejecting renal transplants. Although normal kidneys do not accumulate these materials, the specificity of technetium sulfur colloid for rejection reaction has been called into question, since other complications (acute tubular necrosis, sepsis) have resulted in abnormal renal accumulations of the radiopharmaceutical.

REFERENCES

Sapirstein LA, Vidt DG, Mandel MJ, et al: Volumes of distribution and clearances of intravenously injected creatinine in the dog. Am J Physiol 181:330, 1965

Cohen ML, Patel JK, Baxter DL: External monitoring and plasma disappearance for the determination of renal function: Comparison of effective renal plasma flow and glomerular filtration rate. Pediatrics 48:377, 1971

Freeman LM, Blaufox MD (eds): Radionuclide studies of the genitourinary system. Semin Nucl Med 4 (1 and 2), 1974

DeGrazia JA, Scheibe PO, Jackson PE, et al: Clinical applications of a kinetic model of hippurate distribution and renal clearance. J Nucl Med 15:102, 1974

Shand DG, Mackenzie JC, Cattell WR, et al: Estimation of residual urine volume with ^{131}I-hippuran. Br J Urol 40:196, 1968

McNeil BJ, Varady PD, Burrows BA, et al: Measures of clinical efficacy. Cost-effectiveness calculations in the diagnosis and treatment of hypertensive renovascular disease. N Engl J Med 293:216, 1975

RENAL BIOPSY

Marvin Forland

The development of safe and reliable techniques for the performance of percutaneous renal biopsy has led to the widespread use of this diagnostic method over the past 25 years. The ability to perform serial studies of renal morphologic changes over a period of time has made possible enormous advances in our appreciation of the diversity of renal lesions seen in idiopathic renal disease and the renal manifestations of systemic disease. It has been possible to further characterize their individual natural histories and responses to therapeutic interventions. Thin section light microscopy and electron and immunofluorescence microscopy have been parallel developments making possible more detailed study of the biopsy material. The last technique has been of particular usefulness in the formulation of concepts concerning the pathogenesis of immune-mediated renal disease.

INDICATIONS

The primary goal in renal biopsy is to establish a diagnosis and assess the morphologic severity of a renal lesion. This information will permit both informed therapeutic decision and a stronger foundation for prognostication. The technique is of most assured usefulness in the differential diagnosis of diffuse renal disease (Table 1). Glomerulonephritis or persistent microscopic hematuria of renal origin and nephrotic syndrome or persistent asymptomatic proteinuria are clinical settings in which percutaneous renal biopsy has seen its widest application. The assessment of the renal lesion in systemic lupus erythematosus is another common indication. With prolonged acute oliguric renal failure the question of potential return of renal function or management as endstage renal disease is a frequent issue. The biopsy specimen is a very small sample of renal cortex, usually 5–35 glomeruli, and consequently is most useful in diffuse renal disease, as already described. Since the specimens are predominantly cortex, the technique has limited usefulness in evaluating the early stages of diseases which are predominantly medullary.

CONTRAINDICATIONS

An informed and cooperative patient as well as a skilled and experienced operator are essential for a successful procedure with minimal possibility of complication (Table 2). The performance of percutaneous

Table 1

Indications for Consideration of Renal Biopsy
(Differential Diagnosis of Diffuse Renal Disease)

Nephrotic syndrome or persistent proteinuria
Glomerulonephritis or persistent microscopic hematuria of renal origin
Systemic lupus erythematosus
Prolonged acute oliguric renal failure
Renal complications of pregnancy
Pretransplantation evaluation
Posttransplantation renal deterioration

renal biopsy should be reserved for the specialist who is doing the procedure frequently. Major bleeding complications can be minimized by hematologic evaluation, including a careful family and individual history, platelet count, prothrombin time, and partial thromboplastin time. Hypertension is a factor which correlates directly with postoperative bleeding as well as the development of arteriovenous fistulae and must be well controlled prior to biopsy. Active renal infection should be treated before biopsy is undertaken. The culture of renal biopsy material, even in patients with bacteriuria, has provided low yields in revealing evidence of renal parenchymal infection.

The uremic patient presents a number of risk factors regarding percutaneous biopsy. Hypertension, anemia and coagulation abnormalities are usually present and renal size may be decreased with cortical contraction. The former problems must be ameliorated with dialysis or conservative measures if biopsy information is considered necessary for patient management, and an open biopsy is preferable if renal contraction is demonstrated.

Increased risk of bleeding during pregnancy has been reported, but this has not been a uniform experience.

COMPLICATIONS

Gross hematuria is the most frequent complication and the reported incidence ranges from 5 percent to 40 percent, with the former figure most representative of current experience in major centers (Table 3). Hematuria is usually painless and subsides with bed rest within 24 hours. Surgical intervention is rarely necessary, and epsilon aminocaproic acid has been used with success in incidents of prolonged bleeding.

The development of a perinephric hematoma is accompanied by flank pain, usually with radiation to the groin, fall in hematocrit, and instability in vital signs. This occurred in 1.4 percent of subjects in a recent survey. Surgical intervention and at times nephrectomy may be necessary. An estimated mortality of 0.07–0.17 percent was found in two large surveys totaling over 18,000 biopsies. Laceration of an adjacent organ, including liver, spleen, and bowel, is a potential complication, as is pneumothorax. Infection is an additional rare complication.

PROCEDURE

The technical procedure for renal biopsy has been well described in several publications. The development of proficiency in the procedure requires a period of supervised training and its frequent use to achieve and maintain satisfactory biopsy yields with minimal occurrence of complications. In the original descriptions of the technique, localization of the kidney was initially accomplished by delineating renal outlines on a KUB film or IVP and transcribing them to the patient's back with the assistance of surface landmarks. The accuracy of this method was limited by the renal depth and parallax introduced by the x-ray beams. Subsequently, renal isotope scan was introduced, which avoids parallax distortion and minimizes radiation exposure. Ultrasound localization eliminates radiation and provides an accurate assessment of renal depth. Biopsy under direct vision using image amplification or cinefluoroscopy monitoring is now widely employed and is particularly useful for the obese or heavily muscled patient.

Sterile preparation is accomplished with the patient lying prone on a sandbag or rolled pillow to help immobilize the kidney. Following the introduction of

Table 2

Contraindications to Percutaneous
Renal Biopsy

Untrained operator
Uncooperative patient
Uncontrolled hypertension
Bleeding disorder
Active renal infection
Renal tumor or cysts
Hydronephrosis
Single kidney (relative)
Uremia (relative)

Table 3
Possible Complications of Percutaneous Renal Biopsy

Gross hematuria
Perirenal hematoma
Laceration of adjacent organ (liver, spleen, bowel, etc.)
Arteriovenous fistula
Dissemination of infection

local anesthetic, the operator determines the lateral border of the lower pole of the kidney with an exploring needle, usually a 6-inch, 22-gauge spinal needle. The site is characterized by the resistance of the kidney in contrast to that of the subcutaneous tissue and muscle and the more objective pulsation of the needle ar⁻ᵈ characteristic arc movements upon deep respiratio The depth is measured and used as a guide for tl needle biopsy. The Franklin modification of the Vim-Silverman needle and the Travenol Tru-cut disposable needle are the most commonly used instruments. The yield of specimens adequate for interpretation is approximately 85–95 percent in experienced hands.

HANDLING OF SPECIMEN

If a single core appears of adequate size, it may be processed for light, electron, and immunofluorescence microscopy. A horizontal transection rather than vertical cut of the core is recommended so that a concentration of glomeruli at the superficial end of the specimen may be shared. Often two cores must be obtained for adequate studies.

Immediate fixation of half the specimen in 2 percent buffered glutaraldehyde permits utilization of the tissue for both light and electron microscopy. In the pathology laboratory 1 mm blocks are cut from both ends of the specimen and postfixed in 1 percent osmium tetroxide and subsequently embedded in epon or araldite for electron microscopic study. The remainder is routinely processed for light microscopy and cut in 2–3μm sections. Slides are prepared and stained with hematoxylin and eosin, periodic acid–Schiff (PAS), Masson's trichrome, and methenamine silver stains.

Tissue for immunofluorescence studies must be immediately suspended in an embedding medium and snap-frozen in liquid nitrogen.

Details of these studies are considered in the following three chapters (*Light Microscopy, Electron Microscopy,* and *Immunofluorescence*).

REFERENCES

Bolton WK, Tully RJ, Lewis EJ: Localization of the kidney for percutaneous biopsy. A comparative study of methods. Ann Intern Med 81:159, 1974

Bolton WK, Vaughan ED Jr: A comparative study of open surgical and percutaneous renal biopsies. J Urol 117:696, 1977

Diaz-Buxo JA, Donadio JV Jr: Complications of percutaneous renal biopsy: An analysis of 1,000 consecutive biopsies. Clin Nephrol 4:223, 1975

Kark RM, Muehrcke RC: Biopsy of the kidney in prone position. Lancet 1:1047, 1954

Striker GE, Quadracci LJ, Cutler RE: Use and Interpretation of Renal Biopsy. Philadelphia, W.B. Saunders, 1978

LIGHT MICROSCOPY

George A. Bannayan

The use of light microscopy in the study of biopsy tissue remains the most important tool in the interpretation and evaluation of the various pathologic lesions observed in kidney diseases. A significant limitation of light microscopy is the predominant absence of pathognomonic or specific changes of the various clinical renal diseases. Such a limitation mandates the augmentation and correlation of the light microscopic findings with the clinical, laboratory, electron microscopic, and immunofluorescence observations.

In evaluating a renal biopsy, careful and detailed analysis should be made of all the kidney components, namely, the glomeruli, tubules, interstitium, and blood vessels. This chapter describes generally the various histologic forms of renal disease as well as categorizes the pathologic alterations in a variety of systemic diseases. The reader should use this chapter in association with the section of this book describing Specific Renal Diseases.

ACUTE GLOMERULONEPHRITIS

This lesion most commonly follows infections of the throat and skin with nephritogenic strains of group A beta hemolytic streptococci. Acute glomerulonephritis has also been described with *Staphylococcus* coagulase positive septecemia, *Streptococcus viridans* subacute bacterial endocarditis, *Staphylococcus* coagulase negative infection of ventriculoatrial shunts, pneumococcal infections, and in certain other bacterial, parasitic, and viral infections. Light microscopic examination shows generalized and diffuse involvement of all the glomeruli. The glomerular tufts are swollen, enlarged, hypercellular, and bloodless, and the capillary lumina are narrowed (Fig. 1). The hypercellularity is due primarily to proliferation of mesangial and endothelial cells. Polymorphonuclear cells are found in variable numbers. There is usually no significant increase in the amount of mesangial matrix. Some glomeruli may show proliferation of the parietal epithelial cell lining Bowman's capsule with formation of a few scattered crescents. A few crescents do not denote a worse prognosis. Some cases will have

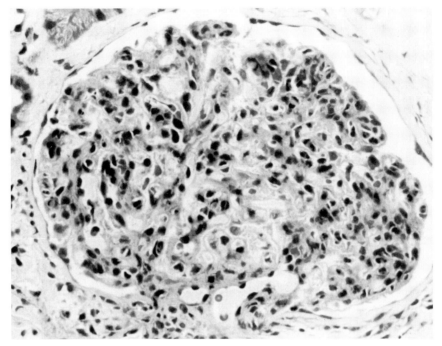

Fig. 1. Acute glomerulonephritis. The glomerulus shows increased cellularity, polymorphonuclear cell exudate, and reduction of capillary lumina. H&E. × 400.

extensive crescent formation and may pursue a rapid and progressive course. Adhesions between the glomerular tuft and Bowman's capsule, capillary luminal thrombi, and necrosis are occasionally observed. Red blood cells as well as leukocytic and hyaline casts are seen in the lumina of the tubules. The interstitium is edematous and may contain an admixture of inflammatory cells. The arteries and arterioles are usually unremarkable but may show fibrinoid necrosis in severe cases.

In the healing phase, cellular proliferation recedes over a period of 3–6 months with progressive opening of the capillary lumina. No definite criteria exists which predict progression to chronicity; however, histologic changes which are frequently found in such cases include necrosis of glomerular tufts, capillary luminal thrombi, numerous crescents, adhesions, and prominent interstitial reaction.

RAPIDLY PROGRESSIVE GLOMERULONEPHRITIS

This type of glomerulonephritis encompasses a number of diseases with diverse etiologies all of which have a rapid and progressive clinical course and essentially similar light microscopic appearance (Table 1). Light microscopy shows the characteristic lesion of epithelial crescent within Bowman's spaces (Fig. 2). These cresencents involve as many as 75–95 percent of the glomeruli. The crescents are formed predominantly by proliferation of the parietal epithelial cells lining Bowman's capsule, with some participation from the visceral epithelial cells. The stimulus for this cellular proliferation is thought to be fibrin leaking from the injured glomerular capillary walls into Bowman's space.

With passage of time the crescents become fibrocellular and eventually fibrous.

The glomerular tufts are compressed and markedly distorted by the crescents. The changes in the tufts include mesangial and endothelial cell proliferation, polymorphonuclear cell exudation, increased mesangial matrix, necrosis, obliteration of capillary lumina, luminal thrombi, adhesions to Bowman's capsule, and varying degrees of sclerosis. The interstitium is edematous and contains an admixture of inflammatory cells. The tubules may show degenerative changes, atrophy, and dropout. The blood vessels may on occasion show fibrinoid necrosis and vasculitis. Rapidly progressive glomerulonephritis is observed in the following conditions:

1. Antiglomerular basement membrane antibody disease.
2. Antiglomerular basement membrane antibody disease with lung hemorrhage (Goodpasture's syndrome). In this disease entity, two histologic patterns are recognized—focal and crescentic glomerulonephritis. The former seems to be the initial lesion which invariably progresses to the latter.
3. In some cases of poststeptococcal glomerulonephritis.
4. In some cases of *Str. viridans* subacute bacterial endocarditis.
5. In a few cases of Henoch-Schönlein purpura with renal involvement.
6. Microscopic variant of polyarteritis nodosa.

Table 1
Summary of Histologic Lesions in Glomerulonephritis

Acute Glomerulo-nephritis	Rapidly Progressive Glomerulonephritis	Focal Glomerulonephritis	Mesangio-Proliferative Glomerulonephritis	Chronic Proliferative Glomerulonephritis	Membrano-proliferative Glomerulonephritis	Epimembranous Glomerulonephritis
Poststreptococcal	Anti-GBM without lung hemorrhage	Goodpasture's syndrome	Idiopathic	Idiopathic	Type I	Idiopathic
Str. viridans subacute bacterial endocarditis	Anti-GBM with lung hemorrhage (Goodpasture's syndrome)	Microscopic variant of polyarteritis nodosa	Poststreptococcal	Poststreptococcal	Type II (dense deposit disease)	Lupus glomerulonephritis
Staphylococcus coagulase positive septecemia	Poststreptococcal	Wegener's granulomatosis	IgA glomerulonephritis	IgA glomerulonephritis	Sickle cell disease	Australia antigenemia
Staphylococcus coagulase negative infection of ventriculoarterial shunt	*Str. viridans* subacute bacterial endocarditis	Lupus glomerulonephritis	Lupus glomerulonephritis	Lupus glomerulonephritis	Neoplasia	Quartan malaria
Pneumococcal infections	Henoch-Schönlein purpura	Henoch-Schönlein purpura	Mixed connective tissue disease	Henoch-Schönlein purpura		Syphilis
Other bacterial parasitic and viral infections	Microscopic variant of polyarteritis nodosa			Hereditary nephritis		Heavy metals
	Wegener's granulomatosis	IgA glomerulonephritis		IgG–IgM cryoglobulinemic glomerulonephritis		Sarcoidosis
	Lupus glomerulonephritis	Mixed connective tissue disease				Neoplasia Mixed connective tissue disease Renal vein thrombosis

110

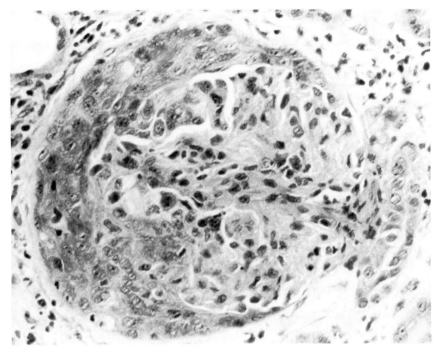

Fig. 2. Rapidly progressive glomerulonephritis. The glomerulus shows an epithelial crescent within the Bowman's space. H&E. × 400.

7. Wegener's granulomatosis.
8. In some patients with diffuse lupus glomerulonephritis.

FOCAL GLOMERULONEPHRITIS

Focal glomerulonephritis is a pathologic lesion which is observed on light microscopy in a variety of renal disorders. In this type of glomerulonephritis only a certain number of glomeruli are affected, with the rest appearing normal (Fig. 3). Within the affected glomeruli the changes are segmental (localized), being confined only to some lobules. The histologic changes that occur in the affected areas include proliferation of mesangial and endothelial cells, increased mesangial matrix, necrosis, nuclear fragmentation, polymorphonuclear cell exudation, obliteration of the capillary lumina, adhesions to Bowman's capsule, and proliferation of both the parietal and visceral epithelial cells with formation of small crescents in certain instances. Focal glomerulonephritis is seen in the following conditions.

1. Initial state of Goodpasture's syndrome.
2. Initial stage of microscopic variant of polyarteritis nodosa.
3. Initial state of Wegener's granulomatosis.
4. Initial stage of hereditary nephritis (Alport's syndrome).
5. In about one-third of patients with lupus glomerulonephritis.
6. Mixed connective tissue disease.
7. *Str. viridans* subacute bacterial endocarditis. The glomerulonephritis associated with this condition is immune complex in origin. Most patients have a focal lesion; however, a small group may have either an acute or crescentic lesion.
8. Henoch-Schönlein purpura. Most patients with glomerular disease have focal glomerulonephritis which is usually nonprogressive but which rarely may transform to chronic proliferative glomerulonephritis. A few may have a crescentic lesion, which pursues a rapid and progressive course. The outcome of the chronic proliferative lesion is unpredictable, but some will progress slowly to chronic renal failure.
9. IgA glomerulonephritis (Berger's disease). About 85 percent of patients have focal glomerulonephritis, which is usually nonprogressive. The rest may have either a mesangioproliferative or chronic proliferative glomerulonephritis. The latter group may pursue a slow course to chronic renal failure.

MESANGIOPROLIFERATIVE GLOMERULONEPHRITIS

This is a poorly defined and understood entity. The histologic lesion is characterized by proliferation of the mesangial cells with either no or some increase in the amount of mesangial matrix. The glomerular capillary walls are thin and delicate, and the lumina are patent. There are no adhesions, necrosis, epithelial cell proliferation, or polymorphonuclear exudation. The etiology of mesangioproliferative glomerulonephritis in most instances is unknown; however, essentially a similar lesion has been described in a variety of conditions, including (1) the resolving phase of poststreptococcal glomerulonephritis, (2) IgA glomerulonephritis, (3) lu-

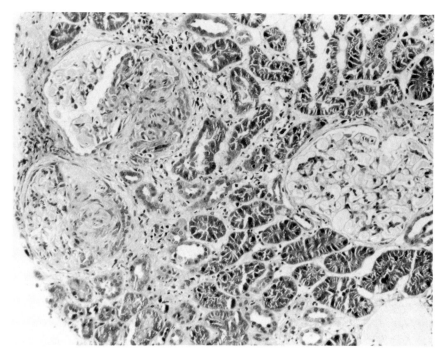

Fig. 3. Focal glomerulonephritis. Three glomeruli are seen; the one on the right is normal, while the two on the left show segmental proliferative changes. H&E. × 150.

pus glomerulonephritis, and (4) mixed collagen tissue disease.

CHRONIC PROLIFERATIVE GLOMERULONEPHRITIS

In this type of glomerulonephritis, there is a sustained and nonresolving inflammation with most patients, progressing slowly to chronic renal failure. The glomeruli show a spectrum of changes which includes proliferation of mesangial and endothelial cells, increased mesangial matrix, obliterations of the capillary lumina, irregular thickening of the glomerular basement membranes, adhesions to Bowman's capsule, proliferation of the epithelial cells with occasional crescent formation, and glomerulosclerosis. Tubular atrophy and interstitial fibrosis are prominent features. There may be arterial and arteriolar nephrosclerosis commensurate with the duration and severity of hypertension. The etiology of chronic proliferative glomerulonephritis in most instances is unknown, without any clearcut time of onset; however, similar histologic appearance is also observed in a large variety of disorders (Table 1).

MEMBRANOPROLIFERATIVE GLOMERULONEPHRITIS

This category of glomerulonephritis is subdivided into two types:

Type I (classic variant). This type is two or three times as common as type II. In this variant the glomeruli are enlarged and hypercellular and have an accentuated lobular pattern. The hypercellularity is due to proliferation of the mesangial and endothelial cells. The glomerular capillary walls are irregularly thickened, and this is accompanied by increased mesangial matrix and

some obliteration of the capillary lumina. Polymorphonuclear cell exudation, adhesions to Bowman's capsule and proliferation of the epithelial cells with formation of occasional crescents may be present. A characteristic feature is the duplication of the glomerular basement membrane, accompanied by circumferential mesangial cell interposition between the true and duplicated membrane. This can be demonstrated by methenamine silver stain, in which the glomerular basement membrane will show a double contour or "tram track" appearance.

This entity seems to be an immune complex type of disease, although the etiologic agent or agents remain obscure. Some cases have followed streptococcal infections. A similar histologic appearance is seen in sickle cell disease and in some cases of neoplasia that have associated glomerular disease.

A closely related condition is chronic lobular glomerulonephritis. In this entity the glomeruli are enlarged and have markedly accentuated lobular patterns due to extensive expansion of the mesangium by waxy, uniform, acellular nodules. This entity most probably represent a progression or a late stage of type I membranoproliferative glomerulonephritis.

Type II (dense deposit disease). This type is characterized by the presence of dense deposits in the glomerular capillary walls. The glomeruli are enlarged and hypercellular and may reveal some accentuation of the lobular pattern. The hypercellularity is due to proliferation of the mesangial and endothelia cells. Some epithelial cell proliferation with occasional crescent formation may also occur. A particular feature is the widespread, rather uniform thickening of the glomerular capillary walls due to the presence of refractile, ribbon-like eosinophilic material within the basement membranes. Duplication of the glomerular capillary basement membranes with mesangial cell interposition between the true and duplicated membranes often is present, but is not as prominent as in type I disease.

EPIMEMBRANOUS GLOMERULONEPHRITIS

This lesion is considered as a form of immune complex disease with trappings of the antigen–antibody complexes along the epithelial surfaces of the glomerular basement membranes, between the foot processes of the visceral epithelial cells and the glomerular capillary basement membranes.

All the glomeruli are involved by a diffuse uniform thickening of the glomerular capillary walls (Fig. 4). There is no cellular proliferation, polymorphonuclear cell exudation, necrosis or adhesions between the glomerular tufts and Bowman's capsule. At an early stage the thickening is slight and the capillary lumina are widely patent. With progression of the disease, the capillary wall thickening becomes more prominent, leading gradually to luminal narrowing and ultimately to glomerulosclerosis. Methenamine silver stain shows the presence of spikes projecting from the capillary basement membranes towards the epithelial side. Interpositioned in between the spikes are the immune complex deposits, which appear red with trichrome stain. At a later stage the tips of the spikes fuse together, giving the basement membranes a double contour appearance. Hyaline droplets and lipids are seen in the cytoplasm of the epithelial cells lining the proximal convoluted tubules. Tubular atrophy, interstitial fibrosis, interstitital chronic inflammatory cell infiltrate, foamy macrophages, and cholesterol granulomas are frequently observed. In most cases the nature of the antigen remains obscure (idiopathic). Specific etiologies have been associated with this lesion and are outlined in Table 1.

NIL DISEASE

In this disease entity, the glomeruli by light microscopy appear almost normal. The capillary lumina are widely patent, and the capillary walls appear fixed and rigid but not thickened. There are no polymorphonuclear exudations, proliferation of any of the cellular elements, increased mesangium, or adhesions. Fat deposition and hyaline droplets are seen in the cytoplasm of the epithelial cells lining the tubules. The interstitium is usually edematous.

FOCAL GLOMERULAR SCLEROSIS AND HYALINOSIS

The etiology of this disease is unknown, although there are reports of its occurrence in heroin addicts. The histologic, laboratory, clinical, and prognostic feature of this disease define it as a separate entity from nil disease. In the initial stages there is focal and segmental glomerular sclerosis involving the glomeruli in the juxtamedullary region. As the disease progresses, glomeruli away from the juxtamedullary region become involved, and gradually all the glomeruli become totally sclerosed. There is no cellular proliferation, although adhesions to Bowman's capsule are frequently observed.

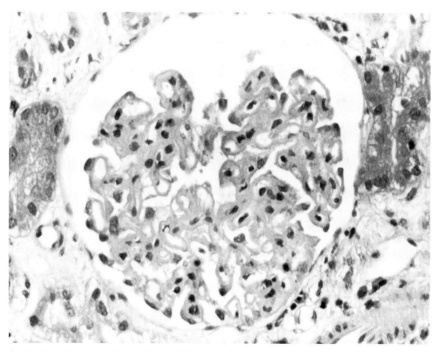

Fig. 4. Epimembranous glomerulonephritis. The glomerulus shows uniform thickening of the glomerular capillary wall with absence of any cellular proliferation. H&E. × 400.

The other feature of this disease is the presence of eosinophilic, acellular refractile hyaline material within the glomerular tufts.

GLOMERULOPATHIES OF NEOPLASIA

Some of the neoplasias that have been associated with glomerular lesions include carcinomas, embryonal tumors, Hodgkin's disease, non-Hodgkin's lymphomas, leukemias, myeloproliferative disorders, plasma cell dyscrasias, and benign tumors. The glomerular lesions observed include epimembranous glomerulonephritis, nil disease, amyloidosis, focal glomerulonephritis, rapidly progressive glomerulonephritis, membranoproliferative and proliferative glomerulonephritis, membranoproliferative and intravascular coagulation.

POLYARTERITIS NODOSA

Two forms of this disease are recognized.

Classic polyarteritis nodosa. In this form the affected blood vessels are the medium sized muscular arteries. The arcuate arteries show vasculitis, fibrinoid necrosis, luminal thrombi, and destruction of the internal elastic membrane. Healing results in microaneurysmal formation.

Microscopic polyarteritis nodosa. In this variant, small blood vessels are involved primarily in the glomerular capillary tufts. Microscopically the lesion is characterized initially by focal glomerulonephritis, which invariably progresses to crescentic glomerulonephritis.

WEGENER'S GRANULOMATOSIS

This kidney lesion has great similarity to the microscopic variant of polyarteritis nodosa. In addition there is a destructive glomerular lesion characterized by periglomerular granulomatous inflammation.

RHEUMATOID ARTHRITIS

The kidney is not frequently involved in this disease. The most significant lesion is vasculitis, similar to that seen in classic polyarteritis nodosa. The other lesions seen in rheumatoid arthritis, namely amyloidosis, epimembranous glomerulonephritis, and chronic interstitial nephritis with papillary necrosis, are due to complications of chronicity, gold therapy, and analgesic abuse, respectively.

MIXED CONNECTIVE TISSUE DISEASE

Renal lesions are rarely observed. Some of the lesions described include focal, mesangioproliferative, and epimembranous glomerulonephritis.

SCLERODERMA

The most significant lesion is in the blood vessels. The interlobular arteries show marked myxoid, collagenous thickening, containing concentrically arranged fibroblastic nuclei, resulting in considerable narrowing of the blood vessel lumina. The afferent arterioles and glomerular capillary tufts show fibrinoid necrosis and luminal thrombi.

SYSTEMIC LUPUS ERYTHEMATOSUS

At least four different glomerular lesions have been described.

Mesangioproliferative lupus glomerulonephritis. The incidence of this lesion is not known exactly. It is usually nonprogressive, but in about one-third of the patients there is transformation to the more severe diffuse proliferative glomerulonephritis.

Focal lupus glomerulonephritis (type I). At least one-third of lupus glomerulonephritis falls into this category. It is usually nonprogressive, but in at least 15–20 percent of the patients there is transformation to diffuse proliferative glomerulonephritis. A much smaller number will undergo transformation to the epimembranous type.

Epimembranous lupus glomerulonephritis (type II). About 15 percent of lupus glomerulonephritis falls into this category. The clinical course is that of slow progression to chronic renal failure. Occasionally transformation to diffuse proliferative glomerulonephritis may occur.

Diffuse proliferative lupus glomerulonephritis (type III). About half of lupus glomerulonephritis falls into this category. In this form there is generalized and diffuse involvement of glomeruli. The glomeruli show accentuation of the lobular pattern, widespread mesangial and endothelial cell proliferation, increased mesangial matrix, necrosis, luminal thrombi, obliteration of the capillary lumina, nuclear fragmentation, adhesions to Bowman's capsule, hematoxylin bodies, capillary wall thickening and some degree of epithelial cell proliferation, which in some instances is marked enough to form extensive epithelial crescents. A characteristic feature is the irregular glomerular capillary wall thickening, which may be localized or widespread. This thickening is due to the presence of massive, acellular, and eosinophilic material along the luminal surfaces of the basement membranes, which corresponds to the subendothelial deposits seen on electron microscopy. This type of capillary thickening is referred to as the "wire loop lesion."

DIABETES MELLITUS

A number of heterogenous lesions are observed which collectively are referred to as diabetic nephropathy.

Diffuse intercapillary glomerulosclerosis. This lesion is characterized by a diffuse increase in the amount of mesangial matrix. This lesion is not specific for diabetes mellitus and is seen in a variety of conditions, including aging, liver cirrhosis, congenital cyanotic heart disease, and glomerulonephritis of heterogenous etiologies. There is good evidence that the Kimmelstiel-Wilson nodule is a progression of this lesion.

Nodular intercapillary glomerulosclerosis. This lesion is called the Kimmelstiel-Wilson nodule and is pathognomonic for diabetes mellitus. By light microscopy these nodules are seen as almost spherical, homogenous, eosinophili acellular masses located near the periphery of the glomerular tufts and surrounded by patent capillaries. The nodules vary in size and number within the individual glomeruli and may be widespread or seen only within a few glomeruli.

Diffuse capillary glomerulosclerosis. This lesion is characterized by uniform thickening of the glomerular basement membrane. Diffuse capillary glomerulosclerosis may be preceded or occur simultaneously with intercapillary glomerulosclerosis. This is probably the earliest, most common, and most significant lesion of diabetic nephrosclerosis.

Capsular drop. This lesion is infrequently observed. The capsular drop is composed of an eosinophilic, waxy, globular material located between the parietal epithelial cells and Bowman's capsule. The lesion is specific for diabetes if it is homogenous and free of cells and collagen.

Fibrin caps. These are eosinophilic, homogenous, spherical or crescentic shaped deposits located at the periphery of the glomerular tufts. Fibrin caps are not specific for diabetes and may appear in other conditions.

Vascular lesions. The muscular arteries show subintimal fibroelastic thickening. The arterioles are extensively hyalinized. This process involved both the afferent and efferent arterioles. The involvement of both arterioles is almost specific for diabetes mellitus.

Tubular lesions. The basement membranes are thickened, with the tubules showing atrophy and dropout commensurate with the degree of interstitial fibrosis. A lesion which is observed in poorly controlled diabetic patients is the Armanni-Epstein lesion, in which the cells of the most distal straight portion of the proximal convoluted tubules are filled with glycogen and which appear empty and plant-like on light microscopy.

GOUT

The most significant lesion is the presence of urate crystals in the lumen of collecting tubules and the interstitium. The crystals are doubly refractile, deep blue in color, and elongated, rectangular, or amorphous in appearance and are surrounded by giant cells. The crystals are best seen in alcohol-fixed tissue.

FABRY'S DISEASE

This lesion on light microscopy is characterized by the presence of fine, foamy vacuoles in all the cells of the glomeruli, tubules, and blood vessels. In the glomeruli the vacuoles are most prominent in the cytoplasm of the visceral epithelial cells. In the tubules, the cells lining the loop of Henle and distal convoluted tubules are most severely affected. In the blood vessels the vacuoles are seen in the endothelial and smooth muscle cells.

AMYLOIDOSIS

Amyloid consists of eosinophilic, acellular material which in the glomeruli is initially deposited in the mesangium and in relation to the basement membrane. The aggregates of amyloid gradually enlarge and coalesce, leading to obliteration of the capillary lumina and ultimately to solidification of the glomeruli. Amyloid is also deposited in the walls of the blood vessels, tubular basement membranes, and interstitium. Amyloid can be demonstrated on light microscopy because of its characteristic staining features. It turns red when treated with methyl violet (metachromatic reaction). Congo red gives a brown-red color to amyloid which becomes apple-green in color when polarized. Amyloid also fluoresces under ultraviolet light when treated with thioflavin T.

MULTIPLE MYELOMA

The most significant renal lesion is the formation of casts within the tubular lumen. These casts are surrounded by syncytial epithelial cells and amyloid. Amyloid in the glomeruli is infrequently observed and when present usually is not massive.

WALDENSTRÖM'S MACROGLOBULINEMIA

The glomerular capillary lumina contain coagulated material almost exclusively composed of IgM. Amyloid deposits are infrequent.

MIXED IgG–IgM CRYOGLOBULINEMIC GLOMERULONEPHRITIS

The glomeruli are hypercellular due to proliferation of mesangial and endothelial cells and exudation of polymorphonuclear cells. There is usually increase in the amount of mesangial matrix. Adhesions to Bowman's capsule and proliferation of the epithelial cells with crescent formation may also occur. The capillary lumina contain coagulated material. The cytoplasm of the mesangial and endothelial cells contain rhomboid crystals which stain blue with PTAH and red with trichrome.

HEREDITARY NEPHRITIS

In the mild forms and especially in female patients, the changes are minimal and nonspecific. In the more severe forms of the disease, the initial lesion is the focal glomerulonephritis which invariably progresses to diffuse chronic proliferative glomerulonephritis and chronic renal failure. The changes in the basement membrane are best seen on electron microscopy. Foam cells are frequently seen in the interstitium but are not specific.

SARCOIDOSIS

The most significant changes are observed in the interstitium and consist of calcium deposition and the presence of noncaseating granulomatous inflammation. Glomerular lesions have also been described. The commonest glomerular lesion is epimembranous glomerulonephritis, with, less frequently, chronic proliferative glomerulonephritis.

SICKLE CELL DISEASE

The glomerular capillaries, the arterioles, the intertubular plexus, and the vasa recta are markedly dilated and engorged with sickle cells. With progression of the disease, there is papillary necrosis, cortical scars, tubular atrophy, interstitial fibrosis, and glomerulosclerosis. Membranoproliferative glomerulonephritis has also been described.

COAGULOPATHIES

Similar histologic lesions are observed with hemolytic uremic syndrome, postpartum acute renal failure, and thrombotic thrombocytopenic purpura. The common underlying pathogenetic mechanism is intravascular coagulation. The characteristic renal lesion consists of thrombi in the glomerular capillary lumina and arterioles, with occasional segmental or diffuse glomerular necrosis. In severe cases cortical necrosis may ensue.

TOXEMIA OF PREGNANCY

The glomeruli are large and bloodless and have reduced capillary lumina. This appearance is primarily due to cytoplasmic swelling of the endothelial and mesangial cells. Irregular thickening of the glomerular capillary walls, luminal thrombi, and hyperplasia of the juxtaglomerular apparatus are also observed.

ACUTE TUBULAR NECROSIS

Histologically two main lesions are recognized.

Nephrotoxic acute tubular necrosis. This is caused by the direct effect of chemicals on the tubules. There is severe necrosis of the epithelial cells lining the tubules, primarily of the proximal tubules. The more specific pathologic changes vary with the etiologic agent.

Tubulorrhectic acute tubular necrosis. This is caused by a lengthy list of conditions, the common mechanism of which is ischemia to the tubules. In this type there is rupture of the tubular basement membranes, but the epithelial necrosis is not very impressive. Unequivocal necrosis of the epithelial cells does not appear with any significant frequency, and when it is present, although it may be found in any part of the nephron, is most frequently seen patchily distributed in the straight terminal portion of the proximal convoluted tubules at the corticomedullary boundary area. Both the proximal and distal tubules are dilated and lined by flattened regenerating epithelial cells, possessing hyperchromatic nuclei and basophilic cytoplasm and showing some mitotic activity. The lumina of the proximal tubules contain eosinophilic casts, while the lumina of the distal tubules contain pigmented casts which are composed of Tamm-Horsfall myoglobin protein, and hemoglobin. The interstitium is markedly edematous and may contain a scattering of inflammatory cells. Of interest is the finding of nucleated red blood cells in the vasa recta of the medulla. The presence of nucleated red blood cells remain unexplained but may be due either to extramedullary hematopoiesis or to stagnation and accumulation of nucleated red cells as they are released from the bone marrow, spleen, and lymph nodes.

ACUTE NONBACTERIAL INTERSTITIAL NEPHRITIS

This form of the disease is usually an adverse reaction of the hypersensitivity type to therapeutic agents, including antiepileptic drugs and antibiotics. Acute interstitial nephritis is most frequently observed as a complication of antibiotic administration, in particular methicillin. The light microscopic appearance, irrespective of the causative agent, is similar. This picture consists of interstitial edema, accompanied by inflammatory cell infiltrate composed of lymphocytes, mononuclear cells, plasma cells, and eosinophils. The tubules may show necrosis, atrophy, and degenerative changes. The glomeruli and the blood vessel are unremarkable.

CHRONIC NONBACTERIAL INTERSTITIAL NEPHRITIS

This denotes a condition in which there is fibrosis of the interstitium accompanied by a scattering of chronic inflammatory cells, tubular atrophy, and glomerulosclerosis. This type of nephritis should be reserved for conditions in which the interstitium is primarily affected rather than secondarily fibrosed by a variety of glomerular, tubular, and vascular diseases. The etiology in most cases is obscure, although such a lesion may be observed in Balkan nephritis, heat stroke, vesicoureteral reflux, radiation nephritis, Sjögren's syndrome, sarcoidosis, medullary cystic disease, urate nephropathy, nephrocalcinosis, and immunologically mediated tubulo-interstitial diseases such as lupus glomerulonephritis, dense deposit disease, and Goodpasture's syndrome.

ACUTE PYELONEPHRITIS

In this instance there is extensive edema of the interstitium, accompanied by a large number of polymorphonuclear cells, with formation of microabscesses. The tubular lumina are filled with polymorphonuclear cells, and their lining epithelium cells show varying degrees of necrosis. The process is patchy, with normal tracts admixed with inflamed areas. The epithelium of the pelvicalyceal system and the submucosa are infiltrated with polymorphonuclear cells.

CHRONIC PYELONEPHRITIS

The histologic observations of the renal parenchyma are nonspecific. For a definitive diagnosis, papillary blunting, deformity and dilatation of the calyceal system with the overlying cortical scars should be demonstrated. The disease has a patchy distribution with diseased tracts admixed with normal parenchyma. In the involved areas, the interstitium is extensively fibrosed and contains a number of chronic inflammatory cells. The tubules show either dropout or atrophy, with the latter being lined by flattened epithelial cells and their lumen containing homogenous eosinophilic casts. The glomeruli show nonspecific changes, including periglomerular fibrosis, collapse of glomerular tufts, deposition of collagen within Bowman's space, cellular proliferation, and glomerulosclerosis. The pelvicalyceal submucosa is infiltrated with chronic inflammatory cells with frequent formations of lymphoid follicles. In the uninvolved areas the kidney parenchyma shows no significant histologic changes.

HYPERTENSION

The histologic appearances of benign and malignant hypertension differ from each other.

Benign hypertension. The changes that will be described may also be observed in aging without a history of hypertension. In this phase of hypertension, changes are observed in both the muscular arteries and arterioles. The interlobular and arcuate arteries show luminal narrowing due to subintimal fibroelastic thick-

lumina. There are massive, homogeneous, dark-staining, electron-dense deposits in the subendothelial location and within the sclerotic regions which correspond to the areas of hyalinosis observed by light microscopy. Myxovirus-like particles have been described in the cytoplasm of the endothelial cells. The visceral epithelial cells show microvillous transformation of the cytoplasmic membranes and fusion of the foot processes. No cellular proliferation is observed.

MICROSCOPIC VARIANT OF POLYARTERITIS NODOSA AND WEGENER'S GRANULOMATOSIS

The electron microscopic observations in both of these diseases are essentially similar. The most significant feature is the extensive proliferation of the epithelial cells within Bowman's space, admixed with some fibrin.

The changes in the glomerular tufts are nonspecific and include increased mesangial matrix, collapsed and irregularly thickened basement membranes, obliterations of capillary lumina, proliferation of mesangial and endothelial cells, and the inconsistent presence of ill-defined and irregularly shaped electron-dense deposits in the mesangium and contiguous to the basement membranes.

SYSTEMIC LUPUS ERYTHEMATOSUS

The electron microscopic patterns vary, depending on the type of lupus glomerulonephritis.

Mesangioproliferative lupus glomerulonephritis. In all instances osmophilic electron-dense deposits are present, primarily in the mesangium. There is usually some increase in the mesangial matrix which is accompanied by some proliferation of the mesangial cells.

Focal lupus glomerulonephritis (type I). In the diseased areas there is limited fusion of the foot process of the visceral epithelial cells, slight thickening and irregularity of the glomerular capillary basement membranes, and some increase in the mesangial matrix accompanied with some proliferation of the mesangial and endothelial cells. Electron-dense deposits are seen in all cases and are located primarily in the mesangium and occasionally in subendothelial and intramembranous locations.

Epimembranous lupus glomerulonephritis (type II). The electron microscopic features are similar to those described under epimembranous glomerulonephritis, consisting of numerous epimembranous osmophilic electron-dense deposits separated by spikes extending from the glomerular basement membranes.

Diffuse lupus glomerulonephritis. The most characteristic finding is the presence of massive subendothelial osmophilic electron-dense deposits which correspond to the ''wire loop lesion'' seen on light microscopy (Fig. 4). Electron-dense deposits may be also seen in epimembranous and intramembranous locations, mesangium, and within the basement membranes of the tubules. There is usually an increased mesangial matrix and hyperplasia of both the mesangial and endothelial cells.

An interesting but not pathognomonic finding in lupus glomerulonephritis is the presence of interlacing,

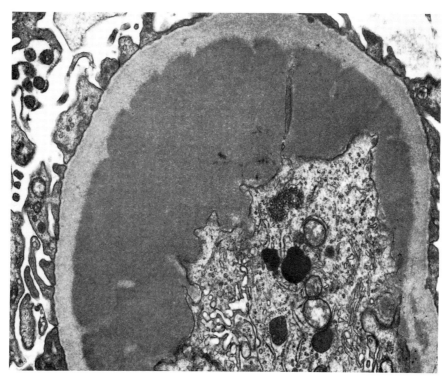

Fig. 4. Diffuse lupus glomerulonephritis, type III. Massive osmophilic electron-dense deposits are seen in the subendothelial location. The cytoplasm of the endothelial cell contains a clump of myxovirus-like particles. Uranyl acetate and lead citrate. Original magnification × 18,000

branching, tubular structures in the cytoplasm of the endothelial cells, which on cross-section resemble myxoviruses. They have not been proven to be viruses, and most likely are composed of phospholipid and glycoproteins. Another feature which is not frequently observed but which when present is pathognomonic of lupus glomerulonephritis is the presence of curvilinear bands, resembling fingerprints, in the glomerular and peritubular capillary basement membranes, the mesangium, and within electron-dense deposits. The significance and the origin of these "fingerprints" are uncertain.

COAGULOPATHIES AND SCLERODERMA

The electron microscopic features of hemolytic uremic syndrome, thrombotic thrombocytopenic purpura, postpartum acute renal failure, and scleroderma are essentially similar.

The glomerular capillary basement membrane may be collapsed and wrinkled and show the presence of a widened rarefied zone in the subendothelial location which contains a collection of numerous granular but irregularly shaped electron-dense deposits. There may be duplication of the basement membranes, giving the glomerular capillary walls a double contour appearance.

The capillary lumina usually contain thrombi, which are composed of fibrin, platelets, and deformed and fragmented red blood cells. The endothelial cells are usually swollen, but there is no significant proliferation of any of the cellular elements.

TOXEMIA OF PREGNANCY

The most characteristic lesion is the marked swelling and cytoplasmic vacuolization of the endothelial and mesangial cells, leading to partial or total occlusion of the capillary lumina. The basement membranes may be focally thickened, but a significant finding is the presence of a widened, rarefied, translucent zone in the subendothelial location containing both granular and fibrillar electron-dense material. The mesangial matrix may be increased and may contain an increased number of mesangial cells.

DIABETES MELLITUS

In the early stages of the disease, there is diffuse increase in mesangial matrix of the glomerular lobules which corresponds to the diffuse intercapillary glomerulosclerosis seen on light microscopy. The excessive mesangial matrix leads eventually to the formation of nodules which correspond to the Kimmelsteil-Wilson lesion. These nodules may contain foci of calcium and incarcerated fragments of degenerated mesangial cells, lipid, and collagen fibers. The nodules are initially surrounded by patent capillary lumina, but with progression of the lesion the nodules obliterate the capillary lumina and merge with the basement membrane. Probably the most significant and earliest lesion observed on electron microscopy is uniform thickening of the glomerular capillary basement membrane due to increased amounts of basement-membrane-like material. Early in the disease the contours of the basement membrane are regular along both the luminal and epi-

thelial surfaces, but in advanced stages the basement membrane develops irregular outlines. Similar thickening is also observed in Bowman's capsule and basement membranes of tubules and peritubular capillaries.

FABRY'S DISEASE

The characteristic feature is the presence of intracytoplasmic glycolipid inclusions in all types of renal cells. These inclusions vary in size from 0.3 up to 10 μm. The inclusions have a coarsley lamellated appearance and may appear either round with concentrically arranged lamellae or ovoid with parallel lamellae.

AMYLOIDOSIS

The electron microscopic appearance of both primary and secondary amyloidosis is similar.

Initially amyloid is deposited in the mesangium and along both surfaces of the glomerular capillary basement membrane. In the early stages the basement membranes are distinct from the amyloid deposits. With progression of the disease, however, the whole glomerulus becomes solidified with amyloid and the basement membranes become incorporated. Amyloid deposits are also seen in the interstitium, blood vessels, and tubular basement membranes.

Amyloid is composed of randomly arranged fibrils each measuring 80–110 Å in diameter and up to 1 μm in length.

IgG–IgM CRYOGLOBULINEMIC GLOMERULONEPHRITIS

The most characteristic finding is the presence of rhomboid crystals in the cytoplasm of the glomerular tuft endothelial cells. The glomeruli also show increased mesangial matrix, proliferation of mesangial and endothelial cells, and the presence of electron-dense and fibrillar subendothelial deposits.

HEREDITARY NEPHRITIS

The most characteristic feature is the thickening of the glomerular capillary basement membranes, which also appear laminated due to splitting of the lamina densa into multiple, thin, electron-dense layers. Electron-lucent areas are noted in the lamina densa containing granules, each 500 Å in diameter. Similar changes are seen in the tubular basement membranes and Bowman's capsule. The basement membrane changes have been considered specific by some but not by others. The glomeruli also show some increase in mesangial matrix and proliferation of the mesangial cells. Rarely electron-dense deposits are observed in mesangial and subendothelial locations.

SICKLE CELL DISEASE

Electron microscopy shows paracrystalline structures in the red blood cells and membrane bound iron deposits in the mesangium. In those cases that have a membranoproliferative glomerulonephritis, the electron microscopic features are similar to those described in type I membranoproliferative glomerulonephritis.

REFERENCES

Baldwin DS, Gluck MC, Lowenstein J, et al: Lupus nephritis. Am J Med 62:12, 1977

Beathard GA, Granholm HA: Development of the characteristic ultrastructural lesion of hereditary nephritis during the course of the disease. Am J Med 62:751, 1977

Gluck MC, Gallo G, Lowenstein J, et al: Membranous glomerulonephritis. Ann Intern Med 78:1, 1973

Gubler MC, Lenoir G, Grunfeld JP, et al: Kidney Int 13:223, 1978

Heptinstall RH: Pathology of the Kidney. Boston, Little, Brown, 1974

Hill GS, Hinglais H, Tron F, et al:Systemic lupus erythematosus. Am J Med 64:61, 1978

Spargo BM: Practical use of electron microscopy for the diagnosis of glomerular disease. Hum Pathol 6:405, 1975

Turner DR, Cameron JS, Bewick M, et al: Transplantation in mesangiocapillary glomerulonephritis with intramembranous dense "deposits:" Recurrence of disease. Kidney Int 9:439, 1976

Watanabe I, Whittier FC, Moore J, et al: Gold nephropathy. Arch Pathol Lab Med 100:6321, 1976

IMMUNOFLUORESCENCE*

Curtis B. Wilson

Antibodies can interact in two ways with glomeruli and/or interstitial renal tissue to cause most incidences of glomerulonephritis and an undetermined amount of tubulointerstitial nephritis in man. That is, antibodies can react either with renal structural components in situ—the glomerular basement membrane (GBM) or tubular basement membrane (TBM)—or with circulating nonglomerular antigens to form immune complexes that are subsequently trapped nonspecifically in the glomerulus or renal interstitium. The anti-basement-membrane antibody mechanism is responsible for perhaps 3–5 percent of glomerulonephritis in man, whereas the immune complex mechanism causes at least 80 percent of the remainder. Either way, when antibody accumulates in the renal tissue, potent mediators of inflammation become activated [including vasoactive amines, complement proteins, the Hageman factor systems (coagulation and kinin-forming proteins)], and polymorphonuclear leukocytes or other such cellular elements are recruited. Antibody deposition and mediator activation by either mechanism results in an often indistinguishable histologic inflammatory response in the glomerular or interstitial tissue.

Although clues as to the specific immunopathologic process involved can be drawn from light or electron microscopic examination, the fluorescence microscope has the greatest value to the immunopathologist in this respect. With it, using fluorochrome-labeled antiimmu-

*This is publication 1587 from the Department of Immunopathology, Research Institute of Scripps Clinic, 10666 N. Torrey Pines Rd., La Jolla, Calif. 92037. This work was supported in part by USPHS Grants AM-20043, AM-18626, and AI-07007 and BRS Grant RRO-5514.

noglobulin (Ig) antisera, one easily sees the discrete linear patterns characteristic of anti-basement-membrane antibodies as they react with antigens distributed throughout the GBM or TBM (Fig. 1). In a contrasting pattern, as one might expect, antibodies that accumulate in the glomerular or tubulointerstitial tissue as part of the random deposition of circulating immune complexes lodge in a distinctive irregular, granular distribution (Fig. 2). In addition, immune complexes may preferentially localize in the mesangial area of the glomerulus or assume a variety of patterns of distribution involving the peripheral glomerular capillary wall and/or mesangium. In a general way, these patterns correlate with the eventual histologic form of glomerulonephritis that the immune complex deposit generates.

Immunofluorescence is additionally useful for identifying mediators of inflammation, such as complement or coagulation proteins, that can amplify the inflammatory process and for locating cell types, such as thymus-dependent lymphocytes (T cells), that can accumulate within cellular infiltrates at the site of inflammation, as in transplant rejection. In human renal disease, immunofluorescence is, then, the key to the immunopathologic differentiation of the anti-basement-membrane and immune complex mechanisms of renal injury. Because of its usefulness and ready availability, immunofluorescence should be used routinely for all kidney biopsies.

IMMUNOFLUORESCENCE TECHNIQUE

Immunofluorescence depends upon the use of fluorochrome (fluorescein isothiocyanate, tetramethylrhodamine isothiocyanate, etc.)-labeled antibodies specific for Ig molecules of various classes or for molecules of the different mediator systems. Experimental studies indicate that about 5 μg of diffuse linear anti-GBM IgG antibody or about 0.25 μg of discrete granular antigen per gram of kidney tissue can be detected by the immunofluorescence technique. A fluorochrome, when exposed to an exciting light of proper wavelength, emits a secondary light of somewhat longer wavelength. Insertion of a barrier filter in the optical path suppresses the exciting light, allowing viewing of the secondary light. Fluorescein, for example, has a usable absorption maximum of 490 nm and emits a secondary light at 517 nm. Fluorescence microscopes use either transmitted or incident illumination, usually from a high-pressure mercury light source, and include excitation and barrier filters to allow maximum excitation and viewing of fluorescein. Various combinations of filters effectively differentiate the nonspecific autofluorescence intrinsic in all tissues from the specific immunofluorescence produced by the fluor-labeled antibody.

Monospecific antibodies conjugated with fluorescein isothiocyanate can be prepared relatively easily or are obtainable commercially. Heavy chain class-specific anti-Ig sera are used for detecting Ig of various classes. Fluoresceinated antisera reactive with Ig light chains have also been used in studying kidneys from patients with some gammopathies and certain forms of amyloi-

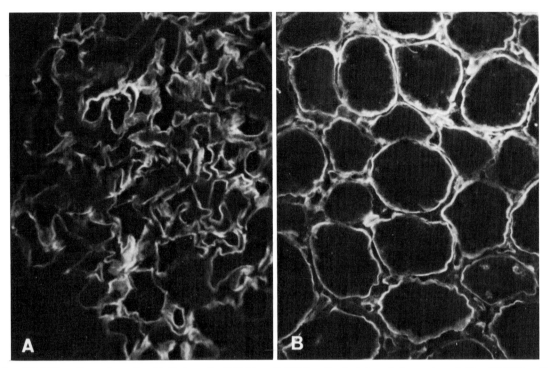

Fig. 1. (A) Diffuse linear deposits of IgG along the GBM in anti-GBM antibody-induced glomerulonephritis. (B) Diffuse linear deposits of anti-TBM antibodies. Fluorescein isothiocyanate conjugated anti-IgG antiserum. Original magnification × 250.

dosis. The specificity of any fluoresceinated reagent is confirmed if prior absorption with the purified antigen of interest blocks its reactivity.

Renal tissues to be studied by immunofluorescence are ''snap-frozen,'' generally by immersion in liquid nitrogen, to reduce the freezing artifact. The thinnest

possible sections are then cut with a microtome in a cryostat and fixed by any of a variety of methods. Stained sections are viewed with attention to the pattern and amount of the fluorescent deposit, rather than to its intensity, which is merely a function of the reagent. The viewer should realize that the fluorescence tech-

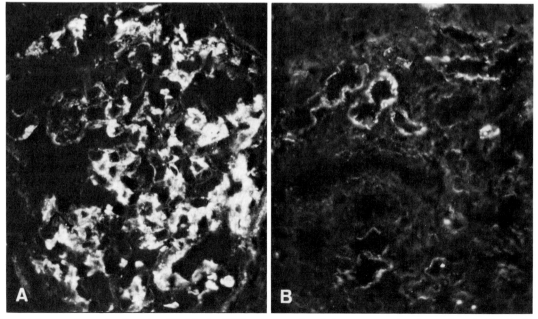

Fig. 2. (A) Scattered granular deposits of IgG in the GBM and mesangium in immune complex glomerulonephritis. (B) Granular immune complex deposits in the TBM. Fluorescein isothiocyanate conjugated anti-IgG antiserum. Original magnification × 250.

nique's greatest usefulness is in localizing material deposited in tissue, not in quantitating it. All structures in the section should be examined for deposits, not only the glomeruli, since tubulointerstitial and vascular deposits may be equally important. Serum proteins in tubular casts and in reabsorption droplets in tubular epithelium from patients with heavy proteinuria must be differentiated from specific immune deposits. Similarly, autofluorescent cellular granules, connective tissue, and elastic lamina of vessels must not be confused with specific deposits; however, unusually striking autofluorescence may hint at a cause of the disease process (for example, calcium deposits). Anti-GBM antibody deposits usually are extremely uniform, so that even a single glomerulus may be adequate for a tentative diagnosis. Immune complex deposits may be very focal, so that many glomeruli may need to be available for meaningful characterization.

ANTI-BASEMENT-MEMBRANE ANTIBODY-INDUCED NEPHRITIS

The hallmark of anti-basement-membrane antibody-induced disease is the linear deposit of Ig along the basement membrane of the glomerulus, tubule, alveolus, or infrequently another structure such as the choroid plexus or intestine. Prior to severe architectural disruption, the GBM deposit is smooth and continuous; however, with increasing damage the GBM and its deposit become corrugated and fragmented as seen by immunofluorescence. IgG is the most common Ig identified, with IgA or IgM only infrequently found in a linear distribution. The third component of the complement sequence (C3) accompanies the IgG deposit in about two-thirds of patients with anti-GBM antibody-induced nephritis. Fibrin deposits are also prominent in the Bowman's space of patients with the crescentic, rapidly progressive form of anti-GBM nephritis. Linear deposits of IgG are found on the TBMs of about 70 percent of patients with anti-GBM antibody disease, indicating the concomitant presence of anti-TBM antibodies. These TBM deposits may be focal, involving only segments of the tubule, or may be diffuse.

Troublesome deposits of IgG (usually with albumin) emit weak but identifiable linear patterns in some normal kidneys, in most kidneys at autopsy, and in kidneys from patients with diabetes mellitus and must be differentiated from specific anti-GBM antibody deposits. The immunofluorescent diagnosis of anti-GBM disease is supplemented by detecting circulating anti-GBM antibodies (indirect immunofluorescence, radioimmunoassay). The best confirmatory study is to elute the antibody from renal tissue with buffers known to dissociate antigen–antibody bonds and then to test the eluate for its anti-GBM specificity in vitro or in vivo in subhuman primates.

The lungs of patients with anti-GBM antibody-induced Goodpasture's syndrome (glomerulonephritis and pulmonary hemorrhage) often contain linear IgG deposits along the alveolar basement membrane when viewed by immunofluorescence (see the chapter on

Goodpasture's Syndrome). Occasionally, patients with pulmonary hemosiderosis but not overt clinical nephritis have evidence of anti-basement-membrane antibody disease found as linear alveolar basement membrane deposits. When evaluated further, these patients also have linear deposits of Ig along the GBM. Presumably a qualitative and/or quantitative difference in the amount of anti-basement-membrane antibody present distinguishes these patients from those with overt anti-GBM antibody-induced nephritis.

Occasional patients develop anti-TBM antibodies in the absence of detectable anti-GBM antibody reactivity. This has been noted most frequently in transplant recipients and is an occasional complication in patients with immune-complex-induced nephritis and with drug-induced tubulointerstitial nephritis. Anti-TBM antibodies are also the suggested cause of primary tubulointerstitial nephritis in a few patients. By immunofluorescence, IgG and usually C3 are bound in a circumferential linear pattern along the TBM. IgA or IgM anti-TBM antibodies are rare. As in the anti-GBM nephritic reaction, the specificity of the anti-TBM reaction should be confirmed by detecting circulating anti-TBM antibodies or by elution studies. [For example, patients with diabetes mellitus often have intense nonspecific staining for IgG (and albumin) in their TBMs.]

Although no examples have been identified with certainty in man, experimental studies in animals suggest that non-basement-membrane glomerular antigens or foreign antigens that are first trapped or "planted" in the glomeruli are occasionally involved in nephritogenic antigen–antibody reactions in situ. Immunofluorescence will be useful in attempting to identify similar reactions in humans.

IMMUNE COMPLEX NEPHRITIS

Granular deposits of Ig, usually accompanied by C3, are believed to be the mark of immune complex renal disease in man. This granular deposition is identical to the deposit in animals with known immune complex nephritis. Analyses of the antigenic components of the granular renal deposits in an increasing number of patients confirm that the deposits are, in fact, immune complexes. Such confirmation should alert the patient's nephrologist to the antigenic source of disease and the possibility of its elimination with therapeutic benefit.

The amount and distribution of granular deposits in glomeruli of patients with immune complex nephritis is variable and may not involve all glomeruli. The granular deposit can be characterized by its size (fine, moderate, coarse) and its distribution (mesangial, segmental GBM, diffuse GBM, etc.). The presence of granular deposits in the tubulointerstitial tissue, TBM, and arteriole walls should also be noted. The granular deposit can be further characterized by identifying its specific Ig classes, which relates to various histologic forms of presumed immune complex nephritis, as summarized in Table 1. IgG is the most profuse and is sometimes found along with IgA and IgM. IgA is

Table 1
Generalizations About Immunofluorescence Findings in Immune Complex
Glomerulonephritis (GN)

	Granular Ig	C3
Diffuse proliferative GN	Diffuse IgG, variable IgA, IgM	Similar to IgG, may be predominant in poststreptococcal GN
Proliferative and crescentic GN	Diffuse IgG, variable IgA, IgM, deposits may be minimal	Similar to IgG
Focal proliferative GN	Segmental and/or mesangial IgG, often prominent IgA or IgM	Similar to IgG
Membranous GN	Diffuse IgG, variable IgA, IgM	Similar to IgG
Membranoproliferative GN	Diffuse, sometimes scant IgG, variable IgA, IgM	Prominent, present without Ig in one-third
Chronic GN	Variable IgG, IgA, IgM, most prominent in least damaged glomeruli	Often more prominent than Ig
Lupus GN	Diffuse or segmental IgG, IgA, IgM	Similar to Ig

particularly prominent in glomeruli of patients with systemic lupus erythematosus. The glomeruli of some patients with focal glomerulonephritis may contain considerable IgA or IgM, largely in the mesangium. Mesangial IgA deposits are also frequent in patients with Henoch-Schönlein purpura. Segmental deposits of IgM have been identified in patients with focal glomerulosclerosis. The Ig deposits are usually accompanied by proteins of the complement sequence, with C3 being the component generally sought.

Once granular Ig deposits suggestive of immune complexes have been identified, the next step is to identify the antigen–antibody system involved to actually confirm that they are immune complexes. The patient's physician must serve as a detective, narrowing the field of potential antigen–antibody systems to a few which can be tested. Immunofluorescence study using fluorescein-conjugated antibody specific for the antigen in question can be used for direct identification of the antigen bound in the glomerular deposit. Elution studies to remove and characterize the antibody in the deposit have also been successful. When eluting antibody from a renal biopsy, it is important to show that the antibody recovered from the glomeruli is more concentrated than that present in serum, indicating its degree of accumulation. Antigens from infectious agents (bacterial, protozoan, and viral) are the most commonly identified to date in patients with immune complex nephritis; however, antigens from endogenous sources, such as DNA, thyroglobulin, and neoplastic tissue, have also been identified.

The frequency of circulating immune complexes in patients with immunofluorescent evidence of immune complex deposits in their glomeruli correlates best with the acuteness of the nephritic process. That is, patients with acute, generally proliferative forms of glomerulonephritis frequently have circulating immune complexes

when tested by one or more assay systems. Patients with more indolent forms of glomerulonephritis, such as membranous or membranoproliferative glomerulonephritis, or chronic glomerulonephritis, generally do not have detectable circulating immune complexes. The serologic studies are then not as useful in confirming the immune complex nature of granular deposits in glomeruli as are immunologic assays for anti-GBM antibodies in confirming the specificity of linear deposits, as described in the preceding section.

Immune complexes may also deposit in renal tubulointerstitial tissues, including the TBM, peritubular capillaries, and arterioles. Such extraglomerular deposits are most frequently identified in patients with systemic lupus erythematosus. Studies of the antigen–antibody systems involved in this extraglomerular deposition suggest that the immune complexes are of similar types to those identified within the glomeruli. Of interest, cells in kidney biopsies from patients with systemic lupus erythematosus may have IgG bound to their nuclei, indicating the presence of antinuclear antibodies. (It is suspected that antibodies present in extravascular fluids combine with the nuclei during the staining process rather than binding in vivo.) The presence of nuclear staining in addition to extraglomerular deposits of Ig and C3 strongly suggest a diagnosis of systemic lupus erythematosus.

COMPLEMENT IN GLOMERULAR DISEASE

Fluorescinated antisera specific for C3 and other complement components are frequently used in studying tissue sections from glomerulonephritic kidneys. As noted earlier, about two-thirds of kidneys from patients with anti-GBM nephritis and nearly all kidneys from patients with immune-complex-induced nephritis have detectable complement deposits. In such kidneys, all nine components of the classical complement sequence are usually identifiable by using reagents reactive with each component. This suggests that the entire classical complement pathway is being activated by the accumulation of anti-GBM antibody or immune complex deposits.

In some patients with membranoproliferative glomerulonephritis, particularly those with the so-called type II or dense deposit form of the disease, the picture of Ig and complement is somewhat different. Many of these patients have no detectable Ig, although striking C3 and terminal complement component (C3–C9) deposition is often observed in their glomeruli (and TBM). The C3 is present in the absence of the early-acting complement components, namely, C1, C4, and C2. Therefore this suggests that the complement may accumulate in these kidneys through activation of not the classical but of the alternative pathway, which begins with C3 and continues through the terminal components. Of interest, some of these patients also have circulating factors capable of activating C3 in normal serum. Recently, these so-called nephritic factors were shown to be Ig with the properties of immunoconglutinin and reactive with complement antigens.

Of additional interest, in perhaps 10 percent of renal biopsies studied (usually those from patients in advanced stages of glomerular injury) C3 and later reacting complement components may be present in glomeruli, TBM, and vessels in the absence of Ig and initial complement components. In a few kidneys of this type biopsied sequentially, an immune complex type of glomerular deposit was noted at first, but later only complement remained. Little is known about the relative disappearance rates of Ig and complement from glomerulonephritic kidneys, but apparently C3 can persist or even increase while Ig becomes undetectable.

This suggests a transition in pathogenesis during which preexisting immune-complex-induced injury to the kidney is perpetuated by continuing complement deposition, possibly activated through the alternative complement pathway.

CONCLUSIONS

The immunopathologist can identify the major immunopathogenic mechanism responsible for a patient's renal injury according to the pattern of Ig deposition seen by immunofluorescence. Patients with immune-complex-induced renal injury can be characterized further by the type of antigen–antibody that comprises the nephritogenic immune complex deposit. Finally, by analyzing the mediators of inflammation, such as the complement proteins in such patients, one can place in perspective the involvement of these amplifying mechanisms in the production of the renal injury.

REFERENCES

Burkholder PM: Atlas of Human Glomerular Pathology. Hagerstown, Harper & Row, 1974

Germuth FG, Rodriguez E: Immunopathology of the Renal Glomerulus. Immune Complex Deposit and Antibasement Membrane Disease. Boston, Little, Brown, 1973

Morel-Maroger L, Leathem A., Richet G: Glomerular abnormalities in nonsystemic diseases. Relationship between findings in light microscopy and immunofluorescence in 433 renal biopsy specimens. Am J Med 53:170, 1972

Wilson CB: Immunohistopathology of the kidney, in Rose NR, Friedman H (eds): Manual of Clinical Immunology. Washington, D.C., American Society of Microbiology, 1976

Wilson CB, Dixon FJ: Diagnosis of immunopathologic renal disease. Editorial. Kidney Int 5:389, 1974

Wilson CB, Dixon FJ: The renal response to immunological injury, in Brenner BM, Rector FC Jr (eds): The Kidney. Philadelphia, W.B. Saunders, 1976

Symptoms of Renal Disease

PROTEINURIA

Marvin Forland

Increased urinary protein loss is a major indication of the presence of primary renal disease or renal involvement in systemic illness. Proteinuria is frequently an early manifestation of a kidney abnormality during an as yet asymptomatic phase and always requires further evaluation and etiologic definition.

Proteinuria was first definitely described in 1694 by Frederik Dekkers of Leiden, who reported the precipitating effect of heat and acetic acid on the urine of certain patients with consumption and other wasting diseases. In 1794 Cotugno described an association between edema and urine "which formed itself into a white mass" when boiled. Richard Bright is credited with the definitive correlations among edema, proteinuria, and renal disease in his exemplary clinical and laboratory studies at Guy's Hospital in the early nineteenth century.

PATHOPHYSIOLOGY

Although approximately 180 liters of plasma containing over 12,000 grams of plasma protein are filtered across the glomeruli each day, the glomerular filtration barrier permits only a very small amount of protein to traverse the glomerular capillary wall. Micropuncture data from experimental animals indicate the proximal tubular fluid may contain 1–10 mg/dl of protein. Since the total renal excretion of protein in normal man is approximately 50–150 mg/day, the renal tubules normally reabsorb most of the approximately 2–20 g which may be filtered.

The glomerular filtration barrier is definable by electron microscopy into three discrete layers (Fig. 1). The endothelium lining the inner capillary surface is comprised of thin, attenuated cells containing multiple fenestrae of 500–1000 Å diameter. They lie adjacent to the glomerular basement membrane, a continuous gel-like structure approximately 3000 Å wide. A central, electron-dense component of the glomerular basement membrane can be discerned, the lamina densa, bound by two relatively electron-lucent layers, the lamina rara interna and externa. Biochemically the glomerular basement membrane is a collagen-like material, high in carbohydrate content, structured into 30–50 Å wide

fibrillar units. Projections of the capillary epithelial cells extend to and interdigitate along the outer surface of the glomerular basement membrane. These cytoplasmic foot processes are separated by filtration slits approximately 240 Å in width. A thin, single-layer membrane 70 Å thick bridges the podocyte extensions. This flat structure has been termed the filtration slit diaphragm.

A glycoprotein coat lining the endothelial and epithelial cell surfaces of the glomerular capillary wall has been identified by histochemical techniques. The coat has a net negative charge due to the carboxyl groups of its high sialic acid component.

Multiple factors influence the permeability of the glomerular capillary wall to macromolecules. The glomerular clearance of uncharged macromolecules decreases with increasing molecular weight and, particularly, effective molecular radius. Glomerular clearance of polymer macromolecules is similar to that of inulin up to a molecular radius of 24 Å and then becomes a sigmoid function when plotted as a percentage of glomerular filtration rate. The membrane approaches impermeability with macromolecules larger than 60 Å in radius. These characteristics are compatible with the diffusion theory, postulating macromolecules diffuse across the glomerular capillary wall at a rate determined by their intramural diffusion coefficient; however, other factors have been found to be operative. Because of the electronegative cell surface coat, molecular charge has been identified as a major factor in studies measuring permeability of dextran and horseradish peroxidase in experimental animals. Negatively charged molecules have lower fractional clearances than neutral molecules (Fig. 2), while cationic molecules have high clearances. Consequently, negatively charged serum albumin has a lower fractional clearance than a neutral dextran of similar molecular weight. Molecular shape is an additional consideration, with proteins being less permeable than flexible linear molecules such as dextran or polyvinyl pyrrolidone. Finally, hemodynamic factors influence filtration. Fractional clearance is inversely related to glomerular filtration rate, and the transient cessation of renal blood flow in experimental animals promotes glomerular permeability.

While the glomerular basement membrane provides a diffusion barrier to larger molecules, the filtration slit is emerging as an additional principal filtration barrier.

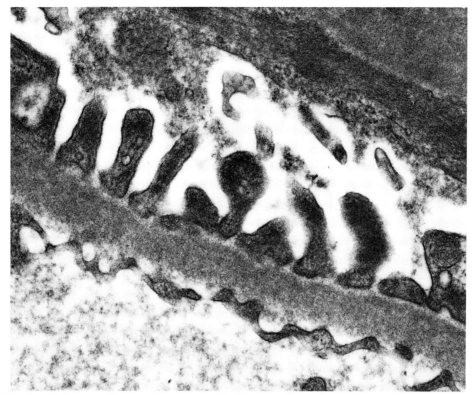

Fig. 1. High-power electron photomicrograph of human glomerular capillary wall demonstrating epithelial cell podocytes abutting superior margin of glomerular basement membrane and fenestrated endothelial cell cytoplasm along the inferior margin. × 28,000. [Courtesy of Dr. George A. Bannayan.]

This has been demonstrated by morphological observations showing smaller electron-dense macromolecules restricted in passage at the site of the pore.

Recent studies indicate the proximal tubule plays a major role in the metabolism of proteins and peptides and their final urinary concentration. The small but critical proportion of larger molecular weight proteins and polypeptides which are filtered, such as albumin, insulin, and growth hormone, are unselectively reabsorbed by the process of endocytosis following binding to the luminal plasma membrane of the proximal tubular cells. Incorporated into newly formed apical vacuoles, the proteins are hydrolyzed following fusion of the vacuoles with primary lyosomes. The remaining peptides and amino acids then diffuse from the cell into the blood. Consequently, the reabsorptive process is a catabolic sequence and does not directly contribute to the restoration of serum albumin levels.

There is evidence that small linear peptides comprised of up to ten amino acids, such as the octapeptide angiotensin II, are hydrolyzed at the luminal surface of the proximal tubule. The activity of hydrolytic enzymes of the brush border results in the reabsorption of breakdown products into and across the tubular cell.

Together these tubular mechanisms help to regulate the plasma levels of circulating hormones, to conserve the amino acids resulting from cell surface or intracell-

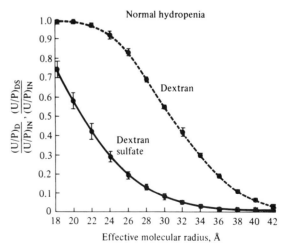

Fig. 2. Fractional clearances of dextran sulfate and neutral dextran, plotted as a function of effective molecular radius, demonstrating greater clearance of uncharged equal-sized molecules. [Reprinted from Kidney International with permission—Chang RLS et al: Permselectivity of the glomerular capillary wall: III. Restricted transport of polyanions. Kidney Int 8:215, 1975.]

ular catabolism, and possibly also to inactivate toxic peptides.

NORMAL URINE

Urine normally may contain up to approximately 150 mg of proteins daily. A portion of these proteins are identical to serum proteins and most likely represent filtered plasma components which have escaped tubular reabsorption. Albumin is the major component of this fraction and represents 10–20 percent of the total excreted protein. Both IgA and principally the secretory form of IgA are present in milligram quantities. The principal urinary protein components, representing approximately a third of the total weight, are large molecular weight glycoproteins believed to be secreted by the more distal segments of the renal tubule. The Tamm-Horsfall glycoprotein, originally isolated from urine as an inhibitor of viral agglutination, is the major component and is also an important constituent of hyaline casts. The remaining urinary proteins are a heterogeneous mixture of as many as 30 components, mainly demonstrating the electrophoretic mobility of globulins.

ABNORMAL PROTEINURIA

Five principal mechanisms can be identified to account for the abnormal presence of protein in the urine: (1) increased concentrations of plasma protein leading to an overloading of the tubular reabsorptive mechanisms by normal filtration, (2) structural or functional abnormalities in the glomerular filtration barrier resulting in increased permeability to proteins, (3) renal tubular impairment leading to alterations in normal reabsorptive function, (4) altered lymphatic permeability with loss of plasma proteins into the urinary tract, and (5) abnormal secretion of renal or lower urinary tract proteins which may accompany inflammatory processes such as infections.

Overflow proteinuria. This is exemplified by the excessive production of light chains by proliferating plasma cells resulting in Bence Jones proteinuria in 50–70 percent of patients with multiple myeloma. Although originally defined by their thermosolubility properties, Bence Jones proteins are now characterized immunologically. In multiple myeloma, the abnormal protein is usually a single type of light chain which can be detected by specific antibodies directed against either kappa or lambda light chains. Using sensitive electrophoretic and immunologic techniques, small amounts of heterogeneous light chains may be found in normal urine. Immunoglobulin fragments similar to the Fc fragment of the IgG molecule are present in the serum and urine of patients with heavy chain disease, a relatively rare form of plasma cell dyscrasia.

Acute renal failure may result from intratubular precipitation of such proteins, and careful attention to hydration is critical in these patients, particularly in association with intravenous pyelography. Light chain proteinuria has also been implicated in the development of a variety of tubular dysfunctions, including Fanconi's syndrome, nephrogenic diabetes insipidus, and gradient-limited renal tubular acidosis. It has been sug-

gested the increased filtration of light chains and their subsequent tubular reabsorption and catabolism interfere with specific tubular transport mechanisms.

Glomerular proteinuria. The principal mechanism of abnormal proteinuria is a structural or functional abnormality in the glomerular filtration barrier resulting in increased permeability to proteins. Evidence to support this contention includes the invariable presence of glomerular abnormalities on electron microscopy of renal biopsies in patients with massive proteinuria. In addition, the earlier discussed inverse relationship between urinary loss and protein molecular diameter suggests transport across the altered glomerulus.

The usual increased thickness of the glomerular capillary wall in conditions associated with marked proteinuria appears contrary to the increase in permeability and indicates the responsible alteration is at a level of resolution beyond that of electron microscopy; however, a recent study of serial electron micrographs demonstrated breaks or gaps in the glomerular capillary basement membrane in patients with proliferative lesions, particularly extracapillary cell proliferation and epithelial crescent formation. Gaps were in association with necrosis, leukocyte-associated lysis, intramembranous deposits, and glomerular sclerosis. Such discontinuities may account for the presence in Bowman's space of large molecular weight plasma proteins and elongated proteins such as fibrinogen.

Alterations in the polyionic glomerular surface coat may also contribute to increased glomerular capillary wall permeability by removing an electrical hindrance to the passage of anionic proteins such as albumin. Reduction in glomerular polyanion has been reported in human lipoid nephrosis, as well as experimental disease models such as aminonucleoside nephrosis and nephrotoxic serum nephritis, all associated with proteinuria (Fig. 3).

Tubular proteinuria. A modest proteinuria, usually less than 2 g/day, accompanies a diversity of renal diseases associated with renal tubular injury (acute tubular necrosis, Balkan nephropathy, chronic cadmium poisoning, cystinosis, Fanconi's syndrome, galactosemia, hypothermia, multiple myeloma, nephronophthisis–medullary cystic disease, potassium depletion, renal allograft rejection, and Wilson's disease). These proteins are of low molecular weight, usually 12,000–45,000 daltons. Electrophoretic mobility includes prealbumin and α, β, and postgamma patterns, in contrast to the predominant albumin and gamma mobilities with glomerular disease. Full biochemical characterization reveals a widely heterogeneous mixture of proteins, with β_2 microglobulin and lysozyme among those most extensively studied.

Chyluria. The lymphatic system may contribute to proteinuria when obstruction increases the permeability to protein of lymphatics within the urinary tract. This is seen with parasitic diseases due to filaria and has been termed tropical chyluria. Chyluria also may

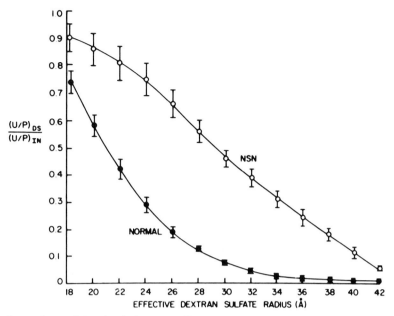

Fig. 3. Comparison of fractional dextran sulfate clearances plotted as a function of effective molecular radius for normal hydropenic rats compared to those with nephrotoxic serum nephritis. [Reprinted with permission from Bennett CM et al: Permselectivity of the glomerular capillary wall: Studies of experimental glomerulonephritis in the rat using dextran sulfate. J Clin Invest 57:1291, 1976.]

occur with obstruction to lymphatic flow in pregnancy, with malignancy, or following trauma.

Lower tract inflammation. Modest proteinuria, usually less than 1 g/day, may be observed with both acute and chronic infection of the renal parenchyma. A poorly or nonselective glomerular pattern of proteinuria has been described with acute pyelonephritis. Mixed glomerular and tubular patterns have been reported with both obstructive and nonobstructive chronic pyelonephritis. Marked increases in urinary excretion of IgG and IgA and an inconstant finding of IgM, not normally present in urine, have been reported with active or recurrent urinary infections. The specificity of urinary antibodies to infecting organisms in the absence of total elevation in urinary immunoglobulin concentrations in some patients supports the local synthesis of antibody within the kidney as a contributor to the measurable proteinuria.

EXERCISE PROTEINURIA

An increase in urinary protein concentration may be seen with marked physical exertion. Excretory rates may rise from a normal 0.03 mg/min to 2.00 mg/min, and values to 5 mg/min have been seen in the recuperative phase. The major increase in urinary proteins is in components of plasma origin, rather than the glycoproteins of renal origin, and no direct relationship between molecular weight and renal clearance of proteins is seen.

It has been postulated the rise in protein excretion is a consequence of exericse-associated renal vasoconstriction with reduction in glomerular filtration rate permitting increased diffusion of plasma proteins across the filtration barrier. The increased excretion in the recuperative phase may be a washout phenomenon. Marked increase in urinary lysozyme excretion without elevation in amylase, a relatively nonreabsorbable protein, indicates the possible coexistence of transient impairment in tubular reabsorption.

ORTHOSTATIC PROTEINURIA

Orthostatic or postural proteinuria is defined as the occurrence of increased urinary protein excretion only with standing or ambulation and its absence during recumbency. It may be intermittent—that is, inconstant from day to day—or fixed—consistently demonstrable on repeated collections. Its presence is established by quantitation of urinary protein on an overnight specimen whose collection is initiated after voiding while recumbent and is completed before arising. This is compared to a collection obtained during normal ambulation and activity. Total protein excretion is usually less than 1.5 g/day, and characterization of the urinary proteins shows a nonselective pattern, including proteins of higher molecular weight.

Orthostatic proteinuria occurs with equal frequency in both sexes and is most common in adolescents or young adults. Association with exaggerated lumbar lordosis has been suggested.

Transient postural proteinuria has been reported in the resolving phases of acute glomerulonephritis, nephrotic syndrome, and active pyelonephritis, and the presence of such definable renal disease must be excluded. Formed elements are usually minimal on urinalysis in patients with idiopathic postural proteinuria, in contrast to the latter syndromes.

A renal biopsy study of young males with fixed and reproducible orthostatic proteinuria showed well defined disease in 8 percent, subtle but definite abnormalities in 45 percent and normal findings in 47 percent. On long-term followup of this group, 70 percent at 5 years and 49 percent of those available for followup at 10 years still had some detectable form of proteinuria. None, however, had laboratory or clinical evidence of progressive renal disease. This study demonstrates that orthostatic proteinuria is often not a transitory condition of adolescence, but it also indicates that its 10 year prognosis is excellent. Whether a small percentage of such patients later develop renal functional impairment remains to be determined. Another followup of college students from 37 to 45 years after the demonstration of "intermittent" proteinuria, defined as proteinuria in less than 80 percent of repetitive routine urinalyses, found no evidence of endstage renal disease.

The mechanism(s) of orthostatic proteinuria remains unexplained. Postural alterations in renal hemodynamics have not been found to differ from control subjects without proteinuria.

MEASUREMENT OF URINARY PROTEIN

A number of methods are available for the detection of proteinuria on routine urinalysis. These range from the time-honored semiquantitative heat–acid test to the use of the simple and rapid dipstick. These are reviewed in detail in the chapter on *Urinalysis*. Most nephrologists prefer the sulfosalicylic acid method. Two or three drops of 20 percent sulfosalicylic acid are added to 3–5 ml of clear urine. The degree of turbidity is estimated. Slight turbidity is reported as trace proteinuria and indicates approximately 4–10 mg/100 ml; the presence of a flocculent precipitate is considered to be 4+ proteinuria and generally indicates in excess of 500 mg protein/100 ml. The intermediate ranges of turbidity are scaled from 1+ to 3+. False positive readings may occur in urines that contain radiologic contrast media, tolbutamide, sulfisoxazole metabolites, or massive doses of penicillin. Highly buffered alkaline urines may give a false negative test. Sulfosalicylic acid will detect Bence Jones proteins, which may not be evident by the dipstick method.

Selectivity. Blainey and associates developed the concept that characterization of the pattern of urinary protein might correlate with the histologic lesion in patients with nephrotic syndrome and hence their response to therapy and prognosis. The serum concentration and renal excretion of reference proteins of varying size are measured by gel diffusion precipitation techniques. The "selectivity" of proteinuria is determined by the log–log relationship between molecular weight and relative clearance of the proteins studied. Selectivity is maintained when the principal urinary protein is albumin with minimal loss of the larger size and higher molecular weight globulins. Initial reports indicated selectivity was best maintained with the minimal change ("nil") lesion and hence indicated a good response to corticosteroid therapy. Decreasing selectivity was observed with proliferative and membranoproliferative glomerulonephritis and epimembranous nephropathy. A number of approaches have been suggested to simplify the determination of differential protein clearances including the use of only two reference proteins, such as the ratio of the clearance of 7S gamma globulin (mol wt 150,000) to the clearance of transferrin (mol wt 78,000), with less than 2.0 indicating highly selective proteinuria.

Further studies have questioned the usefulness of differential protein clearances in characterizing glomerular lesions beyond separation of the minimal change lesion. This may be related to the heterogeneity of glomerular damage as illustrated by the earlier mentioned electron microscopic demonstration of focal gaps or discontinuities in glomerular basement membrane with proliferative lesions.

EVALUATION

When a semiquantitative test for proteinuria is confirmed as positive it is necessary to collect a 24 hour urine to better quantitate the degree of proteinuria. In most laboratories up to 150 mg protein in the urine per 24 hours is considered normal. Values greater than this necessitate further investigation. The 24 hour specimen should be normal in the patient whose casual urine specimen may have contained small amounts of protein related to unusual exertion, acute disease with associated fever, or unusual exposure to cold. The possibility of orthostatic proteinuria must be excluded by the earlier described assessment of association with activity.

The total protein loss is helpful in approaching a differential diagnosis. If the quantity of protein is in the range that may be associated with nephrotic syndrome, that is, generally greater than 3 g/24 hours, five main categories of renal diseases should be considered. The first is renal disease secondary to systemic illness, and possible diagnoses include diabetic glomerulosclerosis, lupus nephritis, periarteritis, amyloidosis, neoplasia, or infections such as malaria or syphilis. A second consideration would be renal disease associated with specific toxins such as the heavy metals (mercury, gold, or bismuth), drugs such as penicillamine or paramethadione, or allergens such as poison oak or ivy. A third category would be renal disease associated with mechanical causes; although these relationships are controversial, the presence of constrictive pericarditis or severe right heart failure must be considered as well as renal vein thrombosis. Recent evidence suggests that renal vein thrombosis is usually a secondary occurrence in patients with a preexisting renal disease. A fourth consideration would be a complication of pregnancy such as preeclampsia, eclampsia, or exacerbation of preexisting hypertensive or renal disease. The final category would be the presence of primary renal disease. Evidence of an active glomerulonephritis of the poststreptoccal or rapidly progressive variety should be found on urinalysis with the presence of red cells and red cell casts. Idiopathic forms of renal disease include lipoid nephrosis, focal glomerulosclerosis, epimembranous nephropathy, proliferative glomerulonephritis, or membranoproliferative glomerulonephritis.

When the proteinuria is less than 2 g/24 hours this may represent a milder expression of the previously considered abnormalities but also may be a result of vascular or interstitial renal disease such as arteriolar nephrosclerosis associated with long-standing hypertension or chronic pyelonephritis. Proteinuria of lower genitourinary tract origin is usually associated with evidence of infection in the vagina, prostate, or bladder.

Very often the most careful medical history and physical examination and skillful utilization of laboratory data do not clearly indicate the particular renal lesion responsible for proteinuria. Then percutaneous or open renal biopsy is necessary to provide a histologic diagnosis which usually has important prognostic and therapeutic implications.

REFERENCES

Bennett CM et al: Permselectivity of the glomerular capillary wall: Studies of experimental glomerulonephritis in the rat using dextran sulfate. J Clin Invest 57:1291, 1976

Chang RLS et al: Permselectivity of the glomerular capillary wall: III. Restricted transport of polyanions. Kidney Int 8:215, 1975

Farquhar MG: The primary glomerular filtration barrier—Basement membrane or epithelial slits? Kidney Int 8:197, 1975

Levitt JI: The prognostic significance of proteinuria in young college students. Ann Intern Med 66:685, 1967

Pollak VE, Pesce AJ: Proteinuria: A review of glomerular permeability in the normal and in various disease states, in Becker EL (ed): Seminars in Nephrology. New York, John Wiley & Sons, 1977, p 155

Rennie ID: Proteinuria. Med Clin North Am 55:213, 1971

Thompson AL, Durrett RR, Robinson RR: Fixed and reproducible orthostatic proteinuria: VI. Results of a 10-year follow-up evaluation. Ann Intern Med 73:235, 1970

Venkatachalam MA, Rennke HG: The structural and molecular basis of glomerular filtration. Circ Res 43:337, 1978

HEMATURIA

H. John Reineck

Hematuria is defined as the abnormal presence of red blood cells in the urine. Addis found that normal healthy individuals, at normal activity, may excrete up to 1,000,000 red blood cells per 24 hours. Translated into the commonly employed semiquantitative urinalysis, this number of red cells results in up to 1–2 cells per high-power field (HPF). In addition, it should be mentioned that vigorous physical exercise and high fever may increase the number of red blood cells excreted without signifying intrinsic genitourinary tract disease. In general, however, the finding of greater than 1–2 red cells per high-power field implies an abnormality and, as such, represents a common clinical problem. Fur-

ther, because hematuria may represent the first manifestation of a serious but potentially curable disease, it it imperative that the physician be aware of its many causes and be aggressive in pursuing an accurate diagnosis.

CAUSES OF HEMATURIA

The causes of hematuria are listed in Table 1. It should be noted that the appearance of blood in the final urine may occur with virtually any condition which results in interruption of normal vascular integrity in a location contiguous with the urinary space. Such lesions may occur at any level of the genitourinary tract. Since most of the entities listed are dealt with in detail elsewhere in this volume, they will not be discussed individually in this chapter. One entity, however, does deserve special mention. Anticoagulant drugs are frequently viewed as a potential cause of hematuria; indeed, hematuria constitutes a complication of these agents. In a recent report, however, significant urinary tract pathology, including three cases of carcinoma, was discovered in 13 of 16 patients evaluated for hematuria noted during anticoagulant therapy. This finding suggests that such therapy often unmasks underlying disease, and hematuria discovered under such circumstances deserves complete evaluation.

DIAGNOSTIC APPROACH TO HEMATURIA

As with any other sign or symptom of disease, the evaluation begins with a thorough history, physical examination, and appropriate laboratory evaluation. In obtaining this fundamental data base, the physician may obtain some clue to the etiology of the hematuria which allows for direct evaluation. In many cases, however, hematuria may be totally asymptomatic. Figure 1 schematically outlines a diagnostic approach to this problem. The urinalysis provides the focal point for the evaluation, and essentially three categories of urinalysis results may be obtained. In patients with hematuria and significant proteinuria or cylinduria, renal parenchymal disease is present and is probably glomerular in nature. A renal biopsy may be performed to obtain prognostically or occasionally therapeutically important information. A second category of urinalysis findings is that of hematuria and pyuria, which suggests an infectious etiology. An intravenous pylegram (IVP) may reveal anatomical evidence of the disease (e.g., genitourinary tract tuberculosis, prostatic disease, or obstructive uropathy). If negative, however, cystoscopy and even retrograde pyelography may be necessary. The third category of urinalysis findings is isolated hematuria. A wide variety of diseases may be apparent on the IVP (e.g., nephro calcinosis, calculi, cystic disease of the kidney, tumors). In many of these cases, more detailed information may be obtained by arteriography or cystoscopy. In those patients with negative pyelography, cystoscopy should be performed and, if negative, arteriography obtained. Finally, if this procedure fails to uncover a source of the hematuria, a renal biopsy may be necessary.

The efficacy of this approach is illustrated by a

Table 1
Causes of Hematuria

Renal causes
  Immunologic mediated disease
    Glomerulonephritis
    Vasculitis (polyarteritis nodosa, SLE)
  Nonimmunologic glomerulopathies
    Diabetic nephropathy
    Amyloidosis
  Vascular disease
    Renal infarction (thromboembolic disease)
    Cortical necrosis (thrombotic thrombocytopenic purpura,
      hemolytic–uremic syndrome)
    Arteriovenous malformations
    Renal vein thrombosis
  Renal calculi
  Hereditary disease
    Chronic interstitial nephritis
    Cystic disease
    Familial benign hematuria
    Hereditary hemorrhagic telangectasia
  Tumors
    Benign or malignant renal tumors
    Metastatic infiltration
  Infectious disease
    Acute pyelonephritis
    Renal tuberculosis
    Miscellaneous infections
  Renal trauma
    Exercise-induced hematuria

Lower urinary tract causes
  Tumors (benign and malignant)
  Infection (cystitis, prostatitis, epididymitis, urethritis)
  Calculi
  Trauma
  Vascular malformations

Systemic conditions
  Coagulopathies
  Thrombocytopenia
  Anticoagulant drugs
  Polycythemia
  Hemoglobinopathy (S-type hemoglobin)

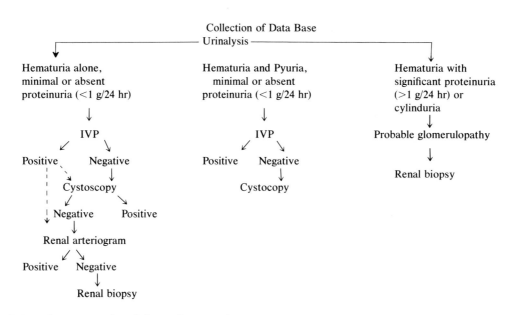

Fig. 1. Schematic representation of diagnostic approach to asymptomatic hematuria. [Adapted from Coe FL: The clinical and laboratory assessment of the patient with renal disease, in Brenner BM, Rector FC (eds): The Kidney. Philadelphia, W.B. Saunders, 1976, p 765.]

recent report that radiologic and urologic evaluation revealed the source of hematuria in 411 of 440 patients. Of the remaining 29 cases, the renal biopsy findings were diagnostic in 19. Thus the cause of hematuria was diagnosed in over 97 percent of the cases.

REFERENCES

Antolak SJ, Mellinger GT: Urologic evaluation of hematuria occurring during anticoagulant therapy. J Urol 101:111, 1969

Coe FL: The clinical and laboratory assessment of the patient with renal disease, in Brenner BM Rector FC (eds): The Kidney. Philadelphia, W.B. Saunders, 1976, p 765

Hamburger J, Richet G, Crosnier J, et al. The principal symptoms, in: Neprology. Philadelphia, W. B. Saunders, 1968, p 119

Northway JD: Hematuria in children. J Pediatr 78:381, 1971

Relman AS, Levinsky NG: Clinical examination of renal function, in Strauss MB, Welt LG (eds): Diseases of the Kidney. Boston, Little, Brown, 1971, p 87

DYSURIA

Andrew K. Diehl

Dysuria is defined as difficult urination and clinically is usually equated with pain or burning on voiding. Frequency, urgency, and hesitancy are commonly associated. The majority of conditions producing dysuria arise in the bladder, urethra, or prostate. The role of vaginitis and cervicitis in the production of these symptoms is less clear, and at present these entities remain to be established as definite causes of dysuria.

The etiologies of dysuria vary somewhat between women and men. Dysuria is, however, more common and troublesome in women, and most studies have concerned female patients.

DYSURIA IN WOMEN

Infections of the bladder. Approximately half of all episodes of dysuria in women are due to urinary tract infection, defined as urine colony counts greater than 10^5 organisms/ml. It is likely, however, that bacterial counts less than 10^5 (and especially those greater than 10^4) result in urinary complaints, and, in fact, many patients with the "urethral syndrome" will on repeated urine cultures show significant bacteriuria. In some women, urinary symptoms may persist for several days after a bacterial cystitis has been cleared by the patient's own host defenses. Thus unless a urine culture is obtained at the onset of symptoms the patient erro-

neously may be considered to have "sterile dysuria."

Infections of the bladder due to viruses, including herpes simplex and adenoviruses, have been described and account for an unknown proportion of patients with dysuria. Gonococci have been grown from centrifuged urine specimens as well as from percutaneous bladder aspirations. Tuberculous cystitis may cause symptoms, probably owing to granulomatous involvement of the bladder. Other infectious agents, including fungi, chlamydia, and trichomonas, are suspected but not established etiologies of symptomatic cystitis.

Infections of the urethra. Since infectious urethritis is common in men, by analogy it would be expected to occur in women as well. Urethral infection, however, usually cannot be demonstrated in symptomatic women. The normal female urethra contains various strains of staphylococci, enterococci, diptheroids, and, in about one-quarter of patients, gram-negative organisms. Approximately half of women with recurrent urinary tract infections have pathogenic gram-negative organisms on urethral culturing. Most women, however, with frequency and dysuria with negative urine cultures do not have common gram-negative pathogens on urethral culturing. Even in those patients in whom gram-negative organisms are isolated, it remains unclear whether the organism is the cause of symptoms or only a colonizer. The appearance of purulent discharge on manual stripping of the urethra occurs only rarely.

Gonococci can be isolated from the female urethra, but almost always in association with positive cultures in other sites, especially the cervix. Chlamydia have been isolated from the urethras of sexual contacts of males with nonspecific urethritis. The clinical implications of such isolations, however, are unknown, and "nonspecific urethritis" remains at present an affliction only of men.

Infections of the vagina and cervix. Although most clinicians accept vaginitis as a frequent etiology of dysuria, there is little direct evidence to support this view. One recent study reported dysuria in 28 percent of women with vaginitis and sterile urine and suggested that the complaint of pain felt in the inflamed vaginal labia as the stream of urine passed ("external dysuria") was especially characteristic. Other causes of dysuria, however, were not excluded, and, since many women with dysuria have neither vaginitis nor bacteriuria, vaginitis as an explanation for dysuria cannot be assumed. The most suggestive evidence for infectious vaginitis or cervicitis as a cause of dysuria occurs with gonococcal infections, in which dysuria is more frequently encountered than in controls. A case may also be made for herpes simplex vaginitis, where burning symptoms may be caused by passage of urine over painful lesions. Trichomonas, *Hemphilus vaginalis,* or monilia vaginitis are sometimes diagnosed in women presenting with dysuria, but their presence does not establish them as the basis for symptoms; When a

Table 1
Differential Diagnosis of Dysuria in Women

Infections
  Infections of the bladder
    Bacteriuria of greater than 10^5 colonies/ml
    Bacteriuria of less than 10^5 colonies/ml
    Intermittent bacteriuria
    Viral cystitis
    Tuberculous cystitis
  Infections of the urethra
    Gonococci
    Other gram-negative bacteria
    Chlamydia?
  Infections of the vagina and cervix
    Gonococci
    Herpes simplex
    Trichomonas, monilia, etc.

Noninfectious causes: The urethral syndrome
  Chemical irritants
  Adjacent inflammatory processes
  Bladder tumors
  Estrogen deficiency
  Urinary outflow obstruction
  "Female prostatitis"
  Chronic interstitial cystitis
  Psychosomatic
  Miscellaneous

patient with lower urinary tract symptoms has vaginitis in the absence of significant bacteriuria, however, the vaginitis should be considered the most likely cause for the symptoms.

Noninfectious causes. The "urethral syndrome" is a term commonly applied to those cases of frequency and dysuria in which the presence of infection cannot be documented. Synonyms include aseptic dysuria, symptomatic abacteriuria, and the frequency and dysuria syndrome. Very common in general urologic practice,, this diagnosis is characteristically applied only to women, and the problem often is chronic or recurrent in nature. It is indistinguishable from urinary tract infection on the basis of symptoms and signs, and may or may not be associated with pyuria. Multiple explanations for this condition have been proposed.

Chemical irritants, such as douches, deodorant aerosols, contraceptive jellies, and bubble baths may cause local inflammation with associated symptoms. Various inflammatory conditions which involve organs lying near the bladder, such as Crohn's disease, diverticulitis, and radium implants of the cervix, can result in urinary tract symptoms if the bladder becomes involved by the adjacent inflammation. Tumors of the bladder can result in symptoms, especially frequency and urgency. In postmenopausal women, estrogen deficiency may result in symptoms related to atrophic mucosa, since the distal urethra is of the same embryologic origin as the genital tract. Often such women respond to replacement estrogen therapy.

Many urologists attribute dysuria and frequency in the presence of negative cultures to urinary outflow obstruction. Such obstruction has been postulated to occur via a variety of mechanisms, including meatal stenosis or stricture, diffuse urethral narrowing due to fibrosis resulting from chronic trauma, or fibroelastosis of the urethrovaginal septum. Others propose alterations in the normal dynamics of urine flow due to spasm of the distal urethral sphincter or to lack of synergy between bladder contraction and sphincter relation. Transient urethral edema following sexual intercourse, masturbation, or motorcycle riding can cause obstruction and subsequent symptoms. Urethral caruncles and diverticuli are thought to cause symptoms due to alterations in urine flow. Unifying all these proposed mechanisms is the assumption that obstruction to urine flow can cause symptoms of dysuria and frequency.

On cystoscopic evaluation of these patients, chronic inflammatory changes are commonly seen in the urethra. Biopsies of these areas show infiltration with chronic inflammatory cells, although cultures are negative. In the bladder, the presence of trabeculation or trigonitis is often taken to be the result of chronic outlet obstruction. Usually the urethra is calibrated with bougies, although recent studies emphasize that such measurements are unreliable. Attempts to measure the dynamics of urine flow have led to contradictory results in patients with recurrent frequency and dysuria, but overall probably less than 10 percent of such patients can be shown via full urologic assessment to have outflow obstruction.

The female urethra is associated proximally with many small paraurethral glands. These glands are homologues of the male prostate and when inflamed are felt to be capable of causing symptoms of "female prostatitis." Chronic stasis, healed infection, and trauma may lead to fibrosis of the paraurethral glands as well, contributing to chronic urinary tract complaints.

Chronic interstitial cystitis, an inflammatory process involving the bladder wall, may be an autoimmune disease. Anti-bladder-muscle and antinuclear antibodies have been described in affected patients, and focal deposits of immunoglobulins have been found in the bladder smooth muscle and connective tissue. Diagnosis is made by distending the bladder at cystoscopy and noting the appearance of punctate bleeding points, known as Hunner's ulcers.

Not surprisingly, many women who complain of recurrent dysuria and frequency in the presence of normal physical findings and negative cultures are felt to have a psychosomatic basis for their complaints. Studies have shown that patients who score high on psychometric testing for depression are less likely to have an identifiable organic basis for their symptoms than those women whose scores fall in the normal range.

Finally, miscellaneous other etiologies of frequency and dysuria have been proposed, including cold weather, food allergy, menstruation, and the ingestion of spicy foods.

DYSURIA IN MEN

In male patients, several additional etiologies of dysuria are accepted. Nonspecific urethritis and postgonococcal urethritis are clearly defined entities. Infection with chlamydia is thought to account for 30–50 percent of nonspecific urethritis and up to 70 percent of postgonococcal urethritis; *Ureaplasma urealyticum*, a mycoplasma, may account for some of the remainder. Acute and chronic prostatitis and seminal vesiculitis account for some cases of dysuria in males. The "urethral syndrome" is rarely applied to men, though some of what is called chronic prostatitis may represent the male equivalent.

EVALUATION OF DYSURIA

A careful history should be taken, noting the duration and persistency of symptoms, history of previous infections of the urogenital tract, previous instrumentation including urethral dilatation, menstrual status, use of local chemical agents, and presence of other disease of the bowel or pelvis. Physical examination should include observation for urethral discharge or meatal abnormality. In women, a pelvic exam is necessary to evaluate for vaginitis or pelvic pathology, and in males a rectal exam should be performed to evaluate the prostate and seminal vesicles. Bacterial cultures of urine may need to be repeated several times to rule out infection, and cultures at the onset of symptoms may provide additional yield. In women, the cervix should be cultured, and any vaginal discharge examined in the usual fashion. Urethral cultures may occasionally be helpful, especially in males without purulent discharges who may harbor gonococci. If the workup to this point is negative, the patient should be scheduled for intravenous pyelography with voiding cystourethrography. The latter procedure can be especially helpful in children, demonstrating vesicoureteral reflux, aberrant ureters, urethral diverticula, strictures, valves, or calculus. Following this, the patient may be referred to a urologist for cystoscopy.

MANAGEMENT OF DYSURIA

The syndrome of frequency and dysuria can often become a chronic condition with exacerbations and remissions, and the physician must be careful not to overdiagnose or overtreat the patient in the absence of careful clinical data collection. Much of the literature to date is hampered by a lack of controlled studies and poor long-term followup of treated patients.

When a specific infectious process is discovered, it should be treated with appropriate agents. Vaginitis should be treated in the expectation that symptoms of dysuria will be relieved as well. If no specific infection is encountered, many authorities suggest an empiric course of antibiotics. Although such treatment has not been proved to be of benefit, a short course of tetracycline, which covers many gram-negative pathogens as well as gonococci and chlamydia, may be useful in this setting. If atrophic vaginitis is encountered in a postmenopausal woman, replacement estrogen therapy may be beneficial. The patient should be counseled regarding the use of bubble bath and deodorant sprays, encouraged to take showers, and reminded to wipe fore to aft. Changes in position for sexual intercourse are probably of no benefit.

When radiologic studies reveal possible obstruction or symptoms persist, referral to a urologist is indicated for cystoscopy and therapeutic evaluation. Urologic approaches employed by some include urethral dilatations or more extensive procedures such as internal urethrotomy or external urethroplasty. Although such procedures are said to be successful at a frequency approaching 70 percent, few studies have been controlled, and several studies question their usefulness. Diazepam has been found useful in some patients and has been suggested to have a regional relaxant effect on pelvic muscles as well as a central action. Finally, phenazopyridine may be tried as a stopgap measure (see the chapter on *Urinary Tract Infections*).

REFERENCES

Brooks D, Maudar A: Pathogenesis of the urethral syndrome in women and its diagnosis in general practice. Lancet 2:893, 1972

Catell WR, Brooks HL, McSherry MA, et al: Approach to the frequency and dysuria syndrome. Kidney Int 8:S138, 1975

Dans PE, Klaus B: Dysuria in women. Johns Hopkins Med J 138:13, 1976

Komaroff AL, Pass TM, McCue JD, et al: Management strategies for urinary and vaginal infections. Arch Intern Med 138:1069, 1978

Rees DLP, Whitfield HN, Islan AK, et al: Urodynamic findings in adult females with frequency and dysuria. Br J Urol 47:853, 1976

POLYURIA

N. Lameire

The term polyuria signifies a larger than normal daily volume of urine. There is considerable variation in the amount of urine passed, but a urinary output of more than 3 liters per 24 hours is nearly always abnormal. As with several other excretory functions, urine flow and urine osmolality exhibit a characteristic diurnal cycle. Flow is lowest and concentration maximal by night, with rapidly rising flow and decreasing concentration during the first hours after awakening.

A classification of polyuric disorders is given in Table 1, based on the lesions in the two major organs involved in the body water regulation, the brain and the kidneys.

Group I. In this group, polyuria is due to a diminished output into the circulation of antidiuretic hormone (ADH). This decrease in circulating ADH is caused by either an impaired ability of its secretion, as in true diabetes insipidus (DI), or by a suppression of its secretion as a physiologic response to excessive

Table 1
Classification of Polyuric Disorders

Diminished cerebral output of ADH
    Primary diabetes insipidus
        Head trauma, skull fractures
        Pituitary surgery
        Craniopharyngioma, cerebral tumors
        Metastatic tumors, e.g., breast
        Granulomas—sarcoid, tuberculosis, syphilis
        Histiocytosis
        Sickle cell
        Encephalitis
        Meningitis
        Vascular aneurysms
        Idiopathic—50%
    Increased thirst or excessive water drinking
        Compulsive water drinking
        Electrolyte disorders—potassium depletion, hypercalcemia
        Lithium therapy
        Drug-induced thirst—insulin, clonidine

Defective renal response to ADH
    Congenital nephrogenic diabetes insipidus
    Acquired nephrogenic diabetes insipidus
        Hypercalcemia
        Hypokalemia
        Postobstructive uropathy
        Renal diseases—chronic renal failure, diuretic-phase acute tubular necrosis
        Drug induced
            Lithium salts
            Demeclocycline
            Methoxyflurane
            Sulfonylureas—glyburide, tolazamide, acetohexamide
            Propoxyphene, colchicine, vinblastine
        Sickle cell disease
        Hypergammaglobulinemic disorders—multiple myeloma, sarcoid, Sjögren's
            syndrome, amyloidosis
        Osmotic diuresis
            Mannitol
            Urea—chronic renal failure, diuretic phase of acute tubular necrosis, successful
                renal transplant, high-protein tube feeding, intravenous hyperalimentation
            Glucose—diabetes mellitus, nonketotic hyperglycemic hyperosmolar
                coma
            Sodium—diuretics, excessive administration of Na^+-containing
                intravenous fluids

drinking of water, as occurs in states of compulsive water drinking, potassium deficiency, hypercalcemia, or lithium therapy.

Group II. This group is characterized by an inability of the kidney to respond to ADH, the hormone being present in sufficient quantity and quality. This group can be divided into a first subgroup with what is called nephrogenic diabetes insipidus and a second subgroup where polyuria is caused by osmotic diuresis.

DECREASED SECRETION OF ADH
Central Diabetes Insipidus

DI is a polyuric disorder in which large volumes of dilute urine are excreted. The disease represents a failure to secrete adequate amounts of ADH. The consequence at the renal level is the inability to con-

centrate the urine adequately by a mechanism to be described later in this chapter.

Physiology of ADH secretion. (See also the chapters on *Water Metabolism* and *Antidiuretic Hormone.*) The mammalian neurohypophysis contains two hormones, oxytocin and either arginine (Arg^8) or lysine (Lys_8) vasopressin, the latter occurring only in the pig and related species. Vasopressin is an octapeptide. Vasopressin, oxytocin, and their associated carrier proteins, called the neurophysins, are synthetized by neurosecretory cells, which have their nerve endings in the neurohypophysis. The neurohypophysis functions as an organ for the storage and release of the hormones, but synthesis is localized primarily in the hypothalamus. Steps in the synthesis of vasopressin involve the incorporation of the peptide in secretory granules and the binding of the peptide to neurophysins within these granules. Cleavage of these macromolecules results in the formation of smaller, biologically active octapeptides. The granules containing the formed polypeptide hormone are then transported down the axons of the neurohypophyseal tract to storage sites in the nerve endings in the posterior pituitary. It is now believed that the neurons of the hypothalamus are stimulated by both osmotic and nonosmotic stimuli. Excitation results in the transmission of nerve impulses, which generates action potentials and depolarizes the axon terminals in the neurohypophysis, causing an influx of calcium ions. This in turn triggers the release of the hormone together with its specific neurophysin by a process of exocytosis.

Pathophysiology of ADH secretion. Central DI can thus be caused by an inappropriately low production, a defective release, or an increased rate of inactivation of ADH. An abnormally low production of ADH is well documented in the Brattleboro rat, a strain with hereditary DI. In humans, DI can occur as a hereditary disease with underproduction of ADH. Postmortem observations in these patients and in a few patients with so-called idiopathic DI reveal a marked decrease in the number of nerve cells in the hypothalamus; however, most cases of human DI fall into the second category, characterized by a defective release of ADH in the circulation. This may occur by neural disconnection between the osmoreceptors and the neurosecretory neurons in the hypothalamus, by damage of the hypothalamoneurohypophyseal tract, or by a direct interference with the process of exocytosis. An unusual form of pure central DI can also be caused by the endogenous production of antibodies to vasopressin. As reviewed in Table 1, many causes of central true DI in man are known, and they include a variety of sytemic and intracranial diseases; however, many cases of idiopathic DI occur in which no explanation is discernable. One to three percent of this idiopathic group is of a familial type. In most of these cases the disease has been transmitted as an autosomal dominant, although a sex-linked recessive form has been described. Presently, surgery in the region of the neurohypophyseal system together with head trauma account for the majority of cases of DI. In the course of surgery (or injury), interruption of the supraopticohypophyseal tract leads to a retrograde degeneration of the hypothalamic nuclei whose axons terminate below the level of the lesion. It is the extent of the degeneration that determines the magnitude and duration of postoperative DI. Permanent, severe DI does not occur until about 90 percent of the cells in the hypothalamic nuclei are destroyed.

Clinical course of idiopathic and postsurgical DI. The onset of polyuria in spontaneous DI is characteristically abrupt. Urine volumes can range from 4 to 8 liters daily. Polyuria and thirst are both intense and present a serious inconvenience for the patient during both day and night. Spontaneous DI usually starts in early adult life, and in some large series male predominance is present. Due to the long-standing and massive polyuria, hydronephrosis may develop in the untreated patient.

The pattern of polyuria in these patients is quite variable. In some patients, polyuria lasts only a few days before the urine concentrating ability returns to normal. In these patients, there is presumably only minor damage to the neurohypophyseal system. This pattern can also be observed after severe head injuries, especially associated with fractures at the base of the skull. Postsurgery central DI is classically associated with a "triphastic" pattern of polyuria. The first immediate postoperative phase is characterized by profound polyuria and polydipsia, which may last from hours to a week. This period is followed by an equal period in which urine volumes are normal. Only then does a third phase of permanent polyuria develop. The development of the antidiuretic interphase is probably due to a discharge of ADH from the injured axons. The third period of DI may, depending on the extent of the injury, be temporary or permanent and complete or partial.

Thirst is a vital compensatory mechanism in DI patients, and as long as DI patients are able to gratify their thirst dehydration and its clinical consequences do not occur. If, however, a DI patient has no water access or if consciousness is altered by anesthetic agents or trauma, serious dehydration with hypernatremia may result.

A number of pharmacological agents inhibit the release of ADH, including ethanol, parenteral diphenylhydantoin, norepinephrine, atropine, and possibly phenothiazines. Their effects are transient, and none of them can produce sustained polyuria. Narcotic antagonists such as oxilorphan, presumably by antagonizing endorphan-induced ADH release, may produce polyuria.

Polyuria as a Consequence of Increased Thirst or Suppression of ADH by Increased Water Intake

This group includes the so called compulsive water drinker and situations where polydipsia is induced by a variety of organic disorders or by thirst-provoking drugs.

The most important physiological stimuli of thirst are cell dehydration and extracellular volume depletion (see the chapter on *Water Metabolism.*) Angiotensin II may also be a major modulator of the thirst mechanism.

Compulsive water drinking. This is a common condition, classically found in psychoneurotic middle-aged females. The polydipsia and polyuria may occur suddenly and fluctuate in severity. Usually these patients do not complain of thirst. Hysterical manifestations and depression are part of the syndrome. In view of the large intake of water, patients with compulsive water drinking can present with polyuria and polydipsia and be initially thought to have complete central DI. In the compulsive water drinker, the onset of polydipsia and polyuria not unfrequently coincides with medical advice to drink more fluid.

Potassium depletion, hypercalcemia, and lithium therapy. There is some evidence that potassium depletion and hypercalcemia directly stimulate the thirst center. Polyuria, observed in rats in the first weeks after induction of potassium depletion or administration of lithium salts, has been recently attributed to be a consequence of polydipsia. Although most cases of primary polydipsia have a psychogenic origin, a few cases have been described where local organic cerebral lesions directly stimulate the thirst center with secondary polyuria.

Drug-induced thirst and resulting polyuria. Numerous drugs and pharmacological agents stimulate the thirst center and provoke abundant drinking. Among the most widely used are insulin and clonidine. Insulin appears to cause increased drinking probably by hypoglycemia-induced renin release. Clonidine, a common antihypertensive drug, provokes intense thirst, leading to increased drinking and polyuria; however, the polyuric action of clonidine can also be mediated by inhibition of ADH release through its alpha adrenergic action on the baroreceptors.

POLYURIA DUE TO DEFECTIVE RENAL RESPONSE TO NORMAL CIRCULATORY LEVELS OF ADH

The effects of ADH on renal water handling cannot be understood without a knowledge of the renal concentrating mechanism (see the chapter on *Water Metabolism*). Briefly, the concentration of the urine is achieved by the osmotic abstraction of water from fluid in collecting ducts into the hypertonic medullary interstitium under the influence of ADH. The high solute concentration results primarily from the action of Henle's loop as a countercurrent multiplier. Consequently, the polyuria in this group of disorders can result not only from inadequate renal response to normal circulating ADH levels but also from interference with the generation and maintenance of the corticomedullary osmotic gradient. Production of a maximal osmotic gradient requires sufficient glomerular filtration, adequate delivery of sodium chloride out of the proximal tubule, normal ascending limb reabsorption of sodium chloride, and medullary trapping of urea under conditions of normal renal perfusion and urine flow. Concentration of the urine requires further utilization of this osmotic gradient, and this is largely accomplished by the action of ADH on the collecting duct. It is thought that ADH is bound to specific receptor sites on the contraluminal side of the collecting duct cells. The receptor hormone complex is then coupled to and activates the adenylate cyclase on the contraluminal membrane, and the production of cyclic AMP from ATP is stimulated. The cyclic AMP is transported to the luminal cell membrane, where it causes activation of membrane bound protein kinase, which causes the phosphorylation of membrane proteins. This reaction increases the permeability of the membrane and allows movement of water along the osmotic gradient. The ADH-generated cyclic AMP is inactivated by cyclic AMP phosphodiesterase, converting cyclic AMP to 5'AMP. The transtubular movement of water depends on the integrity of cytoplasmic microtubules in the interior of the epithelial collecting duct cells.

Congenital Nephrogenic Diabetes Insipidus

This inherited disease, in which the nephron is usually completely unresponsive to ADH, is transmitted by an x-linked recessive gene; however, occurrence of symptomatic disease in females suggests transmission by an autosomal dominant trait. Most of the cases in the U.S. can be traced to descendants of an Ulster Scotsman who arrived on the ship Hopewell in 1761. The polyuria occurs shortly after birth and is intense, and the affected infant can develop mental defects due to severe dehydration if the disease is not recognized. Studies of homogenates of renal medullary tissue of mice with an inherited form of nephrogenic DI suggest impaired activation of the adenylate cyclase system by vasopressin. High levels of ADH in plasma and urine of the affected individuals can be demonstrated; injections of cyclic AMP in these children failed to produce antidiuresis.

Acquired Nephrogenic DI

In these forms, the exact mechanism of the vasopressin resistance at the collecting tubule level is not yet completely elucidated, and a combination of several factors which determine adequate urine concentration is often responsible. The clinically relevant types of these diseases are reviewed below.

Hypercalcemia. The concentrating defect of hypercalcemia may be related to the inhibitory effect of calcium on the generation of adenylate cyclase and cyclic AMP. Hypercalcemia may also inhibit sodium reabsorption in Henle's loop and interfere with the creation of a hypertonic interstitial fluid.

Hypokalemic nephropathy. As already mentioned, increased ingestion of water may be a major determinant of the polyuria, at least in the initial stages; however, a persistent form of nephrogenic DI finally develops. The impaired renal concentrating ability may be due to enhanced proximal tubular sodium reabsorption with resulting diminished sodium chloride delivery in the loop of Henle. Prolonged hypokalemia also interferes with the effects of vasopressin and cyclic AMP on water transport in the toad bladder preparation. In vitro studies indicate that potassium depletion inhibits the adenylate cyclase system.

Postobstructive uropathy. The occurrence of a massive natriuresis and diuresis after relief of complete or partial urinary tract obstruction is referred to as postobstructive diuresis (see the chapter on *Obstructive Uropathy*). Based on animal experiments, the major mechanisms of this polyuria involve an inhibition of proximal and distal tubular fluid reabsorption by urea and other circulating natriuretic factors and a direct effect of the obstruction, causing a marked decrease in reabsorption or a net secretion of salt and water in the medullary collecting duct.

Renal diseases. It is not surprising that polyuria due to a renal defect in the concentrating mechanism is likely to occur in situations in which the structure or function of the distal tubule and collecting duct is affected by the disease process. A number of kidney diseases listed in Table 1 are associated with polyuria. A combination of several factors can be responsible for the polyuria in these states—a reduced water permeability in the distal nephron, unresponsiveness of the diseased collecting duct cells to ADH, changes in medullary blood flow, and disruption of the countercurrent system.

Drug-induced nephrogenic DI. A number of pharmacological agents may produce polyuria by interference with the renal action of ADH.

Lithium. Li salts are frequently used in therapy of manic depressive disorders. Although a central role by its thirst-stimulating effects and interference with ADH release is highly suggestive, the major effect of Li seems to be an inhibition of the activation of ADH-dependent renal medullary adenylate cyclase; however, Li salts increase the polyuria in Brattleboro rats with hereditary DI, suggesting an additional diuretic action unrelated to ADH. In the rat, the antidiuretic action of dibutyril cyclic AMP is inhibited by Li, indicating an inhibition of the action of ADH beyond the activation of adenylate cyclase. On the other hand, toad bladder experiments indicate an inhibition of the ADH but not cyclic AMP. An impairment of proximal tubular fluid reabsorption by Li can also contribute to the polyuria.

Demeclocycline (DMC). Polyuria and polydipsia are prominent side effects in patients treated with very large doses of DMC (600–1200 mg/day). The diuretic action of DMC is based on the inhibition of basal and ADH-stimulated renal medullary adenylate cyclase and AMP-dependent protein kinase. Other tetracyclines are equally effective in inhibiting cyclic AMP and protein kinase but have not produced clinical nephrogenic DI. Differences in lipid solubility, calcium chelating ability, and serum protein binding may explain these differences.

Methoxyflurane. The ADH-resistant polyuric state associated with methoxyflurane anesthesia is related to the marked increase in serum concentration and urinary excretion of inorganic fluoride. Toad bladder studies suggest that ADH-induced water flow is reduced at a site beyond the generation of cyclic AMP. In addition, a reduction in the medullary solute gradient due to the vasodilatory action of fluoride may contribute to the generation of nephrogenic DI.

Sulfonylureas. In contrast to the well known antidiuretic effects of chlorpropamide, three other sulfonylurea agents—glyburide, tolazamide, and acetohexamide—have diuretic actions in normal subjects and in patients with DI and diabetes mellitus. The diuretic action of glyburide is independent of vasopressin, since the drug exerts a diuresis in the Brattleboro rat. Paradoxically, glyburide stimulates the effects of submaximal doses of vasopressin on water transport in the toad bladder. All three sulfonylurea drugs produce water diuresis. The exact mechanism of their diuretic activity is not yet elucidated, but an inhibition of proximal tubular reabsorption of salt and water has been suggested.

Other drugs like phenacetin, propoxyphene, colchicine, and vinblastine may rarely cause polyuria.

Sickle-cell disease. A defect in concentrating ability is commonly seen in patients with sickle-cell disease and may be the only renal functional abnormality. This defect is most probably due to severe medullary ischemia by intravascular sickling and occlusion of the vasa recta.

Osmotic diuresis. Increasing the solute excretion to very high levels interferes with the ability to both concentrate and dilute the urine. Such a defect is commonly seen after administration of mannitol, in diabetic patients with severe glucosuria, and in patients subjected to large urea loads (protein tube feeding). The hyposthenuria and mild polyuria in chronic renal failure is due to an osmotic diuresis per remaining intact nephron coupled with a defect in the water permeability of the distal nephron. The polyuria induced by mannitol can be explained by a combination of a diminished water reabsorption in the proximal tubule and an inhibition of descending limb water reabsorption.

APPROACH TO THE PATIENT WITH POLYURIA

The first step in the approach to the polyuric patient is to differentiate the nonrenal from the renal causes of polyuria. A careful history, physical examination, and selected standard laboratory tests suffice to identify states of osmotic diuresis, drug-induced polyuria, and most causes of acquired nephrogenic DI (Table 1).

The most frequently serious electrolyte disturbance that can be associated with a polyuric disease is the hyperosmolality syndrome, usually reflected by hypernatremia. The normal defense against hyperosmolality and/or hypernatremia is enhanced ADH release and thirst. Even patients with no secretion of ADH are able to maintain near-normal water balance by increasing their water intake. Symptomatic hypernatremia is therefore virtually never seen in an alert patient with a normal thirst mechanism and access to water even in the total absence of ADH.

When the underlying cause of polyuria is not readily apparent, the magnitude of the polyuria itself may point toward the correct diagnosis; urine volumes in excess of 6–8 liters per day suggest a central disorder, psychogenic polydipsia, or congenital nephrogenic DI.

The most difficult step in the diagnosis of polyuria is the differentiation among the several central causes of polyuria, i.e., the distinction between complete or partial central idiopathic DI and psychogenic polydipsia. The few laboratories which have a radioimmunoassay for circulating vasopressin are able to establish in a relatively simple way the etiology of the polyuria by obtaining a simultaneous measurement of plasma vasopressin and plasma and urine osmolalities under conditions of dehydration. In dehydrated patients with primary polydipsia or nephrogenic DI, a normal or elevated vasopressin level will be present, while in the dehydrated central DI patient persistent low circulating vasopressin levels are observed.

Since a sensitive and specific radioimmunoassay for circulating vasopressin is not yet routinely available, the diagnostic approach to the patient with a suspected central cause of polyuria is still based on a large number of indirect diagnostic procedures.

An initial differentiation between compulsive water drinkers and vasopressin-sensitive DI patients can be found in the finding of a chronically low plasma osmolality (<280 mOsm/kg) in compulsive water drinkers, whereas untreated patients with both central and nephrogenic DI generally have a normal or elevated plasma osmolality; however, a wide overlap between the two groups may be found. The simplest reliable method of diagnosing central DI is the fluid deprivation test with vasopressin injection, showing that urinary osmolality, which normally reaches a peak after a 12–18 hour period of dehydration, can be further significantly increased by the intravenous injection of aqueous vasopressin (5 mU/min for 1 hour). Usually, normal patients and patients suffering from psychogenic polydipsia or nephrogenic DI fail to show this further rise of urinary osmolality after the administration of exogenous vasopressin.

Some important practical points must be taken into account in this water deprivation test. At the conclusion of the water deprivation period and before the injection of vasopressin, the urinary osmolality must reach a plateau (defined as less than a 30 mOsm/kg increase in urinary osmolality in two consecutive hourly specimens) and a plasma osmolality should be measured. Failure to reach a plateau in urine osmolality after 16 hours of water deprivation indicates antecedent compulsive water drinking. On the other hand, if the plasma osmolality at the end of the dehydration period is higher than the normal range (281–294 mOsm/kg) an elevated "setting" of the osmoreceptors may be suspected. Patients with psychogenic polydipsia can usually concentrate their urine to the isotonic level after water deprivation. An important clue to the diagnosis of psychogenic polydipsia may be that as in normal subjects a higher urinary osmolality may be achieved

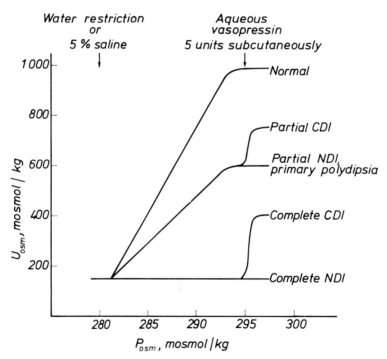

Fig. 1. Effect of the induction of hyperosmolality, either by water restriction or 5% saline, and exogenous vasopressin on urine osmolality in normal subjects and in polyuric states. In normal subjects, as the P_{osm} reaches 285–295 mOsm/kg, there will be a maximum ADH effect on the kidney resulting in a U_{osm} greater than 800 mOsm/kg. Exogenous vasopressin will be without effect. In patients with complete central diabetes insipidus (CDI) or nephrogenic diabetes insipidus (NDI), the urine will remain hypotonic to plasma. Vasopressin increases the U_{osm} only in CDI. Patients with partial CDI (or complete CDI with colume depletion) or NDI show an intermediate response, and only the former will respond to vasopressin. These tests will not differentiate primary polydipsia from mild forms of NDI or partial CDI. [From Rose BD: Clinical Physiology of Acid-Based and Electrolyte disorders. New York, McGraw-Hill, 1977. Copyright 1977, McGraw-Hill. Used with permission of McGraw-Hill Book Company.]

following dehydration than after exogenous vasopressin without dehydration. On the other hand, vasopressin-sensitive DI patients concentrate their urine more effectively following vasopressin. The water deprivation test can be harmful to the patient with DI, since severe volume depletion and vascular collapse can occur. In general, maximal weight loss should not exceed 3–5 percent of body weight.

Infusion of hypertonic saline, resulting in a reduction in urine flow in normals and psychogenic polydipsia patients, as a consequence of the osmotic stimulus, is less reliable than the fluid deprivation test in diagnosing central DI.

Since some forms of nephrogenic DI may be related to a reduced cyclic AMP generation by ADH, it may be useful to measure the urinary cyclic AMP excretion following both ADH and parathyroid hormone infusion in patients suspected of having nephrogenic DI.

The various tests described above will certainly be helpful in distinguishing the normal state from the complete form of either central or nephrogenic DI; however, differentiation between partial DI and primary polydipsia may still be difficult. Both patients with central DI and compulsive water drinkers may have reduced their medullary interstitial osmolality because of the longstanding water diuresis. Therefore the water deprivation test must sometimes be repeated after chronic administration of ADH in central DI and control of water intake in psychogenic polydipsia patients. The different patterns of response to the combination of a water deprivation test with subsequent vasopressin administration in the polyuric syndromes are illustrated in Fig. 1.

REFERENCES

Epstein FH: Disturbances in renal concentrating ability, in Andreoli TE, Grantham JJ, Rector FC Jr (eds): Disturbances in Body Water Osmolality. Bethesda, American Physiological Society, 1977, p 251

Forrest JN Jr, Singer I: Drug-induced interference with action of antidiuretic hormone, in Andreoli TE, Grantham JJ, Rector FC Jr (eds): Disturbances in Body Fluid Osmolality. Bethesda, American Physiological Society, 1977, p 309

Hays RM, Levine SD: Pathophysiology of water metabolism, in Brenner BM, Rector FC Jr (eds): The Kidney, Philadelphia, WB Saunders, 1977, p 553

Maffly RH: Diabetes insipidus, in Andreoli TE, Grantham JJ, Rector FC Jr (eds): Disturbances in Body Fluid Osmolality. Bethesda, American Physiological Society, 1977, p 285

Rector FC Jr: Renal concentrating mechanisms, in Andreoli TE, Grantham JJ, Rector FC Jr(eds): Disturbances in Body Fluid Osmolality. Bethesda, American Physiological Society, 1977, p 179

Robertson GL, Athar S, Shelton RL: Osmotic control of vasopressin function, in Andreoli TE, Grantham JJ, Rector FC Jr (eds): Disturbances in Body Fluid Osmolality. Bethesda, American Physiological Society, 1977, p 125

Schrier RW, Berl T, Anderson RJ, et al: Nonosmolar control of renal water excretion, in Andreoli TE, Grantham JJ, Rector FC Jr (eds): Disturbances in Body Water Osmolality. Bethesda, American Physiological Society, 1977, p 149

Clinical Syndromes of Renal Disease

ACUTE NEPHRITIS

Terry B. Strom and Marvin R. Garovoy

The acute nephritic syndrome results from several morphologic entities which manifest acute diffuse glomerular inflammation. While this syndrome often follows an upper respiratory or cutaneous (pyoderma) infection with group A beta hemolytic streptococci, the acute nephritic syndrome is not synonymous with poststreptococcal glomerulonephritis. The syndrome consists of the abrupt onset of hematuria, often with red blood cell casts, decreased glomerular filtration rate (GFR), edema, circulatory overload, proteinuria, and occasionally oliguria. Since full expression of this syndrome does not occur in each patient with acute glomerulonephritis, the acute nephritic syndrome may be operationally defined as the abrupt onset of hematuria of renal origin coexistent with another indication of acute renal injury such as decreased GFR or proteinuria. Furthermore, the syndrome is transient, although some patients present initially with an identical syndrome but relentlessly develop permanent and progressive renal insufficiency.

CLINICAL MANIFESTATIONS

In the most classical form of the acute nephritic syndrome, a young patient arises in the morning to find facial puffiness. Later shortness of breath and ankle edema develop. In older patients facial edema is often absent despite the accumulation of pedal edema. Urine flow diminishes. The urine is discolored and is often described as smoky or likened in color to cola or weak coffee. Occasionally gross hematuria is noted. About half of the patients with acute nephritic syndrome manifest high blood pressure. While this hypertension is most often asymptomatic, occasionally severe headache, convulsions, or even cerebral hemorrhage develop. In the classical acute nephritic syndrome, diuresis ensues and azotemia remits. Despite remission, microscopic hematuria may persist for many months in patients destined for total remission. The clinical course of patients that present initially with the acute nephritic syndrome is outlined in Fig. 1.

A minority of patients, usually adults lacking a convincing history of streptococcal infection, develop a much more grave course after initial presentation with a similar syndrome. Such patients develop nephritic syndrome and subsequently sustain inexorable loss of renal function culminating in renal failure. This is the syndrome of rapidly progressive glomerulonephritis. Renal biopsy often reveals proliferative glomerulonephritis with epithelial crescents.

Other patients develop the acute nephritic syndrome with hematuria and/or erythrocyte casts and oliguria but also manifest a systemic vasculitis. In children the acute nephritic syndrome may be accompanied by Henoch-Schönlein purpura, while systemic lupus erythematosus, polyarteritis nodosa, and Wegener's granulomatosis are more common in adults.

Finally, a group of patients that develop recurrent hematuria often with red blood cell casts but without oliguria or hypertension should be distinguished from the acute nephritic syndrome. In this syndrome of recurrent hematuria, modest proteinuria can occur on occasion. The patients are usually young males. Hematuria often recurs in association with strenuous exercise or respiratory tract infections. Loin pain may

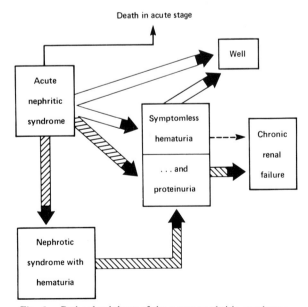

Fig. 1. Pathophysiology of the acute nephritic syndrome.

also occur. The prognosis for patients with this syndrome is excellent.

PATHOPHYSIOLOGY

The pathophysiology of acute nephritis is outlined in Fig. 2.

Hematuria

Hematuria is the cardinal finding of acute nephritis. In the acute nephritic syndrome, erythrocytes presumably enter the urine stream via discontinuities in the glomerular capillary wall created by glomerular inflammation. Since hematuria may result from the entry of blood into the urine stream from any site between the kidney and urethra, hematuria itself does not constitute proof that the blood is of renal origin. Hematuria of renal origin is frequently described as "smoky," while pink or bright red colored urine suggests a lower urinary tract origin for the episode of hematuria. In nephritis, the concentration of red blood cells within a voided urine sample is equally distributed in the initial, middle, and terminal stages of the urine sample. The presence of red blood cell casts are of particular importance, since such casts are unequivocal evidence for the renal origin of hematuria. While erythrocyte casts are most often related to active nephritis, vasculitis (often) and tubulointerstitial nephritis (rare) may also produce red blood cell casts. Red blood cell casts result from the envelopment of erythrocytes within the tubular lumen by Tamm-Horsfall glycoprotein, which gels in the presence of albuminuria.

A voided urine suspected to harbor erythrocyte or other casts should be examined promptly after collection, since urine left standing will alkalinize, resulting in disruption of the casts. Alternatively, addition of acetic acid and sodium chloride to a freshly voided urine sample plus refrigeration will permit short-term storage with preservation of the formed elements.

Hematuria and red cell casts are frequently accompanied by leukocytes and leukocyte casts. The presence of leukocyturia signals inflammation and does not necessarily suggest pyelonephritis.

Proteinuria

Proteinuria is nearly always present in acute glomerulonephritis but is usually of moderate severity, ranging from 200 to 500 mg per day in one-half of the children with poststreptococcal glomerulonephritis, while about one-quarter of adult patients demonstrate proteinuria in excess of 3 g/day. In 1933, Bayliss demonstrated that molecules larger than 60,000 daltons are not normally excreted into the urine. The proteinuria of acute nephritis, the pattern of glomerular proteinuria, consists of urinary loss of large proteins. Nonglomerular proteinuria can result in the urinary excretion of proteins of less than 40,000 daltons, which are normally filtered and subsequently undergo tubular reabsorption. Thus tubular injury may result in the excretion of $\beta 2$ microglobulin, lysozyme, or light chains (mol wt range from 12,000 to 22,000). Increased excretion of albumin, globulin, and other large proteins occurs only in the presence of glomerular alterations. Indeed, the proteinuria associated with glomerular diseases inevitably includes albumin.

Different elements of the glomerulus contribute to this selective barrier impeding transglomerular passage of macromolecules (see the chapter on *Proteinuria*). Glomerular capillary endothelial cells block the passage of cells and particles but do not prohibit filtration of proteins. The glomerular basement membrane itself does not allow passage of molecules larger than 100 Å

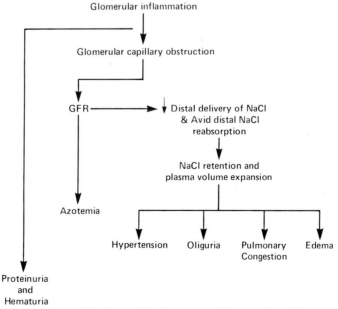

Fig. 2. Natural history of patients with abrupt onset of hematuria and decreased GFR.

in radius, corresponding to an approximate molecular weight of 200,000 daltons. Visceral epithelial cells of the glomerular tuft in covering the basement membrane create small channels that constitute a severe restriction to passage of large proteins.

Nonetheless, size does not constitute the sole property governing solute transfer across the glomerular capillary wall. For example, the fractional clearance of albumin, which has a molecular radius of approximately 36 Å, is 0.11. The vast differences in filtration of albumin and neutral dextran are governed by differences in molecular charge. Thus neutral or cationic molecules are filtered more efficiently than anionic molecules such as albumin. Current evidence suggests the glomerular capillary exerts a charge selectivity that is attributable to fixed polyanionic sialoprotein which coats the epithelial cells and consequently repels the filtration of polyanions. Hence albuminuria may result from the loss of fixed glomerular polyanions.

In addition to size—and charge—selective regulation of transglomerular penetration of proteins, hemodynamic changes resulting in altered glomerular filtration alter the fractional clearance of macromolecules. Afferent glomerular plasma flow is inversely related to the fractional clearance of macromolecules. Thus a reduction in glomerular plasma flow would be expected to result in increased clearance of macromolecules.

The mechanism(s) responsible for proteinuria in clinical acute glomerulonephritis cannot be stated with certainty; however, elegant studies concerning this issue have been conducted in experimental models of immunologically induced glomerular injury. For example, while decreased glomerular permeability to neutral dextrans occurs during experimental acute nephrotoxic serum nephritis, filtration of anionic dextrans is increased. Obviously, the most facile explanation is glomerular inflammation results in disruption of glomerular sialoprotein and a resultant diminution in fixed glomerular anionic charge. This loss of fixed negative charge destroys the charge-selective glomerular impermeability to anionic albumin. Indirect support for this hypothesis derives from the observation that glomerular sialoprotein is decreased in human glomerulonephritis.

It is far from certain that loss of glomerular polyanion is the sole or universal mechanism for glomerular proteinuria. In two experimental models of immunologically induced glomerular injury, passive Heymann nephritis and autologous immune complex nephropathy (active Heymann nephritis), no loss of staining for glomerular polyanion is apparent until after the development of proteinuria. Furthermore, the fractional clearances of anionic, cationic, and neutral forms of a protein tracer, horseradish peroxidase, all about 40 Å in molecular radius, are similarly increased. Thus the proteinuria which results from subepithelial antibody deposits in these models may reflect changes in size selection rather than charge selection. In human acute glomerulonephritis associated with the transglomerular passage of very large protein molecules such as fibrinogen, it is likely that loss of the sieving properties of the glomerular capillary wall permits proteinuria. In contrast, it is probable that in many forms of selective glomerular proteinuria, e.g., albuminuria without excretion of larger proteins, loss of glomerular polyanions causes proteinuria.

Renal Blood Flow

Injury of the glomerular capillary wall is obviously the primary lesion of acute glomerulonephritis, yet there is no evidence that total renal blood flow is significantly diminished during an episode of acute nephritis. In fact, total renal blood flow may actually increase acutely. Relative hyperemia, defined as high blood flow per unit of functional tubular mass, has been determined to be present by a number of investigators. The precise mechanisms underlying relative or absolute hyperemia in acute glomerulonephritis are not certain. Current evidence suggests that afferent arterioles dilate and decrease in resistance. This interpretation is derived from animal experiments revealing increased glomerular capillary hydraulic pressure and glomerular capillary flow in the absence of changes in renal artery pressure or hematocrit.

Glomerular Filtration

Acute glomerulonephritis routinely causes reduced glomerular filtration. Since glomerular filtration rate is compromised while renal plasma flow is minimally altered, the filtration fraction falls. Filtration fraction is defined as clearance of inulin (glomerular filtration rate)/clearance of PAH (renal plasma flow). The precise mechanism causing reduced glomerular filtration in acute glomerulonephritis is ill defined. The primary morphologic alterations in acute poststreptococcal glomerulonephritis include mesangial proliferation and endothelial swelling which probably directly cause decreased filtration. Since the determinants of glomerular filtration rate are the area of the filtering surface, effective filtration pressure, and the glomerular capillary permeability, it seems reasonable to assume that glomerulonephritis results in a decreased filtration rate secondary to endothelial and mesangial cell encroachment on the filtering surface. Direct measurements of single nephron glomerular filtration rate during experimental nephritis also support the hypothesis that GFR falls primarily as a result of a reduction of the surface area available for filtration, although a decline in capillary permeability cannot be excluded as causal. The intraglomerular adaption, as previously mentioned, to falling GFR includes diminished afferent arteriolar resistance. The major possibilities that may govern this change are extracellular volume expansion, reduced sympathetic outflow, or local release of vasodilator agents such as prostaglandins and decreased renin–angiotensin activity.

Tubular Function

While decreased glomerular filtration is the major functional consequence of acute glomerulonephritis, reduction of tubular function also occurs. Nonetheless, tubular function is not as compromised as glomerular filtration.

Circulatory Overload

Sodium and water retention occur in glomerulonephritis solely due to renal disturbances. There is no evidence that increased capillary permeability or that myocardial, adrenal, or hepatic dysfunction contribute to the development of edema during a bout of acute glomerulonephritis. While sodium and water retention occur commonly in glomerulopathic states, the acute nephritic syndrome is accompanied by unusually dramatic sodium retention. Indeed, the predominant clinical problem in severe acute nephritis is often pulmonary edema. Reduction of GFR in nephritis directly produces sodium retention due to a decrease in the filtered load of sodium. In most states associated with increased extracellular plasma volume, initial sodium and water retention is followed by establishment of a new steady state in which sodium intake reequilibrates with renal sodium loss. Hence an "escape" from progressive extracellular volume expansion occurs albeit in the presence of a chronically expanded extracellular volume. For example, in chronic glomerulonephritis, sodium and water retention increase the fractional sodium excretion and often increase GFR. Thus sodium retention is self-limiting. Correction of sodium retention in chronic glomerulonephritis is facilitated by an increased ability per functional nephron to excrete salt. In the acute nephritic syndrome, however, such adaptive changes permitting enhanced salt excretion per nephron do not accur. In fact, experimental acute nephritis is associated with diminished, not enhanced, capacity to increase salt excretion after extracellular volume expansion. Thus in acute glomerulonephritis, avid salt reabsorption results in decreased presentation of salt to the distal nephron, which perpetuates extracellular volume expansion.

A minority of patients with the acute nephritic syndrome will experience a period of massive proteinuria. The resultant hypoproteinemia will contribute to edema formation, since the loss of plasma proteins decreases the plasma oncotic forces and permits transudation of fluid from the vascular compartment to interstitial tissues.

Hypertension

Hypertension usually occurs as part of the acute nephritic syndrome. While other mechanisms may participate, expansion of the extracellular volume due to salt and water retention is primarily responsible for this hypertension. Plasma renin level is not elevated and may be low or normal. Since extracellular volume expansion leads to an increased sensitivity to angiotensin, it is conceivable that angiotensin contributes to hypertension especially in patients with "normal" renin. Even normal renin levels may be inappropriately high considering the volume expanded state. While a deficiency of renal vasodilators such as prostaglandin

might also cause hypertension, there is no direct evidence that such deficiencies are responsible for the hypertension of acute glomerulonephritis.

REFERENCES

Glassock RJ, Bennett CM: The glomerulopathies, in Brenner BM, Rector FC Jr (eds): The Kidney. Philadelphia, W. B. Saunders, 1976

Cameron JS: Bright's disease today: Pathogenesis and treatment of glomerulonephritis—I, II, III. Br Med J 4:87, 4:160, 4:217, 1972

Earle DP, Seegal D: Natural history of glomerulonephritis. J Chron Dis 5:3, 1957

Maddox DA, Bennett CM, Deen WM, et al: Determinants of glomerular filtration in experimental glomerulonephritis. J Clin Invest 55:305, 1975

Merrill JP: Medical progress—Glomerulonephritis (three parts). N Engl J Med 290:257, 290:313, 290:373, 1974

NEPHROTIC SYNDROME

Marvin Forland

The term "nephrotic syndrome" refers to a cluster of clinical and laboratory abnormalities which are the consequences of glomerular disease. The syndrome occurs when the pathologic process produces proteinuria of significant magnitude to result in hypoalbuminemia. As a consequence of decreased plasma oncotic pressure the patient develops edema and usually the findings of hyperlipoproteinemia and lipiduria.

The use of this term as a major category of renal disease has a number of advantages. Although the list of idiopathic glomerular lesions, nephrotoxic agents, and systemic illnesses which may be associated with a nephrotic syndrome grows steadily, definition of the syndrome continues to provide a nosologic framework for the student of renal diseases at all levels of sophistication. Of equal importance is the appreciation that the clinical and laboratory abnormalities which result from massive proteinuria and the consequent hypoalbuminemia, independent of etiology, are associated with an increasingly more clearly defined group of pathologic consequences which contribute greatly to the morbidity and mortality of the underlying disease. Among these complications are the manifestations of malnutrition, possible acceleration of the development of atherosclerosis, increased susceptibility to infection, an increased prevalence of thromboembolic events, and the urinary loss of polypeptides and protein bound hormones.

HISTORY

A relationship between renal disease with nephrosclerosis and edema has been appreciated since the time of the Roman empire. Proteinuria was described in the late seventeenth century and its association with edema recorded by Cotugno in 1764; however, in the early nineteenth century, Richard Bright provided the definitive correlations between the frequent occurrence of renal lesions in patients with dropsy and the coagulability of their urine with heat. Bright, his associates, and students later described hypoproteinemia, urea retention, and lipiduria in some patients with renal diseases.

Bright's name soon became synonymous with glomerulonephritis, but some of his contemporaries appreciated that the eponym was being applied indiscriminately to include a diversity of renal diseases. The term nephrosis was introduced by Müller in 1905 to characterize a renal tubular lesion which he considered a degenerative change, since the accompanying glomeruli appeared normal and inflammatory changes were absent. Soon after, Munk noted fat bodies in the urine of patients with chronic parenchymatous nephritis who had similar fatty tubular changes, and he introduced the term lipoid nephrosis. Volhard and Fahr helped establish the term by including it in their influential monograph on kidney diseases. They characterized nephrosis as a particular category of Bright's disease to be contrasted to the inflammatory form, which they termed glomerulonephritis.

In the subsequent half century the primacy of a glomerular lesion was accepted as well as the diversity of pathologic patterns which could be present. Thus the term nephrotic syndrome gained increasing acceptance, initially in the pediatric literature in the 1930s and in internal medicine in the late 1940s.

The development of techniques for percutaneous biopsy approximately 25 years ago provided an opportunity to draw clinicopathologic correlations concerning the incidence, natural history, and response to therapy of the diversity of idiopathic lesions associated with nephrotic syndrome as well as the systemic diseases which affect glomerular permeability. Technical advances applied to biopsy specimens, including the use of thin sections, special stains, electron microscopy, and immunoflourescence microscopy, have all contributed in major ways to our diagnostic distinctions in this group of patients and hence more rational and effective approaches to therapy.

PROTEINURIA

Proteinuria of sufficient magnitude to result in hypoalbuminemia is the hallmark of nephrotic syndrome. This quantity is usually considered to be approximately 3 g/24 hours (2 g/m²/24 hours) and generally is seen only with diseases of the glomerulus. Proteinuria in the range of 1–2 g daily may be seen in patients with tubulointerstitial disease such as arteriolar nephrosclerosis or chronic pyelonephritis, but the nephrotic range of proteinuria is not characteristic of these disease processes. The overproduction of large quantities of low molecular weight kappa or lambda chains in patients with multiple myeloma may result in proteinuria reaching several grams daily, but serum albumin concentration is usually maintained unless amyloidosis with

renal involvement and a diffuse proteinuria is superimposed.

The normal individual excretes approximately 50–150 mg of urinary protein daily. This is comprised mainly of albumin, a wide range of lower molecular weight globulins, and some glycoproteins of tubular origin. The conventional tests for the qualitative measurement of urinary proteins are normally negative except with a markedly concentrated urine specimen, which may indicate trace proteinuria (see the chapter on *Proteinuria*).

The normal glomerular filtration barrier excludes proteins of greater than 50,000–60,000 Daltons (> 35 Å) and hence the minimal amount of albumin (mol wt 69,000) normally found in the urine. In addition to the basement membrane, a principal barrier to glomerular filtration appears to be the slit pores, the separations between the tentacle-like foot processes of the epithelial cell where they rest upon the basement membrane. Studies employing graded sizes of electron-dense markers indicate this to be the site of inhibition of particle passage with increasing molecular size. Paradoxically, electron microscopic studies of the kidney in patients and experimental animals with proteinuria reveal a thickening of the glomerular capillary wall due to the fusion or effacement of these foot processes, a phenomenon which is reversible with remission of the proteinuria.

A role for the renal tubule in the reabsorption of protein in the normal animal has been supported by the demonstration that proximal tubular fluid contains approximately 1–10 mg/dl of protein. If comparable quantities are filtered in man in the absence of tubular reabsorption, approximately 2–20 g of protein would be lost in the urine each day. The protein reabsorptive mechanism has been found to be localized to the proximal tubule where brush border attachment of the protein is followed by endocytotic engulfment and lysosome mediated breakdown to polypeptides and amino acids. Normally proteins of molecular weights up to approximately 50,000 participate in this catabolic reabsorptive process.

A number of lines of experimental and clinical evidence support the primacy of the glomerular lesion in the development of proteinuria. The earlier cited animal micropuncture data indicate that total inhibition of tubular reabsorption of normally filtered protein could not result in the massive proteinuria frequently observed with nephrotic syndrome. In experimental animal models of nephrotic syndrome, increases in proximal tubular protein concentration approach tenfold, supporting alteration in glomerular permeability. Glomerular abnormalities are invariably present on renal biopsy in patients with nephrotic syndrome, particularly with the resolution of electron microscopy, which permits demonstration of foot process fusion. Volume expansion with intravenous albumin or dextran has been found to increase urinary albumin loss in patients with mild albuminuria. The vacuolar tubular abnormalities emphasized by early pathologists in characterizing "nephrosis" appear to relate to the tubular reabsorptive process.

The mechanism for the altered glomerular permeability remains unexplained. No increase in porosity—rather the converse—usually is observed on examination of the glomerular basement membrane with the resolution of electron microscopy. X-ray diffraction studies indicate molecular rearrangement in the glomerular basement membrane with increase in the intermolecular interstices; alterations in the chemical composition of the glomerular basement membrane have been reported in both experimental and human renal disease.

Recent attention has been directed at the role of the polyanionic glycoproteins, principally sialic acid, which are dispersed along the surface of the glomerular capillary epithelial cells and the foot processes, providing an electronegative barrier. Repulsion of like-charged circulating proteins which penetrate the glomerular basement membrane may contribute significantly to the permeability barrier. It has been demonstrated that negatively charged molecules are far less effectively filtered than positively charged molecules of similar size. Effacement of the epithelial foot processes can be produced experimentally with the infusion of the polycation protamine sulfate and strikingly reversed with administration of a polyanionic molecule such as heparin.

A corticosteroid-reversible reduction in the filtration of smaller molecules (< 40 Å) as measured by ^{125}I-labeled polydisperse polyvinyl pyrolidine excretion has been reported in minimal change nephrotic syndrome. This was attributed to reversible foot process fusion interfering with the normal function of the epithelial slit pore. Inulin clearance decrease was postulated as a consequence of restriction of passage of smaller-sized molecules.

Selectivity of proteinuria is an assessment of glomerular permeability based on the relative urinary loss of lower molecular weight proteins as compared to larger protein molecules (see the chapter on *Proteinuria*). It has been suggested that preservation of selectivity with predominant loss of albumin and minimal loss of larger gamma globulins correlates with the presence of a minimal change lesion and a favorable response to corticosteroids or the possibility of spontaneous remission. Decreasing selectivity is observed with epimembranous nephropathy and with proliferative or membranoproliferative glomerulonephritis. The determination is based on the comparative clearance of reference proteins of varying sizes and necessitates serum and urine measurements by gel diffusion precipitation techniques. A representative method for the measurement of selectivity is determination of the clearance ratio of 7S gamma globulin (molecular weight 150,000) to transferrin (molecular weight 78,000); a ratio of less than 0.2 is indicative of highly selective proteinuria. Overlap in selectivity between histologic

groups is frequent, and patients with congenital nephrotic syndrome and amyloidosis may have preservation of selectivity despite corticosteroid resistance and a grave prognosis.

HYPOALBUMINEMIA

Hypoalbuminemia appears to provide the pathophysiologic stimulus for the appearance of two of the other major findings of nephrotic syndrome, edema and hyperlipoproteinemia. Serum albumin levels are usually below 3.0 g/dl and frequently below 2.5 g/dl. Loss of protein into the urine and protein catabolism in the tubular reabsorptive process are the principal sources of protein depletion. Under normal circumstances the liver has been found capable of replacing approximately 5–10 percent of the plasma albumin pool each day; this is equal to about 25 g. Studies in nephrotic patients uniformly demonstrate the increased fractional catabolism of a decreased total body pool of protein. The hepatic synthesis of albumin has been found to be at least normal or slightly increased.

Since the measurable amount of protein lost each day is usually considerably less than the hepatic synthetic ability, and since there is no evidence to support compromise in liver albumin production, an additional site of protein loss must be postulated. The endocytic lysosomal protein reabsorptive process in the proximal renal tubule appears to be the location of this catabolic activity. This site normally reabsorbs the relatively small amount of filtered protein with molecular weight mainly below 50,000 daltons. With increase in glomerular permeability due to glomerular disease, there appears to be a marked increase in tubular reabsorptive function as demonstrated morphologically and histochemically in the experimental animal. This mechanism results in polypeptide and amino acid reabsorption and contributes to the decrease in serum concentration of albumin and a variety of globulins.

The plasma protein electrophoretic pattern reflects the preferential urinary loss of lower molecular weight proteins and the compensatory increased synthesis and better retention of the higher molecular weight moieties. Serum albumin is markedly decreased; both the lower molecular weight alpha-1 and gamma globulins are low. The alpha-2 globulin component, containing alpha glycoproteins, and the beta-1 globulins, which include the beta lipoproteins, are both elevated. Plasma fibrinogen level is also increased as a reflection of increased hepatic synthetic activity and accounts for the characteristic increase in erythrocyte sedimentation rate. Analysis of specific serum proteins reveals reduced concentrations of low molecular weight proteins of defined biologic importance such as transferrin and ceruloplasmin.

EDEMA

Edema, an increase in the interstitial component of extracellular fluid, is the principal clinical characteristic of nephrotic syndrome. It is present with significant hypoalbuminemia, usually plasma concentrations of 2.5 g/dl or less. This characterization presents a circular argument, since it is the edema which defines the hypoalbuminemia as "significant," and the level of serum albumin at which edema appears may be quite variable from patient to patient. This inconsistency may relate to individual differences in dietary sodium intake, responsiveness of the renin–aldosterone system, or capillary hydrostatic pressure. It is frequently noted that patients with congenital analbuminemia are not edematous; this is attributed to compensatory changes in capillary hydrostatic pressure. The development of edema is the result of disruption in the normal Starling forces across the capillary. Capillary hydrostatic pressure provides a driving force for fluids across the permeable capillary wall and is opposed by plasma oncotic pressure, produced primarily by the plasma albumin, and the interstitial pressure of the surrounding tissues. At the arteriolar end of the normal capillary bed the forces for filtration predominate. At the venous end the increased protein concentration and hence oncotic pressure and tissue pressure are able to overcome the diminishing capillary hydrostatic pressure, leading to fluid reabsorption. With the altered permeability of the specialized glomerular capillary bed present in nephrotic syndrome, the loss of protein into the glomerular filtrate results in hypoalbuminemia and a fall in plasma osmotic pressure throughout the circulatory system. Consequently the outwardly acting forces predominate across the systemic capillary beds, the interstitial volume expands at the expense of the plasma volume, and edema appears.

The consequences of the decreased effective circulating volume may include falls in effective renal blood flow and glomerular filtration rate, which in turn set in motion a series of compensatory mechanisms as described in the chapter on *Disorders of Sodium Metabolism.* Thus despite an increase in total body salt and water, the patient with nephrotic syndrome continues to retain sodium in order to preserve an effective circulation. Studies measuring blood volume in nephrotic patients indicate many achieve a compensated steady state by this relatively crude measurement, with approximately 40 percent showing normal blood volume, 50 percent a decrease, and 10 percent an elevation; however, exaggerated hypovolemia in the upright position despite normal recumbent plasma volume has been reported in some nephrotic patients.

HYPERLIPIDEMIA

Elevation in serum cholesterol, triglycerides, and phosphatides are commonly but not invariably observed with nephrotic syndrome. The magnitude of increase appears to be inversely related to the serum albumin level. Rise in serum cholesterol occurs gradually with falling serum albumin concentration but increases sharply with severe hypoalbuminemia. Triglycerides display a similar pattern of elevation but at lower serum albumin levels. Low-density lipoproteins (LDL) are increased in mild to moderate hypoalbuminemia, while very-low-density lipoproteins (VLDL) predominate with markedly decreased serum albumin levels.

The lipoprotein profiles in adults with nephrotic syndrome have been found to fall into three nearly equal groups—IIa, IIb, and V. No correlation has been observed between the histopathologic lesion and the predominance of a particular lipoprotein type. The prevalence of hyperlipoproteinemia is no less in patients with nephrotic syndrome secondary to systemic lupus erythematosus than other groups, contrary to earlier reports.

Studies of immune-mediated nephrosis in rats implicate increased synthesis of lipoproteins by the liver as the source of the hyperlipemia. The overproduction appears to result from stimulation of hepatic albumin synthesis, which shares common hepatic pathways of metabolic synthesis and secretion with VLDL and other plasma proteins. The central role of hypoalbuminemia and more specifically the decrease in oncotic pressure is supported by several observations. Significant inverse correlations have been found between concentration of serum lipids and serum albumin, but no inverse or direct correlations have been noted with serum lipids and creatinine clearance or 24 hour urinary protein excretion, respectively. Also, dextran infusions as well as albumin administration result in transient falls in VLDL levels in nephrotic subjects.

A number of additional mechanisms have been postulated to contribute to the hyperlipemia (Table 1). These include urinary loss of protein lipid-clearing factors or co-factors (lipoprotein lipase), or impairment in lipoprotein lipase-related lipid removal caused by insulin insufficiency.

LIPIDURIA

The presence of lipid droplets within cells or casts is characteristic of nephrotic syndrome. Significance pertains only when the lipids are within urinary constituents, since free-floating lipids may result from seminal vesicle or vaginal gland secretions. The lipid-laden epithelial cell, termed an oval fat body, is believed to be a degenerated renal tubular epithelial cell containing cholesterol esters. Demonstration of the lipid is facilitated by polarized light revealing the Maltese cross—

Table 1
Possible Mechanisms in the Hyperlipidemia of Nephrotic Syndrome

Hepatic overproduction of lipoproteins secondary to hypoalbuminemia
Impairment in clearance of plasma lipids
Urinary loss of lipoprotein lipase and "activator" apolipoproteins
Insulin deficiency impairing lipoprotein lipase activity

or, more accurately, cross pattée—pattern of birifringence (see the chapter on *Urinalysis*). Phase microscopy and light microscopy with Sudan stains are also useful.

The presence of lipiduria correlates more closely with the magnitude of proteinuria rather than the level of hyperlipemia. It appears to result primarily from degeneration of the lipid-laden tubular cells and in lesser part from filtered and nonreabsorbed lipoproteins.

GLOMERULAR FUNCTION

Glomerular filtration rate as measured by inulin clearance has been found to be increased in some patients with childhood nephrotic syndrome; this was associated with increased diodrast clearance and consequently attributed to increased renal blood flow. Urea clearances have also been found to be elevated, but decreased BUN is more usually related to low protein intake than to increased glomerular filtration rate. Fall in glomerular filtration rate may relate to the progression of glomerular and possibly tubular injury, but hypovolemia must always be excluded and is often related to overzealous diuretic therapy. Impaired clearance of low molecular weight solutes, including inulin, has been attributed to foot process fusion and may give false depressions in the measurement of glomerular filtration rate using inulin clearance.

TUBULAR FUNCTION

Glycosuria and aminoaciduria have been the most commonly reported of the multiple renal tubular defects attributable to impairment of proximal tubular function. Impaired potassium conservation, hyperchloremic acidosis, and hyperphosphaturia have also been observed. Impairment of tubular reabsorptive or secretory mechanisms due to increased protein reabsorption has been postulated as the mechanism, similar to the Fanconi syndrome variants associated with light chain overproduction and resultant light chain proteinuria.

THYROID METABOLISM

The possible role of thyroid deficiency in nephrotic syndrome was raised by early investigators because of the clinical appearance of the patients, the presence of hypercholesterolemia, and the finding of lowered basal metabolic rates. Early efforts at treatment with thyroid extract produced no significant clinical improvement. More sophisticated measurements of thyroid function have produced variable findings, with the PBI and the total T_4 frequently in the hypothyroid range and thyroid binding globulin (TGB) sometimes decreased.

These patients are clinically euthyroid, however; their speed of reflex relaxation is normal, and ^{131}I uptake is normal or increased. Decrease in BMR is common to edematous states and relates to diminution in heat dissipation and possibly shunting of blood from the skin due to decreased effective circulating volume. Hypercholesterolemia is part of the generalized hyperlipoproteinemia postulated to result from hepatic efforts to compensate for hypoalbuminemia. Urinary losses of TBG and T_4 as well as stool loss of T_4 contribute to the decreased PBI; however, decreased levels of TBG do not appear to account entirely for the lowered PBI in all patients studied, and better correlation has been reported with PBI and total plasma protein concentration than with TBG. The preservation of normal free T_4 levels has been postulated to maintain the euthyroid state.

OTHER METABOLIC ABNORMALITIES

A number of electrolyte abnormalities have been reported as occurring with increased frequency in patients with nephrotic syndrome. Most are not clearly of clinical importance but may become significant if other abnormalities are superimposed.

Hypokalemia. The presence of this abnormality has been suggested to result from a combination of secondary aldosteronism, with renal potassium loss, and decreased dietary intake, yet it is quite rare for this abnormality to be present in nephrotic patients not on diuretics. Further, newly diagnosed nephrotic patients may be modestly hyperkalemic.

Hypocalcemia and hypocalciuria. Hypocalcemia results in part from a decrease in protein bound serum calcium which can be estimated as an approximately 0.4 mg decrease per g/dl decrease in albumin. A lowering of serum ionized calcium levels has been attributed to a possible decrease in gastrointestinal calcium absorption. Decrease in blood levels of 25-hydroxyvitamin D and its binding protein, a 58,000 dalton alphalike globulin, has been reported in patients with nephrotic syndrome and normal renal function. Elevated serum levels of parathyroid hormone have been found in some of these patients, as has evidence of enhanced bone reabsorption. Urinary loss of 25-hydroxyvitamin D may be responsible for the decreased intestinal calcium absorption, lowered blood levels of calcium, hypocalciuria, and osteomalacia.

Hypomagnesemia. Hypomagnesemia has been reported as a uniform finding in a small group of children with nephrotic syndrome responsive to corticosteroid therapy. Serum concentrations returned to normal with corticosteroid treatment. A combination of secondary aldosteronism and urinary loss of protein bound magnesium were the suggested mechanisms.

SUSCEPTIBILITY TO INFECTION

A heightened susceptibility to bacterial infection, particularly peritonitis secondary to *Streptococcus pneumoniae*, has long been associated with nephrotic syndrome, particularly in the pediatric age group. Recent studies have demonstrated the increasingly frequent role of gram-negative enteric organisms, particularly *Escherichia coli*, in infectious complications of the nephrotic patient. Before the availability of antibiotics, infection was the leading cause of death in children with nephrotic syndrome, and effective antibiotic therapy has been a major contributor to the improved prognosis in minimal change nephrotic syndrome over the last 25 years. The successful use of glucocorticoid and immunosuppressive therapy in inducing rapid and ultimately sustained remissions in patients with lipoid nephrosis also has contributed to a striking decline of fatal infections in this group; however, in patients with less responsive forms of idiopathic or secondary nephrotic syndrome, prolonged use of glucocorticoids and immunosuppressive therapy may contribute to infectious complications, often with opportunistic organisms.

Impairment in normal humoral defense mechanism has been suggested as the major factor compromising host defenses. Decrease in serum gamma globulin levels has been appreciated since 1940, and more recently decreased serum levels of IgG have been described irrespective of the etiology of the nephrotic syndrome. Urinary loss and catabolic reabsorption have been suggested as the major contributors to the hypogammaglobulinemia. Measurement of specific serum immunoglobulin concentrations has revealed markedly decreased serum IgG and IgA in children regardless of the etiology of nephrotic syndrome; however, children with minimal change nephrotic syndrome had significant and persistent elevations in serum IgM concentrations not found in those with other chronic glomerulonephritides, and these were unaffected by successful corticosteroid treatment. The authors suggested these findings supported an immunopathogenesis of the minimal change lesion and could reflect deficiency in T cell mediated conversion of IgM to IgG synthesis. It was recently reported that patients with lipoid as well as other types of nephrosis could respond to pneumococcal capsular antigens with specific antibody formation in manner similar to controls over a 6 week followup period; however, preimmunization titers were found to be decreased in nephrotic subjects, and this was attributed to urinary loss of protein or increased catabolism rather than increased suppressor T cell activity or dysfunctioning B cells.

COAGULATION

A propensity for venous thrombosis was recognized early in the description of patients with nephrotic syndrome and has been found to occur in most major regional venous systems but with particular frequency in the lower extremities and renal veins. These clinical observations have focused attention on the coagulation mechanism in nephrotic syndrome. A wide variety of laboratory abnormalities have been described, many favoring coagulation and others inhibiting thrombus

formation, but emphasis has been placed mainly on the hypercoagulable state (Table 2). Increase in plasma fibrinogen (factor I) has been the most consistent finding, and both concentration and turnover correlate with the degree of proteinuria and hypoalbuminemia present. Similarly, antithrombin and cholesterol concentrations show inverse correlation with hypoalbuminemia, supporting an increased synthesis in response to renal protein loss and hypoalbuminemia as discussed in the mechanism for hyperlipoproteinemia. Elevations in factors V, VIII, and combined VII and X activity have been reported; the first two are of high molecular weight and minimal urinary loss coupled with a generalized increased protein synthesis could result in increased levels. Increased platelet counts and enhanced platelet aggregation in response to collagen and adenosine diphosphate have also been reported.

A variety of alterations in the fibrinolytic system have been found, some of which favor and others of which inhibit this mechanism. Controversy concerning assays employed has made these data difficult to interpret and often contradictory; however, serum plasminogen may be elevated, and in patients with marked hypoalbuminemia serum antithrombin III levels may be decreased. The latter, an alpha-2 globulin, is the main inhibitor of thrombin, and its inherited deficiency is associated with a thrombotic diathesis. The molecular weight of antithrombin III is similar to albumin, and its renal clearance correlates with the degree of serum antithrombin III deficiency in nephrotic patients.

The occurrence of thromboembolic events also may be promoted by the marked edema and relative immobilization of the severely nephrotic patient. The use of diuretics may ameliorate edema but can contribute to further decrease in plasma volume, leading to hemoconcentration and thus promoting thrombosis. Hypercoagulability also has been associated with the administration of ACTH and corticosteroids, and increase in factor VIII levels has been attributed to the corticosteroids.

Conversely, evidence of impaired coagulation has been found in patients with nephrotic syndrome, often detected in the evaluation preceding percutaneous renal biopsy. Prolongation in partial thromboplastin time due to deficiency of factor IX has been attributed to its

Table 2
Described Abnormalities in Factors Influencing Coagulation in Nephrotic Syndrome

Favoring Coagulation	Impairing Coagulation
Increase in plasma fibrinogen	Factor IX deficiency
Increase in factors V, VIII, combined VII and X	Accelerated plasma disappearance rates for factors II, IX, X
Increase in platelet counts	Decrease in factors XI, XII
Increased platelet aggregation in response to collagen and ADP	Increased fibrinolytic activity
Decrease in antithrombin III	Increased plasminogen
Edema, immobilization, diuretic therapy	
Corticosteroid therapy	

urinary loss. Accelerated plasma disappearance rates for factors II and X, as well as IX, have been shown to follow prothrombin complex administration, and the coagulation defect has improved concomitant with decreased proteinuria following glucocorticoid and immunosuppressive therapy. Low circulating levels of factor XII have been attributed to both urinary loss and increased consumption. The latter mechanism has also been suggested to explain decrease in factor XI concentration.

ATHEROSCLEROSIS

The striking hyperlipoproteinemia, particularly hypercholesterolemia, which usually accompanies nephrotic syndrome might be expected to be a significant risk factor contributing to accelerated atherosclerosis. Published clinical studies differ markedly in their conclusions regarding the prevalence of coronary artery disease in nephrotic patients. Estimates range from a frequency of myocardial infarction 85 times that expected in a comparable nonnephrotic adult male age group to absence of unequivocal myocardial infarction among 212 adults with nephrotic syndrome observed over a decade.

MALNUTRITION

The increasing weight and body mass of the edematous state may mask a progressive loss of lean body weight. This may be particularly striking in growing children and not appreciated until after diuresis is achieved. Edema of the gastrointestinal tract has been implicated as the cause of anorexia and vomiting which may be prominent with nephrotic syndrome. This decreased intake coupled with the catabolic effects of corticosteroid therapy and the contribution toward negative protein balance of the renal protein loss may result in significant malnutrition.

DIFFERENTIAL DIAGNOSIS

The differential diagnosis of nephrotic syndrome does encompass virtually the entire spectrum of glomerular disease (Table 3). It is useful to approach consideration of diagnosis from the perspective of three major clinical categories—(1) systemic disease associated with renal involvement, (2) primarily renal disease of known etiology, and (3) idiopathic renal disease.

The above are among the wide variety of factors necessitating consideration and assisting the physician in focusing the diagnostic approach. Since lipoid nephrosis accounts for approximately 80 percent of nephrotic patients in the pediatric age group, many pediatricians initiate a therapeutic trial of corticosteroids in a child with nephrotic syndrome with a noninflammatory urinary sediment, normal physical examination but with edema, and laboratory findings of normal renal function and serum complement.

In the adult age group, diabetes mellitus is probably the most frequent cause of nephrotic syndrome, and a long history of glucose intolerance, evidence of diabetic retinopathy, preservation of renal size, and a noninflammatory urinary sediment often suffice for a presumptive diagnosis.

Geographic considerations are major factors. The above comments are relevant to practice in the United States and Europe. In parts of Africa, *Plasmodium malariae* is the major etiologic agent associated with childhood nephrotic syndrome; in developing nations amyloidosis related to tuberculosis is the major cause of nephrotic syndrome in adults; in the Near East amyloidosis related to familial Mediterranean fever is a predominant diagnosis.

The outline of differential diagnosis (Table 3) combines the discussed considerations, a histopathologic classification, consideration of the time course of the diffuse and generalized glomerular diseases, and the apparent immunopathologic mechanism.

MINIMAL CHANGE NEPHROTIC SYNDROME

Minimal change or nil lesion nephrotic syndrome is the classical lipoid nephrosis which is found in approximately 80 percent of children presenting with nephrotic syndrome. It accounts for roughly 20 percent of the idiopathic nephrotic syndrome in adults. About two-thirds of childhood patients are males, but the sex incidence is approximately equal among adults. The peak incidence in childhood is between 1 and 5 years, and it may occur at an earlier age than is characteristic for poststreptococcal glomerulonephritis.

Etiology

Evidence for an immune mechanism for minimal change nephrotic syndrome long has been sought. This has been suggested because of its frequent occurrence in children with atopy and the usual prompt response of the patient to corticosteroid or cytotoxic therapy. A history of asthma, eczema, or hay fever has been found to be approximately twice as frequent in these children as in a control group, and seasonal exacerbations associated with atopy have also been reported; however, renal biopsy material has not been characterized by deposition of immunoglobulins or complement, and serum complement levels are normal. The glomerular localization of IgE and elevation in serum IgE concentration have both been reported but not generally confirmed. Several reports recently have appeared of circulating soluble immune complexes found in the serum of children and adults with steroid responsive nephrotic syndrome which do not bind complement. Their role is not understood.

With little evidence for an immune complex mechanism and the occasional occurrence of nil lesion in association with Hodgkin's disease, attention has been directed toward possible disorders in T cell function. Evidence for the production of a circulating lymphokine potentially damaging to the glomerulus has come from a number of studies. A lymphokine-type factor which enhances vascular permeability has been found to be released from cultured peripheral lymphocytes from patients with minimal change lesion. Isolated lymphocytes from these patients, but not from those with proliferative glomerulonephritis, demonstrate significantly greater cytotoxicity against a neonatal human renal cell culture than do lymphocytes from normal

Table 3
Differential Diagnosis of the Nephrotic Syndrome

Generalized and diffuse glomerular involvement
    Acute glomerulonephritis: Immune complex deposition
        Poststreptococcal
        Idiopathic
        Postinfectious—syphilis, malaria, bacterial endocarditis, leprosy
    Rapidly progressive glomerulonephritis
        Immune complex deposition—poststreptococcal, idiopathic
        Anti-glomerular-basement-membrane disease—Goodpasture's syndrome,
            idiopathic
    Chronic glomerulonephritis: Immune complex deposition
        Disorders confined to the kidney
            Idiopathic chronic proliferative
            Poststreptococcal
            Epimembranous nephropathy
            Membranoproliferative and its variants
        Multisystem disorders
            Systemic lupus erythematosus
            Henoch-Schönlein purpura
            Idiopathic mixed cryoglobulinemia
            Polyarteritis
            Neoplasia
    Renal disease without immune complexes: Lipoid nephrosis (minimal change disease;
        nil lesion)
    Metabolic and systemic disease without immune complexes
        Diabetic glomerulosclerosis
        Amyloidosis (primary, secondary, multiple myeloma)
        Neoplasia
        Pregnancy (preeclampsia, recurrent nephrotic syndrome of pregnancy)
        Accelerated hypertension
    Possibly transient, mechanical factors
        Constrictive pericarditis
        Congestive heart failure
        Renal vein thrombosis
    Specific toxins
        Heavy metals (bismuth, gold, mercury)
        Drugs (trimethadione, paramethadione, penicillamine)
        "Allergens" (bee sting, poison ivy, poison oak)

Focal-local glomerular involvement
    Immune complex deposition
        Idiopathic focal glomerulonephritis (IgA nephropathy)
        Systemic lupus erythematosus (Type I)
    Renal disease without immune complexes: Focal glomerulosclerosis and hyalinosis

Miscellaneous disorders
    Renal transplant rejection
    Congenital nephrotic syndrome
    Sickle cell disease
    Thrombotic thrombocytopenic purpura
    Hemolytic-uremic syndrome

controls. Plasma from patients with minimal change nephrotic syndrome inhibits the blastogenic response of lymphocytes to mitogen phytohemagglutinin or to allogeneic lymphocytes, suggesting a role for suppressor T lymphocyte activity. Serum IgM levels have been found to be higher and IgG lower in these patients as compared to nephrotic syndrome secondary to chronic glomerulonephritis, and an impaired T cell mediated conversion of IgM to IgG synthesis has been suggested. Thus the hypothesis postulating an immune mediated alteration in glomerular permeability continues to have increasing suggestive but not yet definitive support.

Clinical Features

Presentation is usually with edema. Initially this may be noted in the periorbital area on arising in the morning. Localization is related to the low tissue turgor in this region and the absence of pulmonary congestion and orthopnea which prompts the cardiac patient to sleep in a more upright position. Adults are frequently first aware of lower extremity edema, more marked toward the end of day and persisting overnight. With increasing fluid retention, pleural effusions, ascites, and vulvar or scrotal edema may develop. Decrease in body mass due to anorexia and protein loss frequently occurs but may not be evident until after diuresis because of the massive edema. Nonspecific symptoms of weakness and malaise may accompany the anorexia. Hypertension is usually not seen except in the relatively rare patient with progressive renal insufficiency. During periods of marked hypoalbuminemia (2.0 g/dl) whitish narrow arcuate bands may develop on the fingernails, parallel to the lunulae. These are located in the nail bed rather than the plate and do not move distally with nail growth. Prompt resolution occurs with return of serum albumin levels to normal. This finding has been termed leukonychia or Muehrcke's lines.

Laboratory Findings

Selective proteinuria is characteristic of minimal change nephrotic syndrome, with albumin the predominant protein. Transient microscopic hematuria is observed in some patients but is not a characteristic feature. Lipiduria, including oval fat bodies, and cylinduria are often marked. Serum complement and antinuclear antibody studies are normal. Decreased serum IgA and IgG and elevated IgM levels have been commented upon. Hyperlipoproteinemia is also usually prominent. The erythrocyte sedimentation rate is markedly elevated, related to increased serum fibrinogen levels.

Pathology

Grossly the kidneys are enlarged, pale yellow, and smooth. The cut surfaces bulge due to interstitial edema.

On light microscopy the glomeruli appear normal with wide patent capillary lumina (Fig. 1). Cellular proliferation is usually not evident, but a slight increase in both mesangial matrix and cellularity may be present, particularly with frequently relapsing lipoid nephrosis. Hyaline droplets are evident in the proximal tubular cells. Birefringent lipid is often present within casts and degenerating tubular cells, and also within occasional clusters of interstitial foam cells. Interstitial edema is frequently present. The blood vessels are normal.

Electron microscopy. Fusion or effacement of the epithelial cell foot processes is often extensive and may create a continuous cytoplasmic layer on the subepithelial surface of the glomerular capillary basement membrane (Fig. 2). Numerous microvilli extend from the swollen podocytes (villous transformation). Slight circumscribed thickening of the capillary basement membrane, particularly the lamina rara interna, is often noted, particularly after frequent relapses. Mesangial changes confirm the light microscopy. Deposits are not seen.

Immunofluorescence studies are negative. A report of glomerular localization of IgE has not been confirmed.

Treatment

A prompt and complete response to corticosteroid therapy occurs in over 90 percent of children and in up to 85 percent of adults, usually within a treatment period of eight weeks or less. Relapse occurs in at least half the childhood responders and in a third to half of adults. Cyclophosphamide or chlorambucil have been used successfully in patients with frequent relapses and those dependent on or resistant to corticosteroids. (See the section on Treatment of Nephrotic Syndrome).

Prognosis

Prognosis for children is favorable for complete remission, and several large series have reported that over 75 percent achieved sustained complete remissions on long-term followup. Mortality rates have been 6–7 percent. A controlled study in adults indicated a slower but similar remission rate without steroid therapy as

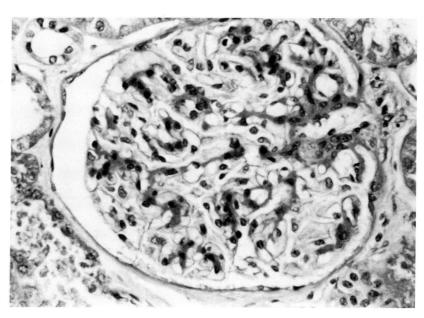

Fig. 1. Light microscopy of normal appearing glomerulus in patient with minimal change nephrotic syndrome. H & E. × 350. [Courtesy of George A. Bannayan, M.D.]

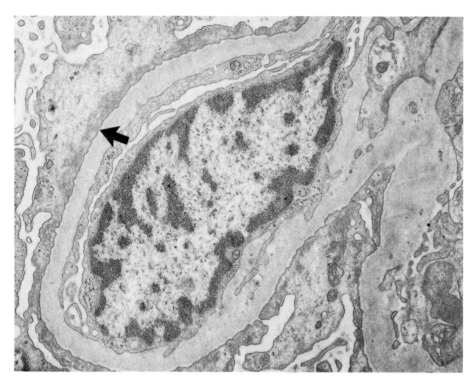

Fig. 2. Electron micrograph of capillary loop in minimal change nephrotic syndrome showing confluent fusion of epithelial foot processes. × 7200. [Courtesy of George A. Bannayan, M.D.]

with treatment and a higher death rate in the prednisone treated patients, usually related to cardiovascular disease. The small percentage of patients progressing to endstage renal disease may represent a failure to diagnose focal glomerular sclerosis, a lesion with an early predilection for the deeper, juxtamedullary glomeruli (see the chapter on *Focal Glomerular Sclerosis*).

MALIGNANCY

Neoplasia (see the chapter on *Renal Lesions in Malignancy*) has been firmly established as an etiology of nephrotic syndrome since the report of Lee and associates demonstrated 11 percent of nephrotic adults had a concurrent malignancy. Epimembranous nephropathy has been the most common histologic finding, most often in association with carcinoma of the lung, but carcinomas of the adrenal, breast, cervix, colon, kidney, ovary, stomach, and thyroid have also been observed. Immune complex deposition is clearly the pathogenic mechanism, and tumor-associated antigens have been demonstrated in the renal lesions of an increasing number of patients. Viral antigens and neoplastic-induced alterations of endogenous antigen have also been postulated as possibly playing a role in the pathogenesis.

Minimal change nephrotic syndrome has been associated particularly with Hodgkin's disease and suggested to result from a T cell abnormality, possibly production of a lymphokine(s) altering glomerular permeability. Remission and exacerbation of the nephrotic syndrome in parallel with response to treatment

of the Hodgkin's disease has been observed. Renal amyloidosis and renal vein thrombosis have also been reported in association with Hodgkin's disease.

The appearance of the nephrotic syndrome may precede or follow diagnosis of the neoplasm. The association is sufficiently well established to necessitate consideration of an underlying malignancy in an adult with nephrotic syndrome, particularly with demonstration of epimembranous nephropathy. Remission of nephrotic syndrome following successful excision of cancer has been observed, but the nephrotic syndrome is usually persistent and the course brief with disseminated carcinomatosis.

RENAL VEIN PRESSURE ELEVATION

A number of cardiovascular abnormalities associated with marked and prolonged elevation in systemic and renal venous pressure have been associated with proteinuria and the nephrotic syndrome. These include congenital heart disease, congestive heart failure, constructive pericarditis, and inferior vena cava obstruction above the renal veins. Amelioration of the proteinuria with correction of the cardiovascular abnormality has been cited to support the causative relationship; however, the experimental induction of elevation in renal venous pressure results in only modest proteinuria, and the pathophysiology of this association remains unexplained. Most patients with nephrotic syndrome attributed to congestive heart failure were treated with mercurial diuretics, themselves identified as capable of inducing nephrotic syndrome.

RENAL VEIN THROMBOSIS

Bilateral renal vein thrombosis in its chronic form has been associated with development of nephrotic syndrome for many years. While this was initially attributed to alterations in renal vein pressure, lack of success in the development of animal models, evidence of bilateral proteinuria in patients with unilateral thrombosis, and its usual association with an epimembranous lesion have cast doubt on that mechanism. The factors operative in nephrotic syndrome which may promote a hypercoagulable state have been reviewed. Autoimmunity to tubular antigens altered due to the thrombosis also has been postulated to account for the immune complex lesion; however, recent prospective studies indicate that thrombosis is a secondary occurrence to a preexisting renal lesion.

Radiologic evidence of thrombosis in about a third of patients with epimembranous or membranoproliferative glomerulonephritis has been reported in several prospective series, while others have found it far less frequently. Amyloidosis has also been associated with a high incidence of renal vein thrombosis. The reasons for these particular predilections are not clear. While the impact of this complication on renal function does not appear to be major, pulmonary and other embolization occurs more frequently, and establishment of the diagnosis merits anticoagulation. Surgical intervention has occasionally been successful with acute episodes, but long-term anticoagulation is the treatment of choice until resolution of the thrombosis.

DRUG-INDUCED NEPHROTIC SYNDROME

The occurrence of nephrotic syndrome concurrent with the use of a variety of drugs has been well documented. Associations with penicillamine, gold, mercury, and trimethadione are among the best studied.

The limited renal biopsy material available has most often revealed an epimembranous nephropathy, supporting an immune-mediated pathogenesis. Postulated mechanisms for immune complex deposition have included a tubular toxicity releasing autologous antigens, as suggested for gold, or a role for the drug as a hapten leading to circulating immune complexes with subsequent renal deposition. Direct toxicity with drug altered glomerular permeability, similar to aminonucleoside-induced nephrotic syndrome in the rat, has not been demonstrated in man.

The proteinuria usually resolves with discontinuation of the drug, and a correlation between duration of administration and glomerular basement membrane thickness has been suggested. Reversibility with cessation of the antigenic stimulus is compatible with the 20–30 percent spontaneous remission rate observed with idiopathic epimembranous nephropathy, presumably also related to termination of complex formation and deposition. Prednisone has been used in the treatment of drug-induced nephrotic syndrome in uncontrolled observations without demonstration of acceleration of resolution.

An association between heroin addiction and nephrotic syndrome has been supported by the frequent finding of a focal and segmental glomerular sclerosis associated with focal glomerular disposition of IgM and C'3. Renal functional deterioration is usually continuous and rapid with the development of focal global sclerosis. The lesion has been suggested as representing an undefined response to heroin, its vehicle, or associated contaminants. Focal separation of podocytes from the basement membrane has been observed in a high percentage of these patients, similar to the ultrastructural lesion found in the aminonucleoside nephrosis of rats.

INFECTIOUS AGENTS

A wide variety of infectious agents, including bacteria, helminths, protozoa, and viruses, has been associated with nephrotic syndrome which is usually self-limited to the course of the infection. When electron microscopy has been performed on biopsy material, dense deposits are frequently evident in the subepithelial or mesangial area, and immunofluoresence has also supported an immune complex deposition pattern.

Hepatitis B infection is one of the better studied associations. Epimembranous nephropathy in one such patient was accompanied by glomerular deposition of IgG, C'3, and hepatitis B antigen in a diffuse granular pattern, indicating the formation of soluble immune complexes with glomerular deposition. Persistent antigenemia has been associated with progressive deterioration in renal function and an epimembranous or membranoproliferative lesion.

The nature of the lesion associated with *Plasmodium malariae* infection has shown regional variability with focal, segmental, and diffuse mesangiocapillary sclerosis observed in Nigeria and epimembranous nephropathy seen in Ugandan adults and mainly a proliferative lesion in children. Coarse granular glomerular IgG, IgM, and C'3 deposition was reported by both groups. Nephrotic syndrome associated with *P. falciparum* infection is associated with a proliferative glomerular lesion, subendothelial and paramesangial deposits, and finely granular immunoglobulin and C'3 deposition. *P. falciparum* antigen has been isolated from biopsy specimens, and immunoglobulin eluates have been shown to have antimalarial activity, strongly supporting an immunopathogenesis.

In approximately 10 percent of patients with acute poststreptococcal glomerulonephritis, proteinuria may be of sufficient magnitude to result in hypoalbuminemia and superimpose a nephrotic syndrome on the nephritic picture. Amyloidosis may be a secondary development in patients with chronic infection, particularly tuberculosis, resulting in nephrotic syndrome.

TREATMENT OF NEPHROTIC SYNDROME

Intravenous Albumin

The efficacy of salt-poor albumin administration in nephrotic syndrome is markedly limited by its rapid urinary loss. This results from increased albumin clearance caused by both elevation in plasma concentration and increase in glomerular filtration rate. The latter appears related to expansion of intravascular volume, since increased urinary albumin loss can also result from intravenous dextran administration. Consequently, the use of albumin is reserved primarily for the treatment of symptomatic volume depletion with evidence of impending shock, as an ancillary measure in the initiation of a diuresis in a patient with symptomatic and refractory edema, or in preparation for surgical procedures, including renal biopsy.

Dietary Sodium Restriction

Excessive salt intake clearly promotes edema, and judicious control of dietary sodium is an effective therapeutic measure. Patient compliance is the limiting factor, and this can usually be achieved with moderate restriction in the range of 2–3 g sodium chloride daily (35–50 mEq sodium).

High-Protein Diet

Increasingly positive nitrogen balance has been demonstrated with increments of protein intake up to 5 g/kg per day in adults with nephrotic syndrome; maximum positive nitrogen balance in children with nephrotic syndrome has been reported at 3.2 g/kg protein daily. Increase in serum protein is usually small and gradual, and increased proteinuria occurs regularly in parallel with the increased protein intake. Maintenance of dietary protein intake in children particularly, at 2–4 g/kg/day as tolerated, is recommended while the nephrotic phase continues.

Diuretics

Diuretics play an ancillary role to dietary sodium restriction in preventing or reversing excessive sodium retention which results in extracellular volume expansion and edema. These agents must be used cautiously with the understanding that the avid renal sodium reabsorption is a homeostatic mechanism operating to maintain effective circulating volume despite hypoalbuminemia. Overzealous use of diuretic agents may result in postural hypotension and fall in renal blood flow and glomerular filtration rate, with elevation in creatinine and BUN or frank shock and oliguric renal failure.

Thiazide diuretics, which inhibit sodium and chloride reabsorption in the distal tubule, are usually the initial agents of choice. In instances of more refractory edema, the loop diuretics, ethacrynic acid or furosemide, both acting to inhibit chloride reabsorption in the ascending limb of the loop of Henle, are capable of achieving considerably greater excretion of filtered sodium.

Since both the thiazides and loop-active diuretics exert their effect proximal to the distal tubular sites of aldosterone-mediated sodium reabsorption and potassium excretion, their efficacy can be markedly compromised by the effects of aldosterone at these sites. Consequently, the addition of spironolactone, a competive inhibitor of aldosterone, or triamterene, active in similar manner but by a noncompetetive mechanism, may be useful supplements in promoting sodium excretion in the absence of renal insufficiency.

While hypokalemia may be a consequence of the thiazides and loop diuretics, the distal site diuretic agents inhibit potassium secretion and may contribute to hyperkalemia. The problem of depletion of intravascular volume has already been mentioned as an area of critical concern in patients with nephrotic syndrome. Detailed discussions concerning complications of diuretic therapy are found in the chapter on *Disorders in Sodium Metabolism*.

Water Restriction

With the proper use of sodium restriction and diuretic agents, water restriction is usually not necessary. Because of their sites of action, both the thiazide and loop diuretics impair clearance of free water, the urinary diluting mechanism of the kidney. Consequently, hyponatremia may result with inordinate water intake in patients on these agents.

Anticoagulation

Prophylactic anticoagulation has been proposed for patients with nephrotic syndrome, particularly those with epimembranous or membranoproliferative lesions, owing to the high incidence of venous thrombosis and embolic phenomena. The very high prevalence figures of these lesions have not been confirmed by all groups, and the risk/benefit margins have not yet been established for patients with nephrotic syndrome. Consequently, efforts to treat the underlying disease when possible and steps to ameliorate factors contributing to thrombosis, such as immobilization, edema, and hemoconcentration due to plasma volume contraction, deserve initial therapeutic attention.

Hyperlipoproteinemia

In patients with nephrotic syndrome refractory to therapy the cardiovascular risks of prolonged hyperlipoproteinemia necessitate consideration. Dietary instructions to assist in the achievement and maintenance of normal lean body mass and a diet prudent in content of saturated fats should be accomplished. When drugs are utilized to assist in the management of hyperlipoproteinemia, attention must be paid to possible alterations in dosage due to the nephrotic syndrome and the level of renal function. Clofibrate has been associated with a severe myopathy in patients with nephrotic syndrome related to high plasma levels of the free drug due to decreased albumin binding. The daily dose of clofibrate should not exceed 0.5 g for each 1 g/dl of serum albumin. Advanced renal insufficiency may result in a similar toxicity, and total weekly dosage of 1.0–1.5 g clofibrate has been adequate to control hypertriglyceridemia in patients with endstage renal failure on hemodialysis.

Corticosteroids

The efficacy of corticosteroids in more rapidly inducing complete remission in patients with minimal change nephrotic syndrome than occurs in untreated patients is well established. Their usefulness in epimembranous nephropathy is more controversial, although recent controlled studies suggest their value in preserving glomerular filtration rate. Most observers have not demonstrated effectiveness of corticosteroids in the treatment of either focal glomerulosclerosis or membranoproliferative glomerulonephritis, although some suggest improvement with long-term alternate day therapy for both lesions. Detailed appraisals of corticosteroid therapy for specific lesions are provided in the chapters devoted to these conditions.

A variety of schedules and protocols have been employed in the administration of corticosteroids. Introduction of 4 day per week dosage and alternate day programs have been very useful in minimizing side effects of the drugs for long-term administration. Daily dosage and duration of therapy have also varied widely among clinical investigators. A representative protocol efficaciously used in adult minimal change nephrotic syndrome is 1 mg/kg body weight prednisone up to 80 mg/day, given in divided dose. This is administered for 4 weeks and then reduced to a similar dose given on alternate days by progressive increases in dosage for the "on day" and reduction for the "off day" over a period of 1–2 weeks. With complete remission, the alternate day dosage is continued for 3–6 months and then tapered and discontinued. With partial remission, tapering is initiated when the urinary protein excretion has stabilized, and then the dosage reduced over 3–6 months. If no response is seen after 8 weeks of treatment, the prednisone is tapered and discontinued. In children, 60 mg/m² is the usual recommended dose of prednisone, given in three divided doses. Response is usually rapid, and alternate day therapy may be initiated when complete remission is attained, tapering to a maintenance dose of 30 mg/m² on alternate days for 3–6 months.

Immunosuppressive Therapy

Both cyclophosphamide and chlorambucil have been found to be highly efficacious when given in combination with prednisone in decreasing the number of relapses in children with minimal change nephrotic syndrome who are frequent relapsers. Azathioprine has not been found to be effective when given in addition to prednisone. Approximately 25 percent of children with this lesion are frequent relapsers (as defined by two relapses within 6 months of their initial successful corticosteroid therapy or four relapses within any 12 month period).

While experience with cyclophosphamide has been more extensive, reports of gonadal toxicity have prompted new caution concerning its use. Azoospermia and oligospermia in pre- and postpubescent males and ovarian failure in pre- and postpubescent females have been reported. Evidence indicating reversibility is encouraging but not yet definitive. It is recommended that cyclophosphamide not be used for patients with minimal lesion nephrotic syndrome who are adrenal corticosteroid sensitive unless they are frequent relapsers and have experienced significant toxicity from their steroid therapy. Guidelines for the clinician include obtaining informed consent of the patient or parent and that the dosage should be limited to 60–80 days at 2.5–3 mg/kg per day for the child. If a patient is steroid sensitive, diuresis should be produced with corticosteroids prior to cyclophosphamide therapy so that the urine flow will minimize the risk of hemorrhagic cystitis. Other potential complications of cyclophosphamide include leukopenia, alopecia, bladder tumors, vomiting, anorexia, and pulmonary fibrosis. The possible long-term influence on carcinogenesis and mutagenesis is an additional consideration. Chlorambucil, given to the point of inducing leukopenia, has also been found to be efficacious in preventing relapse with minimal change nephrotic syndrome in children. Initial doses of 0.1–0.2 mg/kg per day were given in divided dosage and increased to the point of falling white count. In one study an average daily dose of 0.3 mg/kg was given along with corticosteroids for a 6–12 week period. Complications with chlorambucil appear to be less than those reported with cyclophosphamide; however, azoospermia has been reported in patients receiving chlorambucil for the treatment of lymphoid disorders. Restrictions concerning the use of chlorambucil in children with relapsing nephrotic syndrome are similar to those for cyclophosphamide.

Nephrectomy

Rarely patients with nephrotic syndrome and progressive renal insufficiency continue to have massive proteinuria despite levels of glomerular filtration which approach endstage renal disease and even necessitate chronic dialysis. When such carefully documented renal protein loss compounds the nutritional problems of chronic uremia and creates difficulty in preventing symptoms of decreased effective circulating volume, consideration of bilateral nephrectomy arises as an ancillary measure to chronic hemodialysis or transplantation. Surgical nephrectomy, bilateral renal infarction via transarterial embolization, or the administration of nephrotoxic doses of mercaptomerin have all been used to terminate remaining renal function.

REFERENCES

Eagen J, Lewis EJ: Glomerulopathies of neoplasia. Kidney Int 11:297, 1977
Earley LE, Harvel RJ, Hooper J Jr, et al: Nephrotic syndrome. Calif Med 115:23, 1971
Hayslett JP, Kashgarian M, Bensch KG, et al: Clinicopathological correlations in the nephrotic syndrome due to primary renal diseases. Medicine (Baltimore) 52:93, 1973
Lim VS, Sibley R, Spargo BH: Adult lipoid nephrosis. Clinicopathological correlations. Ann Intern Med 81:314, 1974
Rose G: Medical Research Council trials, in Kluthe R, Vogt A, Batsford SR (eds): Glomerulonephritis. New York, John Wiley & Sons, 1977, p 174
Spitzer A: Ten years of activity. A report for the International Study of Kidney Disease in Children, in Kluthe R, Vogt A, Batsford SR (eds): Glomerulonephritis. New York, John Wiley & Sons, 1977, p 201

ACUTE RENAL FAILURE

Peter Smolens and Meyer D. Lifschitz

Acute renal failure (ARF) is a clinical syndrome resulting from the abrupt diminution of renal function. Normally the body's internal environment is rigidly regulated, in large part by the kidneys. When the kidneys fail, this control is lost and dysfunction of other organ systems may result. It is, indeed, the dysfunction of these other organ systems that usually causes the constellation of clinical findings in ARF.

The clinical hallmark of acute renal failure has classically been suppression or urine flow. The amount of this suppression has been characterized by either oliguria (daily urine output less than 500 cc), or anuria (daily urine output less than 50 cc). In recent years a nonoliguric form of ARF with daily urine outputs of 500–1500 cc has been observed with increasing frequency. This observation would suggest that a sizable number of patients with ARF have gone undetected in the past because of the dependence on finding a reduction in urine flow as a diagnostic marker of ARF. Therefore it is necessary that one be aware of the high frequency of ARF in certain clinical settings and routinely screen for this possibility with serial measurements of serum creatinine concentration in addition to following the urine output.

When the clinical syndrome of ARF was delineated in the 1940s and 1950s, it was observed that most of the patients had the entity which was called acute tubular necrosis (ATN). This entity was characterized histologically by varying degrees of tubular necrosis and cast formation without glomerular abnormalities and was often associated with a severe crush injury or other types of trauma. The renal failure was usually reversible with correction of the underlying disease process. It was of interest that despite the name, actual tubular necrosis was not uniformly present in these patients and indeed was usually much less impressive than the degree of functional renal impairment present. Many have subsequently proposed using a more morphologically correct name to describe this entity, but no one name has gained wide acceptance. Because of the confusion engendered by the term ATN the present authors prefer to use an alternative expression, functional renal failure (FRF). This describes the preeminent feature of the entity and avoids the morphologic inaccuracy of calling it ATN.

This chapter is primarily devoted to the etiology, pathophysiology, clinical course, and treatment of FRF. Other causes of ARF will be discussed in the section on differential diagnosis, since the presentations and early clinical course of the renal failure are often the same regardless of the cause. In depth discussion of the other causes of ARF may be found elsewhere in this book.

ETIOLOGY

As may be seen in Table 1, a large number of pathologic processes may be associated with ARF. These are typically broken down into prerenal, postrenal, and renal causes. The prerenal causes include those processes which lead to a decreased effective blood volume and diminished renal perfusion. In these conditions, volume expansion often results in rapid restoration of normal renal function. Examples include hemorrhage, gastrointestinal fluid loss, and third space fluid

sequestration. Impaired cardiac function may also cause prerenal ARF. Postrenal causes include processes which obstruct urine flow such as stones, tumors, and retroperitoneal fibrosis.

The renal causes may best be conceptualized by the pathology involved. The morphologic abnormality may reside primarily in the glomerulus, the blood vessels, the interstitium, or the tubules. The processes may be differentiated into those which involve multiple organ systems (such as thrombotic thrombocytopenic purpura) or those that effect only the kidney (such as pyelonephritis or acute glomerulonephritis). Unlike the above, the last category listed in Table 1, FRF, is not well characterized pathologically; however, it is the most common cause of ARF, and in most studies accounts for over 75 percent of the cases. FRF is usually seen in settings associated with diminished renal perfusion or nephrotoxin exposure. Examples of the former are listed under "hemodynamically mediated renal failure" and examples of the latter under "acute nephrotoxic renal failure."

PATHOLOGIC FINDINGS IN FRF

At autopsy, the kidneys of patients with FRF appear swollen due to increased water content. The cortex is usually widened and pale, the medulla dark and congested. Unlike normal kidneys, whose proximal tubules are collapsed in autopsy specimens, the kidney of FRF has noticeably dilated proximal tubules. The distal tubule commonly displays a widened lumen filled with casts and is lined by flattened tubular epithelium. Mitotic figures may also be seen in this segment; the flattened epithelium is felt to represent regenerating cells. Patchy tubular epithelial necrosis may also be seen, but interestingly only about 20 percent of autopsy specimens actually demonstrate this finding. The glomeruli are usually normal in appearance, even when studied with electron microscopy. Rarely podocyte swelling and/or glomerular capillary thrombi (as in disseminated intravascular coagulation) have been reported. The interstitium is usually widened with edema and may contain a small amount of inflammatory infiltrate.

It should be mentioned that the morphology of biopsy specimens in FRF differs somewhat from that seen at autopsy; however, the major findings of tubular dilatation and flattening of the epithelium with cast formation in the distal tubule are found in biopsies as well. It is important to understand that the morphologic changes described above are characteristic but not diagnostic of FRF. They may be seen in other settings associated with tubular ischemia such as vasculitis and glomerulonephritis; however, these latter entities have other characteristic pathological changes in addition to those of FRF, and the diagnosis should not be confusing.

PATHOGENESIS

FRF is usually preceeded by a hemodynamic or nephrotoxic insult to the kidney. The mechanisms by which the ARF is generated by these insults, and how

Table 1
Classification of ARF

Prerenal failure
  Hypovolemia. Examples—hemorrhage, excess fluid loss from GI tract, skin or
  kidney
  Decreased cardiac output. Examples—myocardial failure, pericardial tamponade,
  vascular pooling

Postrenal failure
  Urinary obstruction. Examples—calculi, prostatic enlargement, pelvic or abdominal
  neoplasm, retroperitoneal fibrosis, ureteral instrumentation with edema or bleeding

Parenchymal renal failure
  Glomerulonephritis
    Rapidly progressive glomerulonephritis
    Poststreptococcal glomerulonephritis
  Vascular lesions
    Inflammatory—polyarteritis nodosa or Henoch-Schönlein purpura
    Large vessel occlusive—thromboembolic, atheromatous, scleroderma
    Small vessel thrombi—disseminated intravascular coagulation, thrombotic
        thrombocytopenic purpura, hemolytic uremic syndrome, cortical necrosis
  Interstitial nephritis
    Infectious—pyelonephritis
    Inflammatory
    Allergic—acute allergic interstitial nephritis
  Functional renal failure
    "Hemodynamically mediated" ARF
      Major surgery—aortic aneurysm repair
      Obstetrical—septic abortion, placenta previa, abruptio placenta
      Trauma—crush injury
      Pigment release—hemoglobin, myoglobin
    Acute nephrotoxic renal failure
      Antibiotics
      Miscellaneous drugs—methoxyfluorane
      Heavy metals—mercury, cadmium, uranium
      Organic solvents—carbon tetrachloride
      Pesticides
      Glycols

the renal failure is maintained even after the insult has been removed, have been the object of intense study for the past several decades. The most widely accepted mechanisms proposed to account for the fall in glomerular filtration in FRF include renal vasoconstriction, tubular obstruction, back leakage of filtrate across the damaged tubular epithilium, and a fall in the glomerular capillary ultrafiltration coefficient (k_f). Although some of these mechanisms have been studied in human disease, most of our information on the pathogenesis of FRF has been derived from observations of experimental animal models. In the following sections some of these observations in human and experimental FRF will be reviewed.

Experimental FRF

FRF has been produced in animals in a variety of ways, including temporary occlusion of the renal artery, administration of norepinephrine into the renal artery, intramuscular injection of hypertonic glycerol, and administration of mercuric chloride and uranyl nitrate. The first three techniques are felt to induce renal failure via ischemia and are representative of hemodynamically mediated renal failure. The last two are representative

of nephrotoxin-induced renal failure. The observations regarding possible mechanisms operative in the renal failure in these models will be summarized below.

Renal vasoconstriction. The initial phase of renal failure in the glycerol model, the norepinephrine model, and the renal artery occlusion model is characterized by a fall in renal blood flow (RBF) and increased renal resistance. Measurement of RBF in nephrotoxic models of FRF has revealed somewhat conflicting data, with some studies demonstrating a fall in RBF while others have not. Of interest, it was possible to induce a fall in glomerular filtration rate (GFR) after uranyl nitrate administration even while maintaining a RBF 50 percent higher than control with the administration of the vasodilator PGE_2. Thus while a decrease in RBF may play a significant role in the initiation of hemodynamically mediated FRF, renal vasoconstriction does not seem important in the initiation of at least some experimental models of nephrotoxic renal failure.

RBF measurements 24–48 hours after renal failure is initiated are usually increased over those seen in the initial phase. This is true in both the hemodynamic and nephrotoxic models. Some investigators have shown that restoration of RBF with volume loading in both hemodynamic and nephrotoxic models was not associated with substantial improvement in inulin clearance (which may not be comparable to GFR in these models). One may conclude from these findings that renal vasoconstriction does not play an important role in the maintenance phase of FRF.

Where the increase in renal resistance is generated remains controversial. Some investigators suggest that in experimental FRF there is an increase in afferent arteriolar resistence and a decrease in the resistence of the efferent arteriole. The resultant fall in glomerular capillary pressure could then explain the diminution of GFR seen. In Munich-Wistar rats, which have glomeruli located on the surface of the kidney, it is possible to directly measure glomerular filtration and plasma flow. When these rats were subjected to partial renal artery occlusion, both GFR and plasma flow were decreased by 50 percent. Afferent and efferent arteriolar resistance, rose in parallel, suggesting, at least in the partial clamp model, that the resistance changes were similar in the pre- and postglomerular vasculatures.

A number of observations have suggested that the renin–angiotensin system might play an important role in the genesis of experimental FRF. Plasma renin activity (PRA) is commonly elevated in the initial stage of FRF. The juxtaglomerular apparatus was found to be enlarged in early histologic studies of kidneys with FRF. In addition, chronic salt loading has been shown to diminish the renal functional impairment induced in some experimental models of FRF, and this was associated with PRA levels that were lower than usual. On the other hand, there are reasons to believe that the renin–angiotensin system may not play a significant role in FRF. First, the PRA levels are only mildly elevated and rapidly return to control values. In other states associated with quite large increases in PRA, such as Bartter's syndrome, cirrhosis, and the nephrotic syndrome, FRF is not commonly seen. Second, investigators have attempted to modify the renin–angiotensin system to evaluate its role in the development of FRF. In these studies some animals received immunization against renin or angiotensin II and others were given inhibitors of either angiotensin II synthesis or action. These modifications of the renin–angiotensin system did not bestow any protective effect on the development of FRF. Thus it would appear that in most cases the renin–angiotensin system does not play an important role in the genesis of FRF, and evaluation of other possible mediators of renal vasoconstriction will be necessary.

Tubular obstruction. Some degree of tubular obstruction has been demonstrated in many of the experimental models. In the total renal artery clamp model, intratubular pressure (measured by micropuncture technique) was markedly increased 1–3 hours after release of the clamp. See Table 2. The kidney histology at this time showed desquamation of proximal tubular cells,

cast filled tubular lumens, and dilated proximal tubules. Intratubular pressures 24 hours after release of the clamp had returned to control levels. When these rats were volume expanded, however, the pressures were noted to rise again. This might suggest that tubular obstruction is important in the genesis of the oliguria in the maintenance phase as well as the initial phase of FRF, yet it should be noted that other investigators have found intratubular pressure to be normal or low in some experimental models. In addition, visual inspection of the tubules in vivo has revealed nondilated and, at times, collapsed tubules. These findings may be a function of the volume status of the animal, since volume loading may permit demonstration of tubular obstruction and dilated tubules. In considering nephrotoxic models, evidence of tubular obstruction has been found with mercuric chloride administration but not with uranyl nitrate.

Leakage of filtrate. Back leakage of filtrate across damaged tubular epithelium has been demonstrated in both ischemic and nephrotoxic models by several different techniques. When lissamine green was injected into the proximal tubule of an animal after renal artery clamping, the dye could be seen exiting from the tubule into the interstitium—a phenomenon not seen in normal tubules. When inulin was infused into the proximal tubule of the postischemic kidney, the inulin was detected after some time in the urine from the contralateral kidney. Since inulin is not reabsorbed by the intact tubule, this finding suggests that back leakage of the inulin across the tubular epithelium must have occurred. Horseradish peroxidase given intravenously was demonstrated in the cytoplasm of isolated tubular cells of ischemically damaged nephrons—evidence that back leakage occurs in ischemic tubules even when the tubules are not punctured or otherwise damaged by the investigator. Although one can demonstrate the presence of back leakage in these models, quantitation of this phenomenon has not been possible. Thus the relative contribution of leakage of filtrate to the functional impairment in ARF is not clear.

Decrease in ultrafiltration coefficient (k_f). The k_f is the product of the glomerular capillary surface area and the hydraulic conductivity across the glomerular capillary membrane. Some investigators have postulated that the fall in GFR seen in FRF might, at least in part, be the consequence of a fall in k_f. This has been suggested in several models, including the intrarenal norepinephrine infusion model and those using uranyl nitrate or gentamicin administration. In the norepinephrine model, scanning electron microscopy revealed impressive glomerular morphologic changes. It should be noted that these glomerular changes have not been demonstrated in human FRF; thus the significance of these experimental findings must remain open to question. It has not been determined whether the fall in k_f (when present) is due to a change in hydraulic conductivity or in capillary surface area.

Table 2
Effect of 1 Hour Unilateral Renal Artery Occlusion

	Before Occlusion: Hydropenia	1–3 Hours After Occlusion: Hydropenia	22–26 Hours After Occlusion	
			Hydropenia	Volume Expansion
Proximal tubular pressure (mm Hg)	11.5	31.2	9.2	18.1
Distal tubular pressure (mm Hg)	5.5	16.4	7.8	—
Glomerular capillary pressure (estimated, mm Hg)	46.5	52.1	31.1	45.1

Adapted from Arendhorst WJ, Finn WF, Gottschalk CW: Pathogenesis of acute renal failure following temporary renal ischemia in the rat. Circ Res 37:558, 1975.

Human Studies

The study of FRF in man has been essentially limited to morphologic study of autopsy and biopsy material, angiographic assessment of the renal vasculature, and measurement of RBF and GFR. The morphologic findings, as noted earlier in this chapter, were often far less impressive than were the functional disturbances noted in the same patient. This discrepancy suggested that the functional changes must, in large part, be due to changes in renal hemodynamics which would not be detected morphologically. Angiographic and hemodynamic assessment of patients with both nephrotoxic and ischemic ARF seemed to confirm this suggestion. Renal angiography has demonstrated markedly attenuated cortical vessels and the absence of the normal cortical nephrogram. When measured, RBF is reduced by 25–50 percent. In other studies, however, the intrarenal administration of vasodilators such as PGE_1, hydralazine, and acetylcholine increased RBF but failed to affect the oliguria. Thus although one can demonstrate vasoconstriction and a reduction in RBF, the importance of these mechanisms in the initiation of maintenance of ARF is not clear.

Whether tubular obstruction and/or back leakage of filtrate play a role in the genesis of human FRF is difficult to evaluate. Morphologic findings such as cast formation and tubular dilatation which are suggestive of obstruction may or may not be present. One study using a multiple indicator dilution technique was undertaken to evaluate the importance of suppression of glomerular filtration versus back leakage of tubular fluid in the genesis of the oliguria. This study was interpreted to show that suppression of glomerular filtration was the major factor causing renal functional impairment.

Conclusion

Results of studies of the experimental models of FRF would suggest that vasoconstriction and tubular obstruction may play a role in the generation of renal functional impairment. Maintenance of the renal failure probably does not depend on persistent vasoconstriction and instead may be a function of tubular obstruction with or without back leakage of filtrate. Back leakage of filtrate is frequently demonstrable, but how much it contributes to the oliguria is unclear. It would appear that the renin–angiotensin system is not an important mediator of ARF. Whether changes in k_f are important will require further investigation. Obviously one should be cautious in extrapolating information from animal models to explain the genesis of human FRF, but it is hoped that these models will allow clarification of some of the questions that have been raised.

DIFFERENTIAL DIAGNOSIS

The differential diagnosis of ARF is most conveniently divided into three categories. First are those processes which may be reversed with specific therapy; these include volume depletion, obstructive uropathy, and vascular obstruction. Because of their therapeutic implications, these disorders must be considered in every patient with ARF. The second cateogy includes those processes which may precipitate FRF; among these are hypotensive episodes, sepsis, nephrotoxin exposure, complications of pregnancy, and tissue destruction with release of heme pigments. The third category encompasses the less common causes of ARF such as glomerulitis, vasculitis, and cortical necrosis.

Clinical Evaluation

The patient's history often allows insight into the cause of the ARF. Obstructive uropathy is suggested if the patient previously has had nephrolithiasis, retroperitoneal fibrosis, pelvic or abdominal cancers, or papillary necrosis. Volume depletion is usually easy to confirm by examining for orthostatic hypotension, tachycardia, or poor skin turgor. Obstructive vascular disease should be considered in the patient with a history of severe atheromatous vascular disease or a thromboembolic diathesis. The history and physical examination should also suggest the diagnosis of a systemic disease such as a necrotizing vasculitis which could cause ARF. In addition, it is necessary to search for evidence of nephrotoxin exposure, circulatory collapse, or muscle or RBC destruction.

The characteristics of the urine output may be quite helpful. Total anuria is most often associated with complete urinary tract obstruction, vascular (renal arterial) obstruction, cortical necrosis, and severe glomerulitis or vasculitis and is uncommonly seen with hemodynamically mediated or nephrotoxic induced ARF. High-output (>500 cc/day) renal failure was initially described in patients with burns or trauma but now is seen in all types of ARF. It is particularly prevalent in nephrotoxin associated ARF. If there is wide variation in urine flow from anuria to polyuria, consideration should be given to intermittent urinary tract obstruction. Indeed this presentation of obstructive uropathy is more common than is anuria.

Urinalysis

Further information may be obtained from examination of the urine sediment. A benign sediment is commonly seen in obstructive uropathy but is rarely present in FRF or glomerulitis. Hyaline and finely granular casts may be seen in the urine of patients with prerenal azotemia; however, one rarely sees coarsely granular casts, WBCs, or RBCs in this condition. The urinary sediment of FRF is often characteristic, containing tubular epithelial cells, cellular casts, proteinaceous debris, and numerous brown colored coarse granular casts. Indeed this type of sediment is observed in 75 percent of patients with FRF. The presence of numerous WBCs and/or WBC casts should suggest interstitial nephritis, pyelonephritis, or papillary necrosis. Allergic interstitial nephritis is suggested by the presence of eosinophils in the urine.

Laboratory Evaluation

Urinary electrolyte composition and osmolality have been described for a number of causes of acute renal failure. The urine sodium concentration and the fractional excretion of sodium reflect the tubular capacity to reabsorb sodium from the glomerular filtrate. In volume depletion and other sodium retaining states, the urinary sodium concentration (U_{Na}) and fractional sodium excretion (Fe_{Na}) are less than 20 mEq/liter and 1 percent, respectively. In FRF, they are typically high. A low U_{Na}, however, is not specific for prerenal azotemia; it can be seen in acute glomerulonephritis as well as in acute obstructive uropathy. The urine/plasma (U/P) ratios for creatinine and urea reflect the ability to both excrete solute and reabsorb water. This ability is markedly impaired in both FRF and acute glomerulonephritis, and the low U/P ratios reflect this. In prerenal azotemia, water is avidly reabsorbed and thus a high U/P ratio is seen. Although a good deal of overlap occurs, the U/P, U_{Na}, Fe_{Na} and urinary osmolality (U_{osm}) may be very helpful in separating FRF from prerenal azotemia. In one recent study, it was concluded that prerenal azotemia was likely if the U_{osm} is >500 mOsm/kg, U_{Na} <20 mEq/liter, U/P urea >8, U/P creatinine>40, and Fe_{Na}<1 percent. Of all these parameters the Fe_{Na} and U_{osm} are probably the best predictive factors. See Table 3.

Radiologic Evaluation

The anatomy of the kidneys and urinary tract may be defined by using a variety of radiologic techniques. These are frequently necessary in patients with ARF in order to detect surgically correctable diseases. Radiologic procedures that are available include the plain abdominal film, intravenous pyelogram (IVP), renal radionuclide scan, renal sonogram, renal angiogram, and abdominal computed axial tomography (CAT) scan.

On the plain film, one may determine renal size and look for calcium. Only one kidney may be visualized, and this might suggest the possibility of a solitary kidney (which, if obstructed, can cause ARF). Large kidneys are suggestive of hydronephrosis or acute inflammation such as may be seen in glomerulonephritis, pyelonephritis, or acute interstitial nephritis. Small kidneys would suggest that underlying chronic renal disease is present. Calcifications seen in the region of both ureters may suggest the possibility of bilateral ureteral stones with obstruction.

The IVP is performed by the intravenous infusion of radiopaque dye. The substances used are excreted almost entirely by glomerular filtration and are not reabsorbed. Along the normal nephron, the bulk of the glomerular filtrate is reabsorbed, leaving behind a concentrated tubular fluid containing contrast media. In FRF, there is a decrease in both GFR and tubular reabsorption of filtrate. Despite this, utilization of high-dose contrast media infusion, nephrotomography, and delayed films usually permits adequate visualization of the nephrogram and ureters. In the experience of some, decreasing the tubular solute load with dialysis less than 12 hours prior to the IVP may allow adequate visualization of a collecting system that could not be previously visualized. The IVP is of particular importance in excluding obstruction and usually obviates the need for retrograde pyelography with its attendant risks of infection and ureteral trauma. The findings in obstruction include (1) an increase in renal size, (2) the presence of large radiolucent spaces (in immediate nephrogram) representing dilated calyces, and (3) opacification of dilated renal pelvis, calyces, and ureter (later films). When these are not present and a good nephrogram is seen, obstruction can be excluded from the differential diagnosis.

The IVP in FRF characteristically shows a prolonged nephrogram of constant density (perhaps rep-

Table 3
Laboratory Evaluation

	Volume Depletion	FRF
U_{osm} (mOsm/liter)	> 500	< 350
U_{Na} (mEq/liter)	< 20	> 40
U/P urea	> 8	< 3
U/P creatinine	> 40	< 20
Fe_{Na}	< 1%	> 1%

Abbreviations: U_{osm}, urinary osmolality; U_{Na}, urinary sodium; U/P urea, urinary urea/plasma urea; U/P creatinine, urinary creatinine/plasma creatinine; Fe_{Na}, fractional excretion of sodium, clearance of sodium/GFR = $(U/P)_{creatinine}$.

Adapted from Miller TR, Anderson RJ, Linas SL, et al: Urinary diagnostic indices in acute renal failure. Ann Intern Med 89:47, 1978.

resenting leakage of contrast medium into the interstitium). If no nephrogram is seen, one needs to consider acute glomerulonephritis, bilateral renal artery occlusion, or other diseases associated with marked impairment of renal perfusion.

During the 1960s it was felt that IVPs could be done without adverse effect even in the patient with ARF. Over the past 10 years, however, radiographic contrast material has been shown to be associated with significant nephrotoxic potential itself. Patients who appear to be at greatest risk are the elderly, those with previously impaired renal function, and those with diabetes mellitus or multiple myeloma. Patients who undergo overnight dehydration prior to IVP probably are at higher risk than those who are not dehydrated.

Thus in the patient with ARF one needs to weigh the risk of contrast medium nephrotoxicity versus the possibility of missing a reversible surgical lesion. This problem may be circumvented in the high-risk patient with the use of the sonogram or renal radionuclide scan. The sonogram, in expert hands, has been shown to be an excellent screening test for obstructive uropathy with a low false negative rate. It does, however, have a high false positive rate; thus when it is positive an IVP should be performed to confirm the diagnosis. The renal scan may also aid in the diagnosis of obstructive uropathy. One may see renal enlargement and/or diminished flow of the radionuclide into the ureters or bladder. Again, if obstructive uropathy is suggested, an IVP should then be performed. In the rare case where the kidneys cannot be well visualized by the above procedures and obstructive uropathy is possible, retrograde pyelography may be necessary. Here, one need demonstrate patency of only one ureter to exclude obstructive uropathy as the cause of ARF.

If thrombosis of the renal arteries is suspected, the renal scan is quite helpful. If early renal perfusion can be demonstrated, thrombosis of the renal arteries as a cause of ARF may be excluded. If bilateral renal artery occlusion is suggested by the scan, the diagnosis should be confirmed with a renal arteriogram. It should be noted that the contrast agents generally used (in the IVP or arteriogram) are rapidly dialyzable, and possible toxicity from either the medium itself or the osmotic load it represents may be readily managed with dialysis.

CLINICAL FEATURES

In the 1940s and 1950s the clinical features of FRF became well recognized. The clinical course was characterized in terms of four stages—onset, the oliguric phase, the diuretic phase, and the recovery phase. Since that time, modifications in the early detection and treatment of FRF have revealed a somewhat different spectrum of patients with this entity. Routine monitoring of serum creatinine levels has permitted the detection of an increasing number of patients with either mild asymptomatic FRF or nonoliguric FRF who probably escaped detection in the past. The early institution of dialysis has eliminated both the large accumulation of solutes during the oliguric phase and the subsequent large osmotic diuresis which followed in the diuretic phase.

Despite these developments, consideration of FRF in terms of the four phases is still conceptually useful and will be utilized here. The onset takes place during the interval of time between the insult to the kidney and the development of clinically detectable renal failure. Its duration may vary from hours to days depending on the type of insult inflicted on the kidney and on any underlying renal pathology which may have been present.

Oliguric Phase

The oliguric phase is usually characterized by a falling urine output and increasing azotemia. This phase may last 1–40 days but typically averages 9–17 days. The amount of urine output constituting oliguria is usually considered to be 400–500 cc/day. This amount is the minimal volume of urine which, when maximally concentrated, is required to excrete the normal daily osmotic load. A smaller daily urine volume would not permit the maintenance of osmotic homeostasis and thus implies that renal function is impaired. (These considerations hold for most adults; different values apply to children.)

Metabolic abnormalities. The excretion of metabolic waste products is usually markedly diminished in FRF. These products, of which urea and creatinine are the most commonly used markers, are retained by the body, and the rate of rise of the concentration of these materials in the blood becomes dependent on dietary intake and the metabolic (catabolic versus anabolic) state of the patient. In uncomplicated patients, the rate of rise of blood urea nitrogen is 10–20 mg/dl/day and of creatinine 0.5–1 mg/dl/day. In the hypercatabolic patient such as the trauma victim, the rate of rise of urea may reach 100 mg/dl/day and creatinine may rise by more than 2 mg/dl/day.

Many patients with FRF are either unable or unwilling to eat during the oliguric phase. Energy needs, which may be quite large at this time, must therefore be supplied by catabolism of body fat and protein stores (or by exogenous administration). This catabolism results in the generation of 400–500 cc of free water per day. This water can serve as a source of the obligatory daily insensible water loss (via the lungs, GI tract, and sweat). This mode of energy production and water loss should result in a daily weight reduction of 0.5–1 kg per day. The patient whose course is complicated by infection or tissue necrosis will experience a greater rate of catabolism, and his rate of weight loss may be even more rapid.

A number of fluid and electrolyte abnormalities result from ARF and cause significant morbidity and, at times, mortality. These include hyperkalemia, metabolic acidosis, hyponatremia, hyperphosphatemia, and hypermagnesemia.

Hyperkalemia. The kidney is normally the route of excretion of most of the potassium presented each day to the body. Many of the settings in which FRF is

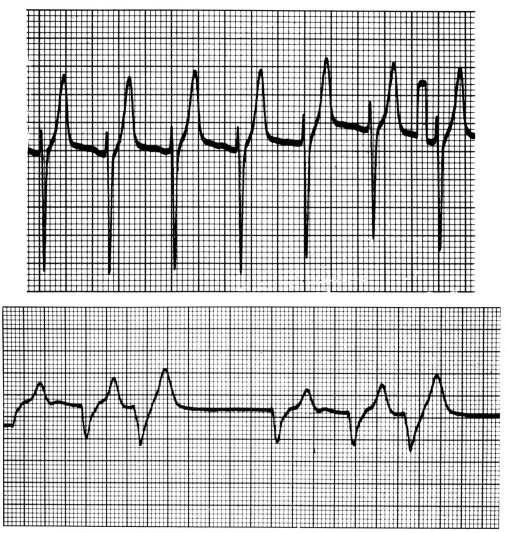

Fig. 1. Electrocardiographic changes of hyperkalemia. The patient in A had a plasma potassium of 6.8 mEq/liter. Note the symmetrical peaking of the T waves. The patient in B had a plasma potassium of 8.6. Here one sees abnormally widened QRS complexes and the loss of p waves.

seen are associated with tissue necrosis (trauma, rhabdomyolysis, burns, blood transfusion) and acidosis, both of which cause a marked release of potassium into the extra-cellular fluid (ECF). Thus in ARF there is both an increased potassium load presented to the body and a diminished capacity to excrete it. The most serious complication of hyperkalemia is its effect on the heart. Manifestations include bradycardia, ventricular fibrillation, and cardiac arrest. Electrocardiogram (ECG) changes (Fig. 1) include peaked T waves, prolonged or absent P waves, widened QRS complexes, and/or QT intervals which may evolve into a "sine wave" rhythm. In earlier series hyperkalemia was frequently seen and was not an uncommon cause of death. Fortunately, over the past two decades, with routine electrolyte monitoring and readily available methods of lowering the potassium level, the morbidity and mortality of hyperkalemia have lessened.

Metabolic acidosis. The kidney normally excretes about 1 mEq of fixed acid/kg body weight per day. The source of these acids (phosphoric, sulfuric) is the catabolism of protein. In FRF, the capacity to excrete these acids is decreased and an anion gap metabolic acidosis develops. Normal compensatory mechanisms used to partially correct the pH include utilization of body buffers found in bone and proteins and hyperventilation (Kussmaul respiration). Severe acidosis may be reflected in cardiovascular dysfunction (arrhythmia and hypotension) and central nervous system dysfunction (impaired sensorium).

Calcium and phosphate. Clinically significant disorders of calcium and phosphate metabolism are sometimes seen in FRF. The most common setting in which this occurs is acute rhabdomyolysis with myoglobinuric renal failure. Here, marked cellular breakdown and release of phosphate may cause deposition of calcium phosphate salts in the traumatized muscle and subsequent symptomatic hypocalcemia. With clinical improvement and healing of the injured tissue, the deposited calcium may be released into the circulation and rebound hypercalcemia may be encountered. Another setting in which FRF may be seen with hypocalcemia and hyperphosphatemia is during cytotoxic therapy of neoplasms. In this condition considerable tissue necrosis with release of large amounts of phosphate also occurs. The significance of the alterations of parathyroid hormone (PTH) seen in FRF is still not clear. With the onset of FRF, PTH levels typically rise; however, the PTH level may be quite variable and when measured during a period of hypercalcemia has ranged from high to subnormal levels. It should be remembered that cell sensitivity to PTH action is often diminished in renal failure, and the increased amount measured may be a consequence of this end organ insensitivity. In addition, the kidney is an important site for PTH catabolism, and diminished PTH catabolism would be expected to occur in FRF.

Hyponatremia. Hyponatremia was felt to have caused a significant amount of morbidity in patients with FRF in the series reviewed in the 1950s. Seizures and obtundation were commonly associated with severe hyponatremia. Improved understanding of the limited capacity of the kidney to excrete free water has led to appropriate restriction in water intake and a decrease in the incidence of clinical hyponatremia.

Hypermagnesemia. In prior years magnesium intoxication was seen on occasion. This was usually due to the administration of magnesium-containing salts in the management of gastrointestinal symptoms such as constipation or epigastric distress which are quite common in FRF. Magnesium, like potassium, is excreted primarily by the kidney. Thus, when administered to patients with FRF, magnesium is retained and symptomatic hypermagnesemia with depression of both peripheral and central nervous system function may develop. Other medications are now substituted for magnesium salts and thus magnesium intoxication is rarely, if ever, seen.

Infections. Infection, one of the most serious complications that may befall the patient with FRF, continues to be the most common cause of death in these patients. In a 1968 review, it was suggested that about one-third of all deaths in patients with FRF were due to infections. More recent series suggest that infections in FRF may be increasing as a cause of death despite the use of newer antibiotics. In one report, infections were the major cause of death in 72 percent of the patients, most of whom had renal failure associated with trauma. In another, more recent series, it was noted that 54 percent of deaths were primarily caused by infection. The presence of sepsis is particularly ominous, since it is associated with a mortality rate of 70–80 percent in patients with FRF. Infections are extremely frequent in FRF, being seen in more than 50 percent of patients. The most common sites are the lungs, urinary tract, wounds, abdomen (peritonitis), and bloodstream. A number of factors contribute to the high incidence of infection. Indwelling vascular and urinary catheters provide convenient portals of entry for microorganisms. In patients with altered sensorium,

aspiration pneumonia is commonly seen. Wound healing in patients with renal failure is impaired and thus postoperative and trauma patients are more prone to wound infection and wound dehiscence. Patients with FRF are commonly volume overloaded. The resultant pulmonary interstitial fluid, pleural effusions, and ascites may provide excellent media in which bacteria may grow. There is a growing body of evidence to suggest that the immune response is impaired in renal failure. Lymphocyte number and activity have been decreased in some studies. Some workers have found that the ability to generate an acute inflammatory response may be impaired. In one study, alveolar macrophage function was found to be defective. Although a number of possible defects in the immune system may be found in FRF, how this relates to the high incidence of infection is presently unclear. The organisms which contribute most to the morbidity and mortality are *Staphylococcus aureus, Streptococcus sp.,* and the gram-negative bacteria. Opportunistic agents such as fungi and unicellular organisms are rarely a problem. In addition to predisposing the patient to overwhelming sepsis and death, the presence of infection also worsens the uremia. Protein catabolism is increased, causing a release of additional nitrogenous waste products and potassium which cannot be readily excreted.

Cardiovascular system. Renal failure may affect the cardiovascular system via volume overload, hypertension, arrhythmias, and pericarditis. With improved fluid management, better control of serum potassium concentration, and the use of prophylactic dialysis, these entities are much less of a problem today than they were in the past; however, they do still occur, and as recently as 1972 congestive heart failure was found in 20 percent, hypertension in 15 percent, and pericarditis in 7 percent of patients in one study. Although pericarditis was reported in 18 percent of a series published in 1955 and continues to be a substantial problem in chronic renal failure, it does not seem to be a common problem in FRF at the present time. The presence of extracellular fluid volume expansion is a consequence of the kidney's limited ability to excrete a salt load in FRF. Despite the high U_{Na} seen, the number of mEq of Na excreted in less than 500 cc of urine is quite small. Therefore if a patient is permitted to eat a normal diet (which may contain over 100 mEq of Na) or is given parenteral NaCl, a positive Na balance will result and manifestations of extracellular fluid volume overload—pulmonary edema, hypertension, etc.—will ensue.

Although the peripheral plasma renin levels in FRF are frequently high, this is usually a transient phenomenona. Renin is usually not felt to play an important role in the hypertension of FRF. Hypertension is most commonly dependent on volume excess, and management is best achieved by removal of the fluid with dialysis or, if possible, diuretics.

Gastrointestinal. Nausea, vomiting, and anorexia are often observed in patients with FRF. Although their precise cause is not clear, mucosal ulcerations in any region of the gastrointestinal tract may occur, and frank ulcers of the stomach and duodenum may also be seen. These problems often result in diminished dietary intake and subsequent nutritional deficiencies.

A more serious problem is gastrointestinal hemorrhage. Some form of gastrointestinal blood loss is found in about 25 percent of patients with FRF. Severe hemorrhage is often fatal and accounts for 5–10 percent of mortality seen in most series. Features of renal failure which may contribute to gastrointestinal blood loss include (1) the mucosal ulcerations noted above, (2) production of ammonia in the gut by urea splitting bacteria, which may foster ulcer formation, (3) decreased wound healing, (4) abnormal platelet function, and (5) possibly depressed levels of vitamin K due to poor dietary intake.

Neurologic. Neurologic manifestations in FRF may be the result of many factors, including hyponatremia, hyper- and hypocalcemia, rapid fluid shifts with cerebral edema, hypertensive encephalopathy, subdural hemotoma, CNS bleeding, and CNS infection. The most common neurologic findings are altered mental state, twitching, and seizures. Neurologic findings are usually minimal when water intoxication is avoided and/or early dialysis is utilized.

Hematopoiesis. Anemia may occur relatively early in FRF, although the presence of severe anemia on admission should suggest the possibility of underlying chronic renal failure or Goodpasture's syndrome. A large number of contributing factors have been identified and include decreased erythropoietin production, bone marrow suppression, shortened RBC survival, deficiencies of folate, iron, or vitamin B_{12}, and hemodilution. Consumptive coagulopathy, malignant hypertension, thrombotic thrombocytopenic purpura, and hemolytic uremic syndrome may all be associated with severe hemolytic anemia and ARF.

Diuretic Phase

The early diuretic phase is characterized by a steady rise in daily urine volume. The magnitude of this volume depends on a number of factors, including the rate of improvement in glomerular filtration and tubular reabsorption and the amount of excess solute and fluid retained by the patient during the oliguric period. Now that dialysis is utilized to remove excess solute and fluid, the massive diuresis noted commonly in earlier series is rarely seen. Increases in urine output of up to 5–6 liters/day may occur, however, so that close monitoring of body weight, fluid intake and output, and vital signs is mandatory during this period to prevent volume depletion or excessive fluid administration.

Generally, the BUN and creatinine levels peak and begin to fall with the onset of the diuresis. On occasion, however, the BUN and creatinine may continue to rise for several days into the diuretic phase. This is usually seen in the markedly catabolic patient who continues to produce urea at a rate faster than it can be excreted. In this setting a week may be required before the patient's metabolic state and glomerular filtration have improved enough to allow a fall in the BUN. It should be noted that during this early diuretic phase, the GFR is still markedly diminished and may well require weeks to months before it will approach the value present prior to the onset of the renal failure.

With increasing urine flow and GFR, marked urinary electrolyte loss may occur, and plasma Na, K, Mg, and PO_4 levels need to be monitored frequently. Hypercalcemia is sometimes seen at the onset of the diuretic phase. As discussed earlier, this is most commonly reported in patients with myoglobinuric renal failure and is felt to be due to the release by healing tissues of calcium salts which had been deposited at the time of injury to muscle.

It should be emphasized that the diuretic phase is a particularly critical time for the patient. Although it suggests that renal recovery is imminent and that the patient will survive, fully one-fourth of the mortality of FRF occurs during the diuretic phase. The potential for hemodynamic instability and serious electrolyte fluctuations is great, and the dangers of infection and gastrointestinal bleeding are still present. Thus continued vigilance is required during this phase. The duration of the diuretic phase is generally about 10 days.

Recovery Phase and Prognosis

After the diuretic phase has terminated, GFR may continue to improve for up to 1 year. In those patients who ultimately have complete recovery, a maximal creatinine clearance is reached in the first 3–6 months after the renal insult. In those who obtain less than complete recovery, the rate of improvement in GFR may be slower and the improvement may continue for up to a year.

In order to clarify the natural history of patients who recover from FRF, the renal function of a group of these patients was reexamined 1–7 years after recovery from the renal failure. The urinalysis, creatinine clearance, urinary concentrating ability and acidification capacity, and the IVP were evaluated. Almost all of the patients were clinically well. Despite this, less than one-third of the patients were normal in all of the parameters measured. Of interest, one group found that ischemic FRF was associated with a diminished GFR in 47 percent of the patients while nephrotoxic FRF caused a diminished GFR in only 25 percent. Also of interest was the finding that 10–20 percent of patients followed for up to 7 years showed a continuing decline in PAH clearance and inulin clearance. The clinical significance of these findings was not clear. Despite the alterations in renal function that were found, most of the patients had no further clinical difficulties with renal function and were not predisposed to recurrent renal failure or urinary tract infection. Some investigators, in fact, feel such patients may be resistant to subsequent episodes of FRF.

There are few useful predictors of how much renal function will return after an episode of FRF. In most series, patients older than 40 years at the time of insult seem to have less capacity for complete recovery. The severity of the FRF (the longer the duration of oliguria) seemed to correlate inversely with potential for recovery in some series but bore no relationship in others.

Mortality

Overall mortality rates have changed little during the interval from the 1950s, when dialysis was first widely used, to the 1970s. If one considers patients with FRF who require at least one dialysis, overall mortality rates of series consisting of surgical and medical patients is still 40–50 percent. Further breakdown of these groups of patients reveal that the cause of the renal failure may be a useful predictor of the outcome. Renal failure caused by nephrotoxic exposure, obstetric complication, or transfusion reaction is associated with a mortality rate of 25–35 percent. That associated with septic or cardiogenic shock may run as high as 60–75 percent. Renal failure associated with cardiovascular surgery, particulary if cardiopulmonary bypass is used, has a mortality of 60–70 percent. Burn victims with renal failure likewise have a very poor prognosis, with mortality rates greater than 90 percent.

What are the causes of death in these patients? In earlier series, significant mortality arose from potassium intoxication, digitalis intoxication, and volume overload with subsequent heart failure, hypertension, and stroke. With the use of early dialysis and more appropriate fluid and electrolyte management, these cause serious problems much less frequently. Unfortunately, the other three causes of death—overwhelming infection, gastrointestinal bleeding, and complications of the patient's underlying disease—continue as before despite the advent of better antibiotics and improved dialytic techniques.

Why present mortality statistics are no better than those noted in earlier series can probably be explained on the basis of a different patient population with renal failure being observed. Older series included relatively large numbers of younger women with acute renal failure secondary to obstetric complications. Excluding those with cortical necrosis, these patients tend to have a lower mortality. More recent series usually include fewer of these low-risk patients and include individuals who are older, have multiple organ system failure, and/ or have undergone major surgery. Several other factors that may affect survival statistics are (1) the severity of renal failure required to be included in the series' statistics, (2) the proportion of patients with nonoliguric renal failure, and (3) the proportion of patients with nephrotoxin induced renal failure. Both the patients with nonoliguric and those with nephrotoxin induced renal failure seem to have better prognoses.

How the mortality rate in a given group of patients with FRF can be improved is not clear. It was hoped that early aggressive dialysis would decrease mortality. It has become evident, however, that although frequent dialysis permits easier management and obviates most of the symptoms of uremia, it has not had a marked effect on wound healing or improving resistance to infection. Since infection continues to be the leading single cause of death in most series, more attention to this area might be worthwhile. Improved efforts at antisepsis (especially in the postoperative patient), the development of more effective antibiotics, and aggressive early diagnosis and management of infection might result in improved survival. In addition, nutritional supplementation in the protein depleted patient may be of benefit in preventing or combating infection. The problem of gastrointestinal bleeding may be diminished through the use of a histamine H_2 blocker such as cimetidine, although this point has not yet been studied. Since magnesium salts are usually contraindicated in FRF and aluminum salts are often not as effective as an antacid or as well tolerated, treatment of the gastrointestinal hemorrhage may be made more effective with newer drugs of this type.

Prophylaxis and Treatment

With the mortality of FRF persisting at about 50 percent, it is clear that the best treatment program is one of prevention. This is possible in many cases. Proper blood banking techniques should virtually eliminate renal failure due to transfusion reactions. Drugs which are nephrotoxins should be identified and avoided whenever possible. If these drugs are deemed necessary, the lowest dose should be used and other drugs which may potentiate their nephrotoxicity should be avoided. IVPs and other studies requiring the use of contrast media should be done only when indicated and avoided whenever possible in the patient with multiple myeloma or diabetes mellitus or when renal impairment is already present. If the study is deemed necessary, the patient should be adequately hydrated beforehand. Renal failure associated with sepsis may be preventable through early diagnosis and institution of appropriate therapy. Overly aggressive diuresis in edematous states such as cirrhosis, nephrotic syndrome, and congestive heart failure should be avoided. Maintenance of an adequate effective blood volume in situations associated with fluid losses is equally important. Appropriate treatment of hypercalcemia and hyperuricemia (particularly in the patient undergoing chemotherapy for neoplasia) should limit the incidence of ARF in these settings.

In addition to the above, it may be possible to modify or prevent the development of FRF in situations known to be associated with it by administering mannitol or furosemide. There is experimental evidence to show that when mannitol is given prior to a hemodynamic insult to the kidney, it may prevent the onset of renal failure. In another experimental model, administration of mannitol after the induction of ischemia resulted in the restoration of glomerular filtration (which was absent prior to the mannitol). This effect was not seen with saline administration. Thus the mannitol must have exerted its effects through a mechanism other than volume expansion. Mannitol has also been reported to be of benefit in human FRF. In the 1950s, a high incidence of postoperative FRF was reported in patients undergoing cardiovascular surgery. Subsequently, it was observed that the use of intravenous mannitol prior to and during aortic surgery was associated with a lower incidence of postoperative oliguria and FRF. This therapy is now used frequently in this surgical setting. Other reports have suggested a beneficial effect of mannitol in the treatment of FRF due to myoglobinuria, acute hemolysis, and burns. Its efficacy in these settings is not well established, but since it is relatively nontoxic and may be effective, a trial of mannitol may be warranted. The administration of mannitol does impose a solute load on the cardiovascular system; thus its use in volume overloaded patients should be discouraged.

The potent loop acting diuretic furosemide has been suggested to exert a beneficial effect in FRF in some clinical and experimental settings. In some animal studies, furosemide has caused an increase in RBF and GFR; however, in others, no increase was demonstrable and indeed GFR and RBF fell if volume depletion was induced. Tubular obstruction with cast formation presumably plays an important role in the generation of FRF. Thus it is possible that an increase in urine flow engendered by furosemide may permit dislodgement of these casts and reversal or modulation of the renal failure; yet there is really no substantial evidence that furosemide can reverse the fall in GFR seen in fixed FRF. Rather, it has been clearly demonstrated that furosemide may cause the conversion of oliguric renal failure to nonoliguric renal failure. In one series nonoliguric renal failure was associated with a lower incidence of hyperkalemia, heart failure, sepsis, gastrointestinal bleeding, and death (regardless of whether the high urine output was spontaneous or induced with furosemide). Others have noted that furosemide administration, while not changing the ultimate outcome of the renal failure, was associated with less hyperkalemia and fluid overload and thus diminished the need for dialysis. It would thus seem reasonable to use a moderate dose of furosemide to determine whether the drug will cause an increase in the urine output and potassium excretion. Only moderate doses of furosemide should be used, since doses greater than 1.5 g/day have been associated with temporary and, on occasion, permanent ototoxicity. If the drug has no effect, it should be discontinued.

Measurement of Established ARF

Once ARF is detected, the principles of treatment center around excluding reversible or treatable causes of ARF and then anticipating and appropriately managing the complications known to be associated with ARF (Table 4). The major reversible causes of ARF were discussed in the section on differential diagnosis.

Potential problems that need to be addressed initially include the state of hydration and the serum Na and K levels. The goal of fluid therapy is to achieve an effective blood volume and avoid water intoxication. The appropriate blood volume may be determined by utilizing the usual parameters such as vital signs, tissue turgor, and assumed dry weight. In the patient with large third space sequestration, such as is seen in the postoperative patient, the trauma victim, or the patient with heart failure, determination of fluid needs may require the monitoring of central venous or pulmonary wedge pressure.

As noted earlier in this chapter, catabolism of body tissues usually generates at least 400 cc of free water per day. Since insensible losses of water average about 500 cc per day, the administration of much more than 100 cc plus the amount excreted in the urine will lead to overhydration. With the generation of free water from metabolism of body tissues and its elimination via insensible losses, the patient should lose about 0.5–1 pound (0.2–0.4 kg) per day. If the patient does not demonstrate this weight loss, he is either not as catabolic as suspected or he is retaining fluid. If the latter occurs, symptomatic hyponatremia may ensue. Ingestion or administration of NaCl in excess of that excreted in the urine and/or lost through the gastrointestinal tract may lead to expansion of the extracellular fluid volume. This may be associated with hypertension, heart failure, or stroke. If volume overload is present, dialytic removal of the excess NaCl will usually be necessary.

Potassium intoxication may cause significant morbidity and mortality in ARF. It is most commonly a problem in the settings of trauma, nontraumatic rhabdomyolysis, extensive surgery, blood administration, and hypercatabolic states. As noted earlier, the major toxic effect is on the heart. Both the electrocardiogram and the serum K need to be closely monitored, since the cardiac toxicity may be more significant than might be predicted by the serum K alone. A serum K of 6.5–7.5 mEq/liter is usually associated with peaking of the T waves. When the serum K is 7.5 mEq/liter, one may see prolongation of the PR interval, loss of the P wave, and prolongation of the QRS complex. Treatment should be instituted prior to development of the latter ECG findings. The mode of therapy to be used depends on the severity of the hyperkalemia. In all cases, potassium removal from the body will be required either through the use of orally administered cation exchange resins or dialysis with a low-potassium bath. If ECG changes are present, rapid lowering of the serum K is required, and this may be achieved by shifting potassium into cells from the extracellular fluid with intravenous administration of glucose and insulin and/or bicarbonate. If serious cardiac dysrhythmias are present, the effect of hyperkalemia on the heart may be counteracted with intravenous calcium gluconate 2 ml/min for a total of 10–20 cc. Calcium chloride is also effective.

Metabolic acidosis usually does not require therapy in the early phases of FRF. The bicarbonate concentration is usually only moderately diminished, and most patients are able to maintain a near-normal pH with respiratory compensation. Bicarbonate administration necessitates simultaneous sodium administration with the attendant problem of volume expansion. Thus when acidosis is severe enough to require treatment, dialysis is the best mode of therapy. Occasionally severe hy-

Table 4
Management of Established Functional Renal Failure

Data base
Monitor daily weight, urine output, fluid intake and output, serum Na, K, Cl, CO_2, glucose
Monitor serial (as needed) CBC, Ca^{2+}, PO_4^{2-}, Mg^{2+}, arterial pH

Diet (if patient not dialyzed)
2 g Na, 20–40 mEq K, 20–40 g protein
Fluids—intake volume should equal urine output plus about 500 cc/day
Nutritional supplementation (see text)

Therapeutic modalities for:
Hyperkalemia
Excretion (when $k>6$), kayexalate (p.o.), dialysis (when necessary)
Redistribution (when $k>7$), glucose and insulin (i.v.), $NaHCO_3$ (i.v.)
Antagonism of potassium effects (in presence of cardiac toxicity), calcium salts (i.v.)
Volume overload—loop acting diuretics, dialysis (when necessary)
Metabolic acidosis—maintain pH>7.25, sodium citrate or sodium bicarbonate, dialysis
Uremic symptoms and/or BUN >100 mg/dl—dialysis
Hypertension—correction of volume overload, antihypertensive medication (if needed after fluid volume corrected)
Hyperphosphatemia—aluminum salts (p.o.), dialysis
Hyponatremia—fluid restriction, dialysis
GI bleeding from peptic ulcer disease—avoid magnesium-containing antacid, may use H_2 blocker such as cimetidine in reduced dose

---

perphosphatemia with hypocalcemia may be seen in patients with marked tissue necrosis. Management of this consists of oral administration of large amounts of phosphate binding antacids. Dialysis may also be utilized for phosphate removal. Intravenous calcium should be given only if the patient develops symptomatic hypocalcemia.

The use of nutritional supplementation was briefly considered earlier. The marked tissue catabolism frequently found in patients with FRF causes release of large amounts of potassium, nitrogenous waste products, and fixed acids into the extracellular fluid. Several studies have shown that this process may be slowed or reversed through the administration of adequate amounts of calories and essential amino acids. The caloric needs of the postoperative or septic patient may thus be met and body protein stores spared. Some workers have suggested that this form of nutritional therapy may allow reutilization of urea nitrogen for protein synthesis, but this issue is presently unclear. Nutritional supplementation may be administered parenterally through a large central vein or may be given via enteral alimentation. Lipid emulsions, unlike the hypertonic glucose mixtures, are isotonic and may be given via peripheral veins. Recommended caloric intake ranges from 35 to 50 kcal/kg/day. Daily protein intake has usually been restricted to 30–40 g in the past, but this limit may be increased to 60 g or more if dialysis is utilized concurrently. Vitamins, including the B complex group, are usually administered at the same time.

When hyperalimentation is employed, some undesired metabolic effects may be encountered, but these can usually be managed without discontinuing the hyperalimentation. For example, supplemental insulin is often needed to control hyperglycemia. Modification of the relative quantities of the carbohydrate, fat, and protein infused may also be required to limit hyperglycemia, hypertriglyceridemia, and worsening azotemia. Metabolic acidosis may be precipitated or worsened by the administration of protein hydrolysates. This may require discontinuation of the infusion or use of another source of amino acids. Hypophosphatemia, hypomagnesemia, and hypocalcemia may all be seen. Supplemental phosphate, magnesium, and calcium are usually necessary. Frequent monitoring of the serum levels of these substances is mandatory. Nonmetabolic complications such as sepsis and pneumothorax secondary to placement of central venous catheters are relatively infrequent in centers experienced in the use of parenteral nutrition.

Hyperalimentation has been demonstrated to be beneficial in FRF, particularly in the surgical setting. In one surgical series, hyperalimentation was associated with a decrease in urea production, a positive nitrogen balance, a lowering of the serum concentrations of potassium, phosphate, and magnesium, and a diminished need for dialysis. In addition, an increase in survival and a shortening of the duration of the FRF were found when hyperalimentation was compared to glucose administration. In a more recent study with both medical and surgical patients with FRF, hyperalimentation was found to have a statistically beneficial effect only when multiple complicating factors were present.

Anabolic steroids have been used in an attempt to induce a positive nitrogen balance, but the results of their use have been equivocal.

Since the 1950s and 1960s the mainstay of the

management of the patient with FRF has been dialysis. Either hemodialysis or peritoneal dialysis may be employed, depending on available facilities. At the present time, it is initiated when the BUN is greater than 100 mg/dl, when volume overload is difficult to manage, or when uremic symptoms develop. It may also be required when medical management of hyperkalemia or acidosis is inadequate. Markedly catabolic patients whose course is frequently complicated by severe hyperkalemia and hyperphosphatemia sometimes are begun on hemodialysis before the above criteria are met, and these patients may require daily dialysis. The use of prophylactic dialysis has simplified management of fluid and electrolyte problems and has permitted patients to ingest a relatively normal diet. In most series, however, its use has not greatly altered mortality rates over the past 20 years, nor does it seem to have directly affected recovery of renal function. Many patients with FRF may be effectively managed with appropriate fluid and electrolyte therapy, administration of adequate doses of diuretics and potassium exchange resins, and careful nutritional supplementation without necessitating dialysis.

REFERENCES

Arendhorst WJ, Finn WF, Gottschalk CW: Pathogenesis of acute renal failure following temporary renal ischemia in the rat. Circ Res 37:558, 1975

Heptinstall RH: Pathology of the Kidney (ed 2). Boston, Little, Brown, 1974, p 781

Levinsky NG, Alexander EA: Acute renal failure in the kidney, in Brenner BM, Rector FC Jr (eds): The Kidney, Vol 2. Philadelphia, W.B. Saunders, 1976, p 806

Levinsky NG: Pathophysiology of acute renal failure. N Engl J Med 296:1453, 1977

McMurray SD, Luft FC, Maxwell DR, et al: Prevailing patterns and predictor variables in patients with acute tubular necrosis. Arch Intern Med 138:950, 1978

Miller TR, Anderson RJ, Linas SL, et al: Urinary diagnostic indices in acute renal failure. Ann Intern Med 89:47, 1978

Stein J, Lifschitz M, Barnes LD: Current concepts on the pathophysiology of acute renal failure. Am J Physiol 234:F171, 1978

Swann RC, Merrill JP: The clinical course of acute renal failure. Medicine (Baltimore) 32:215, 1953

CHRONIC RENAL FAILURE— CLASSIFICATION

Jacques J. Bourgoignie and Allan I. Jacob

Less than two decades ago, renal failure was a terminal and fatal event that physicians could only watch helplessly. Now, life can be supported by chronic dialysis or renal transplantation. Each of these procedures has the potential for reversing the most disabling manifestations of chronic renal failure, and, with both, many patients achieve at least partial physical and emotional

rehabilitation; however, neither of these therapeutic modalities of endstage renal disease is ideal. The most recent transplant registry shows that the expected graft survival rate at 2 years with related transplant donors is approximately 70 percent; with cadaveric donors, this figure is reduced to less than 50 percent. It is distressing, however, that little improvement in graft survival figures has occurred recently in either group of transplant recipients. Similarly, chronic dialysis continues to carry a significant mortality (about 10 percent per year) and a very high morbidity.

Although the victim of progressive renal disease no longer faces death as the result of renal failure, the patient still must experience the suffering and the incapacity that occur during the months to years that the symptoms of uremia advance. As renal function progressively diminishes and dialysis becomes a quickly approaching reality, the patient has difficulties with self-image. Although the patient is instructed to lead as normal a life as possible within the constraints of diet and dialysis schedules and to expect a certain degree of rehabilitation, he clearly remains ill in the traditional sense and requires medical attention and care. Many patients become discouraged and slowly withdraw from the surrounding world. In addition, the financial burden imposed on individual patients and their families by dialysis or transplantation is usually devastating in spite of governmental subsidies. It is estimated that by 1982 nearly 60,000 patients will be undergoing chronic dialysis or renal transplantation with four to five times that number suffering from progressive chronic renal disease. The cost of health care to this group is likely to exceed 2.5 billion dollars annually.

Our understanding of complicating factors that may accelerate the progression of renal failure, such as hypertension, extracellular fluid volume depletion, hypercalcemia, severe hyperuricemia, nephrolithiasis, nephrotoxic agents, and congestive heart failure, has improved greatly. Unfortunately no important therapeutic breakthrough has occurred which would reverse or halt the development of chronic intrinsic renal disease. Moreover, there is the danger of considering chronic dialysis and renal transplantation as final therapeutic modalities and becoming complacent in the workup of patients with chronic renal disease. Thus it behooves the physician to diagnose precisely the underlying etiology of renal disease and to attempt to maintain renal function in patients with chronic renal disease for as long as possible. Many patients when first seen have advanced renal insufficiency associated with small kidneys in whom a biopsy is not performed and a definitive histopathological diagnosis is unavailable. In spite of these difficulties a reliable etiological diagnosis can be made in most patients with renal failure utilizing a detailed family and personal history and minimally invasive techniques of investigation.

A wide variety of intrinsic renal diseases are capable of relentless destruction of the kidneys. In addition, a number of systemic diseases have renal manifestations that can lead to renal failure. With better therapeutic control of systemic disease the incidence of these renal complications is clearly increasing.

Causes of chronic renal failure have been classified on the bases of morphology, etiology, immunology, preventability, response to treatment, clinical presentation, incidence, etc. Since most, if not all, forms of renal disease can result in chronicity and lead to renal failure, we have elected not to develop an encyclopedic review but restrict our comments to some causes of chronic renal disease with particular emphasis on those diseases where prevention may be possible. The major causes of chronic renal failure are listed in Table 1. Some of the diseases listed primarily affect and are restricted to the kidneys; others are systemic diseases with secondary renal involvement.

The most common cause of chronic renal disease is *primary glomerular disease*. Clinical evidence of a glomerulopathy includes erythrocyte casts in the urinary sediment and a protein excretion of 2 g or more daily, but the definitive diagnosis of glomerulonephritis rests with the findings on renal biopsy. The term chronic glomerulonephritis refers to the clinical expression of a broad variety of glomerulopathic states. The early stages are characterized by abnormalities of the urinary sediment, proteinuria, and slight reductions in glomerular filtration rate. The disease may progress rapidly or over several decades into endstage renal disease. Hypertension and the nephrotic syndrome may accompany the course of many chronic glomerulonephritides. In some patients, hypertension may be an early and predominant finding, and such patients may be incorrectly diagnosed as having essential hypertension; however, attention to the findings in the urinary sediment will usually signal the presence of primary renal disease. Other patients may have a past history of acute glomerulonephritis or exacerbations of chronic glomerulonephritis following viral or bacterial infections. A substantial number of these patients present with markedly advanced renal insufficiency that precludes renal biopsy. Nevertheless, a broad pathological view may be constructed. Kidney size is generally grossly reduced, mostly due to cortical atrophy. At this stage, the histological changes often consist of obliterated, obsolescent glomeruli with tubular atrophy, interstitial fibrosis, and vascular disease. A biopsy performed early in the course identifies specific glomerular histopathological abnormalities. In such cases, proliferative and membranoproliferative glomerulonephritis are the most common findings, with focal sclerosis and membranous glomerulopathies occurring less often. Since the natural histories of most primary glomerulopathies span many years, therapeutic interventions are difficult to evaluate; and there is little convincing evidence that therapeutic interventions alter the course of these primary renal diseases.

Another common type of renal disease leading to chronic renal failure is *chronic interstitial nephritis* (see the chapter on *Interstitial Disease*). Clinical and laboratory characteristics typical of interstitial nephritis include sterile pyuria, a urinary protein excretion of less than 2 g daily, and evidence of disproportionately severe tubular dysfunction such as salt wasting, hyperchloremic acidosis, or early hypocalcemia. White blood cell casts may appear during acute exacerbations. Intravenous pyelography reveals asymmetric scarring, calyceal distortion, or papillary necrosis. As the clinical entity of chronic interstitial nephritis has become better defined, it is apparent that a specific etiology can usually be assigned in most patients. The most frequent causes of interstitial nephritis are anatomical abnormalities of the genitourinary tract, analgesic abuse, hyperuricemia, hypercalcemia, hypertensive nephrosclerosis, and nephrolithiasis. Less common causes include sickle cell disease and renal tuberculosis. Interstitial nephritis, previously referred to as chronic pyelonephritis, has received much recent attention directed towards the role that recurrent urinary tract infection may play in its natural history. Early investigators had considered chronic infection as the cause of the pathological abnormalities of interstitial nephritis. More recent data suggest that chronic urinary tract infection may rarely be the primary cause of chronic renal disease in the adult. Infection, when present, is usually the consequence of underlying renal disease and may contribute secondarily to impairment of renal function.

The importance of analgesic abuse as a cause of renal failure has become increasingly evident (see the chapters on *Interstitial Disease* and *Toxic Nephropathy*). Although it has been long appreciated in Australia and in Europe, many North American physicians have only recently become aggressive in considering this

Table 1
Etiology of Chronic Renal Failure

Common	Less Common	Rare
Glomerulonephritis	Polycystic kidney	Acute renal failure without resolution
Interstitial nephritis	Hereditary renal disease	Multiple myeloma
Hypertension	Systemic lupus erythematosus	Amyloidosis
Diabetes mellitus	Sickle cell disease	Gout
Obstructive uropathy		Tuberculosis
		Polyarteritis nodosa
		Wegener's syndrome
		Nephrocalcinosis

important and potentially reversible cause of renal disease. The analgesic abuser is typically a middle aged female with chronic headaches or abdominal pains. She will usually deny taking analgesics, and the history is most often obtained from close relatives. Although such patients represent a diagnostic challenge to the physician, withdrawal from the offending agent may halt or reverse the progressive deterioration in renal function. Removal of phenacetin from both proprietary and prescription medications has been shown to significantly reduced the incidence of chronic interstitial nephritis in Scandinavia and should be implemented in the United States.

Nearly 10 percent of patients with *diabetes mellitus* succumb to renal failure (see the chapter on *Diabetes Mellitus*). As therapy for nonrenal complications of diabetes improves, an increasing number of diabetics survive to develop endstage renal disease. As renal disease progresses, however, they suffer more serious neuropathic and cardiovascular complications. A larger number of diabetics are being hemodialyzed and transplanted, and diabetes is no longer considered a contraindication to these therapeutic modalities; however, the mortality rate for diabetics on hemodialysis approaches 50 percent in the first year.

Hypertension is probably the most common single entity where aggressive therapy and control of blood pressure can result in prevention of renal disease or progression of preexisting disease toward renal failure (see the chapter on *Hypertension*). High blood pressure will lead to renal damage, and, conversely, chronic renal disease of any etiology is often complicated by hypertension. Strict control of hypertension may defer the onset of dialysis. Moreover, in some instances, patients with hypertensive disease and renal failure have been able to withdraw from chronic dialysis with control of the hypertension.

Chronic obstruction of the urinary tract will lead to renal insufficiency, especially in children and in elderly men (see the chapter on *Obstructive Uropathy*). Obstruction may occur alone or as a concomitant event complicating renal failure of other etiologies. Because of the potential reversibility of this insult, obstruction must always be considered and ruled out in the evaluation of a patient with a deteriorating renal function, even when a documented nonobstructive form of renal disease exists.

Another cause of chronic renal failure is *hereditary nephritis*. This broad category of diseases is generally characterized by a progressive course, hematuria, and a well documented familial incidence. The clinical, pathological, and genetic features of this disorder appear to be highly variable. Some families have only renal disease, while others have associated sensorineural deafness, ocular or neurological abnormalities, or thrombocytopathia. When hereditary renal disease is associated with nerve deafness it has been termed Alport's syndrome (see the chapter on *Alport's syndrome*). Microscopic hematuria is the most frequent

and often the only urinary abnormality present. Erythrocytic casts are found in most affected men and about half of affected women. This finding, as well as the characteristic fraying or lamellation of the glomerular basement membrane seen on electron microscopy of biopsy specimens, indicates that hereditary nephritis is a glomerulopathy. The X-linked inheritance explains the clinical observation that men are more severely afflicted than women. In fact, almost all men with this disorder require dialysis before the age of 50 years.

Another form of hereditary renal failure is adult *polycystic kidney disease* (see the chapter on *Polycystic Renal Disease*). Transmitted as an autosomal dominant trait, polycystic kidney is characterized by grossly cystic changes throughout the renal parenchyma. It is frequently associated with recurrent painful hematuria and palpable renomegaly. Progressive renal failure, hypertension, and hyperchloremic metabolic acidosis are characteristic. Intravenous urography is usually diagnostic in this disorder. Most patients develop endstage renal disease at a characteristic age for their family history, but many suffer less anemia and bone disease than patients with renal failure from other etiologies.

About two-thirds of patients with well documented *systemic lupus erythematosus* will have overt evidence of clinical renal involvement (see the chapter on *Systemic Lupus Erythematosus*). A small proportion of these patients, particularly those with membranoproliferative glomerulonephritis, will progress to endstage renal disease requiring chronic hemodialysis. Curiously, most clinical manifestations of systemic lupus may vanish with the development of endstage renal disease or when dialysis is initiated.

Chronic renal failure complicating *multiple myeloma* has become more frequent as survival is improved with chemotherapy (see the chapter on *Multiple Myeloma*). Myeloma kidney, characterized pathologically by diffuse tubular atrophy with dense lamellated casts often associated with multinucleated giant cells in the interstitium, is frequently associated with Bence Jones proteinuria.

Amyloidosis, either primary or secondary, may also contribute to renal failure (see the chapter on *Amyloidosis*). The progression of myeloma or amyloid renal disease may be slowed by chemotherapy, but frequently these patients require hemodialysis.

REFERENCES

Ahlmen J, Gustafsson A, Storm B: Morbidity in azotemia and mortality in uremia. Acta Med Scand 192:113, 1972

Friedman EA, Delano BG, Butt KMH: Pragmatic realities in uremia therapy. N Engl J Med 298:368, 1978

Landsman MK: The patient with chronic renal failure: A marginal man. Ann Intern Med 82:268, 1975

Murray T, Goldberg M: Chronic interstitial nephritis: Etiologic factors. Ann Intern Med 82:453, 1975

O'Neill WM Jr, Atking CL, Bloomer HA: Hereditary nephritis: A re-examination of its clinical and genetic features. Ann Intern Med 88:176, 1978

CHRONIC RENAL FAILURE—
PATHOPHYSIOLOGY

Jacques J. Bourgoignie and Michael M. Kaplan

The normal kidneys in health regulate and maintain external balance for water and a number of solutes.* They also participate in the synthesis and metabolism of a series of hormones. Diseases of the kidneys therefore have their expression and result in derangements of external balance and in endocrine abnormalities. While these manifestations are dramatic and often fatal when renal failure develops acutely, they may remain clinically inapparent during the course of chronic progressive renal disease until renal failure supervenes.

In addition to irreversibility, chronic renal disease differs from acute renal disease in one important aspect: it is insidious, gradual, and relentlessly progressive, developing over a period of years or even decades, often without the patient's awareness. Typically, the patient with chronic renal disease remains asymptomatic and demonstrates only few biochemical abnormalities until 70–80 percent of nephrons have been lost or until the glomerular filtration rate (GFR) has decreased to values of about 25 ml/min. In some instances, such as in patients with polycystic kidneys, survival on a normal diet is the rule, often without symptoms, even at GFR values of 5 ml/min or less.

A great variety of chronic forms of diseases are capable of irreversible nephron destruction. The etiology and pathogenesis of these diseases vary widely, yet as chronic renal failure supervenes, their manifestations in different patients, by and large, are remarkably similar. These similarities make it possible to formulate common principles of pathophysiology that apply to the great majority of patients, irrespective of the underlying pathogenic (infectious, immunological, vascular or other) mechanism responsible for the nephron destruction.** An analysis of the mechanisms and adaptations which allow patients with progressive nephron loss and chronic renal failure to survive is the subject of this chapter. General concepts will be formulated followed by limited comments on specific solutes.

BASIS FOR SURVIVAL: NEPHRON
ADAPTATION

Characteristic of normal kidneys is the tremendous functional reserve available to the nephrons which allows them to adjust and maintain balance in health over very large ranges of water and solute intakes. The normal individual can regulate water excretion to match intake over a range of less than 0.5 liter to as much as 22 liters a day. External balance for sodium is maintained over a range from essentially zero to in excess of 500 mEq/day. Normal kidneys allow the diabetic patient with ketoacidosis to excrete well in excess of 500 mEq hydrogen ions per day, while, under circumstances where alkalosis exists, the same patient may curtail hydrogen ion excretion to zero.

Thus it is apparent that normal nephrons have a marked potential for adjustment and great functional flexibility. They adapt their function to the need of the organism. It appears that the same mechanisms responsible for these functional adjustments in health remain operative in individuals with chronic renal disease.

In contrast, these functional adjustments do not exist, or, if they exist, they cannot be expressed in acute renal failure. For instance, secondary hyperparathyroidism is present in both acute and chronic renal failure and has been viewed as an adaptation to increase phosphorus excretion and restore phosphorus balance. The latter can be achieved in chronic renal failure. In acute renal failure all the nephrons are damaged and the end organ is destroyed without time allowance permitting development of the adaptations at the nephron level.

INTACT NEPHRON HYPOTHESIS
Effect of Disease per se on Kidney Function

Although the various disorders listed in the preceding chapter usually result in some specific anatomical changes that a pathologist can recognize in the early stage of disease, in the advanced stage certain features common to most forms of chronic renal disease develop. Usually the kidneys are small, often weighing less than one-third of normal, the cortical zone is narrowed, and it may be difficult to recognize glomeruli on gross inspection. Microscopically, the morphological changes in chronic renal disease are characterized by heterogeneous alterations. Some glomeruli are hypertrophic; others appear normal or completely atrophic. Tubules are reduced in number; some are atrophic, others normal or hypertrophic. They may show segmental abnormalities of dilatation, atrophy, or hypertrophy. Fibrosis of the interstitium may be dominant.

The functional ability of the patient with chronic

---

*External balance is defined as the equality that exists for water or any given solute between the amounts that have access to and exit from the extracellular fluid volume. For water and solutes primarily excreted by the kidney, balance is maintained when renal excretion is equal to the amount absorbed from the GI tract and/or produced by metabolism.

**Diseases that affect specific segments of the nephrons can have specific functional expressions. In particular, diseases that distort the medullary architecture can interfere preferentially with potassium secretion, ammonium excretion, calcium reabsorption, or urinary concentration. Patients with intersti-

tial diseases or cystic diseases of the kidney do appear to develop defects related to the handling of specific solutes and water earlier in their course and to a more severe degree than patients with glomerular diseases. Usually, these specific defects are not apparent under conditions where external balance exists. They can be evoked and become more readily overt when the system is stressed such as under conditions of acute loading. In advanced stages of renal disease, however, the same functional impairments occur in all forms of renal disease, and group data comparisons then generally fail to differentiate between patients with glomerular disease and those with nonglomerular disease of the kidney.

renal disease often offers a striking contrast with the histological anarchy that seems to prevail in the end-stage kidney. Recognition of this contrast led to a series of clinical and experimental observations which resulted in the formulation of the intact nephron hypothesis. The hypothesis states that in progressive renal disease the residual nephrons function as if they were normal.

Effects of Disease per se on Nephron Function

The original studies designed to examine the patterns in which the composite population of nephrons functions as an integrated whole were performed in experimental animals in which a chronic form of renal disease was induced in one of the two kidneys. The function of each kidney was then simultaneously studied using a clearance methodology to compare a series of tubular functions to the simultaneously measured GFR. When the ratios of various tubular functions in the diseased kidney were compared with those of the intact kidney, closely comparable values were obtained.

This is illustrated in Table 1 for ammonium excretion by each kidney of the same dog before (stage I) and after (stage II) induction of pyelonephritis in one kidney. Ammonium excretion is well suited for an analysis of the functional pattern of the diseased kidney because of the complex metabolic and transport events necessary for ammonium excretion. Because ammonia is secreted both in the proximal and in the distal tubules, any systematically induced defects of nephron function by the disease process per se would be expected to alter the pattern of ammonium excretion by the diseased kidney. At stage I, when both kidneys were normal, GFR and ammonium excretion were similar for both organs. Between stage I and stage II, pyelonephritis was induced in one kidney and the function of both kidneys was reinvestigated 14 days later. The induction of unilateral pyelonephritis resulted in a 65 percent decrease in GFR in the diseased organ but an 11 percent increase in GFR in the normal kidney. The induction of disease resulted in a 56 percent reduction in ammonium excretion in the diseased kidney in association with a 39 percent increase in the control organ. $U_{NH_4}V$/GFR depicts the changes in ammonium excretion in relation

to the simultaneous changes in GFR. The ratio prior to induction of disease (stage I) averaged 131 μEq per 100 ml GFR for both kidneys. After induction of unilateral disease ammonium excretion increased proportionately more than GFR in the control kidney and averaged 159 μEq per 100 ml GFR. Hence the relationship between ammonium excretion and GFR was reset in the nephrons of the control kidney. In the diseased kidney, the value of ammonium excretion per 100 ml GFR was similarly and equally reset. Thus the residual nephrons of the diseased organ appear to respond in an intact fashion to whatever stimuli resulted in a 39 percent increase in ammonium excretion in the normal kidney.

An equality of clearance ratios for tubular to glomerular functions between the intact and the diseased kidney has been observed for a variety of solutes undergoing very different processes in the tubules. Equality pertains for substances mainly reabsorbed in the proximal tubule (glucose, bicarbonate, and phosphate), secreted in the proximal tubule (PAH), reabsorbed in the proximal tubule and secreted in the distal tubule (potassium), or secreted throughout the nephron (ammonium). This finding indicates that the relationship that exists between glomerular and tubular functions remains intact in normal and in diseased kidneys. The equality of ratios also was evident whether the induced disease was of glomerular, interstitial, or vascular origin.

A quantitative analysis of equal clearance ratios indicates that for any given volume of glomerular filtrate the nephrons of the diseased kidney excrete exactly the same number of molecules of the measured solute as do the nephrons of the contralateral intact organ.

These observations establish the fact that in chronic renal disease the residual nephrons function in a highly organized fashion and in a manner similar to that of intact nephrons. They clearly establish that the presence of disease per se does not disrupt the normal patterns of function in individual nephron units. The overall decrease in function of the diseased kidney is related to the loss in the total number of nephron units rather than to the loss of glomerular or specific tubular

Table 1

Effects of Disease per se and Influence of Uremia on Ammonium Excretion in Experimental Dogs With Unilateral Pyelonephritis During Induced Metabolic Acidosis

	Stage I		Stage II		Stage III
	C	E	C	E	E
Kidney GFR (ml/min)	40.5	40.3	44.7	14.7	19.7
Total GFR	80.8		59.4		19.7
$U_{NH_4}V$ (μEq/min)	52.7	53.9	73.1	24.0	42.3
Total $U_{NH_4}V$ (*m*Eq/min)	106.6		97.1		42.3
$U_{UH_4}V$ per 100 ml GFR (*m*EQ/100 ml)	130	132	159	163	226

C, control kidney with pyelonephritis.

Data from Dorhout-Mees EJ, Machado M, Slatopolsky E, et al: The functional adaptation of the diseased kidney. III Ammonium excretion. J Clin Invest 45:289, 1966.

functions only. They also establish that if filtration rate in functioning nephrons changes in either direction, tubular function in the appended tubules changes proportionately. Thus if damaged nephrons contribute significantly to renal function, they neither set nor dominate the patterns of renal function. Rather, they behave as if they were normal.

The data of Table 1 also demonstrate that when the GFR of the experimental kidney was reduced to 45 percent of its value in stage I, that of the healthy, control kidney had undergone a compensatory increase; consequently, the total GFR at stage II was still 82 percent of the value obtained at stage I, and uremia was prevented.

EFFECTS OF UREMIA ON KIDNEY FUNCTION

The observations described so far were obtained in experimental models in which uremia was not present because of the presence of the contralateral intact kidney. Let us now consider the function of the chronically diseased kidney in the presence of uremia. In Table 1, stage III represents this condition after removal of the control kidney. Although there was a 34 percent compensatory increase in the GFR of the diseased kidney, it was not sufficient to prevent uremia, for now total GFR had been reduced to 24 percent of the value in stage I. By as yet largely unknown mechanisms, the uremic environment resulted in an increased ability of the diseased kidney to produce ammonia. The relationship between ammonium excretion and GFR was again reset at a higher value of ammonium excretion per 100 ml GFR; however, although an increase in ammonium excretion per 100 ml GFR took place which resulted in a 75 percent increase in ammonium excretion by the diseased kidney (from 163 to 226 μEq/100 ml GFR between stage II and stage III), total ammonium excretion averaged only 40 percent of stage I values, an amount insufficient to preserve hydrogen balance.

Table 1 illustrates several important points: (1) chronic renal disease and chronic renal failure are not synonymous. During stage II there was chronic renal disease but the animal was not in failure, not only because the number of nephrons had not been reduced markedly but also because there had been a compensatory hypertrophy in the function of the remaining nephrons: (2) These adaptations occur early in chronic renal disease; they were evident during stage II in the contralateral control kidney in the absence of uremia: (3) chronic renal failure arises essentially from a critical reduction in the number of nephrons rather than from damage to nephrons. Even diseased nephrons increased their GFR and their production of ammonia; the uremic state of chronic renal failure did not occur until the number of nephrons had been drastically reduced by removing the control kidney.

Thus chronic renal disease is characterized by orderly adaptations in the remaining nephrons. Ablation of renal mass results in hypertrophy with increase in GFR and simultaneous parallel functional changes in the aggregate of the surviving units. These adjustments

are so finely attuned to the need of the body that external balance for water and a number of solutes is precisely maintained until the very late stages of chronic renal disease.

COMPENSATORY HYPERTROPHY IN CHRONIC RENAL DISEASE

The stimulus for compensatory renal growth in surviving tissue is not known but occurs rapidly after reduction in renal mass. After uninephrectomy in rats an increase in cell membrane production is demonstrable within 5 min. A true increase in kidney weight occurs within 24 hours, and within 1–2 weeks renal mass increases 30–40 percent. This compensatory hypertrophy occurs in the glomeruli and in the tubules. In contrast to the uniform growth patterns which occur after uninephrectomy, the structural changes of chronic glomerulonephritis in man and animals present a pattern of heterogeneity in size and shape of glomeruli and tubules. Nevertheless, as emphasized above, the capacity for functional adaptation exists irrespective of the cause of nephron loss.

The formation of new cells probably plays an important role in the response to nephron loss, although the relative importance of hypertrophy and hyperplasia has not been determined. There is no increase, however, in the number of nephrons after uninephrectomy.

The primary stimulus for compensatory renal growth has not been determined, but changes in renal electrolytes transport and associated energy related processes do not stimulate growth.

CHANGES IN RENAL BLOOD FLOW

Reduction in functioning renal mass following surgery or experimental parenchymal renal disease is associated with striking increases in blood flow to individual nephrons. In animals with glomerulonephritis there is also evidence for an increase in blood flow in the less damaged portions of the kidney. An alteration in the pattern of blood flow distribution with disproportionate increases in flow in the deep portions of the remnant kidney has also been described.

These changes in renal hemodynamics have important functional implications for the excretion of water and solutes. The rise in glomerular blood flow helps maintain or increase glomerular filtration, and the filtered load of water and solutes in the surviving nephron segments favors the excretion of substances derived from tubular secretion.

CHANGES IN SINGLE NEPHRON GFR

Whether single nephron filtration rate (SNGFR) increases or falls with respect to control levels depends on the cause of the reduction in nephron population. Levels of nephron filtration rate have been found by micropuncture to increase two- to fourfold in superficial and in juxtamedullary nephrons of the partially infarcted kidney and in superficial nephrons of the pyelonephritic animals. In contrast, in rats with glomerulonephritis, values for SNGFR are much more heterogeneous than in normal animals and may be low, normal, or high.

The dynamic factors that govern single nephron GFR in animals with surgical reduction in renal mass and in animals with immunologically induced glomerulonephritis have been shown to involve changes in the transcapillary hydraulic pressure difference, the glomerular plasma flow, and the surface area and hydraulic conductivity of the glomerular capillary.

SINGLE NEPHRON GLOMERULAR TUBULAR BALANCE

The homogeneity of balance described above between kidney GFR and tubular function for the aggregate of nephrons has also been observed at the individual nephron level in various forms of experimental renal disease. Glomerular tubular balance characteristically is maintained in chronic renal failure, irrespective of the underlying pathological process and despite the great variation in single nephron involvement. Using the tubule fluid to plasma (TF/P) inulin ratio as an index of fluid reabsorption, it has been found that at any given point along the length of the proximal tubule of superficial nephrons fractional fluid reabsorption remains relatively uniform among different nephrons of the same kidney. Thus despite large differences in the amount of filtrate delivered to the proximal tubule among individual nephrons, the amount of water reabsorbed from it is proportional and varies linearly with the amount of filtrate received. Glomerular tubular balance has also been observed for sodium and glucose reabsorption in the proximal tubule of superficial nephrons of remnant kidneys and kidneys with glomerulonephritis.

Similar data are not available for the juxtamedullary nephrons; however, the maintenance of a balance between GFR and whole kidney tubular functions and between SNGFR and proximal tubular functions of superficial nephrons suggests that a similar balance probably exists for the proximal tubule of the juxtamedullary nephrons in the diseased kidney.

The explanation for this remarkable phenomenon has yet to be established. In the normal kidney, micropuncture studies have provided strong evidence for the importance of peritubular physical factors mediated through alterations in hydrostatic and oncotic pressures in the interstitial space adjacent to the proximal tubule in regulating filtrate reabsorption. Similar influences of physical factors on the proximal tubule of diseased kidneys have been demonstrated. There is also evidence

that intraluminal factors related to filtered load influence fluid transport from the proximal tubule of normal superficial nephrons.

There is no evidence, however, that changes in physical factors are responsible for the chronic adaptation in tubular function that follow the loss of renal mass or for the final adjustments in solute and water excretion that take place in more distal segments of the nephrons and result in the precise modulation of external balance.

COMPLEXITY OF REGULATION OF EXCRETORY FUNCTION

The variability of SNGFR among the individual nephrons of the same kidney and the maintenance of a constant fractional reabsorption among the individual nephrons irrespective of their SNGFR introduces an element of singular complexity in the comprehension of the control mechanisms responsible for the regulated excretion of water and solute by the aggregate of nephrons in chronic renal disease. This is developed for sodium excretion in Tables 2 and 3.

Table 2 compares values for total GFR, filtered sodium load, and absolute and fractional sodium excretion in a normal rat and in two other rats, one with glomerular and the other with nonglomerular kidney disease. All animals are in sodium balance with an intake of 1.44 mEq/day and a urinary excretion of 1.44 mEq/day, and all have a serum sodium concentration of 140 mEq/liter. In the two animals with renal disease, total GFR is only one-eighth that in the normal rat; filtered load therefore is also eight times smaller, but, since all animals are in balance, fractional sodium excretion must be eight times greater in the animals with disease than in the normal rat.

In Table 3 mean SNGFR values of 30, 15, and 60 nl/min have been assigned to the normal rat and to the animals with glomerular and nonglomerular disease, respectively. The filtered load of sodium per nephron thus will vary from 2.1 to 8.4 nEq/min.

As noted above, glomerular tubular balance is maintained in chronic renal disease. Given a 50 percent fractional sodium reabsorption (equivalent to a TF/P inulin ration of 2) at the end of the accessible portion of the proximal tubule in all nephrons,* absolute proximal sodium reabsorption and distal delivery out of the end proximal tubule also vary greatly depending on the value of SNGFR. When SNGFR is low, absolute proximal reabsorption is well below normal. On the other hand, when SNGFR is high, proximal reabsorption is greatly above normal.

A similar pattern is present in the distal nephron (i.e. distal to the puncture site in the accessible late portion of the proximal tubule). With a 50 percent reabsorption in the proximal tubule, to have 0.35 and

Table 2
Kidney Sodium Handling by Normal Rat and Rats With Glomerular and Nonglomerular Disease

Rat	Total GFR (ml/min)	Filtered Na Load (μEq/min)	$U_{Na}V$ (μEq/min)	FE_{Na} (%)
Normal	2.0	280	1.0	0.35
Glomerular	0.25	35	1.0	2.8
Nonglomerular	0.25	35	1.0	2.8

$U_{Na}V$, absolute sodium excretion rates; FE_{Na}, fractional sodium excretion; SN, single nephron.

*Some deviation from normal in end-proximal TF/P inulin has been observed in different experimental models of chronic renal disease; these variations, however, have not always been consistent and do not markedly change our conclusions.

Table 3

Single Nephron Sodium Handling by Normal Rat and Rats with Glomerular and
Nonglomerular Disease

Rat	SNGFR (nl/min)	SN Filtered Na Load (nEq/min)	Proximal Na Reabsorption (nEq/min)	Distal Na Delivery (nEq/min)	Distal Na Reabsorption (nEq/min)
Normal	30	4.2	2.1	2.1	2.09
Glomerular	15	2.1	1.05	1.05	0.99
Nonglomerular	60	8.4	4.2	4.2	3.97

$U_{Na}V$, absolute sodium excretion rates; FE_{Na}, fractional sodium excretion; SN, single nephron.

2.8 percent of the filtered load of sodium enter the final urine requires that 99.3 percent and 94.4 percent of the distally delivered sodium be reabsorbed in the normal animal and in the diseased animals, respectively. Thus with mean SNGFRs of 60 nl/min and 15 nl/min the distal reabsorptive rates will vary from a mean of 3.97 nEq/min to a mean of 0.99 nEq/min in the representative nephrons of the animals with nonglomerular and glomerular disease, respectively (as opposed to a mean value of 2.09 nEq/min for the normal nephron). The fourfold difference in absolute excretory rate per nephron indicates the participation of four times less nephrons in the former than in the latter to achieve balance. The difference in reabsorptive and excretory rates among representative individual nephrons of different animals occurs while all animals maintain balance for sodium on the same sodium intake with their aggregate of nephrons excreting the same absolute amount of sodium and the same percentage of filtered sodium.

The differences depicted above between representative nephron units of different animals can also be developed for different nephrons of the same animal. A similar spread of values will exist when the same segmental analysis of sodium reabsorption is applied to nephron units with high, normal, and low SNGFRs.

The mechanisms whereby the activities of the different nephron units are integrated remain unknown; however, before considering these, the patterns of adaptation for water and solute excretion and the limitations to these adaptations will be discussed.

PATTERNS OF ADAPTATION FOR WATER AND SOLUTE EXCRETION

During the course of chronic progressive renal failure, homeostasis for different solutes is characterized by three general patterns of adaptation which are reflected in their serum concentrations. These patterns are depicted in Fig. 1 by the change from normal in serum concentration that develops for different solutes as glomerular filtration rate falls from normal (100 percent) toward zero. Changes in filtered load, excretion rate per nephron, and fractional excretion rate are also indicated for each category of solute. For all three types of solutes, as GFR falls, excretion rate per surviving nephron increases and external balance is maintained.

Solute A is one for which there is "no tubular regulation." As GFR falls a reciprocal rise in serum concentration occurs. Retention in body fluid occurs when GFR decreases. With each wave of nephron loss the serum level rises and filtered load in the remaining nephrons increases. Kidney filtered load (GFR times plasma solute concentration) remains constant and external balance is maintained without changes in fractional excretion. Solutes in this category are exogenous inulin and, to a lesser extent, endogenous urea and creatinine.

While urea undergoes a variable amount of tubular reabsorption, particularly at low flow rates, and creatinine some degree of tubular secretion, the plasma concentration of these solutes will approximately double each time GFR halves. As long as the net acquisition rate remains constant, external balance is maintained and the inverse relationship between serum urea or creatinine concentration and GFR is sufficiently predictable to serve as a clinical index of GFR. The accuracy is particularly valid in chronic renal disease when the correlation between serum creatinine (e.g. 2.0 mg/dl) and creatinine clearance (e.g., 60 ml/min) has been determined at some point during the course of disease in an individual patient. In the preceding example a rise in the serum creatinine concentration to 4.0 mg/dl would represent a 50 percent fall in GFR to about 30 ml/min. A further increase to 8.0 mg/dl would reflect a GFR of 15 ml/min.

Solute B is one that undergoes "tubular regulation with limitation." In contrast to solute A, serum levels of solutes in this category remain constant throughout most of the course of the renal disease. As a consequence, filtered load progressively decreases. External balance is maintained because of a progressive increase in excretion rates per nephron resulting from a progressive increase in fractional excretion (or decrease in fractional reabsorption). This adaptation requires continual modulation of tubular transport processes; however, the ability to increase excretion per nephron at normal serum concentration is limited when GFR falls below a critical level. Serum levels then begin to rise to increase the filtered load per nephron. Thus when GFR is low external balance is maintained through a decrease in net tubular reabsorption or increase in net tubular secretion and a concurrent increase in filtered load per nephron. Phosphate and urate are two solutes with very

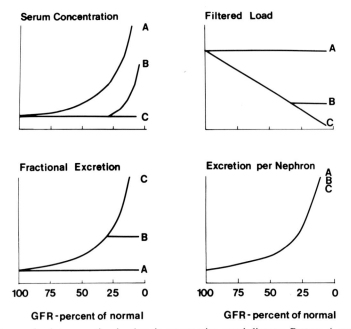

Fig. 1. Patterns of solute excretion in chronic progressive renal disease. Pattern A represents "no tubular regulation," pattern B "regulation with limitation," and pattern C "complete tubular regulation." For each category of solute, balance is assumed and 24 hour excretion is constant at all levels of GFR. For each solute, changes in serum concentration, filtered load, fractional excretion, and excretion rate per nephron are depicted as a function of GFR. For schematization purposes a similar point of origin is presented for all categories of solutes.

different tubular transport processes which undergo "regulation with limitation."

Phosphate is primarily handled by glomerular filtration with subsequent tubular reabsorption. Regulation in the sense of a well maintained fasting serum phosphorus concentration is observed until GFR falls to approximately 25–30 ml/min. To accomplish this, the phosphate biological control system must undergo marked adaptation (see the Phosphorus section). If GFR continues to decrease, the serum concentration of phosphorus will rise. Urate, in contrast to phosphorus, is handled by filtration, tubular reabsorption, and tubular secretion. Like phosphorus, the plasma urate level is well maintained until late in the course of chronic renal disease.

Solutes C undergo "complete tubular regulation." The biological control systems for solutes in this category show remarkable adaptations to maintain normal serum levels virtually throughout the course of chronic renal failure. The residual nephrons have a greater capacity of tubular adaptation for solutes C than for B at GFRs below 25 ml/min. Sodium, potassium, and water fall into this category.

CHANGES IN FRACTIONAL EXCRETION

It is worth emphasizing that as the number of functioning nephrons progressively decreases the adaptations for the maintenance of external balance are achieved for all solutes (and for water) through a progressive increase in absolute excretion per surviving nephron. Excretion per nephron, however, is not synonymous with fractional excretion.

Fractional excretion of a solute (or excretion per unit of solute filtered) reflects the aggregate changes made by the different segments of the functioning tubules to the filtered solute in its transit between Bowman's space and its appearance in the ureter. The changes in fractional excretion are not identical for different solutes in the course of chronic renal disease.

For solute C or for water with complete tubular regulation, fractional excretion and excretion rate per nephron increase in parallel as GFR falls. With each 50 percent reduction in GFR, with no change in diet, a reciprocal doubling in fractional excretion and in excretion per nephron takes place to maintain external balance for that solute or for water. For solute A without tubular regulation, fractional excretion remains constant at 100 percent. Changes in fractional excretion for solute B initially follows the regulated pattern depicted for solute C until fractional excretion reaches a maximum. Then, further increase in excretion per nephron occurs through an increase in filtered load that follows the pattern discussed for solute A, and fractional excretion remains constant.

"MAGNIFICATION PHENOMENON"

The progressive increase in fractional excretion that takes place during the course of progressive renal disease for solutes of category B and C illustrates what has been called the "magnification phenomenon." In the maintenance of sodium balance, for instance, any reduction in GFR will require progressively larger and predictable readjustments in fractional excretion of sodium that vary in inverse proportion to the level of

maximum volume increases only to 1850 ml per day. It is readily apparent that addition of 345 ml of solute-free water will reduce very little the osmolality of 1500 ml of isotonic urine—thus the limitation on urinary diluting ability in chronic renal failure.

In contrast, the limitation in excreting a minimal volume and the inability to maximally concentrate the urine are related to an abnormality in concentrating ability which occurs early in renal insufficiency and is already apparent following uninephrectomy. A normal person can achieve a maximal urine osmolality of 1200 mOsm/kg. This person needs a minimum volume of only 375 ml per day of maximally concentrated urine to excrete a solute load of 450 mOsm. In contrast, a patient with chronic renal failure and a GFR of 2 ml/min has a maximal urine osmolality of no more than about 350 mOsm/kg. To excrete the same 450 mOsm of solute will therefore require a maximum daily urine volume of 1285 ml.

The nature of the defect in renal concentrating ability in chronic renal disease is not known. Over the years it has been ascribed to a variety of etiologies. It probably results from a combination of factors including the osmotic effect of an increased solute load per nephron and increased flow rate per nephron, the existence of anatomic distortion betweeen the different tubular and vascular constituents of the countercurrent system, an increase in renal medullary blood flow with dissipation of the interstitital solute gradient, a decrease in intrarenal recycling of urea, and an acquired impaired responsiveness of the collecting tubule to antidiuretic hormone. Some relationship has also been described between the concentrating defect and the regulation of sodium excretion in chronic renal disease, since prevention of the adaptations necessary for sodium excretion in rats by reduction of dietary sodium intake in proportion to the decrement in GFR is accompanied by an improvement in the ability to concentrate urine.

There are several consequences of practical importance to the clinician resulting from the limited range in water excretion that exists in chronic uremia. The range of fluid intake should be monitored, and both forced fluids and excessive fluid restriction are inappropiate. Hyponatremia in a uremic patient always results from excessive water intake. Because of isosthenuria, the hourly rate of urine formation is constant at night and during the day and nocturia is a consistent and early symptom of chronic renal disease. The sudden subsidence of nocturia should be an ominous sign to the physician, since it signifies either urinary retention or a fall in GFR.

REFERENCES

Bricker NS: On the pathogenesis of the uremic state: An exposition of the "trade-off hypothesis." N Engl J Med 286:1093, 1972

Bricker NS, Bourgoignie JJ, Licht A, et al: Pathophysiology of chronic renal failure, in Edelman C (ed): Pediatric Kidney Disease. Boston, Little Brown and Co, 1978 p 205

Bricker NS, Bourgoignie JJ, Weber H: The renal response to progressive nephron loss, in Brenner B, Rector FC Jr (eds): The Kidney. Philadelphia, W.B. Saunders, 1976, p 703

Dorhout-Mees EJ, Machado M, Slatopolsky E, et al: The functional adaptation of the diseased kidney. III Ammonium excretion. J Clin Invest 45: 289, 1966

Finkelstein FO, Hayslett JP: Structural and functional adaptation after reduction of nephron population. Yale J Biol Med 52:271, 1979

Hayslett JP: Functional Adaptation to reduction in renal mass. Physiol Rev 59:137, 1979

CHRONIC RENAL FAILURE—CONSEQUENCES

Michael H. Humphreys

The two previous chapters have dealt with the classification of chronic renal failure and its pathophysiology. In contrast to the rather specific pathogenetic mechanisms and histologic involvement of the kidneys caused by various forms of renal disease, the consequences of renal failure are nonspecific and give little if any clue to the underlying disease process. The uremic syndrome is the term applied to the multiple signs and symptoms of organ involvement which occur as a result of renal failure, regardless of cause. Many of these signs and symptoms are cured or dramatically improved by chronic dialysis treatment, while others persist in the well dialyzed patient. New symptoms and signs develop in the patient undergoing regular dialytic treatment. Table 1 lists the consequences of chronic renal failure according to their response to dialytic treatment.

CONSEQUENCES OF CHRONIC RENAL FAILURE THAT IMPROVE WITH DIALYSIS

Fluid, Electrolyte, and Acid–Base Abnormalities

One consequence of chronic renal failure is the impaired ability to maintain a constant internal environment. As a result, derangements in fluid, electrolyte, and acid–base balance may occur which are responsible for symptoms. The ability to excrete water is diminished, so that excessive water ingestion will result in hyponatremia. Renal ability to maintain sodium balance is also impaired, so that overly severe restriction of salt intake may result in negative sodium balance and symptomatic volume depletion; often, this will also be accompanied by hyponatremia. Rarely, some patients have difficulty in maintaining salt balance even on a normal (>100 mEq/day) salt intake (salt-losing nephritis); such patients may require frank supplementation with NaCl tablets. Symptoms attributable to hyponatremia per se, whether due to water excess or to sodium depletion, in the patient with chronic renal failure include nausea, vomiting, anorexia, headaches, confusion, and lethargy. As will be seen later, however, these can also be manifestations of the uremic state and thus are not specific for hyponatremia.

Hypokalemia may occur in the patient with chronic

Table 1
Consequences of Chronic Renal Failure Resulting in Uremic Symptoms and Their
Response to Dialysis Therapy

Consequences that improve with dialysis
 Consequences resulting from disorders of fluid, electrolyte, and acid–base metabolism
  Volume excess or depletion
  Electrolyte imbalance: sodium, potassium, calcium, magnesium, phosphorus
  Acidosis
 Consequences of cardiovascular abnormalities in uremia
  Hypertension
  Congestive heart failure
  Uremic lung
 Consequences of chronic renal failure without identifiable etiology
  Neurological
  Gastrointestinal
  Hematological
  Endocrine–metabolic
  Dermatological
  Cardiovascular
  Ocular

Consequences of chronic renal failure that persist or progress despite adequate dialysis
 Circulatory abnormalities producing symptoms in the dialyzed patient
  Refractory hypertension
  Pericarditis
  Accelerated atherosclerosis
 Other consequences of chronic renal failure in the dialyzed patient
  Hematologic
  Endocrine–metabolic
  Renal osteodystrophy

Consequences of chronic renal failure that develop during the course of chronic dialysis
 treatment
 Hepatitis
 Refractory ascites
 Hypersplenism
 Dialysis dementia or dyspraxic syndrome

renal failure as a consequence of long-term diuretic administration and in certain forms of renal disease associated with renal tubular acidosis and potassium wasting. Symptoms possibly caused by hypokalemia, such as muscle cramps, weakness, anorexia, drowsiness, and lethargy, are usually attributed to other factors in the uremic patient. Hyperkalemia develops in chronic renal failure only as a preterminal event usually associated with the onset of oliguria. Fecal potassium excretion is increased in uremia, which may help in the maintenance of potassium balance in the face of dwindling renal function. However, patients with renal failure handle potassium loads poorly and may develop hyperkalemia as a consequence of excessive intake. The acidosis of chronic renal failure may contribute to the development of hyperkalemia, and patients with renal tubular acidosis (RTA) associated with mineralocorticoid deficiency (type IV RTA) may also have chronic hyperkalemia due to the low level of circulating aldosterone and the consequent impairment of potassium secretion into urine and feces. Symptoms caused by hyperkalemia are uncommon and not diagnostic even at levels of serum potassium which produce clearcut electrocardiographic changes.

Hypocalcemia is a common occurrence in chronic renal failure, resulting from impaired metabolism of vitamin D and parathyroid hormone. Since the development of hypocalcemia is gradual and is usually accompanied by mild metabolic acidosis, the hypocalcemia is asymptomatic for the most part; however, rapid correction of acidosis by alkali administration decreases serum ionized calcium and may precipitate symptomatic hypocalcemia, manifested by carpopedal spasm and positive Chvostek's and Trousseau's signs. Hypercalcemia is a much less frequent occurrence in the patient with chronic renal failure; it occurs as a result of underlying disease such as malignancy or multiple myeloma or as a consequence of calcium supplementation or vitamin D administration given in an effort to prevent the development of renal osteodystrophy. Symptoms of hypercalcemia include anorexia, nausea, constipation, fatigue, and mental depression. Phosphate retention is a cardinal consequence of renal failure and may contribute to hypocalcemia through elevation of the Ca–PO_4 product. Prolonged elevation of this product above 60 is associated with significant extraosseous deposition of calcium salts. This occurs in skin, blood vessels, myocardium, joints, eyes, lungs, and other tissues. Skin calcification may underlie the intense and distressing pruritis which some uremic patients experience, and calcification along the medium- and large-sized arteries of extremities may lead to ischemic necrosis and gangrene. Hypophosphatemia occurs uncommonly in patients with chronic renal failure, usually in conjunction with excessive administration of oral phosphate binding antacids. Magnesium retention also is a consequence of chronic renal failure and may result in hypermagnesemia. If excessive magnesium loads are given to these patients, as through magnesium-containing antacids, then severe and potentially fatal hypermagnesemia may develop. Symptoms heralding this occurrence include peripheral vasodilatation, nausea, vomiting, and CNS depression; at a serum magnesium concentration above 6 mEq/liter, deep tendon reflexes disappear, and higher levels result in respiratory paralysis, coma, and cardiac arrest.

Chronic renal failure is associated with impaired ability of the kidneys to excrete acid. As a consequence, nonvolatile acids derived from metabolism accumulate in the body and result in the picture of renal acidosis, a form of metabolic acidosis associated with an increased anion gap and depression of the serum bicarbonate concentration. The acidosis is mild because of respiratory compensation, and serum bicarbonate may stabilize at 16 mEq/liter or more. The acidosis itself is seldom responsible for symptoms at rest, although dyspnea may occur on exertion.

Symptoms related to these fluid, electrolyte, and acid–base disturbances are readily corrected by dialysis, and the chronically dialyzed patient will have blood electrolyte concentrations which do not deviate markedly from normal; however, the absence of significant renal function in the interval between dialyses means that the patient with endstage renal disease must carefully restrict intake of water, sodium, and potassium so that marked changes in body water and electrolyte concentrations do not occur.

Cardiovascular Consequences of Chronic Renal Failure

Hypertension is a nearly universal finding in patients with advanced renal failure and may cause complications by itself over and above the other manifestations of uremia. Accelerated or malignant hypertension may develop, leading to encephalopathy, seizures, and further worsening of renal function. Retinal vascular changes and papilledema may be present. Prompt treatment of this abnormality will decrease morbidity and help to spare residual renal function. Fluid retention in uremic patients will often result in circulatory overload and congestive heart failure. Pulmonary edema can develop in this situation, sometimes occurring without elevations in pulmonary vascular pressures. This observation has led to postulates of a capillary permeability defect induced by the uremic state which results in this picture of "uremic lung."

Consequences of Chronic Renal Failure Without Identifiable Etiology

In contrast to the signs and symptoms which occur in the azotemic patient that can be ascribed to specific aberrations of fluid, electrolyte, and circulatory regulation, there exist a host of abnormalities for which no specific etiology has been found. By default, these have been attributed to the retention or elaboration of a uremic toxin or toxins, the nature of which is unknown; however, these consequences of chronic renal failure all share in common the facts that they develop when renal function is markedly impaired (GFR less than 20 ml/min and often less than 10 ml/min) and that they improve in part or completely once regular dialysis therapy is initiated. Figure 1 is a composite representation of this class of abnormalities.

The earliest and most subtle uremic symptoms involve the central nervous system. Mild behavioral changes can often be appreciated, sometimes only retrospectively, and disturbances in sleep patterns are common, whether manifested as nocturnal insomnia or increased need for sleep. Attention span may be diminished, and mild memory impairment, mood swings, and irritability develop; performance of routine tasks such as simple arithmetic calculations may become difficult. As renal insufficiency progresses, more distinct abnormalities appear. These include evidence of neuromuscular irritability—twitching, fasciculations, tremulousness, and asterixis. Drowsiness and lethargy become common. As the patient approaches a near-terminal state, stupor and coma develop and seizures may occur. The electroencephalogram mirrors these changes, showing a pattern of diffuse slowing and a predominance of brain waves in the frequency range of 3–5 cycles per second.

Symptoms of a peripheral neuropathy are encountered as a late consequence of the uremic state. The "restless leg syndrome" is such a manifestation; it is an ill-defined sensation of discomfort in the feet and lower legs which can only be relieved by frequent movement of the lower extremities. Subsequently, paresthesias develop in the feet, which may progress to involve the fingers, and ultimately the motor nerves, if dialytic therapy is not instituted. Loss of distal reflexes and position and vibratory sense are further signs of progression, and foot drop may occur. Rarely, flaccid quadriplegia may result. The presence of any sign of peripheral neuropathy is now taken as a strong indication to commence regular dialytic treatment.

Gastrointestinal symptoms are among the most common clinical consequences of chronic renal failure. Anorexia may occur well before the advanced stages of uremia and result in poor caloric intake. This may contribute to the poor nutritional status that many uremic patients have prior to the onset of dialysis. Early morning or postprandial nausea is common and may be completely reversed after vomiting. These symptoms do not correlate well with the severity of the azotemia, and they may respond dramatically to restriction of dietary protein intake. An unpleasant, metallic taste is also a common complaint, and production of ammonia from urea by oropharyngeal bacteria is held responsible for the uremic fetor which some patients have. Uremic gastroenteritis is characterized by nausea, vomiting, and diarrhea, frequently accompanied by gastrointestinal hemorrhage. While radiographic con-

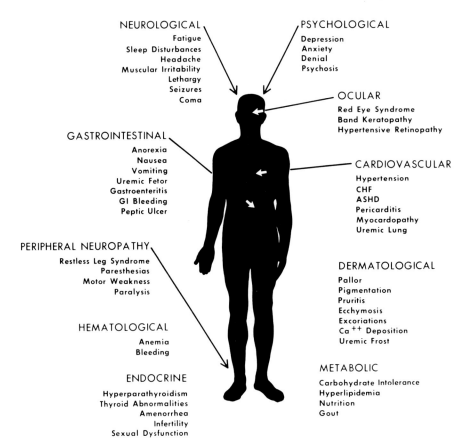

NEUROLOGICAL
Fatigue
Sleep Disturbances
Headache
Muscular Irritability
Lethargy
Seizures
Coma

PSYCHOLOGICAL
Depression
Anxiety
Denial
Psychosis

OCULAR
Red Eye Syndrome
Band Keratopathy
Hypertensive Retinopathy

GASTROINTESTINAL
Anorexia
Nausea
Vomiting
Uremic Fetor
Gastroenteritis
GI Bleeding
Peptic Ulcer

CARDIOVASCULAR
Hypertension
CHF
ASHD
Pericarditis
Myocardopathy
Uremic Lung

PERIPHERAL NEUROPATHY
Restless Leg Syndrome
Paresthesias
Motor Weakness
Paralysis

DERMATOLOGICAL
Pallor
Pigmentation
Pruritis
Ecchymosis
Excoriations
Ca^{++} Deposition
Uremic Frost

HEMATOLOGICAL
Anemia
Bleeding

METABOLIC
Carbohydrate Intolerance
Hyperlipidemia
Nutrition
Gout

ENDOCRINE
Hyperparathyroidism
Thyroid Abnormalities
Amenorrhea
Infertility
Sexual Dysfunction

THE UREMIC SYNDROME

Fig. 1. Uremic syndrome. [Reproduced with permission from Schoenfeld PY, Humphreys MH: A general description of the uremic state, in Brenner BM, Rector FC Jr (eds): The Kidney. Philadelphia, W.B. Saunders, 1976, p 1432.]

trast studies are usually negative, gastroscopy or sigmoidoscopy may reveal shallow, punctate ulcerations in the mucosa. There is also an increased incidence of peptic ulcer disease in patients with chronic renal failure. Acute pancreatitis and parotitis can also be seen in severely ill uremic patients.

Anemia is a virtually universal consequence of chronic renal failure. The anemia is variable in severity and correlates poorly with the degree of azotemia. It is normochromic and normocytic in type, and it results from decreased erythropoiesis and increased red cell destruction. The former abnormality is related in part to diminished levels of erythropoietin, while the latter results from some aspect of the uremic environment, since cells from a normal donor will also have a shortened lifespan when transfused into a uremic patient. Red blood cells exhibit a characteristic burr cell appearance in the peripheral blood smear. The anemia is well tolerated in most patients; however, patients with ischemic heart disease or peripheral vascular disease may require frequent transfusions in order to reduce symptoms exacerbated by the anemia. Dialysis produces an improvement in hematocrit within several months, but anemia still persists.

Uremic patients also exhibit impaired function of white cells. Leukocyte migration is decreased in azotemic individuals and frequently returns to normal after dialysis. Immune responsiveness is decreased in uremia—lymphopenia, reduction of antibody response to certain antigens, and impaired response to intradermal antigens have all been demonstrated. Many of these abnormalities improve with dialysis. Another important consequence of chronic renal failure is the appearance of a bleeding abnormality characterized chiefly by a defect in platelet function. Functionally, this is manifested by diminished platelet factor 3 availability, abnormal platelet aggregation, and poor clot retraction. Clinically, patients show easy bruising, develop spontaneous ecchymoses, and bleed readily from mucous membranes. More serious bleeding can occur into the GI tract, from the vagina, and into the pericardium; spontaneous subdural hematomas and intracerebral hemorrhage may take place. The abnormal platelet function is reversed after dialysis and has been correlated with serum levels of guanidinosuccinic acid, phenol, and parahydroxyphenylacetic acid, although definite proof that one of these agents is responsible for the platelet abnormality is still lacking.

The endocrine and metabolic consequences of chronic renal failure are numerous. Carbohydrate intolerance, manifested by abnormal glucose tolerance, is present in many azotemic patients, while fasting hyperglycemia is a much less common occurrence. Severe hyperglycemia is not seen; if present, it suggests that underlying diabetes may be the cause. The basis for this carbohydrate intolerance in uremia is not clear; evidence demonstrates the presence of insulin antagonism as well as abnormal peripheral glucose utilization, and elevated fasting levels of growth hormone may also contribute to this metabolic derangement. Whatever the etiology, dialysis results in an improvement in carbohydrate intolerance. Another important metabolic consequence of chronic renal failure is the occurrence of hyperlipidemia. This is characterized by an increase in triglyceride-rich very-low-density lipoproteins and results in hypertriglyceridemia with normal or only slightly elevated cholesterol. It can be detected in about 50 percent of patients prior to initiation of dialysis and in about 75 percent of patients on regular dialytic therapy. The etiology of this abnormality may lie in reduced triglyceride removal, reflected in subnormal postheparin plasma lipolytic activity, and increased hepatic triglyceride synthesis due to hyperinsulinemia and increased free fatty acid delivery.

The patient with endstage renal disease resembles a malnourished individual in many ways. Tissue-wasting may be present, and serum albumin and transferrin concentrations are low; plasma amino acid profiles are similar to those seen in starved individuals. These abnormalities may be caused in part by anorexia leading to poor dietary intake, to overly vigorous restriction of protein in the diet, and to urinary albumin loss; however, it is clear that a defect in hepatic albumin synthesis exists in the uremic patient which is in large part responsible for the hypoalbuminemia. With the onset of dialysis, nutritional status improves, the patient feels better and is no longer anorectic, dietary protein restrictions are liberalized, and increases in serum albumin concentration and in dry weight occur; however, dialysis does not correct the abnormal plasma amino acid profile, and impaired synthesis of histidine in uremic man makes this amino acid an essential one in dialyzed patients.

Abnormalities in numerous endocrine systems are also consequences of chronic renal failure. Foremost among these is the development of hyperparathyroidism, which generally occurs by the time GFR has been reduced to 30 ml/min or less. This is due to at least two factors: Phosphate retention, which occurs as a result of a reduction in renal function, causes an increase in the Ca–PO_4 product, thereby favoring a lowering of the serum calcium. At the same time, GI absorption of dietary calcium is diminished due to the low levels of 1,25-dihydroxycholecalciferol, the active metabolite of vitamin D_3 normally made in the kidney cortex. Both these causes of hypocalcemia serve to stimulate release of parathyroid hormone. In addition, adequate levels of

vitamin D metabolites appear necessary for the calcemic action of PTH on bone. Thus the closed feedback loop regulating PTH secretion is interrupted. The resultant hyperparathyroidism is an important factor in the development of renal osteodystrophy and plays a role in extraosseous calcification, the consequences of which have already been discussed. Through its effects on calcium metabolism, bone, skin, brain, lipid metabolism, and sexual function, excess PTH has been called a uremic toxin.

Other endocrine abnormalities also occur. Elevated plasma renin activity may contribute to the hypertension of chronic renal disease. Gonadal dysfunction in males is reflected in loss of libido, decrease in testicular size, and abnormal spermatogenesis; serum testosterone levels are low without an associated increase in gonadotropin levels. In females, amenorrhea or menorrhagia may occur early in the course of chronic renal failure, and infertility is the rule. Thyroid functional abnormalities are reflected in an increased T_3 resin uptake and decreased total T_4 levels, while free T_4 levels are normal. These findings suggest an abnormality in binding of thyroid hormones to plasma globulins. Clinically, uremic patients are euthyroid. One center has reported a high incidence of diffuse goiter in its dialysis population.

The skin can manifest many of the underlying abnormalities of chronic renal insufficiency. A generalized pallor, more evident in palms and conjunctivae, is an indicator of anemia; the presence of ecchymoses and hematomas attests to the underlying bleeding disorder of uremia. Diffuse hyperpigmentation, exacerbated by sunlight, is a frequent finding in patients with longstanding renal failure; it probably results from retention of pigmented metabolites normally excreted in the urine. The pruritus of chronic renal failure may be related to hyperparathyroidism; in severe cases, excoriations may result, particularly where calcium deposits in the skin occur. Such patients may experience relief after subtotal parathyroidectomy. The abnormal nutritional state of the uremic patient may be revealed by the presence of white, transverse bands across the nails (Terry's nails). Uremic frost was formerly seen as a result of precipitation of urea following evaporation of water from eccrine sweat gland secretion; with current standards of nursing care and dialytic treatment, it should never be seen. Most of these dermatologic consequences of chronic renal failure improve with dialysis, although the pallor and pigmentation persist to variable degrees.

The major cardiopulmonary consequences of chronic renal failure relate to the fluid retention and hypertension which are hallmarks of the uremic state; these were discussed above. On the other hand, pericarditis is a common consequence which appears to be a result of uremic toxicity. Clinically, the presentation of uremic pericarditis includes chest pain frequently relieved by sitting up, fever, and a pericardial friction rub. The heart is characteristically enlarged, and a variable degree of pericardial effusion may be present as assessed radiographically, by echocardiography, or at right heart catheterization. Evidence of cardiac tamponade may develop, as seen by neck venous distention, Kussmaul's sign, pulsus paradoxicus, hypotension, and a low cardiac output state. Pericardiocentesis yields hemorrhagic fluid which does not clot, and autopsy examination reveals a thickened, fibrinous pericardium with loculations of fluid caused by bands of fibrinous material adherent to pericardium and epicardium. This picture occurs most typically as a manifestation of uremic toxicity in patients with advanced renal failure, but it can also occur in patients on chronic dialysis therapy; in this latter group, the pericarditis may develop following infections or surgical procedures, although cultures of pericardial fluid are almost always sterile. Treatment in either setting consists of intensive dialysis, with avoidance of systemic heparinization to minimize the risk of further bleeding into the pericardial space. Patients who develop significant cardiac compromise as a result of tamponade require needle aspiration of the pericardial fluid or, preferably, surgical creation of a pericardial window or stripping of the pericardium to prevent further accumulation of fluid. Antiinflammatory agents such as indomethacin, aspirin and corticosteroids have been recommended for symptomatic relief. A small number of patients may go on to develop chronic constrictive pericarditis 10 weeks to 1 year following an acute episode. This complication requires surgical pericardiectomy for treatment.

The entity of uremic lung was mentioned above. Uremic pericarditis has an analogue in uremic pleuritis, in which the pleura is involved in a fibrinous reaction similar to that seen in the pericardium. The pleural fluid is serosanguinous or hemorrhagic and contains elevated protein and lactic dehydrogenase levels characteristic of an exudate. This entity is seen more commonly in chronically dialyzed patients and responds to continued dialysis in 4–6 weeks.

A picture of uremic cardiomyopathy has also been described in patients with endstage renal failure. Although the presence of anemia, fluid overload, hypertension, and arteriosclerotic heart disease makes it difficult to substantiate such an entity, the possibility clearly exists that additional consequences of the uremic state, coupled with these background abnormalities, may combine to produce a specific picture of cardiac dysfunction which is improved by the institution of chronic dialysis. Finally, the murmur of aortic insufficiency has been described in uremic patients in the absence of discernible aortic valvular disease at autopsy. More recent studies suggest this sound may in actuality be a pericardial knock.

Ocular involvement in uremia occurs as a result of hypertensive retinopathy; retinal edema may occur, occasionally accompanied by frank retinal detachment. A form of cortical blindness called uremic amaurosis can also be seen. Uremic neuropathy may involve the cranial nerves as well to produce nystagmus, miosis, and pupillary asymmetry. The abnormalities in calcium metabolism can result in corneal calcium deposition, causing band keratopathy. When calcium deposition occurs in the conjunctivae, hyperemia ensues, producing the "red eyes" of chronic renal failure.

The psychological stresses of any chronic illness pose severe demands on adaptive abilities, and coping with chronic renal failure is no exception. Anxiety develops over the course of the renal failure and the occurrence of uremic symptoms, and the use of denial as a defense mechanism is the rule in most patients. The interaction of central nervous system manifestations of uremia—drowsiness, lethargy, decreased mentation, etc.—and the psychological responses to these distressing symptoms poses a therapeutic challenge to the physician: on the one hand, the patient must be counseled as to the origin of these symptoms, and on the other, he must be supported during the progression of the disease to the advent of dialysis. For many, the exposure to regular dialysis constitutes the first real confrontation with the reality of their illness; in some patients, this may prove so overwhelming that a transient psychotic reaction occurs. Fears concerning vascular access, the dialysis process itself, and death can be successfully dealt with by the physician provided that he maintains a warm and supportive role during this stressful period.

CONSEQUENCES OF CHRONIC RENAL FAILURE THAT PERSIST OR PROGRESS DESPITE DIALYSIS

Many of the consequences of chronic renal failure described above are treated wholly or in large part with regular dialysis; however, certain abnormalities persist even in the well dialyzed patient. Three important consequences of chronic renal failure discussed in this section relate to the circulation (Table 1). The first is persistent, severe hypertension. In most dialyzed patients, moderate hypertension occurs and appears related primarily to fluid retention in the interdialytic interval. In a small number of patients, severe, refractory hypertension, often accompanied by markedly elevated plasma renin activity and clinical manifestations of malignant hypertension, presents as a characteristic syndrome. Potent antihypertensive drugs and vigorous fluid removal during dialysis seem unable in such patients to prevent a rapidly deteriorating course of weight loss, congestive heart failure, and visual disturbances, and the usual treatment has been to perform bilateral nephrectomy, a treatment which can be dramatically effective in arresting this syndrome. Recently, more effective antihypertensive agents have been introduced which offer the hope of controlling the hypertension without resorting to nephrectomy.

Another circulatory consequence of chronic renal failure which occurs in the dialyzed patient as well is pericarditis. The clinical signs and symptoms of pericarditis in this setting are no different from those in the nondialyzed uremic. It is not understood why symptomatic pericarditis can develop in patients who are well dialyzed when judged by usual criteria, and it has been proposed that an infectious etiology may be present; however, this has not been substantiated. Treatment is the same as has already been discussed. A final circulatory abnormality seen as a consequence of renal failure in the dialyzed patient is the occurrence of an accelerated rate of atherosclerosis. The causative factors in this process may include hyperlipidemia, abnormal glucose tolerance, hyperuricemia, hypertension, and vascular calcification. Symptoms related to this process are those of vascular insufficiency to coronary, cerebral, and peripheral vascular trees. In some patients, impaired vascular access for hemodialysis may become a major problem. No currently available treatment appears to influence this abnormality; frequent transfusions to maintain hematocrit above 25 vol% may offer relief of some symptoms of vascular insufficiency.

OTHER CONSEQUENCES OF CHRONIC RENAL FAILURE IN THE DIALYZED PATIENT

Hematological abnormalities persist in the chronic dialysis patient. Mention was made above that the anemia of chronic renal failure improves after institution of dialysis but still persists. In some patients, particularly those with bilateral nephrectomy, symptomatic anemia may remain a severe problem. Contributing factors may include iron deficiency resulting from blood loss in the dialyzer, vitamin deficiency, hemolysis, and hypersplenism. Regular vitamin supplementation, parenteral iron therapy, and, rarely, splenectomy may be appropriate therapeutic maneuvers, but some patients may maintain high transfusion requirements, particularly if symptoms of vascular insufficiency occur. Anabolic steroids have been advocated to improve anemia in dialyzed patients, but their precise role remains to be established. Coagulation disturbances may also persist; the need to anticoagulate the patient during hemodialysis may result in untoward bleeding from the GI tract or elsewhere. Conversely, some patients develop a hypercoagulable state, requiring large amounts of heparin during dialysis and needing to take oral anticoagulants (platelet antagonists, warfarin derivatives) to prevent clotting of external shunts or arteriovenous fistulas. Abnormal fibrinogen metabolism has been reported in dialysis patients and may be responsible for some of these clinical manifestations.

The endocrine and metabolic consequences of chronic renal failure described in the previous section by and large persist in the well dialyzed patient. These include thyroid functional abnormalities, hyperlipidemia, and carbohydrate intolerance. Dialysis may slightly improve gonadal function; menses may reappear, although the menstrual cycle may be prolonged. Fertility remains reduced, and only a few successful pregnancies have been reported in dialyzed women.

Although the development and pathogenesis of uremic hyperparathyroidism were described briefly above, the full manifestations of renal osteodystrophy usually occur in the chronically dialyzed patient. Persistent hyperparathyroidism leads to the development of hyperparathyroid bone disease, osteitis fibrosa cys-

tica, whereas impaired vitamin D metabolism results in the histologic picture of osteomalacia. Bone biopsies in dialysis patients usually show mixtures of these two lesions, although one or the other may predominate. Symptoms of bone disease are more common in patients with osteomalacia and consist of dull, aching pains in pelvis, femora, and shoulders; depression and lassitude may be present. With more severe disease, traumatic or spontaneous fractures occur, particularly in pelvis, femora, and ribs, and may heal very slowly. A proximal muscle myopathy may also occur in patients with this form of bone disease. Symptoms are much less frequent in patients with osteitis fibrosa; the most common are bone pain, pathological fractures, and such psychological disturbances as anxiety, sleeplessness, and emotional lability. This form of bone disease is also associated with metastatic calcification, described earlier, and with a high incidence of nontraumatic aseptic necrosis of bone, particularly of femoral head and knee. Figure 2 illustrates the severity of extraosseous calcification which can occur in some chronic dialysis patients.

Treatment of renal osteodystrophy is based on a multipronged attempt to control secondary hyperparathyroidism and overcome the defect in vitamin D metabolism. Dietary calcium intake should be at least 1–1.5 g/day; if not, then supplemental calcium should be administered as calcium carbonate. This enhances dietary calcium absorption. The serum phosphate should be controlled by reduction of dietary intake and the use of oral phosphate binding antacids. Experience with the newer analogs of vitamin D, particularly 25-hydroxy- and 1,25-dihydroxyvitamin D, show promise of improving calcium balance and decreasing serum parathyroid hormone levels. Finally, a few patients may have severe secondary hyperparathyroidism refractory to these measures and require subtotal parathyroidectomy.

CONSEQUENCES OF CHRONIC RENAL FAILURE THAT DEVELOP DURING THE COURSE OF DIALYSIS THERAPY

The patient treated with chronic hemodialysis is subject to additional complications besides those already mentioned (Table 1). These include viral hepatitis, refractory ascites, hypersplenism, and so-called dialysis dementia. These are discussed more fully in the chapter on *Dialysis* and will be described here only briefly.

Hepatitis in dialysis patients is usually due to hepatitis B virus infection; a national cooperative study recently showed that about 17 percent of dialysis patients and 2.4 percent of dialysis staff had antigen of this virus in their blood, and a much higher percentage had antibody. This high incidence of infection with hepatitis B virus is much greater than in the general population and reflects the widespread use of blood transfusions in dialysis patients and spread of infection between patients and staff. Symptoms of hepatitis in dialysis patients are mild; jaundice is uncommon, and mild to moderate elevations of serum enzymes occur.

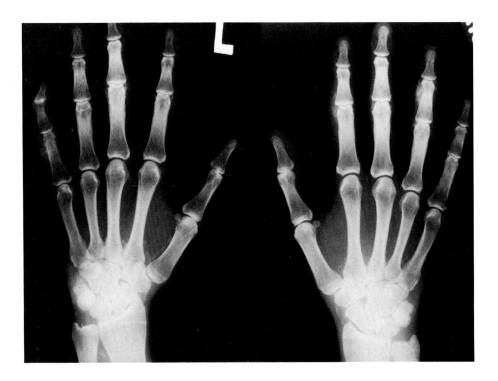

Fig. 2. Hand x-rays from a chronic hemodialysis patient showing extensive periarticular and soft-tissue calcifications of the fingers and calcification along the arteries in the hands. The patient had a persistently elevated serum phosphate concentration and abnormal calcium–phosphorus product as well as an elevated serum parathyroid hormone concentration.

The acute illness subsides after 3–4 weeks, but occasional patients may have a prolonged course lasting several months. Persistence of circulating antigen to hepatitis B virus is common after resolution of the acute episode. It is possible that chronic liver disease may result as a sequelum of hepatitis infection in some dialysis patients.

A less common development in dialysis patients is the picture of refractory ascites which occurs in a small number of patients, usually without liver function abnormalities or infectious or malignant disease. The ascitic fluid commonly contains a high protein concentration. The etiology of this condition is obscure; many patients who develop this ascites have a history of antecedent peritoneal dialysis, suggesting that this treatment may in some way have altered peritoneal permeability. Therapy of this puzzling problem has been disappointing, and no single maneuver tried to date has been uniformly effective except for transplantation, following which the ascites resolves.

A few dialysis patients may develop hypersplenism, manifested by worsening anemia and increased transfusion requirements, leukopenia, and thrombocytopenia. Splenomegaly can usually be detected on physical examination. Studies with chromium-labeled red blood cells show shortened red cell survival and increased splenic sequestration in some patients, and splenectomy has resulted in improvement in hematocrit, white count, and platelet count. Lymphoid hyperplasia is observed in spleens removed for this problem, and many patients also have abnormal liver histology. The relationships of these findings to the underlying etiology of the hypersplenism remains to be established.

An even more puzzling entity occurring in dialysis patients is that of dialysis dementia. This is a bizarre syndrome of central nervous system degeneration characterized by encephalopathy, speech dyspraxia, myoclonus, and tremor, as well as personality changes; it progresses to dementia, seizures, and psychosis, and it culminates in death. It occurs in patients who have been on chronic dialysis for 2–6 years, and striking variations in incidence of the syndrome around the country have been noted. Abnormal EEGs and altered cerebrospinal fluid dynamics are characteristic findings. The etiology of this syndrome is obscure; a growing body of circumstantial evidence has raised the possibility that it may result from aluminum toxicity, although further studies will be required to substantiate this. No treatment is currently available for this condition.

FACTORS INFLUENCING THE DEVELOPMENT OF UREMIC SYMPTOMS

The symptoms of uremia which have been described in this chapter may develop in any patient with severe renal insufficiency; however, a number of factors may alter the presentation of symptoms in an individual patient, such as: rate of progression of renal disease; nature of the underlying renal disease; age of the patient; acute deterioration superimposed on chronic renal insufficiency; presence of extrarenal disease; and therapy of renal disease. Chief among these is the rapidity with which renal failure develops. Patients with acute renal failure are particularly prone to problems of electrolyte imbalance, acidosis, and volume overload; symptoms in these cases are usually related to the underlying cause of the renal failure (trauma, sepsis, hemorrhagic hypotension, etc.) or to the associated electrolyte disturbances, and the toxin-mediated uremic symptoms are less prominent. Patients with rapidly progressing glomerulonephritis of any cause will show a subacute clinical course, with uremic symptoms occurring in rapid progression or appearing in concert; hypertension and its attendant symptoms may be particularly marked, and oliguria with resultant hyperkalemia troublesome. On the other hand, patients with slowly progressive renal disease may show a remarkable ability to accommodate to renal failure, owing not only to the adaptive mechanisms of the remaining functioning nephron units, but also to the slow rate of progression itself, permitting extrarenal adaptive mechanisms to take place.

A second factor which may influence the development of uremic symptoms is the nature of the underlying renal disease. Patients with renal failure from polycystic kidneys have long been felt to develop uremia late in the progression of the disease. True salt-losing nephritis is noted for the rarity of hypertension despite advanced azotemia. Amyloid renal disease also has been said to produce hypertension only infrequently. Vascular and hypertensive complications may be minimal in patients with chronic pyelonephritis or prominent and serious in patients with glomerulonephritis.

The age of the patient may likewise influence the manifestations of uremia, younger patients being able to tolerate more severe degrees of renal insufficiency before becoming symptomatic. Systemic illness may play a major role in the development of the uremic syndrome. Mention was made above of the deleterious effects acute volume depletion caused by diarrhea or vomiting may have on the patient with renal insufficiency. Congestive heart failure may accelerate symptoms in a similar fashion through impairment of residual renal function, and other forms of acute deterioration in renal function (obstruction, acute pyelonephritis, drug toxicity, metabolic derangements) may produce the picture of uremia in a previously well compensated patient with chronic renal disease. The extrarenal effects of systemic illnesses may also confuse the presentation of uremic symptoms; included in this category would be hematologic and central nervous manifestations of lupus erythematosus, the neuropathy, retinopathy, and vascular disease of diabetes mellitus, and the encephalopathy of malignant hypertension in the patient with renal insufficiency. Finally, the treatment of systemic or renal disease may itself alter the development of uremic symptoms. Diuretic administration, if overly vigorous, may lead to electrolyte disturbances, volume

depletion, a fall in GFR, and acceleration of the uremic state. Aldosterone antagonists may produce fatal hyperkalemia in patients with renal insufficiency. The antibiotic tetracycline stimulates catabolism and exacerbates azotemia; its use is contraindicated in patients with renal insufficiency. Steroid therapy is associated with a number of complications which may cloud the interpretation of uremic symptoms; nausea and vomiting may result from peptic disease secondary to steroid treatment; tissue catabolism is promoted by these compounds, so that muscle breakdown and elevated urea nitrogen concentrations are observed; and long-term usage results in osteoporosis and potential exacerbation of renal osteodystrophy. Immunosuppressive agents with or without steroid therapy depress bone marrow function, resulting in increased risk of infection, particularly opportunistic infection, and leading to aggravation of anemia and platelet-related bleeding abnormalities.

REFERENCES

Eknoyan G: Pathophysiology of chronic renal failure and the uremic syndrome, in Kurtzman NA, Martinez-Maldonado M (eds): Pathophysiology of the Kidney. Springfield, Ill., Charles C. Thomas, 1977, p 842

Feldman HA, Singer I: Endocrinology and metabolism in uremia and dialysis: A clinical review. Medicine (Baltimore) 54:345, 1974

Massry SG: Is parathyroid hormone a uremic toxin? Nephron 19:125, 1977

Massry SG, Sellers AL (eds): Clinical Aspects of Uremia and Dialysis. Springfield, Ill., Charles C. Thomas, 1976

Giordano C (ed): Uremia. Kidney Int 7:S267, 1975

Schoenfeld, PY, Humphreys MH: A general description of the uremic state, in Brenner BM, Rector FC Jr (eds): The Kidney. Philadelphia, W.B. Saunders, 1976, p 1423

RENAL STONES

Charles Y.C. Pak

Urolithiasis is a common medical disorder, with a reported incidence of 0.1–1 percent in the United States. Today, virtually all stones are those originating in the kidneys; bladder stones are rarely encountered except in association with a foreign body.

Stones of renal origin may be broadly categorized on the basis of their chemical composition into those containing calcium and those which do not. Calcareous renal stones account for 80–90 percent of stones and are principally composed of calcium oxalate (dihydrate or monohydrate) and calcium phosphate (apatite or rarely brushite and whitlockite). Noncalcareous renal stones include those containing uric acid, cystine, or magnesium ammonium phosphate (struvite).

CALCAREOUS RENAL STONES

Many physiological or metabolic derangements have been associated with the formation of calcium-containing renal stones. These derangements, which may be used as the basis for the classification of calcium urolithiasis (Table 1), include hypercalciuria, hyperuricosuria, hyperoxaluria, defective renal acidification, and impaired renal excretion of inhibitors of stone formation. Although each derangement is not the sole cause, it probably contributes to stone formation. Each category of calcium urolithiasis will be considered with respect to pathogenetic mechanisms, diagnostic criteria, and management.

Hypercalciuria

Hypercalciuria is probably the most common abnormality found in patients with calcium urolithiasis. It probably contributes to stone formation by rendering urinary environment supersaturated with respect to calcium salts.

Pathogenesis

Hypercalciuria has been subdivided into three major forms on the basis of the location of the primary abnormality in calcium transport. In *resorptive* hypercalciuria, typified by primary hyperparathyroidism, the initial event is the excessive resorption of bone from the hypersecretion of parathyroid hormone. The ensuing hypercalcemia may cause hypercalciuria by augmenting the renal filtered load of calcium. The intestinal calcium absorption may also be increased consequent to parathyroid-hormone-dependent stimulation of the renal synthesis of 1,25-dihydroxyvitamin D. Thus hypercalciuria of primary hyperparathyroidism may also be "absorptive" secondarily. The occurrence of hypercalciuria in primary hyperparathyroidism seems paradoxical, since the primary renal action of parathyroid hormone is the stimulation of renal tubular reabsorption of calcium; however, hypercalciuria is often encountered in this condition because the augmentation of renal tubular reabsorption of calcium by parathyroid hormone is "overcome" by an increased renal filtered load of calcium and by a suppressive effect of hypercalcemia on calcium reabsorption.

In *absorptive* hypercalciuria, the basic abnormality is the intestinal hyperabsorption of calcium. The consequent increase in the circulating concentration of calcium augments renal filtered load of calcium and may suppress parathyroid function. Hypercalciuria ensues from the increased renal filtered load of calcium

Table 1
Classification of Renal Stones

Calcareous renal stones
    Hypercalciuria—resorptive, absorptive, renal
    Hyperuricosuria—overproduction, dietary
    Hyperoxaluria—primary, secondary
    Renal tubular acidosis
    Defective inhibitor excretion
    Structural abnormalities
Noncalcareous renal stones
    Uric acid stones
    Cystinuria
    Struvite stones

and the reduced renal tubular reabsorption of calcium resulting from parathyroid suppression. The excessive renal loss of calcium compensates for the high calcium absorption and maintains serum concentration of calcium in the normal range.

The cause for the increased calcium absorption in absorptive hypercalciuria is not known. Two schemes have been presented. One scheme implicates renal phosphate wastage as the primary event. The ensuing hypophosphatemia was then believed to stimulate the renal synthesis of 1,25-dihydroxyvitamin D and to increase absorption and excretion of calcium; however, hypophosphatemia and high serum 1,25-dihydroxyvitamin D are found only in some patients with absorptive hypercalciuria, and no significant correlation has been reported between serum phosphorus and intestinal calcium absorption. Another scheme implicates a vitamin-D-independent process—a selective increased absorption has been shown, involving jejunum and not ileum, and calcium and not magnesium. The diversity of these findings indicates that there may be different pathogenetic mechanisms for absorptive hypercalciuria.

The primary abnormality in renal hypercalciuria is the impaired renal tubular reabsorption of calcium. The consequent reduction in the circulating concentration of calcium stimulates parathyroid function. There may be an excessive mobilization of calcium from bone from the parathyroid hormone excess. The intestinal calcium absorption may also be increased, consequent to parathyroid-hormone-dependent stimulation of 1,25-dihydroxyvitamin D synthesis. These effects restore serum calcium toward normal. The cause for the impaired renal tubular reabsorption of calcium is not known. There need not be any other obvious abnormality in renal function.

The absorptive and renal hypercalciurias probably represent the two major variants of the condition previously termed idiopathic hypercalciuria.

Diagnostic criteria. The nature of parathyroid function distinguishes the three forms of hypercalciuria. Primary hyperparathyroidism is suggested by parathyroid stimulation in the setting of hypercalcemia, absorptive hypercalciuria by normal or suppressed parathyroid function with normocalcemia and hypercalciuria, and renal hypercalciuria by parathyroid stimulation with normocalcemia and hypercalciuria. Reliable measures of parathyroid function may be obtained from serum immunoreactive parathyroid hormone, urinary total cyclic AMP, or nephrogenous cyclic AMP. Hypercalciuria should be defined with respect to the particular diet during which urinary calcium is determined. The normal upper limit for urinary calcium is generally regarded as 250 mg/day for women and 300 mg/day for men on a random diet, 300 mg/day on a diet of 1000 mg calcium/day, and 200 mg/day on a diet with a daily composition of 400 mg calcium, 100 mEq sodium, and 800 mg phosphorus.

Fasting urinary calcium is invariably increased in

renal hypercalciuria and is frequently elevated in primary hyperparathyroidism, whereas it is typically normal in absorptive hypercalciuria. Intestinal calcium absorption is always increased in absorptive hypercalciuria and is often high in the other two forms of hypercalciuria. Clinically, primary hyperparathyroidism may be associated with other symptoms, such as peptic ulcer disease and bone disease (osteitis, subperiosteal resorption, osteoporosis). Renal hypercalciuria is sometimes associated with osteoporosis. Calcium urolithiasis is the only recognized clinical presentation of absorptive hypercalciuria. There is female preponderance in primary hyperparathyroidism, whereas there is male preponderance (particularly middle aged white) in absorptive hypercalciuria. The two sexes are equally affected in renal hypercalciuria.

Treatment. The initial treatment program consists of a dietary restriction of calcium and/or oxalate and increased fluid intake. If hypercalciuria and stone formation persist, a more specific medical therapy may be required, including sodium cellulose phosphate, thiazide, or orthophosphate. While all drugs have been used indiscriminately in all forms of hypercalciuria regardless of cause, it is apparent that certain drugs may be more appropriate for a particular form of hypercalciuria.

Sodium cellulose phosphate is a nonabsorbable ion-exchange resin with a high affinity for the calcium ion. When given orally, it complexes calcium; the complex of resin and calcium is then excreted in the feces. This drug therefore inhibits intestinal calcium absorption by limiting the amount of luminal calcium pool available for absorption. In absorptive hypercalciuria, it has been shown to restore normal urinary calcium and reduce urinary saturation of calcium salts, particularly that of brushite, without overly stimulating parathyroid function or causing bone disease. Sodium cellulose phosphate is contraindicated in primary hyperparathyroidism and renal hypercalciuria because of the danger of further stimulating parathyroid function and producing or aggravating bone disease.

Thiazides (and related compounds such as chlorthalidone) are unique among diuretics in their ability to augment renal tubular reabsorption of calcium. They represent the treatment of choice for renal hypercalciuria. Physiologically, thiazides have been shown to correct the "renal leak" of calcium, restore normal parathyroid function and the circulating concentration of 1,25-dihydroxyvitamin D, and correct the intestinal hyperabsorption of calcium. Physicochemically, these drugs typically reduce the urinary saturation of calcium salts by lowering urinary calcium. Moreover, they increase urinary inhibitor activity against crystallization of calcium salts; part of this action may be ascribed to the stimulation by thiazides of renal excretion of pyrophosphate and zinc.

Thiazides are equally effective in the control of hypercalciuria in absorptive hypercalciuria; however,

they may cause hypercalcemia in resorptive hypercalciuria.

Orthophosphates, as soluble salts of sodium and/or potassium, are potentially absorbable from the intestinal tract, unlike sodium cellulose phosphate. When given orally, they decrease urinary calcium, probably by directly affecting the renal tubular reabsorption of calcium. Whether or not they modify the intestinal absorption of calcium is unsettled. Physicochemically, they reduce urinary saturation of calcium oxalate, although they increase that of brushite. Moreover, urinary inhibitor activity, as measured by limit of metastability of calcium oxalate and brushite, is increased, consequent to the increased renal excretion of inhibitors, including pyrophosphate, citrate, and "phosphocitrate." Theoretically, orthophosphates are optimally indicated in the management of hypophosphatemic absorptive hypercalciuria because of the possibility that they may correct the renal leak of phosphate and restore normal circulating concentration of 1,25-dihydroxyvitamin D. Moreover, they may be useful in the treatment of normocalciuric patients who suffer from calcium urolithiasis because of a presumed deficiency of urinary inhibitors (to be discussed). Potential complications include extraskeletal calcification and bone disease. It is contraindicated in primary hyperparathyroidism, chronic renal failure, and urinary tract infection.

The surgical removal of abnormal parathyroid tissue is clearly the treatment of choice for calcium urolithiasis of primary hyperparathyroidism. Following parathyroidectomy, intestinal absorption and renal excretion of calcium decline towards normal. Urinary saturation and propensity for crystallization of calcium oxalate and brushite are reduced. Parathyroidectomy is contraindicated in renal and absorptive hypercalciurias, however.

Hyperuricosuria

Although hyperuricosuria may be found in some patients with hypercalciuria, it may be the only discernible biochemical abnormality in certain patients with calcium urolithiasis.

Pathogenesis. It is believed that hyperuricosuria may be etiologically important in the formation of calcium-containing renal stones, especially when it is present alone. In patients with hyperuricosuria, urinary environment is frequently supersaturated with respect to monosodium urate, principally because of high urate concentration in urine. Thus either colloidal or crystalline monosodium urate could potentially form. Once formed, monosodium urate may remove inhibitors of crystal aggregation or of nucleation by adsorption and thereby facilitate crystallization. Alternatively, monosodium urate may directly induce heterogeneous nucleation or "crystalline overgrowth" of calcium oxalate. This scheme has not yet been completely validated.

The cause for the hyperuricosuria is usually the result of dietary overindulgence of purine-rich foods. A "primary" overproduction of uric acid may be disclosed in some patients.

Diagnostic criteria. Clinical spectra of hyperuricosuric calcium urolithiasis in its pure presentation are as follows: First, the patients suffer from recurrent passage of calcium-containing renal stones, composed principally of calcium oxalate. Second, they have normocalciuria and no obvious abnormality of parathyroid function or of calcium metabolism. Third, they have a persistent hyperuricosuria of at least 600 mg/day. Finally, urinary pH is greater than 5.5, unlike patients with gout and uric acid stones (see Uric Acid Stones). There is probably no defect in renal acidification, since urinary pH is not significantly different from that of control subjects maintained on a similar diet. (The pH 5.5 approximates the pK for the first proton of uric acid; when urinary pH is greater than 5.5, urate salt is the stable phase, whereas uric acid is stable below this pH).

As in absorptive hypercalciuria, middle aged white males are particularly susceptible to this condition. Calcium urolithiasis is usually the sole presentation; gouty arthritis is uncommon. This condition may coexist with hypercalciuria (resorptive, renal, or absorptive).

Treatment. A low-purine diet is not generally recommended because it is difficult to maintain or may be detrimental to good nutrition. An avoidance of a high sodium intake may be desirable because such a regimen would probably reduce the urinary saturation of monosodium urate. Allopurinol, at a dosage sufficient to restore normal urinary uric acid, has been reported to reduce the urinary saturation of monosodium urate, inhibit spontaneous nucleation of calcium oxalate in urine, and decrease the frequency of new stone formation. The value of allopurinol therapy in patients with combined hyperuricosuria and hypercalciuria has not been clearly established.

Hyperoxaluria

Hyperoxaluria is either primary consequent to an accelerated in vivo synthesis of oxalate or secondary to an increased availability of substrate for oxalate synthesis or to an enhanced oxalate absorption. It may contribute to renal stone formation by increasing the urinary saturation of calcium oxalate.

Pathogenesis. In primary hyperoxaluria, the oxalate synthesis from glyoxalate is stimulated because of the disturbance in the enzymatic conversion of glyoxalate to alternate metabolites. Oxalate biosynthesis and renal excretion of oxalate may also be increased in the absence of enzymatic disturbance when substrates for oxalate synthesis are increased. These substrates include ascorbic acid, ethylene glycol, and methoxyflurane. These causes of hyperoxaluria are rare.

More commonly, hyperoxaluria results from an increased oxalate absorption from the intestinal tract. Normally, an ingestion of excessive amounts of oxalate-rich foods may slightly increase oxalate excretion but rarely cause frank hyperoxaluria because of a limited bioavailability of oxalate in foodstuffs; however, an exaggerated absorption and renal excretion of oxalate may be encountered in patients with an increased intestinal calcium absorption and in those with ileal disease.

In patients with increased calcium absorption, such as those suffering from absorptive hypercalciuria, a slight to moderate increase in oxalate excretion is sometimes found and may be explained by increased calcium absorption → reduced luminal calcium content → reduced calcium–oxalate complexation → increased available oxalate → increased absorbed oxalate → increased urinary oxalate.

Frank hyperoxaluria, often exceeding 100 mg/day, may be found in ileal disease (ileal resection, jejunoileal bypass surgery, inflammatory disease of small bowel). It is now recognized that hyperoxaluria is the consequence of an increased oxalate absorption. The high oxalate absorption may simply reflect an increased availability of luminal oxalate as is encountered in absorptive hypercalciuria. Under normal circumstances, much of dietary oxalate is probably unavailable for absorption because of complexation by calcium and magnesium. When there is malabsorption of fat, as is characteristic of ileal disease, intraluminal content of divalent cations may be reduced consequent to complexation of divalent cations by fatty acids. Thus less divalent cations would be available to limit oxalate absorption. Oxalate absorption may be increased because of an enlarged free oxalate pool. In addition, there is some evidence that oxalate absorption may be stimulated primarily in ileal disease from the action of bile acids on the oxalate permeability of the intestinal mucosa.

Diagnostic criteria. In primary hyperoxaluria, urinary glycolate or glycerate may be increased in addition to oxalate, unlike in secondary hyperoxaluria. Moreover, oxalosis (tissue deposition of calcium oxalate), anemia, and renal failure are common in primary hyperoxaluria.

In secondary hyperoxaluria of ileal disease, urinary calcium is typically low (<100 mg/day) and urinary oxalate high (often > 100 mg/day). Serum calcium and magnesium may be low or low normal, and parathyroid function may be stimulated.

Treatment. Calcium urolithiasis of primary hyperoxaluria may be responsive to treatment with orthophosphate by mechanisms not entirely understood. In stone-forming (nonhyperoxaluric) patients with hyperabsorption of calcium, a moderate dietary restriction of both calcium and oxalate may be advisable. In any stone-forming patient, an excessive ascorbic acid intake should be discouraged.

Oral administration of large amounts of calcium or magnesium has been recommended for the control of calcium urolithiasis of ileal disease. Although urinary oxalate may decrease, the concurrent rise in urinary calcium may obviate the beneficial effect of this therapy, at least in some patients. Cholestyramine does not cause a sustained reduction in oxalate excretion. A limitation of dietary oxalate intake and partial replacement of dietary fat with medium chain triglycerides may be helpful.

Defective Renal Acidification

Nephrocalcinosis (calcification in renal parenchyma) is commonly associated with classic (distal) renal tubular acidosis; however, calcium nephrolithiasis (stones in collecting system) is also encountered. An incomplete renal tubular acidosis may be found in a minority of patients with absorptive and renal hypercalciurias; the importance of this partial defect in renal acidification in the pathogenesis of calcium urolithiasis has not been clarified.

Pathogenesis. The exact cause for stone formation in renal tubular acidosis is not known. Acidosis may cause hypercalciuria by impairing renal tubular reabsorption of calcium, at least during the early stages of the disease before a significant renal impairment ensues. Because of high urinary pH, more phosphate is dissociated. Thus urinary environment may become supersaturated with respect to calcium salts, particularly to calcium phosphate. There may be a defective renal excretion of citrate and other inhibitors; this defect may therefore cause a reduced retardation of crystallization process in urine.

Diagnostic criteria. Biochemically, distal renal tubular acidosis is characterized by a reduced serum carbon dioxide and potassium, hyperchloridemia, and high urinary pH ($\sim$ 7). In late stages, the glomerular filtration rate may be significantly reduced. Urinary tract infection may supervene. Stones composed of calcium phosphate are more commonly encountered than in conditions previously enumerated.

Treatment. Oral administration of citrate or bicarbonate may reduce urinary calcium and augment citrate excretion, even though it does not alter urinary pH.

Defective Inhibitor Excretion

In approximately 10 percent of patients with calcium urolithiasis, no discernible metabolic abnormality may be found. Thus these patients form calcium stones despite normal renal excretion of calcium, uric acid, and oxalate and normal renal acidification.

Pathogenesis. Because of their disdain for drinking water, urinary output is considerably reduced in some of these patients. The consequent urinary concentration renders urinary environment supersaturated with respect to calcium salts and probably contributes to stone formation. In other patients without metabolic abnormality, however, urine output is adequate. It is theoretically possible that these patients may form stones because they lack inhibitors of stone formation in urine. Deficient renal excretion of inhibitors is probably also present in some patients with metabolic abnormality. This fact probably accounts for reduced inhibitor activity, as shown by low limit of metastability of calcium oxalate and brushite, in the urine of some patients with calcium urolithiasis, both those with and those without metabolic abnormality. Although direct experimental verification is lacking, there is preliminary evidence that certain stone-forming patients, particularly male subjects, excrete reduced amounts of pyrophosphate in urine.

Treatment. In patients with presumed deficiency in urinary inhibitors, therapy may be directed at stimulating the renal excretion of endogenous inhibitors or at providing exogenous inhibitors which would appear in urine. Treatment with thiazide (for example, hydrochlorothiazide 50 mg twice a day) may promote renal excretion of pyrophosphate and zinc, whereas that with orthophosphate (500 mg P three or four times per day) may augment excretion of pyrophosphate, citrate, and phosphocitrate.

Alternatively, an inhibitor such as diphosphonate may be given exogenously. Diphosphonate is a synthetic analogue of pyrophosphate. Unlike pyrophosphate, it is not hydrolyzed in vivo. Approximately 5 percent of the oral dose of diphosphonate is absorbed. After saturation of bone, the absorbed diphosphonate eventually appears in urine in an unaltered form. A sufficient amount of diphosphonate may be excreted to inhibit crystallization process and retard stone formation. Unfortunately, the usefulness of the commercially available diphosphonate, disodium etidronate, for the control of calcium urolithiasis is limited because of the potential for the induction of osteomalacia.

Stones Associated With Renal Structural Abnormality

Renal lithiasis may be found in patients with ectopic kidney, polycystic disease, and horseshoe kidney. Stones are typically radiopaque and consist usually of apatite or struvite. It is generally believed that stones form secondarily to the urinary tract infection.

Medullary sponge kidney is often associated with renal stones containing calcium oxalate and/or calcium phosphate (see the chapter on *Medullary Sponge Kidney*). The cause for the stone disease is not known. Certain patients demonstrate metabolic abnormalities, such as hypercalciuria, renal tubular acidosis, or primary hyperparathyroidism.

NONCALCAREOUS RENAL STONES

Uric Acid Stones

In the United States, the incidence of uric acid lithiasis has decreased in recent years, in part as the result of improved treatment programs for gout, with which this condition is frequently associated. Stones of uric acid composition probably account for less than 5 percent of stones. While some stones are composed solely of uric acid, they are more often present as mixtures with calcium oxalate or calcium phosphate.

Pathogenesis. The pK for the first proton of uric acid is 5.47. Thus below this pH uric acid and not its salt is the stable phase. Uric acid is sparingly soluble in this acid environment. The formation of the uric acid stone is typically associated with the persistent passage of urine of low pH (<5.5) and/or hyperuricosuria. The conditions are therefore favorable to the formation of uric acid stones because of the stability of uric acid and because the urinary environment is usually supersaturated with respect to this phase.

Diagnostic criteria. Clinically, uric acid lithiasis is frequently found in primary gout, a fact not too surprising, since passage of unusually acid urine (pH $<$ 5.5) and/or hyperuricosuria may accompany this disease. Secondary causes of purine overproduction which may lead to the formation of uric acid stones include myeloproliferative states, glycogen storage disease, and malignancy. Chronic diarrheal syndromes (ulcerative colitis, regional enteritis, jejunoileal bypass surgery) may be associated with uric acid lithiasis. The frequent occurrence of metabolic acidosis and low urine output probably contributes to stone formation by lowering urinary pH and increasing urinary concentration of uric acid. Theoretically, chronic ingestion of excessive amounts of meat products may cause uric acid lithiasis. Because of high purine and acid-ash contents of these products, urinary uric acid may be increased and urinary pH reduced, conditions favoring crystallization of uric acid.

It should be emphasized that patients with ileal disease or with dietary overindulgence with purine-rich foods may form calcium stones rather than uric acid stones, as previously discussed. The pH in a 24-hour urine sample is often useful in the differential diagnosis, since it is usually less than 5.5 with uric acid lithiasis and greater than 5.5 with calcium urolithiasis. Moreover, uric acid stones are typically radiolucent, whereas calcium stones are radiopaque.

Treatment. Oral administration of soluble salts of bicarbonate or citrate may increase urinary pH and create an environment in which uric acid is unstable. Unfortunately, some patients may form calcium stones following alkali therapy. Theoretically, this complication may result because overaggressive alkali therapy increases urinary uric acid, raises urinary saturation of monosodium urate or other urate salts, and promotes urate-induced crystallization of calcium oxalate. Moderate amounts of alkali sufficient to increase urinary pH to a range of 6–6.5 may be helpful in the management of uric acid lithiasis without producing a significant risk for calcium stone formation.

Allopurinol may be used to control hyperuricosuria; a dose of 300 mg/day in three divided doses is generally sufficient to restore normal urinary uric acid. Dietary purine restriction is seldom practical. Probenecid is contraindicated because of its uricosuric action.

Cystinuria

Cystinuria is due to an inborn error of metabolism, characterized by a disturbance in renal and/or intestinal handling of dicarboxylic acids, including cystine.

Pathogenesis. Some patients with cystinuria, albeit a minority, may develop cystine stones. Stone formation is probably the result of an excessive renal excretion of cystine and a low solubility of this dicar-

boxylic acid in the normal acid pH of urine. Cystine solubility is pH dependent; at pH 5 only 300 mg cystine may be dissolved per liter of urine, whereas at pH 7.5 as much as 500 mg cystine may go into solution. Some patients with cystinuria often excrete more than 300 mg cystine/day. In the normal acid environment, their urine may be supersaturated with respect to cystine, a condition favoring the formation of cystine stones.

Diagnostic criteria. In cystinuria, urinary cystine is increased (>100 mg/day). The cyanide–nitroprusside test provides a qualitative measure of cystine content; if positive, a quantitative test should be performed. Cystine stones are radiopaque, though less so than calcium stones. Moreover, they often grow to a large size and bear uniform density radiographically.

Treatment. Initial treatment program includes a high fluid intake to promote an adequate urine flow and oral administration of soluble alkali (bicarbonate or citrate) at a dose sufficient to raise urinary pH above 7. If this program is ineffective, D-penicillamine (2 g/day in divided doses) may be used. Vitamin B_6 (50 mg/day) should be added to avoid pyridoxine deficiency. Potential side effects of D-penicillamine include nephrotic syndrome, dermatitis, and pancytopenia.

Struvite Stones

Urinary tract infection sometimes accompanies nephrolithiasis. When it results from non-urea-splitting organisms, the stone typically contains constituents other than struvite (magnesium ammonium phosphate). It is not known whether infection caused the stone or developed as a complication of stone. When urea-splitting organisms (proteus, certain species of staphylococcus, pseudomonas, klebsiella) are responsible for infection, stones typically contain struvite with varying amounts of apatite.

Pathogenesis. In some patients, struvite stones may have formed de novo as a consequence solely of infection. In others, specific metabolic disorders associated with the formation of other types of renal stones could be identified; these derangements include hypercalciuria, hyperuricosuria, hyperoxaluria, and cystinuria. Struvite stone formation in the latter instance probably results from metabolic disorder $\rightarrow$ formation of nonstruvite stone $\rightarrow$ urinary tract infection with urea-splitting organisms $\rightarrow$ formation of struvite stone.

The physicochemical basis for struvite lithiasis is probably the same whether such stones form primarily or secondarily. The initial event is the formation of ammonia in urine upon enzymatic degradation of urea by bacterial urease. The ammonia undergoes hydrolysis to form ammonium and hydroxyl ions. The resulting alkalinity of urine stimulates the dissociation of phosphate to form more trivalent phosphate ions and lowers the solubility of struvite. The activity product or the state of saturation of urine with respect to struvite ($MgNH_4PO_4 \cdot 6H_2O$) is therefore increased. Stone formation ensues when sufficient oversaturation is reached.

Diagnostic criteria. In the presence of infection

with urea-splitting organisms, urinary pH often exceeds 7.5. There may be a moderate impairment in glomerular filtration rate and in renal concentrating ability. Struvite stones are radiopaque and sometimes may attain a large (staghorn) size. The diagnosis is confirmed by the demonstration of urea-splitting organisms in urine culture.

Treatment. If a longstanding effective control of infection with urea-splitting organisms can be achieved, there is some evidence that new stone formation can be averted or some dissolution of existing stone may be achieved. Unfortunately, such a control is difficult to obtain with antibiotic therapy. If there is an existing struvite stone, it is difficult to completely clear the infection because the stone often harbors the organisms within its interstices. Even if "sterilization" of urine has been achieved by antibiotic therapy, reinfection could occur by harbored organisms. For these reasons, it has been customary to recommend surgical removal of the struvite stones.

In recent clinical trials, acetohydroxamic acid, an urease inhibitor, has been shown to reduce urinary saturation of struvite and to retard stone formation.

REFERENCES

Coe FL: Nephrolithiasis: Pathogenesis and Treatment. Chicago, Year Book Medical, 1978

Pak CYC: in Avioli LV (ed): Calcium urolithiasis: Pathogenesis, Diagnosis, and Management. New York, Plenum, 1978

Pak CYC: Disorders of stone formation, in Brenner BM, Rector FC Jr (eds): The Kidney. Philadelphia, W.B. Saunders, 1976

Pak CYC: Symposium on urolithiasis. Kidney Int 13, 1978

Thomas WC Jr: Renal Calculi. Springfield, Ill., Charles C. Thomas, 1976

HYPERTENSION

David A. McCarron and George A. Porter

Hypertension, or an abnormal increase in systemic arterial pressure, is the most common disorder of the cardiovascular system encountered in the human species. Despite this acknowledged prevalence, our fragmentary understanding of the pathogenesis and natural history compromises rational therapy of hypertensive disorders.

Prevalence

All age groups are affected, since well documented, persistent elevation of the arterial pressure afflicts 3–10 percent of individuals from 10–50 years of age. In addition, transient elevations, or "labile hypertension," occurs in another 5–10 percent, half of whom will ultimately demonstrate fixed increases in arterial pressure. While the prevalence of hypertension is similar for pediatric and adult populations, there is a disturbingly high prevalence of systolic hypertension in the geriatric segment of our society. It is unclear whether this age-associated prevalence of hypertension has the same pathologic implication we ascribe to hypertensive patients under the age of 50. Despite these uncertainties, hypertension must be considered a lifelong ailment.

Predisposing Factors

In 95 percent of the cases of documented hypertension, a precise etiology cannot be defined. Such patients are categorized as "essential" or "primary" hypertensives. For the remaining 5 percent an identifiable cause is discovered, and these are classified as secondary hypertensives. In point of fact, however, any pathologic increase in the arterial pressure is likely related to multiple factors. This multifactorial influence probably explains the failure to achieve a unified concept concerning the etiology of essential hypertension. Based upon experience to date, the separation into primary and secondary hypertension has not provided enlightenment as to the etiology of essential hypertension and may actually hamper the search for identifiable factors that contribute to the development of sustained blood pressure elevations.

Genetic, cultural, dietary, environmental, and metabolic factors are the best documented as influencing the development of hypertension in humans. A strong family history raises the risk of developing arterial hypertension two- to fivefold. It can be argued that the genetic factor in hypertension reflects survival benefits bestowed to the hypertensive individual. This apparent selection which favors hypertensives may be explained by the studies of Page, who demonstrated increasing mean arterial pressure with increasing level of acculturation. It is apparent that further unraveling of the pathogenesis of hypertension will be aided by investigations which minimize the number of variables, thereby allowing some quantification of the impact of single, isolated factors.

In addition to a strong family history of hypertension, a familial propensity to develop coronary artery disease, cerebral vascular disease, congestive heart failure, thyroid disorders, obesity, or diabetes mellitus increases the chances of a family member becoming hypertensive. Furthermore, obesity, plasma lipid abnormalities, poor physical conditioning, or excess dietary sodium may predispose any individual to hypertension. Finally, as a prognostic sign, approximately 50 percent of subjects with transient or labile elevations of the arterial pressure eventually develop sustained hypertension.

Anatomic and Pathophysiologic Complications

The heart in hypertension undergoes a number of pathologic changes which are progressive and often lethal. Even before blood pressure elevation becomes distinctly pathologic, an increase in the heart rate can be detected. Associated with the accelerated heart rate, cardiac output, ventricular filling pressures, and myocardial oxygen consumption are increased. Prolonged elevation of the blood pressure causes destructive anatomic changes in the myocardium, the coronary arteries, and the valves. In any given patient, the influence of concurrent risk factors often determines which of the three anatomical abnormalities predominates (Table 1). The first two are much more common.

Congestive heart failure. In the spontaneously hypertensive rat, hypertrophy of the myocardium may antedate the blood pressure increase. With sustained elevations of the pressure, hypertrophy of myocardial cells causes a concentric and uniform thickening of the left ventricular wall. Dilitation of the chamber is a late occurrence, heralding the onset of decompensated congestive failure. The manifestations of heart failure in subjects with longstanding hypertension vary. Early changes include electrocardiographic and radiologic evidence of cardiac hypertrophy, while later physical

Table 1
Complications of Chronic Hypertension

Cardiac disease
  Left ventricular failure
    Hypertensive myocardiopathy
    Postinfarction
  Coronary artery insufficiency
    Main coronary lesions
    Small vessel disease
  Aortic valvular dysfunction
    Calcification—stenosis
    Dilatation—insufficiency

Cerebral disease
  Carotid artery stenosis
    Transient ischemic attacks
    Acute brain infarction
  Intracranial Hemorrhage
    Spontaneous
    Aneurysm rupture
  Lacunar infarction
  CNS dysfunction
    Small vessel disease
    Drug related
    Malignant hypertension

Renal disease
  Renal artery stenosis
    Atherosclerotic
    Fibromuscular
  Rapidly progressive renal insufficiency—malignant
    hypertension
  Chronic renal insufficiency
    Accelerated progression of primary disorder
    Nephrosclerosis
    Atheroembolic
    Segmental infarction

Large vessel disease
  Aortic aneurysm
    Thoracic—dissecting
    Abdominal
  Ilial–femoral obstruction
  Peripheral vascular disease

Miscellaneous
  Retinal hemorrhages
  Mesenteric insufficiency

signs will include lateral displacement of the apical pulse, the presence of a gallop rhythm, and tachycardia. When cardiac decompensation occurs in hypertensive heart disease, x-ray evidence of pulmonary vascular congestion is present, as are abnormal values for the BUN, creatinine, and liver enzymes, and decreased arterial pO_2 and pH values. Associated physical signs of biventricular involvement include rales, jugular-venous distension, hepatomegaly, lower extremity edema, and eventually intractable ascites and cerebral hypoxia.

Coronary artery disease. The most frequent initial manifestation of coronary artery involvement associated with hypertension is acute coronary insufficiency. Hypertension initiates the process by inducing lateral wall stress on the vessels, causing endothelial cell injury. The endothelial injury triggers a proliferative response by intimal cells, the rate being accelerated by concurrent risk factors. Evidence of a "silent" myocardial infarction by ECG may be the initial evidence of coronary artery disease in a hypertensive patient, although less dramatic presentations such as angina and/or rhythm disturbances are frequently encountered. Physical examination may be normal or reveal arteriosclerotic retinal vessels or diminished peripheral pulses. Cardiomyopathy complicating hypertensive heart disease is evident when overt signs of congestive failure are observed.

Valvular disease. Aortic valve dysfunction can be associated with systemic hypertension. Progressive calcification of the aortic valve with subsequent stenosis is accelerated by elevated systemic blood pressure after dilatation of the aortic ring complicates prolonged hypertension. While the hemodynamic consequences of these valvular lesions do not usually require surgical intervention, they do compromise cardiac performance by increasing left ventricular afterload and magnifying any symptoms attributable to coronary insufficiency.

Atherosclerotic vascular disease. Large vessel disease. While atherosclerosis can develop in the absence of hypertension, the greater shearing forces associated with hypertension speed the rate of intimal disruption of the arterial wall and augment the development of atherosclerotic plaques. In addition, extension of intimal tears is promoted in the presence of elevated blood pressure, as is calcification of the plaques. The most dramatic demonstration of this pathologic cycle occurs in dissecting aortic aneurysm, a lethal sequel of atherosclerotic disease that virtually never occurs in the absence of hypertension. When either abdominal or thoracic aneurysms show progressive, rapid expansion, acute hypotensive therapy is the only practical treatment currently available. The preferential distribution of atherosclerotic plaques in vessel bifurcations explains the high incidence of carotid, aortoiliac, and ileofemoral stenosis. Clinically, large vessel narrowing is manifested by either intermittent claudication and eventual ischemic necrosis of the involved extremity or cerebral vascular disease culminating in cerebral atheroembolism and infarction. Although the former complication is not likely to be fatal, its occurrence will be associated with major morbidity in hypertensive patients. Conversely, atheroembolic cerebral vascular disease is a major cause of death in hypertensives. Fragments arising from plaques located at the bifurcation of the carotid system seed the distal cerebral circulation. Furthermore, long standing hypertension results in a rightward displacement of the autoregulatory curve of cerebral blood flow. Thus hypertensive subjects become dependent upon a sustained elevation of the mean arterial pressure and will develop symptoms of cerebral ischemia at higher mean blood pressure as compared to normotensive patients.

Small vessel disease. For the majority of individuals who are hypertensive, the development of end-organ complications is insidious, often requiring 20 or more years to become clinically evident. End-organ damage to the heart, brain, kidneys, and eyes develops because small vessel damage results in a decreased blood flow, causing permanent damage.

The rate at which atheroslerosis and occlusive peripheral vascular disease develop in hypertensive patients is accelerated when combined with other risk factors such as cigarette smoking, lipid abnormalities, and/or diabetes. Although occlusive peripheral vascular disease rarely causes death, dissection of an aortic aneurysm in a hypertensive patient is often lethal. Arterioloslcerosis involving the heart, brain, kidney and/or eye is both a more serious and a more frequent consequence of sustained hypertension.

Since hypertension can be a major contributing factor in the development of congestive heart failure, it is of interest that aggressively treating the early phase of experimental hypertension not only stabilizes myocardial failure but actually improves cardiac function. In the case of coronary artery disease, hypertension is an independent risk factor whose contribution is in direct proportion to the level of the blood pressure. Furthermore, as a risk factor, hypertension probably exceeds heredity, smoking, obesity, diabetes, or lipid abnormalities. Myocardial infarction is the most common fatal event in hypertensives, while a cerebral vascular accident, specifically atheroembolic brain infarction, is the second leading category. Although hemorrhagic events in the brain may appear to have a closer correlation with the level of the blood pressure than brain infarcts, in reality the incidence of both types of stroke are equally influenced by the presence of hypertension. Being more frequent, atheroembolic brain infarction is a prime contributor to hypertensive morbidity and mortality. Atherosclerosis involving the carotids is the usual precursor of embolic infarction. Lacunar infarcts, classically involving the basal ganglia or subcortical region of the brain, are common pathologic manifestation of cerebrovascular disease in hypertensive subjects.

Hypertension often complicates the course of many types of renal disease. The hypertension associated with glomerulopathies, diabetic nephropathy, renal vas-cular disease, and other causes of endstage renal disease is causally correlated with more rapid deterioration of renal function. While the overall incidence of malignant transformation of benign essential hypertension is decreasing, accelerated hypertension still occurs most typically in the patient whose impaired renal function is the result of a glomerular disorder. Hypertension in the posttransplant setting affects up to 50 percent of successful graft recipients. Since it is unusual for the hypertension to be caused by the allograft, these patients deserve the same thoughtful evaluation as the newly identified hypertensive patient.

Stenosis of one or more of the main renal arteries is a recognized late complication of chronic hypertension, most often in males. Since these vascular lesions are atheroslcerotic in origin, the resulting renal ischemia intensifies the preexisting elevations in the mean arterial pressure. Involvement is usually bilateral and diffuse, but the rate of progression is dependent upon the adequacy of blood pressure control. Occasionally, stenosis of the renal artery is a chance finding in the elderly hypertensive, and no pathologic significance can be ascribed. In addition to large vessel disease of the kidney, diffuse, progressive arteriolar nephrosclerosis can be expected in most patients subject to longstanding poorly regulated hypertension. Atheroembolic renal disease is a poorly appreciated late complication of severe generalized atherosclerosis. Small portions of larger vessel plaques embolize and become lodged distally in many organs, including the kidneys. In the kidneys, this form of occlusive vascular disease manifests itself as a rather precipitous, often symmetrical reduction in renal size and function.

PATHOGENESIS

The gradual increase in arterial pressure which characterizes systemic hypertension leads to predictable alterations in vascular hemodynamics (see Fig. 1). These changes include disturbances in peripheral resistance, cardiac dynamics, endocrine function, and the central nervous system. Based upon population and animal model studies, one or more of the alterations summarized in Fig. 1 are assumed to initiate the change in vascular resistance which characterizes sustained blood pressure elevations.

In both humans and genetic strains of hypertensive rats, the earliest and most consistent hemodynamic abnormality is an increase in cardiac output with a subsequent rise in peripheral resistance. The stimulus to the myocardium and the resistance vessels has been ascribed to an increased adrenergic nervous system activity. Furthermore, it has been suggested that these changes in catecholamine metabolism are brought about by as yet undefined central nervous system influences. Alternatively, the increase in the adrenergic system activity may be the result of heightened responsiveness or reactivity rather than a true increase in overall activity.

As a consequence of the adrenergic stimulation, peripheral venous constriction leads to the redistribu-

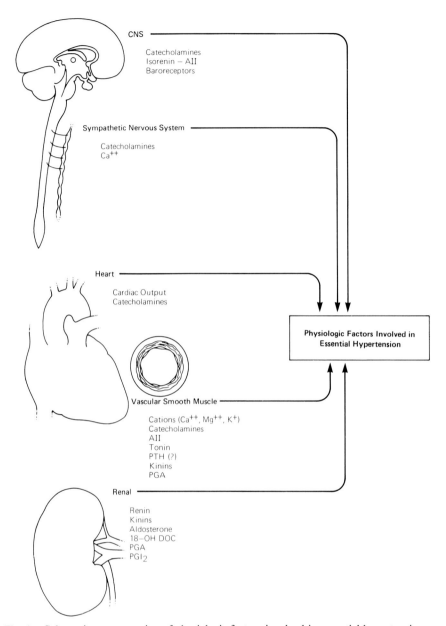

Fig. 1. Schematic representation of physiologic factors involved in essential hypertension.

tion of blood into the central vasculature, with a net increased cardiac output, as both heart rate and stroke volume rise. If peripheral resistance measured at this stage is normal, then autoregulatory vasoconstriction has not occured. Early vascular resistance increases are associated with selective changes in regional blood flow in that myocardial flow is proportionally increased while renal flow is decreased. As hypertension becomes established, regional differences in blood flow are further magnified.

A great deal of attention has also been directed to changes in plasma volume, extracellular fluid volume, and exchangeable sodium and potassium in hypertensive states. While individual studies vary, the bulk of the data indicates these parameters to be either near or at normal levels in persons with primary hypertension. Whether the existence of normal volumes with increased arterial pressures is an abnormal relationship remains to be defined. The reported inverse correlation between arterial blood pressure and plasma volume is usually ascribed to increased hydrostatic pressure at the capillary level. In summary, gross disorders of body fluid volume and electrolyte composition have not been implicated in the early pathogenesis of hypertension; however, that small and as yet unmeasurable differences in the volumes of various body spaces may exist between established hypertensive subjects and normotensive controls remains a possibility.

Vascular Smooth Muscle

Alterations in catecholamine metabolism and/or vascular sensitivity characterize the early phase of hypertension in man. Whether the measured increase in vascular resistance is a response to enhanced production of endogenous vasopressors or an increased vascular smooth muscle sensitivity to these various stimuli is unresolved. It is well documented that the vascular system of hypertensive subjects is more sensitive to both norepinephrine and angiotensin II infusions. This hyperreactivity to endogenous vasoconstrictors may arise from abnormalities of vessel structure and/or smooth muscle cell function. The former explanation is supported by studies demonstrating an increase in the mass of contractile tissue in the vessel wall. Because of the altered geometry of the vessels, a proportionately greater reduction in cross-sectional area occurs for comparable degrees of vasoconstriction induced by norepinephrine infusion. The latter speculation gains support from the many reports of abnormal fluid and electrolyte composition of the vascular smooth muscle cell of a hypertensive animal compared to normal tissue. Intracellular concentrations of Na^+, Ca^{2+}, Mg^{2+}, and water are increased, while K^+ is reduced. Since the catecholamine response of normal smooth muscle cells is cation dependent, and since the norepinephrine content of vascular tissue from hypertensive subjects is reduced, one can speculate that the increased concentration of these cations play a prominent role in the heightened reactivity of hypertensive smooth muscle to reduced amounts of norepinephrine. Furthermore, the altered composition of the vascular smooth muscle cell in the hypertensive state is an attractive explanation for the treatment-induced reversibility of vascular resistance, since structural changes would be more permanent.

The rate of sodium flux is an important determinant of smooth muscle tone. Potassium, calcium, magnesium, and trace metals are also vital. Calcium's role is to modulate the fluxes of both Na^+ and K^+ across the cell membrane. Small changes in membrane bound Ca^{2+} alter the smooth muscle response to vasoconstrictive stimuli induced by norepinephrine, angiotensin II, and K^+.

Humoral Mediators

Similarities between the relationship of Na, K^+, Ca^{2+}, and Mg^{2+} in vascular smooth muscle and their interactions in the kidney exists. This parallelism has lead to speculation on the influence of humoral factors such as catecholamines, aldosterone, parathyroid hormone prostaglandins, and the kinins on vascular cell composition. Stated in another way, the known effect of these compounds on the renal handling of these various electrolytes may be shared by vascular smooth muscle.

Catecholamines. Altered central and peripheral activity of the adrenergic nervous system has long been suspected to contribute to the development of arterial hypertension. Recently this concept has been strengthened by the measurement of increased plasma catecholamine concentrations in nearly 50 percent of essential hypertensives. Their assigned role in pathogenesis relates to the direct action of catecholamines on the heart and vascular smooth muscle, plus the release of renal renin and induction of a natriuresis. Recently, it has been reported that catecholamine levels decrease with age and thus may become less of a factor in long-established essential hypertension.

Renin. Unlike plasma catecholamine, plasma renin activity is within the normal range in the majority of patients with primary hypertension. Attempts to divide hypertensive subjects according to their plasma renin activity has largely failed, at least in terms of identifying pathogenetic mechanisms; however, the failure to demonstrate predictable changes in plasma renin in essential hypertension does not eliminate a central role for renin in the genesis of increased arterial pressure. Most attention has been directed at renin release from the kidney juxtaglomerular cell in response to changes in physical, humoral, and ionic signals. Renin, once released, then governs angiotensin I generation and conversion to the potent vasoconstrictor angiogensin II. Angiotensin II also causes adrenal aldosterone synthesis and secretion with subsequent enhanced sodium reabsorption in the distal nephron.

Renin modulation of blood pressure may not be limited to the peripheral cirulation, since it also acts on the central nervous system. Besides the brain and vessel walls, adrnenal glands, salivary glands, and the genital tract have been identified as tissues producing enzymes similar to renin (isorenins). In the brain, isorenins appear to be directly involved in the central mechanism of blood pressure control. The brain isorenin levels correlate both with central norepinephrine concentrations and the systolic blood pressure of laboratory animals.

The renin–angiotensin system acts on both the vasoconstrictor and volume components of blood pressure regulation. Renin-stimulated angiotensin II is a potent vasoconstrictor, while renal sodium retention, resulting from renin-mediated increase in aldosterone, raises intravascular volume. The former response is usually stipulated as the pathogenic means by which renin contributes to the early phase of essential hypertension. Conversely, in established hypertension, normal plasma renin values suggest that a new renin–volume relationship has developed such that normal renin concentrations coexist with a small but significant increase in intravascular volume. Such a resetting of the renin–volume relationship has been demonstrated in experimental hypertension due to coarctation of the aorta and in the hypertension of chronic renal failure. The difficulty in assigning renin a unified role in the genesis of hypertension may involve the critical importance of local concentrations of the enzyme in the kidney, smooth muscle, and brain rather than the systemic concentrations frequently measured.

Antiotensin II. It is impossible to separate the

effect of renin from that of angiotensin II (A II) on blood pressure control. Renin release is itself inhibited by A II. A II affects blood pressure control not only through vasoconstriction but also by stimulation of central thirst and activation of the sympathetic nervous system. Ultimately, the sustained effect of A II on hypertension may well be the volume expansion resulting from sustained aldosterone secretion. Finally, the response of the vascular smooth muscle to A II (as with catecholamines) is modulated by the sodium, calcium, and potassium concentrations in the vascular tissue. Alterations in membrane and/or intracellular concentrations of these cations account for some of the variability in the pressor response to A II which has been reported in normal and hypertensive subjects.

Tonin. A new enzyme, tonin, has been characterized recently. This compound acts on a naturally occurring protein substrate (toninogen), renin substrate, and/or A I to directly produce A II. Tonin activity is completely inhibited by a variety of plasma protein inhibitors. Alterations in or absence of these inhibitors could result in enhanced tonin activity and a consequent increase in A II formation. The precise role and importance of tonin in blood pressure regulation awaits further study.

Aldosterone. Aldosterone along with 11-deoxycorticosterone (DOC), 18-hydroxy-11-deoxycorticosterone (18-hydroxy-DOC), and dehydroepiandrosterone (DHEA) comprise the most frequent adrenocortical steroids implicated in the pathogensis of human hypertension. The synthesis and secretion of aldosterone appears to be regulated by four factors, including ACTH via adenylcyclase, large changes in plasma sodium concentration, potassium balance, and the renin–angiotensin system. The role of ACTH is finite and limited, since it stimulates aldosterone synthesis by increasing the conversion of cholesterol to pregnenolone. Plasma sodium concentration, independent ot simultaneous changes in the renin–angiotensin system, is of minor significance, since major alterations in sodium concentration are required to vary the aldosterone secretion rate. In contrast, the effect of an abnormal plasma potassium concentration on aldosterone production is striking. Small increases in the serum potassium will stimulate aldosterone synthesis, while declines in serum potassium inhibit it. This effect of potassium has been shown to be independent of any change in either sodium balance or the renin–angiotensin system. Thus changes in either volume or the sympathetic nervous system affect aldosterone production by activating the renin–angiotensin system. Changes in sodium balance are largely responsible for the volume mediated influences. Increased sodium content of vascular smooth muscle cells represents one common pathway whereby elevation of A II and/or aldosterone would reduce vascular cross-sectional area and hence increase peripheral resistance.

Evidence that increased aldosterone activity is involved in essential hypertension comes from two types of studies. In one, plasma aldosterone levels were increased and metabolic clearance rates were decreased in mild, essential hypertensives as compared to normals. In the second type of investigation, several authors have demonstrated that the expected increase in plasma aldosterone in hypertensive patients is blunted following severe sodium restriction and incomplete suppression of either the plasma aldosterone level or secretion rate of aldosterone following salt loading. In summary, data from essential hypertensives seem to suggest that aldosterone, or the sum of aldosterone 18-OH-DOC or other steroids, contributes to the genesis and maintenance of elevated arterial pressure.

Renin–angiotensin–aldosterone system. Many and, at times, seemingly unrelated abnormalities of the expected renin–angiotensin–mineralocorticoid relationship have been described in various populations of hypertensives. Of the many disorders postulated, four appear to have been reasonably documented. First, older subjects show an impaired PRA response to maneuvers designed to stimulate renin release—i.e., salt depletion, diuretic challenge. Second, many hypertensives manifest a delayed or suboptimal suppression of the renin–angiotensin–aldosterone axis with either acute or chronic sodium loading. Third, hypertensives with low renin values often have normal plasma aldosterone concentrations, compatible with an exaggerated responsiveness of A II mediated aldosterone synthesis. Lastly, a significant percentage of hypertensive subjects with normal plasma renins will not increase aldosterone secretion appropriately with acute stimulation of the renin–angiotensin system, implying an altered sensitivity to angiotensin II. These seemingly disparate findings do not negate the importance of the renin–angiotensin–aldosterone axis in the development of elevated arterial pressure but likely reflect the heterogeneous nature of the humoral steady-state which exists in patients with essential hypertension.

Prostaglandins. Interest in a vasodepressor effect of the normal kidney prompted the search for and isolation of substance(s) synthesized in the kidney that cause vasodilation. Prostaglandins (PGE, PGA, and PGI_2) have been the focus of this research. Both PGE and PGA have been shown to have species specific effects on systemic hemodynamics. In general, they lower blood pressure via arteriolar vasodilation. Evidence indicates that locally generated PGE affects vascular smooth muscle function by induced changes in Na^+ K^+ ATPase.

Controversy still exists as to the physiologic significance of PGA (or medullin, as it was initially called). It is produced primarily in the renomedullary interstitial cell of the kidney. It differs most dramatically from PGE in its longer time course of onset and its ability to pass through the pulmonary circulation without being metabolized. PGA function in blood pressure regulation in humans is uncertain, since it has not been found to be detectable in measureable amounts. Prostacyclin (PGI$_2$), the newest prostaglandin to be investigated, has been shown to be ten times more potent than PGA in terms of renin release. Whether this compound or other prostaglandins play a role in the regulation of mean arterial pressure is not established.

Kinins. The kallikrein–kinin system has recently been reconsidered as a possible important humoral component in the regulation of normal blood pressure. The similarities of the enzymatic actions of renin and kallikrein in the generation of vasoactive polypeptides has prompted much of this new interest. The existence of urinary kallikrein activity has been known for over 50 years, but its potential as a regulator of either blood pressure or renal hemodynamics has come from investigations of the past 15–20 years.

Kallikreins are enzymes that act to liberate from kininogens (substrates in the plasma) kinins, of which bradykinin is the best characterized. In the kidney, kallikrein activity and kinin generation have been identified and related to sodium excretion. Urinary kallikrein excretion is proportional to renal production of this enzyme, though some of the activity may come from the filtration of plasma kallikrein. Differences in urinary kallikrein exist in both hypertensive man and experimental animals, when their basal secretory rates and their response to NaCl loading are compared to normotensive controls. Kallikrein excretion is reduced in humans with essential hypertension and in most animal model systems that have been studied. The importance of this suppression of the endogenous renal kallikrein–kinin system in the pathogenesis of elevated arterial pressure and its relationship to prostaglandin and renin production await further investigation.

Parathyroid hormone. An association between parathyroid hormone and the development of hypertension is based upon the unusual frequency of elevated blood pressures in subjects with proven hyperparathyroidism. The basis for a role of parathyroid hormone in blood pressure regulation involves regulation of calcium balance and the inhibition of proximal tubular sodium reabsorption in the kidney. In addition to the natriuretic properties of parathyroid hormone, it has also been implicated in the control of renal renin release. Although early clinical reports implicated either PTH and/ or hypercalcemia in the genesis of the hypertension associated with hyperparathyroidism, more recent data ascribe a vasodepressor effect to acute increases in either endogenous or exogenous PTH and a pressor effect when endogenous PTH is suddenly reduced. Although unproven, an attractive hypothesis is that PTH is involved in the modulation of smooth muscle tone via its influence on ionized calcium.

Central Nervous System

Our understanding of the central nervous system's role in the development and maintenance of hypertension remains largely speculative because of the limited accessibility of the brain to clinical and experimental investigation. There is little doubt that stimulation of specific regions of the brain raises systemic blood pressure or that the CNS modulates systemic pressure through hormonal mediation.

The best evidence to support a primary role for the CNS in arterial hypertension comes from observations using various antihypertensive agents. Propranolol, clonidine, and methyldopa are believed to exert a portion of their antihypertensive effect through an action on midbrain and hypothalamus. Besides reducing blood pressure, the frequency of drug-induced psychological side effects is consistent with a role for the CNS in the pathogenesis of human hypertension. In laboratory animals, acute stimulation of hypothalamic and midbrain structures will initiate an increase in heart rate, cardiac output, and blood pressure. These increases are transient but similar to those observed in humans and animals during emotional stress and/or fright. An explanation by which these acute increases might translate into fixed increases in arterial pressure is missing at present.

Perturbations of the brain's distinct isorenin–angiotensin system will change systemic blood pressure. Angiotensin II directly stimualtes sympathetic nervous activity and has been considered as one way in which CNS function could influence blood pressure regulation. Renin release by the juxtaglomerular (JG) cell is partially under the influence of sympathetic fibers that terminate directly on the JG apparatus. Stimulation of midbrain structures results in renin release that can be inhibited by simultaneous administration by propranolol. By stimulation of the sympathetic nervous system and thus causing renal renin release, the brain isorenin–angiotensin system may contribute to systemic hypertension.

Another important central neural mechanism in hypertension maybe the baroreceptors. Baroreceptor reflexes are a vital negative feedback loop in CNS regulation of arterial blood pressure. Since their description over 50 years ago, numerous hypotheses have been advanced that ascribed a primary role to these pressure-sensing receptors in the development of hypertension. A decreased sensitivity of the baroreceptors and consequent lessening of the negative feedback input have been the basis for these theories. While resetting of baroreceptors has been an attractive idea, data support only a minor role for this speculation in the genesis of most forms of experimental and clinical hypertension. The resetting would appear to be a secondary phenomenon, occurring only after arterial hypertension is established.

The sympathetic nervous system mediates many of the physiologic events which contribute to both regulation and deregulation of systemic blood pressure. Through release of catecholamines from presynaptic cells, alpha and/or beta receptors (depending on the tissue) are stimulated. Alpha stimulation increases arterial resistance and enhanced venous tone, while beta stimulation elevates both heart rate and cardiac output while causing renal renin to be released. As detailed previously, substantial circumstantial evidence points to increased sympathetic nervous system activity or reactivity as the earliest physiologic aberration in the labile hypertensive. Attesting to this is the fact that the highest levels of plasma and urinary catecholamine excretion occur in "labile hypertension." Once increased arterial pressure becomes established, catecholamine concentrations normalize, though at levels which are inappropriately high for the mean arterial pressure; however, catecholamine plasma concentrations and excretion rates are not sufficient to assess the role of the autonomic nervous system. Adrenergic receptor sensitivity and rates of catecholamine release and reuptake must also be evaluated. Unfortunately, at the present time, the reliability of the measurement of these parameters is poor, and yet they are probably extremely important to complete our understanding of the role of the sympathetic nervous system in essential hypertension.

In summary, the basic tenet concerning the pathophysiology of essential hypertension is that this disorder arises from multiple etiologic factors—genetic, environmental, dietary, emotional, humoral, ionic, metabolic, and/or renal. Whatever the primary pathogenetic process, the late changes which accompany the fixed elevation of the arterial pressure often include an increase in peripheral vascular resistance, decreased vascular compliance, a defect in renal sodium excretion, and left ventricular hypertrophy with increased cardiac work but diminished efficiency. Intravascular volume and endocrine function, while apparently normal, are often inappropriately reset. The central and peripheral cardiovascular system is increasingly taxed and ultimately begins to fail, manifesting as coronary artery disease, congestive heart failure, cerebral vascular insufficiency, stroke, renal insufficiency, and/or peripheral vascular disease.

CLASSIFICATION AND CHARACTERISTICS
Primary Hypertension

Ninety-five percent of new patients with confirmed hypertension are ultimately categorized as having primary hypertension. In other words, there is no clearly defined factor(s) that, if corrected, will result in normalizing the blood pressure. Most of these individuals are identified during the fourth and fifth decades of life. Males are affected more often than females, though this disparity is less apparent with advanced age. The new hypertensive is likely to be overweight, a smoker, in poor physical condition, and suffering from at least one other chronic medical disorder. Typically, there is a family history of hypertension, cardiovascular disease, and/or premature death. The subject is often aware of some previous blood pressure readings that were borderline or frankly abnormal which may date back to adolescence. It is unusual for the new patient with primary hypertension to give a past history of entirely normal blood pressure readings. The blood pressure elevations are usually detected during routine physical

examinations, or in the course of an evaluation for another medical problem. It is atypical for the new hypertensive to be symptomatic, although the patient may relate symptoms such as dizziness, nervousness, and headaches. Once hypertension is documented a slow rise in the blood pressure with time is the rule, unless treated. Table 1 includes key historical information which allows for the evaluation of the consequence of hypertension in each patient.

With primary hypertension, the physical examination is rarely revealing. Early physical evidence of increased sympathetic nervous system activity (tachycardia, flushing, dynamic precordium, and sweating) is the only positive finding. With increasing duration of hypertension funduscopic changes appear, manifested as increased light reflex, tortuosity of the retinal vessels, and, rarely, hemorrhages and exudates. Left ventricular enlargement along with the development of diminished peripheral pulses and vascular bruits occurs, and late in the course of hypertension serious end-organ damage will be evident, including congestive failure, cerebral vascular compromise, renal insufficiency, and/or peripheral vascular insufficiency.

Routine laboratory studies in the young hypertensive are typically unremarkable, including the serum electrolytes and creatinine, CBC, urinalysis, EKG, and chest x-ray. In older subjects electrocardiographic and radiographic evidence of left ventricular hypertrophy are the two most frequent abnormalities noted. Less common is biochemical evidence of renal insufficiency. In elderly hypertensives the incidence of associated medical disorders such as diabetes and chronic pulmonary disease are increased. Unless the patient's history, physical examination, and/or routine studies suggest a secondary cause for the hypertension, as outlined in Fig. 2, the initial laboratory evaluation of a new hypertensive patient should be limited. Additional studies should be selected judiciously and only when they are likely to alter diagnosis, therapy, or prognosis.

Spurious Hypertension

Confirmation of the diagnosis of systemic hypertension rests on accurate and repeated blood pressure determinations. Spurious or false elevations of the arterial pressure are a chronic, recurrent problem in the diagnosis and management of hypertension. Because obesity is so prevalent, strict attention must be paid to the appropriate blood pressure cuff size. Use of an undersized cuff can result in an error of as much as 30 mm Hg in the indirect measurement of arterial pressure. Ideally, the bladder of the cuff should be centered over the brachial artery and encircle 70 percent of the arm, with the circumference of the arm fitting within the lines marked on the cuff. A common cause of spurious recordings is patient stress or anxiety. While the measured blood pressure in this situation may be technically satisfactory, it often does not accurately reflect the subject's blood pressure profile. Patients must be relaxed during the blood pressure measurement, familiar with the surroundings, and comfortable with the ob-

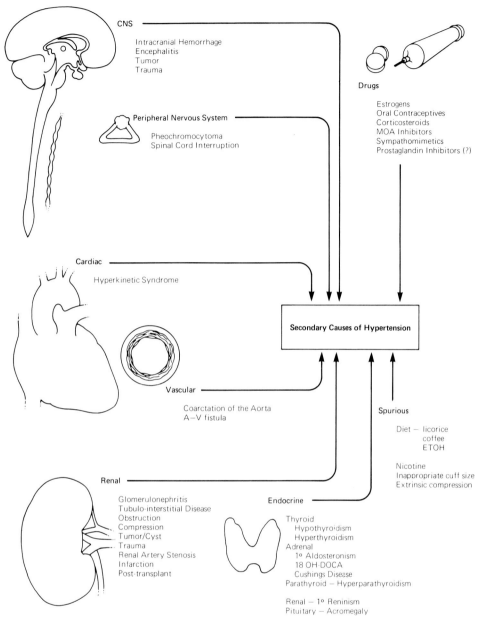

CNS

Intracranial Hemorrhage
Encephalitis
Tumor
Trauma

Drugs

Estrogens
Oral Contraceptives
Corticosteroids
MOA Inhibitors
Sympathomimetics
Prostaglandin Inhibitors (?)

Peripheral Nervous System

Pheochromocytoma
Spinal Cord Interruption

Cardiac

Hyperkinetic Syndrome

Secondary Causes of Hypertension

Vascular

Coarctation of the Aorta
A–V fistula

Spurious

Diet — licorice
            coffee
            ETOH

Nicotine
Inappropriate cuff size
Extrinsic compression

Renal

Glomerulonephritis
Tubulo-interstitial Disease
Obstruction
Compression
Tumor/Cyst
Trauma
Renal Artery Stenosis
Infarction
Post-transplant

Endocrine

Thyroid
     Hypothyroidism
     Hyperthyroidism
Adrenal
     1º Aldosteronism
     18 OH-DOCA
     Cushings Disease
Parathyroid — Hyperparathyroidism

Renal — 1º Reninism
Pituitary — Acromegaly

Fig. 2. Schematic representation of the secondary causes of hypertension.

server. When these criteria are met and repeated de-terminations are made, recorded pressures fall in many individuals. This has been best demonstrated in large-scale screening projects where the percentage of ele-vated readings falls dramatically with as few as 10 percent of the group with initially abnormal readings ultimately meeting criteria for hypertension. Besides stress and anxiety, individuals should be free of acute pain and recent ingestion of stimulants such as caffeine and/or nicotine. Compression of the extremity by gar-mets, jewelry, or orthopedic devices should be avoided.

Secondary Hypertension

Secondary hypertension must be considered in every new hypertensive patient; however, detailed evaluation should be limited to those subjects in whom clinical suspicion is great. The following section cate-gorizes the various causes of secondary hypertension.

Drug-induced hypertension. Other than antihyper-tensive drugs, little is known about the effect of most pharmaceutical agents on arterial pressure. As a rule, any medication should be viewed as possibly effecting the blood pressure adversely. Estrogens and steroids are the compounds most often implicated as causing hypertension. Sympathomimetics used for pulmonary and ocular disorders, psychotropic agents administered to psychiatric patients or taken illicitly, and nonsteroidal prostaglandin inhibitors all influence the blood pressure. Thus a careful, detailed drug-ingestion history is im-portant.

Estrogens and oral contraceptive agents increase

the blood pressure in most women, although the effect is quite small in the majority, with a 4–8 mm Hg increase in mean arterial pressure occurring after 1–2 years; however, the magnitude of the blood pressure increase and the percentage of patients who then meet standard criteria for hypertension appears to rise in proportion to the length of continuous use. The mechanism of the estrogen-induced increase in blood pressure is unclear. A hyperactive renin–angiotensin–aldosterone system is evident in some women; however, the magnitude of increased activity does not adequately account for the changes in arterial pressure observed. Withdrawal of the oral contraceptives or estrogens returns the blood pressure to pretreatment levels in approximately 85 percent of the subjects over 6–12 months, with the majority normalizing within 1–3 months. Women whose mean arterial pressures increase more than 15 mm Hg should have the hormone withdrawn. If end-organ compromise or serious increases in the blood pressure have occurred (BP > 160/105 mm Hg), discontinuation of the drug cannot be delayed. Reassessment of the need for antihypertensive treatment should be made monthly following hormonal withdrawal. In order to avoid this serious complication, women who (1) are already hypertensive, (2) became hypertensive with prior administration of these agents, (3) have strong family histories for hypertension, or (4) have chronic renal disease should be prescribed alternate methods of birth control.

Glucocorticoid-induced hypertension is usually mild and reverses with discontinuation of the drug. The mechanism relates to inherent mineralocortocoid activity of most of these compounds, and treatment with antihypertensives is rarely necessary. Spironolactone is very effective in counteracting the volume expansion when the clinical situation precludes stopping the steroid treatment.

The frequent use of sympathomimetic agents in treating reactive airway diseases and ocular disorders makes them a potential cause of iatrogenic hypertension. This action is transient but sufficient to complicate the evaluation of suspected hypertensives. The impact on blood pressure with chronic administration is unknown.

Many of the psychotropic drugs will raise arterial pressure—e.g., amphetamines, tricyclics, and monoamine oxidase inhibitors. Parenteral amphetamine abuse can result in an arteritis with permanent renal damage and chronic hypertension, even after abstinence.

Inhibitors of prostaglandin synthesis, such as aspirin and other nonsteroidal antiinflammatory agents, are potential pressor substances. Unfortunately, laboratory and clinical evidence to support this contention is fragmentary at present.

Another category of pharmaceutical agents that must be regarded as pressor substances include the antihypertensive drugs. Sudden discontinuation of antihypertensive agents such as clonidine or methyldopa

can result in a paradoxical rise in pressure. In addition, potentially paradoxical responses exist with virtually all antihypertensive agents. Patients who have abruptly stopped blood pressure medications should be monitored carefully for 5–7 days following the cessation of therapy. Long-term diuretic use increases the activity of the renin–angiotensin system and, in some subjects, is associated with an increase in blood pressure. In young, labile hypertensives, beta adrenergic blockers have been implicated in causing a pressor effect that is mediated through unopposed alpha adrenergic activity. Concurrent administration of either clonidine or methyldopa with a beta blocking agent has, on rare occasions, been associated with a paradoxical pressor response.

Endocrine disorders. Thyroid. Thyroid dysfunction (see Table 2) is associated with an increased mean arterial pressure in over 50 percent of afflicted patients. In hyperthyroid states the increase occurs in both systolic pressure and pulse pressure. Conversely, hypothyroidism tends to raise the diastolic component. Observed increases are usually mild in both conditions, and treatment of the thyroid disease leads to an improvement, if not normalization, of the blood pressure. Beta adrenergic blockers are particularly useful in managing hyperthyroid subjects, since they reduce blood pressure while blocking hypermetabolic effects of excess hormone.

Adrenal. Abnormal adrenal function (see Table 2) is a well recognized cause of secondary hypertension, although such disorders are not as common as once thought. Primary aldosteronism is the best characterized disease in this category. New onset of hypertension with associated hypokalemia, mild metabolic alkalosis, and suppressed plasma renin are its hallmarks. Plasma and urinary aldosterone concentrations remain elevated even on a high-sodium diet, while plasma renin is unresponsive to the challenge of a 10 mEq sodium diet. The hypertension encountered can be mild (150/100) to severe (200/140) and pathophysiologically is attributed to increased blood volume. In approximately 85 percent of the patients the source of the increased aldosterone is a single adenoma, found slightly more often on the left side. In the remainder, diffuse, bilateral adrenal cortical hyperplasia is present. A 5:2 predominance

Table 2
Causes of Endocrine Hypertension

Aldosteronism—spontaneous serum K^+ < 3.5 mEq/liter
Pheochromocytoma
   Blood pressure lability, symptomatic paroxysms
   Head pain, palpitations, pallor, and perspiration
   Hypermetabolism
   Abnormal carbohydrate metabolism
   Accelerated hypertension, paradoxical response to drugs
Hyper/hypothyroidism
Hyperparathyroidism/MEN types 1 and 2
Cushing's syndrome
Acromegaly/Turner's syndrome

favors females, and the disease has been reported in all age groups. Differentiation and localization of adenomas is challenging. Adrenal venography and adrenal photoscanning after intravenous injection of ^{131}I-19-iodocholesterol offer the best chance of lateralization. Surgical removal of the adenoma cures both the hypertension and electrolyte disturbances in 70–80 percent of cases. Bilateral hyperplasia is best treated with spironolactone 300–400 mg daily. After several months, the dose can usually be reduced, thus avoiding bilateral adrenalectomy.

When correlated with 24 hour urinary sodium excretion, plasma renin activity is disporportionately low in about 20 percent of unselected essential hypertensives. Since primary aldosteronism does not seem to account for this finding, attention has focused on 18-hydroxydeoxycorticosterone (18-OH-DOC) and 16,18-DOC as steroids responsible for the hypertension. Convincing evidence supporting the hypersecretion of either of these steroids is lacking.

Two rare forms of congenital adrenal hyperplasia can also present with hypertension and hypokalemia. Both disorders result from enzyme deficiencies, 11-β-hydroxylase and 17-hydroxylase. Preferential deoxycorticosterone synthesis is the metabolic consequence in both conditions, causing the elevation in blood pressure.

Excess production of cortisol and related steroids, secondary to an adrenal adenoma (Cushing's syndrome) or to hypersecretion of ACTH from either the pituitary (Cushing's disease) or an ectopic site, is associated with hypertension in over 85 percent of the cases. The postulated mechanisms include changes in peripheral resistance, cardiac output, sensitivity to catecholamines, and plasma renin substrate. Diagnosis is dependent upon classic physical findings of hypercorticism and elevated cortisol levels without the typical diurnal variation. Treatment of the adrenal abnormality often cures the hypertension. Unfortunately, the primary disease is occasionally resistant to therapy, and chronic antihypertensive treatment with diuretics and beta blockers is required.

Excess and prolonged ingestion of licorice can induce a clinical and biochemical syndrome resembling primary aldosteronism. Glycyrrhetinic acid, a derivative of licorice extract, produces physiologic effects similar to aldosterone. Profound hypokalemia may occur, and in elderly patients CHF has developed simply from excessive consumption of licorice candy. Symptoms, physical abnormalities, and electrolyte disturbances clear with abstinence from the candy.

Pheochromocytomas and the related tumors (ganglioneuroma and neuroblastoma) arising from neural crest tissue produce either a sustained or episodic form of hypertension. All these tumors release large quantities of both catecholamines and dopamine into the peripheral circulation. Besides hypertension, glucose intolerance, hypercalcemia, hyperuricemia, tachycardia, and weight loss are frequently associated with these tumors. Pheochromocytomas account for less than 0.5 percent of the hypertension in an unselected population, which makes routine screening in all hypertensive patients impractical. When clinical presentation indicates, diagnostic evaluation should include measurement of plasma concentrations and/or urinary excretions of catecholamines, as well as urinary VMA and metanephrines. Computerized axial tomography may be valuable in locating these tumors. Between 10 and 15 percent are extraadrenal, and surgical exploration is required for localization in these cases. Excision is the treatment of choice, since approximately 10 percent of pheochromocytomas are malignant. All individuals with a pheochromocytoma should also be screened for concurrent hyperparathyroidism and medullary thyroid carcinoma (MEN—type II). Ganglioneuromas, which may develop in any sympathetic ganglion, are usually nonmalignant and symptomatic (including hypertension) only from compression on local structures. Conversely, neuroblastomas are uniformly malignant and are seen almost exclusively in infants and children. Hypertension, when present, develops secondary to pressure on adjacent vessels in the kidney.

Renal. Primary reninism due to renin-producing tumors of the juxtaglomerular cells is typically mistaken for aldosteronism. The hypertension is often severe, though transformation into malignant hypertension has not been reported. Hypokalemia and high aldosterone concentrations coexist with this high renin state. Polyuria, perhaps secondary to the potassium depletion, has been a prominent clinical feature in most cases. Approximately half of these tumors can be visualized during renal arteriography. Surgical removal is curative of both the hypertension and metabolic derangements. Because of the coexisting vasoconstriction and volume depletion, repletion of blood volume during the paraoperative period is mandatory.

Parathyroid hormone. Hypertension is found in over 50 percent of patients with primary hyperparathyroidism. Hypertensive subjects have a 4- to 20-fold increased risk of developing hyperparathyroidism when compared to a normotensive population. The mechanisms involved are unclear, though the finding of minimally increased PTH concentrations in essential hypertensives suggests that the elevation of arterial pressure is the initial event. Since about 50% of the hypertensives with concurrent hyperparathyroidism will demonstrate improvement in their blood pressure following removal of the adenoma, the diagnosis should be pursued in any hypertensive with documented hypercalcemia (thiazide related or not). Such evaluation should include simultaneous measurements of ionized calcium, PTH, and/or nephrogenous cAMP. Beta blockers must be withheld during diagnostic studies, since they suppress parathyroid function and raise the serum phosphate concentration, thus masking the diagnosis.

Renal disease. Renal disorders are the most commonly diagnosed cause of secondary hypertension (Table 3). The majority of the cases are due to either

Table 3
Indications to Search for Renal Cause of Hypertension

Age < 30 years or > 50 years
Diastolic BP > 120 mm—any age
Abdominal bruit
Accelerated hypertension
Palpable kidney(s)
History of acute flank pain, renal trauma, and/or hematuria
Drug-resistant hypertension

chronic renal insufficiency or atherosclerotic renovascular disease. Acute and chronic glomerulopathies have a high incidence of associated hypertensive disease. The hypertension is caused by increased renin activity and/or intravascular volume expansion. The more rapid the progression of the underlying glomerular disease, the more severe the hypertension. The deterioration of renal function is accelerated by inadequate blood pressure control. In advanced renal insufficiency due to glomerular disease, volume expansion is responsible for the maintenance of the hypertension. Replacement therapy in the form of dialysis and/or transplantation frequently normalizes the blood pressure.

Hypertension is less common in the setting of chronic tubulointerstitial renal disease. Many of these patients have normal arterial pressures even in states of advanced renal insufficiency. This is probably a reflection of their tubular dysfunction and associated salt-wasting tendency with depletion of extracellular volume. Transient hypertension in subjects with underlying tubulointerstitial disease usually indicates a complication such as urinary tract infection, obstruction, hypercalcemia, or volume expansion. Treatment of these acute complications improves the blood pressure.

Compression of renal tissue by retroperitoneal masses, renal tumors, subcapsular hematomas, perinephric abscesses, intrarenal cysts, or suprarenal tumors has been associated with hypertension. Treatment of the hypertension is directed toward relief of the compression.

Renal trauma, blunt or penetrating, can cause hypertension. Transient increases are related to tissue swelling and associated hematomas. Persistent hypertension can develop secondary to small AV malformations following penetrating wounds to the kidney.

Renal vascular disease may either be diffuse, affecting primarily the smaller arteries and arterioles, or focal, involving the main renal arteries. Generalized atherosclerosis is the pathologic process in both of these conditions. Small vessel disease is also encountered in patients with vasculitis, diabetes, drug abuse, and atheroembolism. Because of renal ischemia, most of these disorders cause stimulation of renin release and blood pressure increases. Since these are progressive diseases, renal mass is compromised and renal insufficiency develops, further worsening the hypertension. Treatment is directed toward control of the blood pressure and the underlying medical disturbance.

Large vessel disease of the kidneys is divided into two distinct categories—fibromuscular and atherosclerotic. The former is found primarily in young females (20–40 years old) and is a local disorder, though it may be bilateral and recurrent following surgical correction. Atherosclerotic renovascular disease afflicts males more frequently (2:1) than females and is but one manifestation of generalized atherosclerosis. Typically, the diagnosis is made in the sixth decade of life with unilateral stenotic lesions. Renal vein renin is increased on the affected side. Renal arteriography defines the anatomy of the vascular lesion, while lateralization by renal vein renin measurement provides critical data concerning predictability of surgical success.

The young hypertensive with fibromuscular disease is a good candidate for endarterectomy or bypass of the stenotic site. Surgery for these patients is not mandatory, though, since a substantial percentage of such lesions do not progress and the hypertension is often mild and responsive to beta blockers. Surgery is curative in 80–90 percent of these cases, provided that the hypertension has been present for less than 3 years.

Considerable debate exists as to the appropriate management for the older patient with atherosclerotic renovascular disease. Bypassing the stenosis will cure one-third and improve an additional one-third of these individuals initially; however, 2–3 years after surgery, there is no difference in blood pressure control or in survival between surgically and medically treated patients. This seeming paradox reflects the systemic nature of the underlying atherosclerosis and the simultaneous involvement of the smaller vessels of the kidney. The natural history of stenotic lesions that are not surgically corrected is unclear, in part because of the shortened life expectancy. A small percentage eventually occlude the main renal artery, and the loss of renal mass severely compromises function. In others, asymptomatic segmental infarction of the affected kidney occurs due to distal embolization from the main renal artery.

In over 50 percent of renal transplant recipients, hypertension persists or develops independent of graft function. In many of the subjects, the hypertension is the legacy of chronic elevated arterial pressure associated with their renal disease. In others, the hypertension has been attributed to exogenous corticosteroids, abnormalities of the renin–angiotension system, stenosis at the site of the renal artery anastomosis, urinary obstruction, chronic rejection, or hypercalcemia due to persistent hyperparathyroidism. In all cases an etiology should be pursued and treated appropriately.

Vascular. Untreated coarctation of the aorta is associated with systemic arterial hypertension. While most cases are diagnosed within the first 2 years of life, some individuals escape detection until adulthood. The most likely pathophysiologic explanation for this form of hypertension is increased renin activity followed by sodium retention and extracellular volume expansion.

In pediatric cases, surgical excision and repair of the coarctation cure the hypetension.

When congenital or acquired arterial–venous malformations cause hypertension, they usually involve the major vessels of an extremity. Congenital AV defects manifest as differential growth of extremities, while acquired malformations are preceded by penetrating trauma or a fracture at the site. The hypertension is secondary to the increased cardiac output, and successful closure of the shunt usually cures the hypertension.

Neurologic disorders. Diseases of the central nervous system can induce a rise in arterial pressure. Although increased intracranial pressure from any cause (hemorrhage, tumor, trauma, edema) is the most common etiology of CNS hypertension, encephalitis, poliomyelitis, and Guillain-Barré syndrome are also associated with hypertension. Acute and chronic emotional stress is perhaps the most fundamental of all forms of secondary CNS hypertension. Traumatic or congenital interruption of the spinal cord is associated with a unique form of hypertension characterized by widely fluctuating blood pressure induced by change of position, bladder distention, or emotional stress. The pathophysiology is uncertain and treatment difficult.

THERAPY OF HYPERTENSION

The management plan of hypertension begins with the establishment of an accurate, baseline blood pressure (see Table 4). Blood pressures measured in the recumbent and upright positions by the same observer on three separate occasions should be the minimum standard in a new patient. When doubt exists that the office recordings accurately reflect the individual's blood pressure profile, home readings should be obtained and decisions regarding evaluation and therapy postponed. The distinct, sharp first sound of the pulse is designated as the systolic pressure, and complete disappearance of sound (fifth phase) corresponds to the diastolic pressure. The latter is modified if more than a 10 mm Hg difference exists between the muffling (fourth phase) and complete sound disappearance. In that situation, both measurements should be recorded. The importance of proper cuff size in obese patients has been emphasized. Technically, the cuff should be carefully centered over the brachial artery and inflated until the pressure is approximately 30 mm Hg above the point where the palpated pulse disappears, followed by deflation. Accurate standards for commercial, automated blood pressure machines have not been established, thus readings so obtained must be interpreted with caution.

When measured blood pressures are graphically recorded, trends are more apparent, thus facilitating management. Each graphically recorded pressure should be correlated with the treatment regimen, weight and pulse.

Once it is confirmed that an individual's arterial pressure is increased (systolic > 150 mm Hg and/or

Table 4
General Therapeutic Principles

Establish accurate baseline BP
Use appropriate cuff size
Record BP graphically
Set realistic goals with patient
Encourage weight loss and Na^+ restriction
Minimize laboratory studies
Employ simple (one drug) regimens whenever possible
Minimize drug side effects
Change therapeutic modalities one at a time

diastolic > 90 mm Hg), the decision to treat with pharmacologic agents must be addressed, since not every hypertensive requires medications. All patients should be encouraged to achieve their ideal weight, reduce salt intake, stop smoking, and develop an exercise program. These general health measures should be strongly promoted in any hypertension program.

Because hypertension is a lifetime disorder, patient education must include not only the natural history of the disease but also therapeutic goals. The patient must be persuaded that the ultimate success of any treatment requires his or her active, complete commitment. Return visits should be arranged to minimize lost time from work, with the same physician or nurse-practitioner providing long term care. Laboratory monitoring should be kept to a minimum.

Nonpharmacologic Therapy

The introduction of diuretics some 20 years ago ushered in the era of effective pharmacologic treatment of hypertension, yet controversy persists as to who should receive drugs to treat their hypertension. As renewed interest and confidence in nonpharmacologic treatment modalities grow, the indications for drug management have become more conservative.

Dietary. Weight reduction and sodium restriction are potentially complementary and remarkably successful in borderline or mild hypertensives. Over 70 percent of new patients with hypertension are significantly overweight, and numerous studies have concluded that obesity is a significant risk factor. More recent work has provided good evidence that substantial weight reduction, without simultaneous changes in salt intake, can result in a 20–30 mm Hg reduction in MAP. It is estimated that for every 5–7 pound (2–3 kg) decrement in weight, MAP will fall 1 mm Hg. Accordingly, dieting will have the greatest effect in lowering blood pressure in patients who are more than 20 percent overweight. Unfortunately, the long-term efficacy is dependent on maintenance of the weight loss—a goal achieved by less than 50 percent of the patients who are initially successful.

For years, the antihypertensive effects of weight reduction were attributed to concurrent decreases in sodium intake. This is not the case. Weight reduction and salt restriction are complementary but not interdependent. Lowering salt intake has been a cornerstone of antihypertension therapy for many years. As with diuretic therapy, reducing dietary sodium is more effective in older subjects than the young, labile hypertensive. Reducing sodium intake to 2 g/day may be quite effective in controlling the mildly hypertensive patient (diastolics < 105 mm Hg). Measurement of a 24-hour urinary sodium excretion provides a simple check on compliance. Except for beta adrenergic blockers, the effectiveness of all other antihypertensive agents is enhanced by simultaneous sodium restriction. Because of the reliance on prepared foods in our society, limitation of dietary sodium is becoming increasingly difficult to achieve.

Physical conditioning. Regular exercise programs and improved physical conditioning are beneficial adjuncts to weight and blood pressure reduction. The failure of acceptance of this as a primary mode of therapy is largely due to the difficulty in separating the effects of improved cardiovascular performance from simultaneously occurring reduction in weight and sodium intake. Recent short-term studies confirmed that much of the benefits of regular exercise are related to the concurrent weight loss, but they also documented a previously unrecognized benefit. Individuals utilizing dynamic exercise programs alter their cardiovascular response to emotional and physical stress. Pulse rates and blood pressure do not increase as much following stress in subjects who are physically fit. This modulation of cardiovascular responsiveness without significant changes in resting blood pressure may be of significant long-term benefit, particularly in the younger, labile hypertensive. Dynamic rather than static exercise should be encouraged.

Behavior modification. Meditation and the "relaxation response" have been explored as primary forms of therapy in hypertension. Their effectiveness has been attributed to a reduction in the hypertensives' response to stress. As with all forms of antihypertensive therapy, patient motivation and compliance is crucial to the success or failure of behavior modification. Use in younger, labile or mild hypertensives is the most logical setting for this therapeutic modality. Additional benefits include aiding the patient in concurrent efforts to lose weight.

Pharmacologic Agents

The decision to prescribe antihypertensive agents is becoming more complex at a time when the number and effectiveness of pharmacologic compounds are proliferating. This seeming paradox can be attributed to many factors. First, the number of new classes of drugs has increased dramatically. Second, the advantages to each drug vary with the patient. Third, the complementary versus competitive action of separate agents to be used in multiple drug regimens must be considered. Finally, considerable disagreement still exists as to which hypertensive patients should be treated and how aggressively.

This last factor is the most perplexing. There is no question that elevation of the arterial pressure shortens

life expectancy; however, the reverse—i.e., that lowering blood pressure to near normal improves survival—has been difficult to establish for individuals with mild to moderate hypertension (BP < 170/105). In part, this dichotomy probably relates to nonreversible changes in the heart and circulation. Awareness of the benefits and risks have prompted critical evaluation of the previous recommendation that hypertensives be treated with a goal of reducing blood pressure to 150/95. In addition, the rigid adherence to the "step-care" approach can also be questioned. Today, individualized therapy involves consideration of the patient's age, sex, family history, coexisting risk factors, concurrent medical disorders, and extent of end-organ involvement. In general, young males should be treated more aggressively than young females, but for the same level of hypertension the older female is likely to derive more benefit from drug therapy than her male counterpart. Any individual with a strong family history of hypertension and premature death from cardiovascular complications warrants tighter blood pressure control, as do patients with diabetes, renal disease, and/or heart disease. Without this attention to individual patient needs, some hypertensives will be undertreated, but more likely many will be overtreated and subjected to aggressive therapy that has a marginal benefit to risk ratio.

To arrive at the appropriate drug regimen, there are basic tenets which deserve recognition. First, whenever possible use only one antihypertensive agent. If the first agent employed fails, do not automatically add a second agent. Consider stopping the first one, unless it is a diuretic, in which case the next drug to be added will likely require such an agent. Second, change only one drug at a time so as to determine effectiveness of a single modification of the treatment plan. Third, prescribe the medication using the simplest schedule possible, e.g., once or twice a day. Current antihypertensive medications rarely need to be taken more often than twice a day. Fourth, keep patient visits and costs to a minimum, since treating a lifelong ailment has significant cost implications. These fundamental principles, which appear to be of secondary therapeutic importance when compared to the drugs themselves, may ultimately be of the greater value in the long-term success of any antihypertensive treatment program.

Diuretics. Diuretics can be divided into three categories (see Table 5). The benzothiadiazines are the largest and most commonly used groups. The loop diuretics (furosemide, extracrynic acid) are substantially more potent, though they share many characteristics with the thiazides. The third class is the potassium-sparing diuretics (spironolactone, triamterene), which are the least natriuretic but have the advantage of minimizing potassium depletion. All these agents cause initial intravascular volume contraction, which contributes to their acute hypotensive effect. With chronic use, sodium balance is nearly restored while the lowering of the blood pressure is maintained. The mechanism of their persistent hypotensive action remains

Table 5
Oral Antihypertensive Drugs

Category	Name	Initial Dose	Incremental Dose	Maximal Dose	Side Effects
Diuretics-Thiazide	Thiazide	125 mg qd	125 mg	500 mg BID	Postural hypotension Muscle cramps Skin rashes Acute gout Hypokalemia
	Hydrochlorothiazide	25 mg qd	25 mg	100 mg qd	Hypercalcemia Hyperglycemia Hyperlipidemia
	Chlorthalidone	25 mg qd	25 mg	100 mg qd	
	Metalozone	2.5 mg qd	2.5 mg	20 mg qd	
Diuretics-Loop	Furosemide	20 mg qd	20–40 mg	80 mg BID	Severe volume depletion Hypokalemia Skin rashes
	Ethacrynic Acid	25 mg qd	25–50 mg	100 mg BID	Acute gout
Diuretics-Potassium-Sparing	Triamterene	50 mg qd	50 mg	100 mg BID	Hyperkalemia Nausea Skin rashes
	Spironolactone	25 mg qd	25 mg	200 mg BID	
Beta Adrenergic Blockers	Propranolol	40 mg BID	40 mg	200 mg BID	Fatigue GI upset Vivid dreams Sweating
	Metoprolol	50 mg BID	50 mg	250 mg BID	
Alpha Adrenergic Blockers	Prazosin	1 mg BID	1 mg	10 mg BID	Postural hypotension G.I. upset Fatigue
	Phenoxybenzamine	10 mg BID	5 mg	30 mg BID	Same as Prazosin plus Sexual dysfunction Weakness
Vasodilators	Hydralazine	10 mg BID	25 mg	100 mg BID	Headache Tachycardia Angina Rashes Positive ANA
	Minoxidil	5 mg BID	5 mg	30 mg BID	Na$^+$ retention Tachycardia Body hair growth Pericardial effusion

Table 5
(continued)

Category	Name	Initial Dose	Incremental Dose	Maximal Dose	Side Effects
CNS Agents	Clonidine	.1 mg BID	.1 mg	1 mg BID	Dry mouth Nasal congestion Fatigue Mild Na^+ retention
	Methyldopa	250 mg BID	250 mg	1250 mg BID	Same as Clonidine plus Sexual dysfunction

Parenteral Antihypertensive Drugs

Category	Name	Initial Dose	Incremental Dose	Maximal Dose	*Adjunctive Therapy*
Diuretics	Furosemide	40 mg I.V.		400 mg I.V. qd	Use alone or with vasodilators
Beta Adrenergic Blockers	Propranolol	1 mg I.V.		2 mg I.V. q 6°	Use with vasodilators or alone
Alpha Adrenergic Blockers	Phentolamine	5 mg I.V.		5 mg I.V.	Use with beta blockers and diuretics cautiously
	Trimethaphan	3–4 mg/min			Use alone or with diuretics
Vasodilators	Hydralazine	5 mg I.V.		40 mg I.V. q 4–6°	Beta blockers and diuretic
	Diazoxide	300 mg I.V.		300 mg I.V. q 6°	Diuretic and/or beta blockers
	Sodium Nitroprusside	0.5 µg/Kg/min I.V.		8 µg/Kg/min	Beta blocker
CNS Agents	Methyldopa	250 mg I.V.		500 mg I.V. q 6°	Diuretic

uncertain. Speculation has centered on either a direct vasodilatory action on vascular smooth muscle or indirectly by changing the intracellular electrolyte content of vascular tissue. Thiazide-induced increases in ionized Ca^{2+} may also be antihypertensive, since small increases in membrane Ca^{2+} cause a decrease in smooth muscle responsiveness to A II and catecholamines.

Thiazides are the most often prescribed diuretics for treating elevated blood pressure. While the loop diuretics are more natriuretic, their shorter duration of action action and enhanced kaliuretic response make them less desirable as antihypertensive agents. The potassium-sparing diuretics are substantially less effective, except in patients with mineralocorticoid excess, where spironolactone often causes a substantial reduction in arterial pressure. Except for the loop diuretics, the half-life of diuretics is sufficiently long to justify once-a-day administration.

Diuretics produce few intolerable side effects. Generalized weakness, postural hypotension in older patients, cramps, sexual dysfunction, skin rashes, and acute gouty arthritis are the complications which may be noticeable. There are many metabolic side effects from chronic diuretic use, such as hypokalemia, hyperureicemia, hypercalcemia, hyperglycemia, and hyperlipemia. The clinical importance of each of these alterations remains to be defined. At a minimum they increase the need for frequent monitoring of blood chemistry levels, a requirement not encountered with other antihypertensives.

Since their introduction, thiazide diuretics have enjoyed wide acceptance as the initial drug for managing mild to moderate hypertension. The promotion of the "step-care" management scheme further solidified this view. The development of newer agents and review of long experience raise questions concerning perpetuation of this treatment philosophy. In line with more individualized treatment, the prescribing of thiazides is becoming more restricted. Older patients (> 60 years) respond better than younger patients. It should be emphasized, however, that with the exception of beta blockers the maximum pharmacologic effect of all other antihypertensive agents is enhanced by the concurrent use of diuretics. The dose of diuretic in combination therapy is usually less than that needed when it is the sole agent.

Beta adrenergic antagonists. Propranolol is the most widely prescribed beta blocker used in the management of hypertension. Newer compounds include sotalol, metoprolol, acebutalol, and atenalol, the last three of which have more specific β_1 receptor antagonistic properties. Cardioselectivity of the β_1 agents makes them advantageous in subjects with significant reactive airway disease. The introduction of beta adrenergic blockers represents a major advance in the pharamacologic management of clinical hypertension.

The mode of action of beta adrenergic blockers in reducing arterial pressure is still unclear. Proposed and investigated mechanisms include reduction in cardiac output, inhibition of renin release from the kidney, altered baroreceptor sensitivity, and an effect on the vasomotor center of the midbrain. To date, no one mechanism completely explains propranolol's antihypertensive action, and all four probably contribute.

Currently prescribed beta blockers are well tolerated, with mild fatigue, a slight decrease in exercise tolerance, gastrointestinal cramps, and vivid dreams the more common complaints of patients. Compared to the other antihypertensive agents, propranolol and its related compounds rarely cause sexual dysfunction or postural hypertension. In contrast to the changes associated with diuretics, serum potassium rises slightly and plasma renin activity falls in virtually every individual administered beta blockers. While propanolol has multiple potential effects on endocrine function (thyroid, pancreatic, parathyroid, and adrenal), these alterations have little clinical significance.

Oral administration of a beta blocker leads to a gradual fall in blood pressure which plateaus after 3–5 days. This slow onset is attributed to rapid hepatic inactivation of the drug and saturation of tissue stores that must precede establishing therapeutic plasma concentrations. A much more rapid action occurs with intravenous administration. Doses of 20–200 mg propranolol twice daily represent the usual dosage for treating patients with hypertension. While the occasional patient may respond to much larger doses (1000–2000 mg twice daily), their use is rarely justified. Diuretics need not be routinely used with beta blockers. The vasodilator hydralazine or alpha adrenergic blocker prazosin compliment the action of beta blockers where additional hypotensive action is needed.

Beta adrenergic agents are particularly effective and well tolerated in the young hypertensive and thus improve compliance. Older hypertensive patients also respond well to beta blockers; however, caution must be exercised in patients with congestive heart failure, bradyarrhythmias, reactive airway disease, and serious peripheral vascular disease. The initial theoretical concern that beta blockers would mask hypoglycemic symptoms in insulin-dependent diabetics has not proven to be a significant clinical problem. $Beta_1$ agents can be used in patients with asthma and chronic reactive airway disorders provided they are observed closely during the initial treatment period and minimum to moderate dosages are used.

Alpha adrenergic blockers. Three compounds presently compromise this group of antihypertensives. Phentolamine (regitine) is a short-acting competitive alpha adrenergic blocker whose use is limited to emergent clinical situations where severe hypertension results from sympathetic or sympathomimetic overactivity (MOA inhibitor toxicity, sudden withdrawal of antiadrenergic agents such as clonidine or methyldopa, sympathomimetic overdose). Phenoxybenzamine (dibenzyline) is a noncompetitive alpha blocker with a long duration of action. Side effects have limited its routine use to the medical management of pheochromocytoma (10–30 mg twice daily) and, occasionally, to young labile hypertensives with signs of increased sympathetic activity.

Prazosin represents a new alpha adrenergic blocker. Originally marketed as a vasodilator, subsequent investigation suggests that it is a unique, specific blocker of postsynaptic alpha adrenergic receptors. Prazosin carries the added benefit of reducing venous tone, so there is little or no increase in cardiac output. The most bothersome side effect is the first dose response, which consists of postural hypotension, dizziness, and tachycardia, which can be prevented by giving the initial dose at bedtime. Concurrent sodium restriction, diuretic use, or beta blockade may intensify this phenomenon. Dosage increments should begin at 1 mg twice daily and be advanced in 1 mg increments until a total dose of 10 mg/day is achieved. Fatigue, sodium retention, gastrointestinal upset, and sexual dysfunction are occasional limiting side effects. While effective as a single agent, combining prazosin with either a beta blocker and/or a diuretic represents the optimal mode of administration. Preliminary studies suggest that prazosin may be particularly beneficial in treating patients with congestive heart failure and severe hypertension.

Vasodilators. Hydralazine, minoxidil, diazoxide, and sodium nitroprusside induce vasodilation by a direct effect on vascular smooth muscle. Hydralazine, while the least potent, is the most widely prescribed. Diazoxide and sodium nitroprusside are parenteral agents reserved for emergent situations where rapid reduction of blood pressure is necessary. Minoxidil is the most effective oral vasodilator available for long-term therapy. Hydralazine and minoxidil are both concentrated in the vascular smooth muscle cells and produce relaxation by undefined mechanism. By causing dramatic falls in peripheral resistance these two compounds stimulate a reflex tachycardia and a resultant increase in cardiac output which may be distressing to the patient (as well as unmasking occult coronary artery disease).

Hydralazine has enjoyed a resurgence in use through its combination with beta blockers in multiple drug regimens. Alone, oral hydralazine is relatively ineffective and may produce cardiac side effects, headaches, and flushing, which are poorly tolerated by many patients. When added to a beta adrenergic antagonist, it can cause a substantial, additional reduction in blood pressure without these distressing side effects. Hydralazine can be used in small to moderate doses (25–100 mg twice daily). Greater doses add little therapeutic benefit and increase the likelihood of a lupus-like syndrome developing. Conversely, parenteral hydralazine, used alone, is a remarkably effective antihypertensive agents that remains a cornerstone of therapy for hypertensive emergencies. Given in 5–10 mg increments every 45 min until the desired blood pressure control is achieved, the total dose of hydralazine can then be repeated every 4–6 hours.

Minoxidil is a very potent oral antihypertensive

when administered (10–30 mg twice daily) with a beta blocker and a loop diuretic. Severe, resistant hypertension associated with chronic renal insufficiency is the setting in which minoxidil has proven to be of greatest value. Diuretics and beta blockers counteract the majority of side effects. Hirsutism and pericardial effusions, however, may lead to withdrawing the drug.

Diazoxide is usually very effective, provided the dose is injected rapidly into a well functioning intravenous line. The initial 300 mg dose can be repeated after 30–60 min if the desired response has not been achieved. The reduction in blood pressure may last anywhere from 6 to more than 24 hours. Ideally, a loop diuretic should be given some 15–30 min prior to diazoxide. Propranalol (1 mg IV) can also be added to the regimen to potentiate Diazoxide's effect and block any reflex tachycardia. Initial enthusiasm for diazoxide focused on its ability to normalize blood pressure without producing hypotensive episodes or requiring constant monitoring after the first 20–30 min. Unfortunately, the inability to titrate the hypotensive effect of this drug has proven to be a major deficiency. For many patients in whom the risk of an uncontrolled reduction in arterial pressure may result in either myocardial and/or cerebral ischemia, sodium nitroprusside, parenteral hydralazine, and trimethaphan remain the preferred agents. It should be noted that any serious hypotension resulting from diazoxide administration is most likely to occur in the setting of concurrent intravascular volume depletion and/or adrenergic blockade.

Sodium nitroprusside is the most potent and consistently effective parenteral antihypertensive drug. The need to titrate and closely monitor its hypotensive effect is considered a liability in some situations. The ability to titrate the blood pressure response, however, can be advantageous in many hypertensive crises. The dosage of this drug varies between 0.5 and 8 μg/kg/min as a continuous intravenous infusion diluted in 5 percent dextrose in water. The hypotensive effect is apparent within 30–60 sec, with the offset over a similar time interval. Side effects are extremely rare, provided that blood pressure is reduced slowly. Toxicity from the thiocyanate metabolite of nitroprusside is rare and limited to patients with renal insufficiency. Supplemental therapy with parenteral propranolol (1 mg iv every 4–6 hours) may permit a reduction in the dose of sodium nitroprusside.

CNS agents. Clonidine and α methyldopa are representive antihypertensives of this category. Clonidine, an imidazoline derivative, has intrinsic sympathomimetic activity. By stimulating β adrenergic receptors in the vasomotor center of the lower brainstem, clonidine is believed to reduce peripheral sympathetic nervous system activity. The reduction of blood pressure by the drug involves both a decrease in cardiac output and peripheral vascular resistance. Side effects include dry mouth, mild sedation, and sodium retention. Sexual dysfunction is relatively uncommon. Concern about "rebound hypertension" has not been justified from clinical experience. "Rebound hypertension" has been occasionally described with almost all antihypertensives. Most patients respond to 0.1 mg–0.4 mg of clonidine twice daily, though rare subjects may require up to 1 mg twice a day for adequate control. A thiazide diuretic should be prescribed with clonidine in order to counteract sodium retention and to maximize the hypotensive effect of this drug. The effectiveness of once a day administration at bedtime limits side effects and makes the drug particularly useful in many patients.

Methyldopa, after 15 years of widespread clinical use in treating mild to severe hypertension, is being replaced by many of the newer agents. Methyldopa's antihypertensive action is mediated primarily through direct sympathomimetic activity in the vasomotor centers of the brainstem. Methylnorepinephrine, a methyldopa metabolite, is the responsible compound. The side effects are similar to those of clonidine, although depression and sexual dysfunction are more frequently encountered with methyldopa. Coombs' test becomes positive in 10–20 percent of patients on long-term therapy, but hemolytic anemia rarely develops. A drug fever may develop 2–4 weeks after initiating therapy in 1–2 percent of patients, while methyldopa-induced hepatitis must be considered in all patients on the medication chronically. These side effects and the success of newer agents account for the declining use of methyldopa. Patients respond to 250–1250 mg twice daily, and a thiazide diuretic should be added in order to reduce sodium retention and improve the long-term blood pressure control.

Pre- and postganglionic blockers. This category comprises a large number of drugs, many representing the initial agents used in the pharmacologic management of hypertension. Only reserpine, guanethedine, and trimethaphan are still used, although to a limited extent because of their adverse effects. Reserpine acts to deplete catecholamines from the peripheral sympathetic nervous system. As an antihypertensive agent, it can be useful in small dosages (0.1–0.25 mg/day) and because its long duration of action may counteract poor patient compliance; however, patient acceptance of the drug is limited by the side effects such as depression (suicidal at times), exacerbation of peptic ulcer disease, sexual dysfunction, and somnolence.

Guanethedine reduces blood pressure by inhibiting the postganglionic sympathetic neurons. This is accomplished by guanethedine's replacing norepinephrine in the storage granules of the neurons. It is a potent agent causing diffuse impairment of peripheral sympathetic nervous system function. The latter accounts for most of its adverse reactions, including severe postural hypotension, sexual dysfunction, diarrhea, fatigue, and muscle tremors. Recently, renewed interest has been shown in small doses of guanethedine (10–30 mg/day) used in multiple drug regimens.

Trimethaphan is an extremely short-acting ganglionic blocker which prevents acetylcholine's postsynaptic depolarization, thus affecting both sympathetic and parasympathetic nerves. This produces the side effects of postural hypotension, urinary retention, constipation, ileus, and mental obtundation. Even with these numerous adverse reactions, trimethaphan has a limited but valuable role in the management of hypertensive crises, particularly associated with dissecting aortic aneurysms. It is given by continuous iv infusion at an initial rate of 0.5–1 mg/min.

New agents. The most promising category of investigational antihypertensives includes the angiotensin I converting enzyme inhibitors. These small polypeptides competitively block the conversion of A I and A II in the lung. Based upon results from studies utilizing SQ 208801 and SQ 14225, recommended use will likely be limited to patients with severe hypertension that is angiotensin dependent and unresponsive to other antihypertensives. Their role in diagnosing renin–angiotensin mediated forms of secondary hypertension remains to be defined.

Clinical Management

Essential hypertension. With the introduction of newer antihypertensives, the notion that the initial drug should be a diuretic in all hypertensives is changing, since the beta blockers offer an attractive alternative (see Table 6). The beta adrenergic antagonists are more effective than diuretics and are well tolerated because they possess few adverse side effects. When the cost of the required laboratory monitoring and often prescribed potassium supplementation is added to the cost of the diuretic, the claim that diuretics are less expensive than the other antihypertensive agents is debatable. For the mild (diastolic < 105 mm Hg) hypertensive with a strong family history, significant risk factors, and/or early organ compromise (eg., CAD), a beta blocker is the drug of choice. In more severe hypertension, multiple therapeutic options are available. Prazosin or clonidine combined with a small dose of a thiazide diuretic are well tolerated effective initial regimens. Equally successful is the addition of a diuretic, prazosin, or hydralazine to a beta blocker. It is the rare, severe essential hypertensive who cannot be controlled by some combination of beta blocker, prazosin, hydralazine, clonidine, and a diuretic.

Athletes. With increased awareness of elevated blood pressure occurring in adolescents and young adults, more hypertensive athletes are being identified. Of the antihypertensives available, beta blockers cause the least number of unacceptable side effects, although some patients notice a decrease in exercise tolerance with these drugs. If diuretics are employed, the electrolyte disturbances induced by exercise will be magnified.

Pregnancy. Despite substantial improvement in the drug treatment of systemic hypertension of most etiologies, little progress has been made in the treatment of either the young, female hypertensive who becomes pregnant, or the women who develop hypertension during pregnancy. Except for methyldopa and hydralazine, little is actually known about the safety of the various antihypertensives (beta blockers, prazosin, or

Table 6
Optimal Use of Antihypertensive Drugs

	Thiazide Diuretics	Loop Diuretics	K+-sparing Diuretics	Clonidine	Methyldopa	Propranolol	Metoprolol	Prazosin	Phenoxybenzine	Hydralazine	Diazoxide	Sodium Nitroprusside	Minoxidil	Guanethedine	Trimethaphan	Reserpine
Essential hypertension	1	2	1	1	1	1	1	1	4	3	4	4	4	3	4	3
Athletics	2	4	2	1	2	1	2	2	4	3	4	4	4	4	4	4
Diabetes	2	3	2	1	1	2	2	1	4	3	4	4	4	3	4	2
Pregnancy	3	4	3	2	1	2	2	3	4	1	3	4	4	4	4	4
Coronary artery disease	3	3	3	2	2	1	1	2	4	4	4	1	4	3	4	2
CHF	2	1	1	1	1	3	3	1	4	1	4	1	3	3	4	2
COPD	1	2	1	1	1	4	2	1	4	3	4	1	4	3	4	3
Chronic renal disease	4	3	4	1	2	1	2	2	4	3	2	1	1	3	4	4
Cerebral vascular disease	1	2	1	2	4	1	2	2	4	3	4	1	3	4	4	4
Malignant hypertension	3	1	4	2	2	1	2	2	3	3	1	1	1	3	2	4
Aortic aneurysm	3	3	3	2	2	2	2	2	4	4	4	4	4	3	1	3
Pheochromocytoma	4	4	4	3	3	3	3	2	1	3	2	2	4	4	4	4
CVA	1	3	2	2	4	1	2	4	4	2	4	1	4	4	4	4

Explanation: 1, preferred; 2, alternate; 3, adjunct; 4, avoid.

clonidine) in pregnancy. As for diuretics, the debate continues as to their indication in pregnant subjects. At present, the recommendation is to treat mild hypertension with sodium restriction and methyldopa, later adding small doses of diuretics. If this is unsuccessful, then hospitalization and institution of parenteral hydralazine may be required. Failure to adequately control the blood pressure during pregnancy typically leads to either spontaneous abortion or the development of toxemia. The use of the other antihypertensives may be necessary if the limited, traditional agents are inadequate. When toxemia develops, parenteral hydralazine and propranolol should be used to lower the blood pressure while labor is induced. Occasionally diazoxide or sodium nitroprusside may need to be employed. Diazoxide causes cessation of labor in approximately 50 percent of the cases where it has been utilized.

Hypertension complicating specific disease. Diabetes. Over 50 percent of juvenile-onset diabetics ultimately develop hypertension as a consequence of their generalized atherosclerosis and nephropathy. In general, diuretics should be avoided as a first drug in these patients as the potassium depletion, glucose intolerance, and elevated lipids are unacceptable metabolic effects. Beta adrenergic drugs were originally thought to be contraindicated in these patients; however, propranolol and related compounds have proven to be safe and effective, especially when renal insufficiency is also present. The use of prazosin or clonidine with a small dose of a diuretic is an excellent alternative in the diabetic subject.

Coronary artery disease. Beta adrenergic antagonists are the obvious drugs of choice in patients with symptomatic or suspected coronary artery disease.

Prazosin, either alone or in combination with beta blockers, is a good alternative drug. Diuretics, because of the associated potassium depletion, should be used cautiously, since hypokalemia may predispose the patient to tachyarrhythmias. Hydralazine and diazoxide are contraindicated in patients with acute and chronic coronary insufficiency, since they increase myocardial oxygen requirements by raising the heart rate and cardiac output.

Congestive heart failure. When congestive heart failure complicates hypertension, aggressive hypotensive treatment can significantly improve cardiac function. Drug therapy should include a diuretic (with adequate K^+ supplementation) and either prazosin or the combination of hydralazine and a beta blocker. These regimens not only reduce blood pressure, but their combined effect on preload and afterload will restore myocardial function toward normal. If congestive failure is stable, beta adrenergic blockers can be employed, since the likelihood of precipitating acute cardiac decompensation is small while the added benefits may be substantial.

Reactive airway disease. When asthma or chronic obstructive pulmonary disease complicates the course of a hypertensive patient, beta blockers should normally be excluded from therapeutic regimens. The new β_1 cardioselective agent metoprolol can be used cautiously, when the addition of such an agent is necessary to achieve adequate control. In subjects with chronic respiratory acidosis, potassium depletion from diuretics may be masked by the reduced systemic pH.

Chronic renal disease/renal transplantation. Hypertension is a common complication of underlying renal disease. Depending on the etiology of the renal disease and the magnitude of renal functional impairment, increases of intravascular volume, renin activity, and/or fixed peripheral vascular resistance will be of primary importance in sustaining the elevation of the arterial pressure. Volume excess is usually more important in the later stages of chronic renal failure or in dialysis patients. Excess renin tends to contribute more to the hypertension of subjects with renal artery disease or glomerulopathies. The drug therapy employed should reflect the relative importance of these various contributing factors.

In general, a beta blocker, clonidine, or prazosin, either alone or in combinations, will be effective in most patients. Diuretics should be added as indicated, remembering that thiazides are relatively ineffective at a creatinine clearance less than 20 ml/min. Potassium-sparing diuretics are contraindicated in subjects with even mild renal insufficiency, since life-threatening hyperkalemia may occur. Minoxidil is required in the rare patient unresponsive to other agents. Bilateral nephrectomy for control of the blood pressure has virtually been eliminated with the introduction of minoxidil. The increases in serum potassium and phosphrus concentration caused by propanolol are without significance except for some chronic dialysis patients where the increase may erroneously suggest dietary noncompliance.

Cerebral vascular disease. Hypertension, particularly systolic, is a common accompaniment of cerebral vascular insufficiency. Caution must be exercised when lowering blood pressure in these patients. Postural hypotension should be avoided, since it can precipitate acute cerebral vascular insufficiency. For this reason methyldopa and clonidine may be relatively contraindicated. Initiating therapy with prazosin may be difficult because of the severe hypotension that can be associated with the first dose and the unpredictability of this adverse effect. Many of these subjects are sensitive to even small doses of diuretics which cause postural drops in the blood pressure. Beta adrenergic agents will assure the best chance of reducing the blood pressure without causing postural symptoms. In addition, they will cause less fatigue and depression as well as offering prophylaxis against coronary insufficiency that is frequently present in these patients.

Hypertensive emergencies. Hypertensive crises (Table 6) can develop in the setting of rapidly progressive renal failure (malignant hypertension), acute myocardial infarction, pulmonary edema, dissecting aortic anuerysm, acute brain infarction, increased intracranial pressure (trauma or infection related), or the postoperative period. Sodium nitroprusside is the treatment of choice for hypertensive crises related to malignant hypertension. Diazoxide is the reasonable alternative for treating severe hypertension related to renal disease provided that there is no evidence of coronary artery disease. Diazoxide should not be used in acute, dissecting aortic aneurysm or left ventricular failure. Trimethaphan is the preferred drug for treating dissecting aortic aneurysms; sodium nitroprusside, which was once promoted for this situation, is no longer recommended.

Controversy exists today as to whether to aggressively treat the severe hypertension that accompanies an acute brain infarction. Conservative management with bedrest and the initiation of oral antihypertensive therapy is usually sufficient to lower the blood pressure without risking the possibility of further compromising cerebral perfusion. If an immediate reduction of the blood pressure is indicated, nitroprusside should be used, since it will not influence CNS function and the blood pressure control can be titrated. Reductions of mean pressure by 20 percent are well tolerated without a corresponding decrement in cerebral blood flow. The same therapeutic approach can be applied to the treatment of severe hypertension related to increased intracranial pressure.

REFERENCES

Genest S, Koiw E, Duchel O: Hypertension. New York, McGraw-Hill, 1977

Kannel WB: Role of blood pressure in cardiovascular mobidity and mortality. Prog Cardiovasc Dis 17:5, 1974

Laragh JH: Modern system for treating high blood pressure based on renin profiling and vasoconstriction-volume analysis: A primary role for beta blocking drugs such as propranolol. Am J Med 61:797, 1976

McMahon FG: Management of Essential Hypertension. Mount Kisco, N.Y., Futura, 1978

Rabkin SW, Mathewson FAL, Tate RB: Predicting risk of ischemic heart disease and cerebrovascular disease from systolic and diastolic blood pressures. Ann Intern Med 88:342, 1978

Sokolow M, Werdigar D, Kain HK, et al: Relationship between level of blood pressure measured casually and by portable recorders and severity of complications in essential hypertension. Circulation 34:279, 1966

Taylor DW, Sachett DL, Haynes RB, et al: Compliance with antihypertensive drug therapy. Ann NY Acad Sci 304:390, 1978

Wallac JM: Hemodynamic lesions in hypertension. Am J Cardiol 36:670, 1975

URINARY TRACT INFECTIONS

Marvin Forland

Urinary tract infections are among the more common problems seen in medical practice. Approximately 10–20 percent of American women will develop a urinary tract infection at some time. It has been estimated that 10 percent of all hospital outpatient department visits relate to urinary tract disorders, particularly infections.

Both symptomatic cystitis and acute pyelonephritis are more common among women, with the peak prevalence between ages 18 and 40 years. This coincides with the childbearing years. The prevalence of asymptomatic bacteriuria increases with age to 10–12 percent in elderly women. In males, urinary tract infections are most common after age 40 and are usually associated with prostatic obstruction or renal calculi.

Two-thirds of urinary tract infections in newborns occur in males, probably related to the higher incidence of congenital urinary tract abnormalities; however, females predominate by age 2 years. Kunin has reported and others have confirmed an approximately 1.2 percent prevalence of bacteriuria among schoolgirls, with a 0.04 percent prevalence in schoolboys. Approximately 5 percent of schoolgirls will have bacteriuria at some time during elementary or high school.

MICROBIOLOGY

Enterobacteriaceae and *Escherichia coli* in particular are the most significant pathogens in acute urinary tract infection.

The organisms are usually serologically identical to the *E. coli* identifiable in the patient's stool flora. With recurrent infection, more resistant strains of gram-negative organisms appear, including *Klebsiella, Enterobacter, Pseudomonas,* and *Proteus sp.* Gram-positive microorganisms are responsible for 5–10 percent of urinary tract infections and *Streptococcus fecalis (enterococci)* and *Staphylococcus aureus* are the most common organisms isolated.

Identification of *E. coli* by a number of cell wall associated antigens has been useful in epidemiologic studies of urinary tract infections in determining whether recurrent infection is associated with the same organism as before (relapse) or represents infection with a new organism (reinfection). The heat-stable "O" antigen is a lipopolysaccharide component of the cell wall. Approximately 150 types have been identified with specific sera, but only a limited number are frequently occurring urinary pathogens. These include the O4, O6, O75, O1, O25, O17, and O18 antigens. It is still uncertain whether these antigens are associated with particular pathogenic features or whether they simply are found more commonly in the gastrointestinal tract. The heat-labile "H" antigen is associated with the flagella of motile strains, and approximately 50 types have been classified. The "K" antigen is of capsular origin and overlies the "O" antigen of the cell wall. It is also heat labile, and approximately 90 "K" types have been identified in *E. coli*. In a study of bacteriuria during pregnancy, a correlation was found between "K"-rich strains and evidence of renal parenchymal involvement. It was suggested the "K" antigen may render the organism relatively resistant to phagocytosis and destruction by complement.

PATHOPHYSIOLOGY

The establishment of lower tract infection generally is believed to be the initial step in the development of infection in the kidney. Renal involvement—pyelonephritis—occurs with the ascendancy of bacteria to the kidney through the collecting system. The principal alternate routes are bloodstream or lymphatic transmission. The kidney may develop a miliary type of infection as a result of bacteremia, and this is most characteristically seen with staphylococcal and candida sepsis. The transmission of organisms from the bowel via the lymphatic system to the kidney has been postulated but is of doubtful significance.

As noted, the organisms most frequently responsible for urinary tract infection are the enterobacteriaceae, with *E. coli* comprising the single most significant pathogen. These organisms are usually serologically identical to *E. coli* isolated in the patient's stool flora. The means by which these pathogens reach the urethra and enter the bladder has been the topic of extensive investigation.

The introital carriage of enterobacteriaceae has been found in some, but not all, studies to occur with greater frequency in women with recurrent urinary tract infection and usually to precede their episodes of symptomatic or asymptomatic bacteriuria. The nature of the normal resistance to bacterial colonization in this area and its possible alteration in susceptible women is being clarified. Higher colony counts of pathogens are found when the pH of the vaginal introitus is above 4.4. *E. coli* have been shown to adhere more readily to vaginal cells obtained from women with recurrent urinary tract infection than to similar cells from women without a history of genitourinary infection. The nature of the defect that appears to promote bacterial adherence is unknown. It has also been demonstrated that women with recurrent urinary tract infection are less likely to produce cervicovaginal antibody to enterobacteriaceae that colonize the vaginal vestibule. In contrast, control subjects demonstrated the presence of cervicovaginal antibody to their own fecal bacteria. Since the adherence studies were done on subcultured and therefore uncoated organisms, immunoglobulins could not be the principal factor accounting for the difference in bacterial adherence between the two groups.

One means of promoting ascendancy of the organisms from the perineal area is mild urethral trauma. It has been shown that gentle outward milking of the urethra is often associated with the recovery of small numbers of bacteria from the bladder upon suprapubic aspiration. These organisms are frequently nonpathogens and persist only for a short period. It has also been demonstrated that sexual intercourse can be associated with an increase in urinary colony counts of more than one log. This occurred in 30 percent of coital episodes and in approximately half of the women studied. The organisms were often pathogens but more frequently nonpathogens, and the increases were generally transient. These studies, coupled with the evidence of introital colonization, delineate a possible sequence for the establishment of lower tract infection. The roles of residual urine volume, other bladder dysfunction, or vesicoureteral reflux in compromising the normal defenses of the bladder are additional considerations.

Bladder Defense Mechanisms

A dual capacity of the bladder to protect against infection has been described. Vesical emptying reduces bacterial counts but appears to be inadequate to completely rid a simulated bladder of bacteria. While random voided urine permits the in vitro multiplication of bacteria in a manner similar to nutrient broth, under experimental conditions the normal bladder is able to rid itself of large numbers of bacteria within 72 hours after introduction by catheter. This intrinsic bladder antibacterial factor not present in voided urine appears to combine with the mechanical emptying to protect against infection.

Vesicoureteral Reflux (VUR)

Vesicoureteral reflux, the retrograde flow of urine from bladder to ureter, has been considered to be both the cause and consequence of urinary tract infection. From cystogram studies done in premature infants and neonates, VUR is not normally present in infancy. Its congenital presence appears related to trigonal weakness or intrinsic defects of the submucosal ureter. While the rare familial occurrence of VUR has been recognized, it is more often seen in association with underlying ureteral abnormalities, including complete ureteral duplication, an ectopic ureteral orifice, or a ureterocoele. It has been suggested that cystitis will compromise only a previously "borderline" vesicoureteral valve through the development of local edema. With cure of infection, the valve quickly regains competency.

The presence of VUR encourages infection of bladder urine through the presence of a residual urine resulting from the return of refluxed urine to the bladder. It also provides access for bacteria to ascend from the bladder to the kidney. A possible damaging mechanical ("water hammer") effect upon renal tissue independent of infection has been suggested. Hodson and associates have demonstrated the development of intrarenal reflux in the multipapillary kidney of miniature pigs in which partial urethral obstruction has been created to produce critical voiding pressures. These animals develop renal scars morphologically identical to chronic pyelonephritis in areas of intrarenal reflux independent of infection; however, such an occurrence may be peculiar to the pig model because of the relative difficulty of occluding circular openings of the collecting ducts in their upper and lower polar papillae. The importance of reflux alone in the absence of infection in the development of the scarring characteristic of chronic pyelonephritis remains controversial.

Vesicoureteral reflux has been found to be present in 35–50 percent of children with urinary tract infection and has been noted particularly in younger children and those most critically ill. Reports of its occurrence in adults have been variable, ranging from 8 percent in a bacteriuric population to as high as 50 percent in patients with recurrent urinary tract infection. Approximately one-third of children and adults with VUR have evidence of renal scarring, but the de novo development of scarring is almost never observed in adults and appears to be a residual manifestation of infection in the still-growing kidney. When parenchymal scarring is observed in childhood, VUR is almost invariably present.

In the absence of ureteral dilation, VUR will remit in the majority of children if infection can be prevented. It has been suggested that the submucosal ureteral segment may lengthen with age and its muscle cells proliferate and mature to strengthen its action. The principles of conservative management of VUR include maintaining the urinary tract free of infection with long-term low-dosage prophylactic antibacterial therapy and instituting a triple voiding program at 2 min intervals to help minimize residual urine. Normal renal growth without scarring has been achieved in approximately 90% of children maintained with this regimen. The indications for surgery include reflux with ureteral dilation, the presence of scarring in association with marked reflux, infection that cannot be controlled medically, diagnosis in the first 3 years of life, particularly in males, and evidence of a periureteral diverticulum. Surgery generally achieves its immediate goal of correction of reflux in over 90 percent of patients. Approximately 4 percent develop obstruction, which often necessitates reoperation. A reinfection rate of 10–15 percent has been described, but this has been considered to be benign in the absence of VUR.

Medullary Localization

The medulla usually has been found to be the initial site of bacterial proliferation in experimentally induced renal infection. It is the area of most extensive involvement in human infection. A number of factors have been described which may impair the intrinsic defense mechanisms of this region of the kidney against bacterial invasion. The delivery of polymorphonuclear cells and development of an inflammatory response may be adversely affected by the relatively low blood flow of the papillary region as compared to the cortical area. The low pO_2 of the deep medulla, 20 mm Hg, as compared to the outer cortex (100 mm Hg) possibly may impede phagocytic activity. Phagocytosis is also impaired at pH below 6.0. The hypertonicity of the medulla impairs phagocytic ability, inhibits complement activity, and also promotes protoplast survival. Ammonia formation by the kidney may also inactivate the fourth component of complement and locally impair immunologically mediated defense mechanisms.

Prostatic Antibacterial Factor (PAF)

The lower frequency of urinary infections in males has been attributed to the protective effect of the longer male urethra and hence isolation of the bladder from perineal organisms. In addition, a factor with bactericidal activity against a variety of both gram-positive and gram-negative organisms was originally described in canine prostatic fluid and subsequently demonstrated in normal human prostatic fluid and semen. Isolation and purification studies of PAF have demonstrated that a zinc compound represents the entire antibacterial effectiveness of the fluid. Males with active bacterial prostatitis have been shown to have decreased concentrations of prostatic fluid zinc but comparable serum levels to normal controls. Oral zinc supplements did not influence the diminished prostatic fluid zinc levels. Preliminary studies indicate that men with recurrent prostatic infection continue to have lower prostatic fluid zinc concentrations between episodes of infection and suggest this may play a role in the natural resistance of the male urinary tract to infection.

Catheterization and Instrumentation

Almost half of normal subjects subjected to indwelling urethral catheterization will have bacteriuria after 72 hours. The figure exceeds 90 percent in a hospitalized population subjected to prolonged catheterization. The risk of single catheterization for bladder emptying varies widely with the type of patient and the clinical setting. Persistent bacteriuria following such catheterization may be as low as 1 percent in young women in an outpatient setting, 4 percent in nonpregnant women in a hospital, and 20 percent in patients on medical wards or in individuals catheterized prior to delivery. The care with which the procedures are performed is critical, as is the status of the patient's normal defense mechanisms.

Calculi

Renal calculi may be either the cause or consequence of urinary tract infection. Their presence results in areas of localized intrarenal obstruction and apparent decreased resistance to bacterial proliferation. Consequently, renal calculus disease associated with such diverse etiologies as primary hyperparathyroidism, idiopathic hypercalciuria, cystinuria, renal tubular acidosis, and urate nephropathy is often complicated by acute episodes of symptomatic urinary tract infection as well as chronic pyelonephritis.

Renal infection may result in calculus formation when associated with urea-splitting organisms such as *Proteus mirabilis,* which create a persistently alkaline urine. The precipitation of calcium magnesium ammonium phosphate (struvite) is promoted by the alkaline urine, and stones can consequently be formed. Such ''infection stones'' can be formed by other urea-splitting bacteria, including *Klebsiella sp.* and certain *E. coli.* Organisms often can be cultured from the interstices of removed stones, and this lack of accessibility to treatment may account for the frequent recurrence of infection following therapy. Struvite stones may be minimally radiopaque, and tomography is indicated in patients with recurrent *P. mirabilis* infection to ascertain the possible presence of such calculi.

Surgical intervention frequently is necessary to control recurrent infection by removing struvite calculi. The use of long-term prophylactic antibacterial therapy has been shown to maintain sterile urine, prevent symptoms, and stabilize or improve renal function in some patients with idiopathic stone formation; however, stone growth may continue, and infection recurs during or shortly after stopping prophylaxis in most patients.

Pregnancy

The incidence of asymptomatic bacteriuria in pregnancy has been extensively studied, and most surveys have indicated a 6–7 percent incidence with a range extending from approximately 2–10 percent. The majority of affected women will present with bacteriuria at their first antenatal examination. Less than 2 percent will subsequently develop bacteriuria during pregnancy after initial negative cultures. Approximately 25–40 percent of women with covert bacteriuria will become symptomatic before delivery if untreated. Studies using a variety of localization techniques have demonstrated that 20–50 percent of pregnant women with asymptomatic bacteriuria have upper tract involvement.

A number of factors have been implicated in the seemingly high incidence of urinary tract infection during pregnancy and its symptomatic manifestations. Dilation of the renal calyces, pelves, and ureters is usually evident by the second trimester and is accompanied by decreased ureteral peristaltic movement. This has been attributed to a combination of progesterone effects and obstruction by the enlarging uterus. Alterations in the chemical composition of urine during pregnancy have also been described which appear to promote bacterial proliferation. Diminution in host resistance has been suggested in relationship to dehydration with first trimester vomiting and decreased total body potassium.

Lower birthweights and a higher incidence of prematurity in children of untreated bacteriuric women have been reported by some workers but not confirmed by all. A recent study has reported a higher incidence of intrauterine growth retardation in women with urinary infections associated with antibody coating of their infecting organisms and hence parenchymal infection.

An increase in serum creatinine and decrease in creatinine clearance has been found to accompany asymptomatic bacteriuria associated with antibody-coated organisms. A 10–14 year followup of patients after the finding of bacteriuria during pregnancy demonstrated significant bacteriuria in approximately one-quarter of both the sulfonamide-treated women and the placebo-treated group. Five percent of the originally nonbacteriuric group had significant bacterial growth at followup. Mean maximal urinary osmolality was lower in the bacteriuric patients, and intravenous pyelograms showed radiologic changes of chronic pyelonephritis in 29 percent of the initially bacteriuric group available for study. No difference in creatinine clearance was noted among the groups.

Evidence of chronic pyelonephritis has been reported on intravenous pyelography in 8–33 percent of women with bacteriuria during pregnancy. Radiologic studies appear clearly indicated in such patients who have a history of previous urinary tract infection, acute pyelonephritis during pregnancy, or persistent or recurrent bacteriuria in the postpartum period. Pyelography should be delayed until at least 12 weeks postpartum to permit resolution of the collecting system changes of pregnancy.

It has been estimated that screening in the early antenatal period followed by prompt therapy will eliminate 70–80 percent of all episodes of symptomatic prenatal pyelonephritis. Pregnancy, particularly late pregnancy, necessitates certain restraints in the prescription of antibacterial therapy. Ampicillin, cephalosporins, and sulfonamides are usually the agents of choice in the earlier stages of pregnancy. Sulfonamides should be avoided in the last 2 weeks of pregnancy because of their competitive binding with albumin leading to the possibility of hyperbilirubinemia and resultant kernicterus. The teratogenic risk of the trimethaprim–sulfamethoxazole combination remains to be established. Tetracyclines may be associated with staining of fetal teeth and rarely with the development of maternal hepatic toxicity manifested by fatty necrosis of the liver. Nitrofurantoin should be avoided in the last weeks of pregnancies due to the possible development of hemolytic anemia. Chloramphenicol has been associated with the development of a potentially fatal "gray syndrome" of cardiovascular collapse, coma, and cyanosis in newborns related to inability to glucuronidate the parent compound. Gentamicin and tobramicin should be avoided unless the need is critical because of uncertain effects of aminoglycosides on the fetal inner ear.

Sickle-Cell Anemia

A twofold increase in the prevalence of asymptomatic bacteriuria has been reported in pregnant women with sickle-cell trait as compared to women with normal hemoglobin. A similar twofold increase in autopsy evidence of pyelonephritis has been found in sickle trait patients as compared to normals. The prevalence of pyelonephritis was not increased in patients with HbSS, perhaps due to their relatively early demise. Changes in the microvasculature, most marked in the vasa recta of the medullary area, are considered responsible for progressive renal scarring and tubular atrophy and probably increased susceptibility to bacterial proliferation.

Diabetes Mellitus

In contrast to early clinical and postmortem studies indicating a high incidence of pyelonephritis in patients with diabetes mellitus, the reported prevalence of urinary tract infections among diabetic women has varied markedly in studies published since the introduction of quantitative microbiology. Virtually all investigators have found no difference in the prevalence of urinary tract infections in diabetic and nondiabetic men. While a number of studies have shown no substantial difference in incidence between diabetic women and control groups, a number of investigators report as much as a threefold increase, with a 16–19 percent prevalence of urinary tract infections in diabetic women as compared to a 5–8 percent prevalence in nondiabetic women. Studies utilizing bladder washout techniques and antibody coating of urinary bacteria indicate that more than half the asymptomatic infections involve the upper tract, and studies using the latter technique indicate rapid development of parenchymal involvement.

Explanations for the possible high prevalence of urinary tract infections and parenchymal involvement in women with diabetes mellitus are not yet established. Earlier suggestions, including instrumentation of the urinary tract, age of the population, and glycosuria, have not been supported in recent studies Additional contributing factors may include bladder dysfunction related to diabetic neuropathy, diabetic nephropathy impairing intrinsic renal defense mechanisms, impairment in leukocyte function, and recurrent nonbacterial vaginitis.

The functional consequences of renal infection and its contribution to progressive renal insufficiency in diabetic patients are uncertain. Impaired concentrating ability has been noted in diabetic patients with upper tract infection, but no difference in BUN was observed in a group with prompt and sustained response to therapy as compared to those with rapid recurrence. Reinfection has been reported as the major pattern of recurrence with both upper and lower tract infection in this population.

Papillary necrosis, perinephric abscess, and the postmortem changes of acute pyelonephritis are well described as increased hazards in this group and are considerations in prompting early diagnosis and treatment.

LABORATORY FINDINGS

Abnormalities on urinalysis may provide presumptive evidence for the presence of urinary tract infection. Pyuria, greater than 5 WBC/HPF, is a nonspecific indication of urinary tract inflammation. Its presence does not establish nor absence exclude significant infection. The persistence of pyuria in the absence of positive bacterial cultures or evidence of glomerulonephritis is an indication for special cultures for *Mycobacterium tuberculosis*. The presence of bacteria on microscopic examination of an unspun, clean catch specimen using carefully cleaned glassware correlates well with culture growth of 100,000 organisms/ml and is a useful initial screening procedure. Gram staining facilitates detection of small numbers and identification of the organism.

Confirmation of a diagnosis of urinary tract infection is dependent upon growth of a significant number of organisms from a properly collected urine specimen. Quantitative microbiology is now routinely employed and provides uniformly accepted diagnostic criteria to distinguish between contamination versus infection with enterobacteriaceae. Using voided, clean catch, midstream specimens, Kass and associates found that more than 95 percent of patients with clinical acute pyelonephritis had urinary bacterial counts of 100,000 colonies/ml or greater. In survey studies, urine specimens with bacterial counts below 100,000/ml usually contained saprophytic organisms and were from patients without histories of urinary tract infections. A second culture rarely grew the same organism. In contrast, where bacterial counts were 100,000 or more colonies/ml, the organisms were usually pathogenic, the majority of patients had a history of urinary symptoms, and repeat culture usually yielded the same organism.

The reproducibility of findings from a clean catch, midstream specimen is approximately 80–85 percent and rises to 95 percent if the same organism is found on two consecutive specimens. Consequently, the clean catch, midstream specimen has become widely employed as the collection method of choice. In a symptomatic patient significant growth from a single specimen is generally considered adequate; in the asymptomatic patient a second, confirmatory specimen is usually sought. Immediate culture or refrigeration of a collected urine sample is necessary to prevent bacterial proliferation and misleadingly high colony counts. The properly handled negative culture is a definitive finding. When borderline results are obtained or problems arise concerning the reliability of the collection, a bladder aspirate or catheter-obtained specimen can resolve the problem.

Growth of 100 or more colonies/ml of pathogenic organisms from a catheter-obtained specimen or suprapubic or transvaginal aspirate is also evidence of infection.

A number of chemical tests are available commercially to facilitate the office diagnosis of urinary tract infection (summarized in Table 1). None are ideal, and a number of simplified culture techniques, commercially produced, make adequate bacterial quantitation available conveniently and at reasonable cost for office use. Dip slide techniques—using a glass slide coated with agar medium—and the filter paper method are easily performed and interpreted with the availability of a small incubator.

RADIOLOGY

The diagnosis of acute urinary tract infection is rarely facilitated by radiologic studies. The principal functions of x-ray evaluation are to seek evidence of potentially reversible underlying anatomic abnormalities predisposing to infection and to observe changes indicative of chronic inflammation and scarring.

Acute Pyelonephritis

Intravenous pyelography is usually normal. Renal enlargement with narrowing and elongation of the collecting system is occasionally seen. Impairment or delay of contrast material excretion is less common. If response to appropriate antibiotic therapy does not occur within 48–72 hours, intravenous pyelography is useful for identifying the possibility of underlying obstruction, or the occurrence of abscess formation or papillary necrosis.

Chronic Pyelonephritis

The asymmetrical renal contraction and scarring associated with chronic pyelonephritis may occur with a variety of other causes of chronic interstitial nephritis. The characteristic irregular cortical scar, often polar in location, with an underlying dilated calyx is usually a consequence of childhood renal infection with subsequent impairment in renal growth (Fig. 1). The clubbed calyx results from shrinkage and flattening of the papilla with consequent dilatation and loss of sharp definition of the calyceal fornices. The role of ureterovesical reflux in the production of these childhood lesions recently has been emphasized.

LOCALIZATION

The ability to simply and accurately distinguish between infection of the kidney and infection confined to the bladder and urethra would appear to provide important assistance to the clinician in several areas. It would enable him or her to define better the extent of diagnostic evaluation necessary and could influence the nature and duration of therapy. Symptomatology is often misleading, with lower tract complaints frequently predominant in patients with upper tract involvement. Fever is the most reliable of the clinical signs indicating parenchymal disease but is, of course, not invariably present. In a number of series evidence of upper tract involvement was present in up to half of patients with asymptomatic bacteriuria.

Bilateral ureteral catheterization for upper tract sampling is the definitive direct technique for localization, but time, cost, patient discomfort, and risk limit its routine clinical application. The bladder washout technique necessitates bladder catheterization, irrigation with antibiotic and debriding enzyme solutions, cleansing irrigations, and serial collection of specimens then representing newly formed urine of upper tract origin. Cost and discomfort again limit the application

Table 1
Chemical Tests to Screen for Urinary Bacteria

Test	Principle	First Morning Urine Required	False Positives	False Negatives
Catalase	Enzyme catalase present in urinary bacteria releases bubbles of oxygen when mixed with hydrogen peroxide	No	Yes	Yes
Nitrite reduction (Griess test)	Urinary bacteria reduce nitrate to nitrite, which can be measured colorimetrically	Yes	No	Yes
Tetrazolium reduction	Triphenyl tetrazolium is reduced by urinary bacteria to bright red colored triphenyl formazan	No	Few	Yes
Urinary glucose concentration	Urinary bacteria metabolize the small amount of glucose normally present in urine	Yes	Yes	No

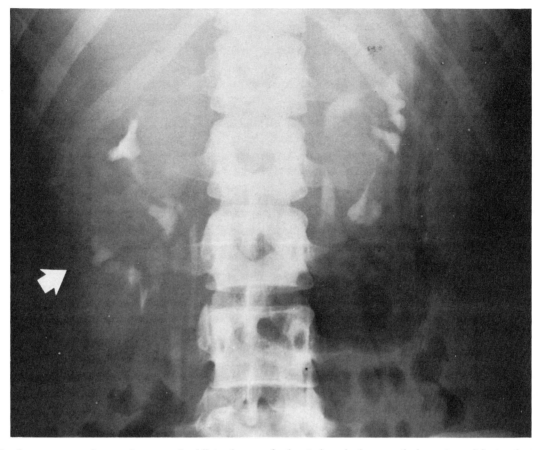

Fig. 1. Intravenous pyelogram demonstrating bilateral areas of calyectasis and a large cortical scar (arrow) in a patient with a history of ureteral reimplantations for severe bilateral ureterovesical reflux.

of this technique. Renal biopsy is not useful due to the spotty and usual medullary distribution of the early lesions and the potential risk of dissemination.

Of the indirect methods, pyelography is useful to ascertain underlying abnormalities or residual scarring but provides little assistance for localization of a specific episode. Impairment in maximal concentrating ability is an early and sensitive indicator of parenchymal infection and interstitial nephritis, but changes may be transient or, with scarring, persist as a residual from earlier episodes. Hence this technique appears useful in defining populations but is of limited help in evaluating the individual patient. Elevation in serum antibody titer against the specific organism is an indication of parenchymal infection but is found in only approximately half of such patients and is useful only when elevated. Antibody coating of urinary bacteria as demonstrated with fluorescein-conjugated anti–human globulin is found with renal parenchymal involvement and prostatitis. It is independent of and more sensitive than increase in serum antibody levels or elevation of urinary immunoglobulin levels Improperly collected specimens may yield small numbers of organisms coated with antibody of cervicovaginal origin, and a delay in anti-

body formation may be observed in patients with early pyelonephritis of acute onset. Urinary LDH isoenzyme 5 has been reported elevated in childhood renal infection but not in bladder infection.

Response to single dose of kanamycin or high single dose oral agents has been reported with lower tract infection but not pyelonephritis. Hence response to therapy may indicate localization, as well as localization techniques suggesting therapeutic approaches.

ACUTE, UNCOMPLICATED INFECTION

When a patient presents with an initial episode of lower urinary tract symptoms—urgency, frequency, dysuria, and hesitancy without fever or flank pain—*E. coli* is almost invariably the responsible organism if the culture is positive. If the organism was not acquired in the hospital or did not follow instrumentation, it usually will respond promptly to therapy with a sulfonamide. A culture is of value in such patients in that several recent studies have demonstrated the presence of significant bacterial growth in only half of women presenting with such complaints, and the "urethral" or "frequency and dysuria syndrome" may require other considerations (see the chapter on *Dysuria*). When the patient is symptomatic, therapy can be initiated before the return of the culture report. Sulfonamide therapy has the advantages of general efficacy at both minimal cost and minimal risk of side effects.

An initial lower tract infection in a male should be followed by radiologic studies. Such infections are frequently accompanied by underlying anatomical abnormalities in the child or young man and calculi or prostatic hypertrophy with obstruction in older men. A carefully performed intravenous pyelogram with both voiding and postvoiding films may reveal a correctible lesion. Abnormalities on the screening study may prompt urologic consultation for cystoscopy and/or a voiding cystourethrogram.

A careful pelvic examination should be part of the evaluation of every woman with urinary tract symptoms. Common conditions which may mimic or predispose to urinary tract infection include trichomonal or monilial infections, Bartholin and Skene gland infection, urethral caruncle, meatal stenosis, or postmenopausal atrophic vaginitis.

Followup cultures are necessary to insure adequacy of therapy. Urine cultures should be sterile within 48–72 hours after the initiation of treatment, and this can provide a useful form of in vivo sensitivity testing. Followup cultures at 2 weeks, 6 weeks, and 6 months after completion of therapy permit detection of asymptomatic relapse or reinfection.

ACUTE PYELONEPHRITIS

The clinical presentation of acute pyelonephritis is usually characterized by fever, chills, and flank pain which may or may not be associated with lower urinary tract symptoms. Therapy with a bactericidal agent which achieves significant renal and urinary concentration is necessary. Oral ampicillin is effective against most of the common gram-negative pathogens and is a reasonable initial choice for the patient with an apparently uncomplicated infection; however, if the patient develops acute pyelonephritis while in the hospital or has underlying functional or structural urinary tract abnormalities or evidence of possible gram-negative shock, with extremely high fever, unstable blood pressure, or decreasing renal function, parenteral medication is necessary. Blood cultures should always be obtained prior to the initiation of the treatment to help ensure adequate bacterial identification.

Gentamicin intramuscularly is the drug of choice in this situation because of its broad bactericidal spectrum against gram-negative organisms, including *Pseudomonas,* and its lesser, though still present, degree of ototoxicity and nephrotoxicity as compared to kanamycin. Ampicillin may be given as a second drug to ensure coverage against enterococci. If the clinical response is prompt and cultures indicate the organism is sensitive to ampicillin, the latter may be continued for the 10–14 day course and gentamicin discontinued.

RECURRENT INFECTION

The importance of organ identification and sensitivity testing is increased in patients with recurrence, since the more resistant gram-negative organisms emerge as the infecting agents and are more difficult to eradicate. The practical usefulness of the concepts of relapse (rapid recurrence with the same organism) versus reinfection (different organism at variable time interval) is undergoing reevaluation because localization studies have not supported a major association of the former with upper tract infection and because reinfection appears to be the predominant recurrence pattern independent of the initial site of infection. Radiologic and urologic evaluation is necessary to make certain the infection is not complicated by a correctable anatomic abnormality of the collecting system. The value of sustained therapy beyond 2 weeks for patients with parenchymal infection has not been established.

Frequent recurrences of infections accompanied by lower tract symptoms may occur, although evaluation may reveal no anatomic or functional lesion or association with sexual activity. Cultures are usually positive with varying serotypes of *E. coli* or species of gram-negative organisms. While the nature of the altered local resistance to infection is still not fully understood, prophylactic therapy and regular perineal cleansing with antibacterial-treated swabs may be useful.

Prophylactic therapy as first described consisted of the long-term use of methenamine mandelate or hippurate in association with an acidifying agent such as ascorbic acid. Dosage was established to maintain urinary pH at 5.5 or lower. This approach has the advantages of not promoting the emergence of restant strains of organisms or altering fecal flora; however, considerable success has been achieved with the use of nitrofurantoin or trimethaprim–sulfamethoxazole in a single bedtime dose. This program makes minimal demands upon patient compliance and is usually well followed and successful.

Nonspecific measures including the avoidance of potentially irritating bubble bath preparations, the regular use of showering rather than tub baths, and the substitution of vaginal tampons for sanitary napkins lack the support of controlled studies.

When frequent episodes of cystitis are directly associated with sexual activity, a number of relatively simple measures are often effective. Voiding regularly following intercourse and then rinsing the urethral area with soap solution may be effective in eliminating potentially ascending organisms. If this is not effective alone, it can be combined with the postcoital use of a single dose of a sulfonamide, ampicillin, or nitrofurantoin.

ASYMPTOMATIC BACTERIURIA

The reproducible finding of significant bacterial growth on urine cultures obtained in screening studies or in the evaluation of patients with nonrenal complaints is not unusual. Elicitation of a careful history may reveal minimal symptoms, and some investigators have preferred the term covert bacteriuria to asymptomatic bacteriuria. The prevalence is considerably higher among women than men and ranges from 1.2 percent among schoolgirls to 6–7 percent in early pregnancy to as many as 10–12 percent of women over age 60. Its occurrence is frequently associated with gynecologic abnormalities in older women and prostatic hypertrophy in men.

The significance of this finding is related to the possibility of underlying anatomical abnormalities which may be associated with progressive renal impairment and, secondly, the development of symptomatic infection. The latter is particularly characteristic of pregnancy (see Pregnancy). In Kunin's study of schoolgirls, 22 percent had reflux on cystourethrograms. Recurrence followed the initial course of therapy in 80 percent, but approximately 20 percent went into long-term remission after each successive course of treatment. Careful followup and repeated treatment achieved what Kunin has termed successful "fractional extraction" of a portion of patients with each course of therapy. This is a desirable goal for patients in this age group who have a higher risk for recurrences after marriage.

Other studies have demonstrated evidence of renal parenchymal invasion in a significant proportion of patients with asymptomatic bacteriuria. This includes a threefold greater prevalence of IVP abnormalities than in a control group, impairment in urinary concentrating ability, development of serum antibodies to bacterial components, and disputed findings of higher mean arterial blood pressure and an increased incidence of hypertension.

Patients with asymptomatic bacteriuria should be treated with a 10–14 day course of antibacterial agents selected by sensitivity testing. A diagnostic evaluation should be pursued in a manner similar to the patient with recurrent urinary tract infection.

CHRONIC BACTERIURIA

A group of patients emerges in most experiences who fail to respond to conventional courses of therapy, develop resistant organisms during prophylactic or suppressive treatment, or quickly recur following cessation of long-term treatment. Such patients usually have discrete anatomical or functional abnormalities of the urinary tract—calculus disease, cystocele in the elder female, or the protracted use of an indwelling catheter. If the underlying abnormality in such patients cannot be resolved, it is usually best to consider them to have chronic bacteriuria and to reserve the potent and potentially toxic antibiotics for symptomatic episodes which may go on to life-threatening sepsis.

INDWELLING CATHETERS

An indwelling urethral catheter is a major contributor to the estimated 40 percent of hospital acquired infections originating in the urinary tract. Preventative systemic antibiotic therapy is not recommended for routine use in the patient with an indwelling catheter. Such treatment encourages the emergence of resistant organisms, and antibiotics should be reserved for the development of urinary symptoms or other evidence of sepsis arising from the urethral focus.

The septic risk of long-term catheterization can be minimized by a number of simple steps. Sterile closed drainage systems appear to help alleviate the problem of infection for the bedridden patient. The collection bag should always be positioned below the level of the bladder, and external drainage should be from the bottom of the bag to minimize postemptying residua and the possibility of back flow. Washing of the urethral meatus and perineal area twice daily with soap and water can help minimize bacterial colonization and ascending infection. Sampling of the urine for cultures and other purposes should be accomplished by aspiration of freshly flowing urine from the distal end of the catheter with a 21 gauge needle after thorough cleansing of the catheter segment with an alcohol sponge.

Intermittent irrigation with saline or antibiotic solutions is of little value in the prevention or treatment of urinary tract infection. Continuous bladder irrigation with a three-way catheter system using neomycin–polymyxin solutions has been suggested as a useful adjunct to a closed drainage system. A recent controlled trial of neomycin–polymyxin irrigation through closed urinary catheters showed no significant difference between treatment and control groups, with a mean daily increment in infection of 5 percent in each group. The organisms from patients with irrigation were more resistant to antibiotics. The lack of effect of irrigation was thought to be related to the increased rate of disconnections due to the extra junction used for irrigation. This counteracted the suppressive role of the irrigation solution and led to more resistant strains.

ANTIBIOTIC THERAPY

The determination of the antibiotic agent of choice is governed initially by the patient's clinical condition and setting as reviewed earlier. Sensitivity studies provide useful guidelines when treatment may be deferred as with asymptomatic bacteriuria or when response to treatment is not prompt. The physician must be cognizant of local variations in bacterial antibiotic sensitivities, particularly in hospitals. Also, patterns of sensitivity may alter with time in response to local preferences for antibiotic use. Table 2 is a summary of characteristic patterns of antibiotic sensitivities based on both personal experience and the literature. Sensitivity testing of the infecting organism becomes mandatory with recurrent infections or in the acutely ill patient because of regional and individual variations.

The importance of the renal excretory route is a major consideration in selecting antibiotic agents in the patient with urinary tract infection and renal insufficiency. Attention must be directed at selecting an agent that achieves effective renal and urinary concentrations while avoiding potentially serious side effects due to impaired renal excretory function. Selection of antibiotic agents and modification of their dose with renal insufficiency is considered in the chapter on Conservative Therapy.

The availability of more easily performed tests of localization has led to reassessment of our standard 10–14 day course of treatment. Preliminary studies

Table 2
Characteristic Antimicrobial Sensitivities of Common Urinary Pathogens

Organisms	Sulfonamides	Nitrofurantoin	Ampicillin	Cephalosporin	Tetracycline	Kanamycin	Gentamicin	Tobramycin	Carbenicillin	Nalidixic Acid	Sulfatrimethaprim
E. coli	+	+	+	+	+	+	+	+	+	+	+
Klebsiella	±	±	−	+	+	+	+	+	−	+	+
Enterobacter	±	±	−	−	±	+	+	+	+	+	+
Proteus mirabilis	±	−	+	+	−	+	+	+	+	+	+
Proteus indole positive	−	±	−	−	−	+	+	+	+	+	±
Pseudomonas	−	−	−	−	−	−	+	+	+	−	−
Enterococcus	−	+	+	±	±	−	−	−	±	−	−

Legend: +, > 75% of isolates sensitive; ±, 60%–75% sensitive; −, < 60% sensitive.

suggest a high single dose course of treatment may be equally efficacious to the standard course in infections limited to the bladder and urethra.

ANCILLARY THERAPEUTIC MEASURES
Fluid Intake

Clinical studies demonstrating the efficacy of water diuresis in treating urinary infections are lacking. Experimental models show wide species variations with results ranging from prevention to increased susceptibility and more severe progression. Theoretically the creation of a water diuresis and more frequent voidings should minimize bladder dwell time, lower the concentration of organisms, and facilitate intrinsic bladder defenses. Lowering the tonicity of the medullary area should assist migration and phagocytosis by leukocytes and possibly facilitate complement activity.

Urinary Analgesia

Phenazopyridine hydrochloride is a useful oral urinary analgesic for the symptomatic relief of dysuria, frequency and urgency. Frequently it is prescribed in subeffective doses; the recommended dosage is 200 mg three times daily. It colors the urine a vivid red-orange, and staining of clothing is difficult to remove. Its use is contraindicated in patients with renal or hepatic failure.

Alteration of Urinary pH

Manipulation of urinary pH can promote the local effectiveness of some antibacterial agents. Acidification is mandatory for the effectiveness of methenamine salts, which act by the release of formaldehyde into the urine at low pH. Mandelic and hippuric acid are also most inhibitory of bacterial growth in an acid urine. The effectiveness of tetracycline and nitrofurantoin are increased by urinary acidification. Ascorbic acid, 500 mg four times a day, or methionine in divided dosage of 2–12 g daily are both effective and usually well tolerated acidifying agents. The patient should be instructed in the use of pH indicator paper to help establish individual dosage.

The effectiveness of the aminoglycoside antibiotics—streptomycin, kanamycin, gentamicin, and tobramicin—are promoted by urinary alkalinization. The antibacterial spectrum of erythromycin can be broadened to include most of the enteric bacteria associated with urinary infection by maintaining urinary alkalization. Sodium bicarbonate in divided dosage of 4–12 g daily can accomplish this. Such manipulation is not necessary in all patients but may be helpful in a refractory therapeutic situation. A 20 percent increase in therapeutic success was achieved by one group through more careful management of urinary pH.

COMPLICATIONS OF URINARY TRACT INFECTION
Septicemia

Transient bacteremia is common in patients with acute pyelonephritis. Blood cultures will be positive in approximately 30 percent and should be obtained in hospitalized febrile patients to aid in bacterial identification and sensitivity studies. The clinical picture of gram-negative sepsis is far less common, although urinary tract infection is the most frequent underlying infectious process in most reported series, accounting for approximately one-quarter to two-thirds of patients. Urologic instrumentation or surgery is a frequent antecedent. Both the frequency and risk of gram-negative sepsis is greatly increased in patients with urinary tract infections who have underlying diseases such as diabetes mellitus, cirrhosis, carcinomatosis, or therapeutic regimens resulting in immunosuppression.

Fever, chills, leukopenia, circulatory collapse, and evidence of the generalized Schwartzman phenomenon are all consequences of endotoxemia related to the release of the lipopolysaccharide components of the gram-negative bacterial wall.

Principles of therapy include maintenance of blood pressure with the administration of intravenous fluids; colloids are often necessary for sustaining intravascular volume. Following the obtaining of blood cultures, intravenous antibiotics are started; an aminoglycoside is the agent of choice for treatment of gram-negative sepsis. If an associated staphylococcal infection is suspected, a penicillinase-resistant agent is added. The use of pharmacologic doses of steroids is controversial, but early bolus administration of 3 mg/kg dexamethasone or 30 mg/kg of methylprednisolone has been suggested to be associated with an improved survival rate. Acid–base abnormalities require careful attention, and the possible development of disseminated intravascular coagulation must be considered.

PERINEPHRIC ABSCESS

Perinephric abscess is a relatively rare complication of urinary tract infection. It is a consequence of the rupture of a renal parenchymal abscess into the perinephric area. The majority occur as a direct extension of pyelonephritis and are associated with *E. coli* and *Proteus* and other gram-negative organisms. The hematogenous spread of gram-positive organisms, particularly *Staphylococcus aureus,* from a skin site to the kidney and then to the perinephric tissue is now a relatively rare occurrence and accounts for approximately 5 percent of cases.

Predisposing factors are found in the majority of patients and most commonly include diabetes mellitus and renal calculi. Other conditions associated with recurrent urinary tract infection are seen, including neurogenic bladder, lower tract obstruction, and polycystic kidney disease. Renal biopsy and flank trauma have also been described as antecedent events leading to the development of a perinephric abscess.

Clinical Presentation

The classical picture of perinephric abscess is the development of a symptomatic genitourinary or cutaneous infection followed by the occurrence of flank pain and persistent fever; however, this is seen in less than one-quarter of patients, and the abscess more commonly presents with unilateral flank pain and fever. Onset is frequently insidious with symptoms of several weeks duration. Fever is present in most but not all patients. Complaints of flank pain or the presence of tenderness is characteristic and a flank or abdominal mass will be found in approximately half the patients. Dysuria is commonly present.

Laboratory Findings

Leukocytosis with neutrophilia and elevated ESR are usual. Urinalysis will usually show pyuria; minimal proteinuria and hematuria are less common, and a negative urinalysis does not exclude the diagnosis. Urine cultures will be positive in approximately 80 percent of patients, and blood cultures have been reported as positive in 20–40 percent.

Abnormalities of the chest x-ray on the side of the abscess occur in approximately 20 percent. Unilateral abnormalities in the plain film of the abdomen may be observed in about half of the patients. Retrograde pyelography or intravenous pyelography will demonstrate abnormalities in 65–85 percent of patients. These include poor or nonvisualization of the affected kidney or calyceal distortion. Assessment of renal mobility has been found to be a highly reliable indication of perinephric abscess with minimal movement of the involved kidney in approximately 90 percent of patients. Normal movement with inspiration–expiration or change from the supine to upright position is approximately 2–6 cm or the height of a vertebral body. Impairment in this mobility may be demonstrated with the latter two maneuvers or on fluoroscopy. With angiography, spreading, stretching, and displacement of intrarenal vessels are characteristic.

Patients may present with fever of unknown origin or generalized sepsis without indication of renal localization. The diagnosis has been made post mortem in as high as 30 percent of reported series. The prognosis depends on the rapidity of diagnosis and effective establishment of surgical drainage, as well as the underlying anatomical and metabolic abnormalities. Drainage of the perinephric space is usually mandatory, and in a recent series 46 percent of the patients necessitated nephrectomy as well.

In contrast to uncomplicated acute pyelonephritis, patients with perinephric abscess tend to have a longer duration of symptoms, usually in excess of 5 days, and their fever tends to continue for 5 days or longer after the initiation of antibiotic therapy, in contrast to relatively rapid resolution with pyelonephritis.

Mortality in reported series ranges from 45–59 percent.

PAPILLARY NECROSIS

Renal papillary necrosis, the partial or total loss of papillae and the adjacent medullary region, may occur as a consequence of renal infection. The disorder is virtually always a consequence of localized ischemia due to preexisting renal disease and which is further complicated by a secondary infection.

Urinary obstruction and diabetes mellitus have long been appreciated as the most frequent coexisting processes (Table 3); however, in recent years analgesic abuse nephropathy with papillary necrosis and interstitial nephritis has assumed a commanding position in etiologic listings. It has been estimated that about one-third of these patients will have secondary infections. Other associations include fulminant acute or active chronic pyelonephritis, sickle cell anemia, alcoholism, Balkan nephropathy, and aging. In a recent review over 90 percent of patients with papillary necrosis were age 50 or older and over 75 percent were age 60 or older. Autopsy prevalence is 1–1.5 percent and is slightly higher in males. With the increasing importance of analgesic abuse, the frequency in women should be rising.

Table 3
Conditions Associated With Renal Papillary
Necrosis

Renal infection and/or urinary obstruction,
  usually with:
    Diabetes mellitus
    Analgesic abuse
    Sickle cell anemia
    Balkan nephropathy
    Alcoholism
    Aging

The clinical manifestations are highly variable, but three patterns may be recognized. Papillary necrosis may present as an acute febrile illness, with chills, renal colic, progressive azotemia, and, if the process is bilateral, ultimately oliguria with renal failure. This usually occurs in a setting of obstruction or diabetes mellitus or as a terminal complication of severe acute pyelonephritis. It may be recognized as a chronic recurrent renal disease with infection, gross hematuria, intermittent colic, and ureteric obstruction due to papillary sequestration. Finally, a picture of progressive chronic renal insufficiency with anemia may be observed with analgesic abuse in the absence of symptomatic secondary infection or urinary passage of papillae.

Diagnosis is based on recognition of the clinical setting and presentation and confirmed by passage of tissue; however, in approximately one-third of patients the tissue passage may not be recognized. Intravenous or retrograde pyelography may reveal characteristic filling defects or the so-called "ring sign" of a sequestered papilla (Fig. 2).

In the chronic disease mild proteinuria, polyuria associated with a concentrating defect and normal blood pressure are usually found.

Antibiotic and fluid and electrolyte therapy must be vigorous in seeking to control the infectious process. The presence of obstruction must be excluded or remedied. Endoscopic surgery with a Dormia ureteric stone basket frequently has been found effective in removal of ureteric impaction with a sloughed papilla.

CHRONIC PYELONEPHRITIS

The role of chronic or persistent urinary tract infection as a forerunner of renal insufficiency secondary to chronic pyelonephritis has been clarified in recent years. The appreciation that chronic pyelonephritis is only one form of interstitial nephritis and the recognition that a variety of etiologic factors may result in the latter histologic and clinical picture has been of major importance. An increasing number of studies have demonstrated the relative benignity of urinary infection in relationship to renal function in the absence of associated metabolic and/or anatomic abnormalities. Obstructive chronic pyelonephritis rather than uncomplicated renal urinary tract infection appears clearly to be the antecedent in the association between renal infection and renal insufficiency. Nonetheless, the possible occurrence of stone formation and sepsis and the major loss of working hours among women due to

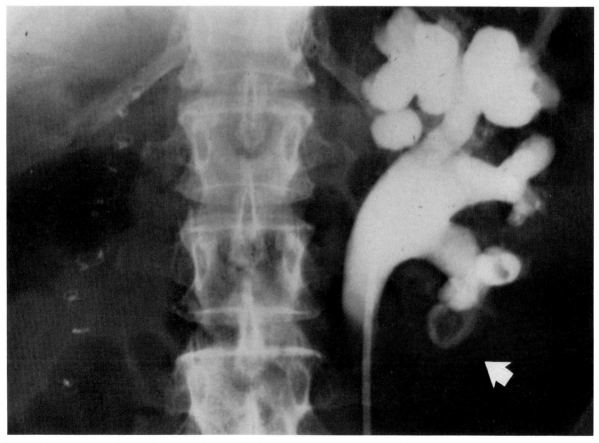

Fig. 2. Retrograde pyelogram in a patient with diabetes mellitus, chronic pyelonephritis, and left ureteral obstruction due to papillary necrosis. A sloughed papilla is present in the lower calyx (arrow).

recurrent infection justify a vigorous approach to both therapy and prevention in nonobstruction infection. (See chapter on Interstitial Disease)

GENITOURINARY TUBERCULOSIS

Although the incidence of pulmonary tuberculosis has decreased sharply in recent years, the occurrence of genitourinary tuberculosis has remained relatively stable. This is most likely attributable to the frequent long latent period between the primary, usually pulmonary focus of disease and the subsequent manifestation of tuberculosis of the genitourinary tract as a consequence of the hematogenous spread of the bacilli. A high index of clinical suspicion is necessary to establish an early diagnosis because of the frequent silent progression of renal involvement.

Renal tuberculosis may present as sterile pyuria, persistent hematuria, symptomatic urinary tract infection resistant to usual antibiotic management, radiologic abnormalities including calyceal distortion, and/or renal calcification or recurrent prostatitis, orchitis, or epididymitis. Genitourinary tuberculosis may be seen at any age but its peak occurrence is usually between ages 20 and 40 years.

Pathophysiology

Following hematogenous spread of the tubercle bacillus from a primary pulmonary or gastrointestinal site, seeding occurs initially in the renal cortex and spreads to the glomeruli. The medullary area becomes involved via the tubules and organisms subsequently proliferate and form foci of caseating granulomata. Localized obstruction with areas of necrosis and excavation develop with later involvement of the ureter, bladder, and male genitalia. Clinical manifestations may consequently include segmental renal destruction, obstructive hydronephrosis, and bladder contracture with chronic cystitis and prostatitis, orchitis, and epididymitis. The disease may be unilateral at its early stages, but approximately 50 percent of patients show evidence of bilateral involvement at the time of diagnosis.

Diagnostic Studies

Pyuria and/or hematuria may be minimal but are critical clues, and one or both are usually present in the majority of patients. Concurrent pyrogenic infection is not unusual.

Culture of first morning urine specimens for recovery of *M. tuberculosis* provides results comparable to 24 hour urine collections and is the preference of most laboratories. Approximately 80 percent of patients will grow organisms from repeated urine cultures; in the remainder the diagnosis is established on the basis of positive skin tests, biopsy results, and intravenous pyelography; however, changes on IVP are nonspecific in the absent of calcification, and less than 20 percent of patients will demonstrate the characteristic calcifications. Urine smears and stains are not helpful in the diagnosis because of the frequent occurrence of acid-fast organisms in the genital region.

Therapy

Recommended drug regimens have varied with the introduction of new therapeutic agents. Isoniazide is a basic agent and usually administered in combination with ethambutol or rifampin for a 2 year period; some centers continue to prefer the addition of streptomycin for an initial 4–12 month period. Latimer has reported an advantage of triple drug therapy over a two drug regimen, with a combination of three oral agents as efficacious as regimens including streptomycin.

The reported frequency of the development of ureteral strictures during therapy has varied widely, but some clinical investigators emphasize the importance of repeated intravenous pyelography at 4–6 month intervals for early detection and treatment of stricture development Relapse is rare and usually associated with the development of drug resistance and is the rationale for combined drug therapy. Nephrectomy is now rarely performed, even with large nonfunctioning kidneys, but cure of hypertension in patients with renal tuberculosis has been reported following unilateral nephrectomy.

REFERENCES

Christensen WI; Genitourinary tuberculosis: Review of 102 cases. Medicine (Baltimore) 53:377, 1974

Fang LST, Tolokoff-Rubin NE, Rubin RH: Efficacy of single-dose and conventional amoxicillin therapy in urinary-tract infection localized by the antibody-coated bacteria technic. N Engl J Med 298:413, 1978

Harding GKM, Ronald AR: A controlled study of antimicrobial prophylaxis of recurrent urinary infection in women. N Engl J Med 291:597, 1974

Kunin CM: A ten year study of bacteriuria in schoolgirls: Final report of bacteriologic, urologic and epidemiologic findings. J Infect Dis 122:382, 1970

Murray T, Goldberg M: Chronic interstitial nephritis: Etiologic factors. Ann Intern Med 82:453, 1975

Smellie JM, Normand ICS: Bacteriuria, reflux, and renal scarring. Arch Dis Child 50:581, 1975

Stamey TA, Condy M, Mihara G: Prophylactic efficacy of nitrofurantoin macrocrystals and trimethoprim-sulfamethoxazole in urinary infection. N Engl J Med 296:780, 1977

Thomas V, Shelokov A, Forland M: Antibody-coated bacteria in urine and the site of urinary tract infection. N Engl J Med 290:588, 1974

Disorders of Water and Electrolyte Metabolism

WATER BALANCE

Richard E. Weitzman

Body fluid tonicity is a critical determinant of intracellular volume (see also the chapter on *Water Metabolism*). Elevations of plasma and extracellular fluid tonicity produce an osmotic gradient across semipermeable cell membranes which leads to rapid outward fluxes of water and produces cellular dehydration. Conversely, ingestion of large quantities of solute-free water has the opposite effect. Water loading causes a reduction of plasma and extracellular fluid tonicity which results in an osmotic dysequilibrium across cell membranes and produces cellular overhydration. Under normal conditions intracellular volume is maintained within very narrow limits by a physiological control system that closely balances water intake with water excretion and, as a consequence, regulates plasma osmolality within very narrow limits. If the portion of this system that controls water conservation is selectively disrupted (as in diabetes insipidus) and the thirst mechanism remains intact, then the functioning portion of the regulatory system compensates for the water losses and plasma osmolality is maintained within the normal range, albeit at considerable social discomfort. In other circumstances the organism is unable to compensate for malfunctions of the control system and substantial alterations occur in plasma osmolality. Such alterations produce marked disturbances of cellular function. This is particularly apparent in the central nervous system, where cellular overhydration causes symptoms ranging from headaches and muscle cramps to stupor, seizures, or coma and cellular dehydration causes irritability and ataxia. It therefore can be seen that diseases of the water balance control system can cause a spectrum of disorders ranging from relatively benign polyuria to cellular overhydration and death.

Body fluid tonicity or osmolality is usually regulated by two main mechanisms—thirst and secretion of antidiuretic hormone (also known as arginine vasopressin or AVP). Elevations of plasma osmolality trigger an increased firing rate of osmosensitive cells in the anterior hypothalamus, which, in turn, bring about a sensation of thirst and water-seeking behavior. At the same time there is an increased rate of synthesis and secretion of AVP, which, acting upon the renal collecting ducts, enhances the reabsorption of free water from glomerular filtrate. Thirst (and not AVP release) is the major defense against dehydration. Under usual conditions of hydration, man normally reabsorbs more than 99 percent of glomerular filtrate. After dehydration and stimulation of maximal AVP release, renal water losses are further reduced about 50 percent with an additional saving of only 0.5–1.0 liters of water. This saving would be insufficient to maintain water balance under environmental conditions associated with greatly enhanced evaporative water losses. Under such conditions the thirst mechanism may lead to 20-fold or greater increases in water intake and maintenance of water balance. On the other hand, maximal suppression of thirst has relatively little value in adopting to chronic overhydration inasmuch as persistent water intake remains as a social convention in the absence of osmotic stimulation. In contrast, suppression of AVP release can produce a 20-fold increase in renal water excretion, which is of major importance in preventing overhydration. Thus the AVP system is most effective in defense against overhydration. In contrast, the thirst system is relatively unresponsive to overhydration but is particularly effective in defense against dehydration.

CONTROL OF AVP SECRETION AND THIRST

AVP is synthesized in neurosecretory neurons of the supraoptic and paraventricular nuclei of the hypothalamus and is carried in neurosecretory granules down the pituitary stalk to the neural lobe, where it is released into the circulation. The firing rate of the neurosecretory neurons (and, as a consequence, AVP synthesis and release) is under the influence of many different neural control mechanisms. One major influence on AVP secretion is plasma osmolality, as mediated by the osmosensitive centers of the anterior hypothalamus. Baroreceptors located in the carotid sinus and aortic arch and volume receptors in the left atrium also have important effects on AVP secretion. Diminished blood pressure or central blood volume result in significant increases in AVP secretion. Other influences on AVP secretion include pain and noxious stimuli, emesis, hypoglycemia, hypercapnea, and the renin–angiotensin system as well as many drugs and hormones.

Thirst is also regulated by osmotic and volume stimuli and, in addition, is influenced by the renin–angiotensin system, hypokalemia, and possibly hypercalcemia.

DISORDERS OF BODY WATER REGULATION
Polyuric Disorders

Polyuria (see also the chapter on *Polyuria*) is defined as urine volumes in excess of 2.5–3 liters per day. Massive urinary volumes do not necessarily represent a defect in water conservation per se. Some polyuric patients may be undergoing a solute diuresis due to glucose or sodium or due to various pharmacologic agents such as mannitol or radiographic contrast material. In such instances the urine is usually isotonic to plasma ($U_{osm}/P_{osm} = 1$) and the osmolar clearance ($C_{osm} = U_{osm} \times$ volume$/P_{osm} \times$ time) is in excess of 3 ml/min. In contrast, polyuric patients having a water diuresis have distinctly lower ratios of urine to plasma osmolality (0.7 or less), with urine osmolalities frequently less than 100 mOsm/kg. There are three possible defects in such patients—diminished release of AVP due to disease of the hypothalamic neurohypophyseal system (central or vasopressin sensitive diabetes insipidus), renal resistance to AVP (nephrogenic diabetes insipidus), or diminished release of AVP due to hypoosmolality of body fluids following greatly increased water intake (psychogenic polydipsia). In the first two groups renal water losses result in elevations of plasma osmolality which, in turn, stimulate thirst and water ingestion, which then further enhance polyuria.

Central diabetes insipidus rarely occurs as an inherited disorder with either autosomal dominant or sex-limited inheritance (Table 1). Also, in a few patients diabetes insipidus occurs in early childhood with no discernible cause (idiopathic diabetes insipidus). In all other instances central disturbances of AVP release are acquired in association with other intracranial diseases. One common cause of diabetes insipidus is damage to the neural lobe and pituitary stalk sustained after either head trauma or a neurosurgical procedure. Under such circumstances a triphasic pattern of diuresis may be seen, with an initial period of polyuria due to localized edema of the pathways for neurosecretion in the pituitary stalk, an interphase lasting up to 5 days when previously synthesized AVP is released from the nec-

rotic neural lobe, and a final period of unremitting polyuria when the stores of previously synthesized AVP are exhausted. Intracranial neoplasms are important causes of diabetes insipidus, particularly in children, where polyuria may be a presenting symptom of craniopharyngiomas. Sarcoidosis, histiocytosis, and infectious processes, particularly tuberculous meningitis, are also important causes of central diabetes insipidus. Not all cases of central diabetes insipidus necessarily cause massive polyuria; frequently there is only limited destruction of the neurohypophysis producing mild impairment of maximal urinary concentration.

Impaired ability to maximally concentrate the urine may also be due to an inherited or acquired renal defect. This can have many different etiologies. Renal concentrating ability is dependent on the coordinated function of several different nephron segments, and disease in any one of them can lead to less than maximally concentrated urine. Table 2 lists various types of concentrating defects on the basis of the underlying pathophysiological abnormality. In some instances there is a normal increase in water permeability of the collecting duct in response to AVP but the urine cannot be concentrated because of a defective osmotic gradient at the medullary tip. In other instances, the cellular response to AVP is impaired either by interference with renal medullary adenylate cyclase or by a more distal lesion such as an impaired cellular response to cyclic AMP. The precise pathophysiologic basis for many of these lesions is at present unclear. The common denominator in all these situations is an impaired ability to maximally concentrate the urine even in the presence of maximal endogenous or exogenous AVP. The severity of the lesions range from severe unremitting polyuria of up to 10 liters a day, as in familial nephrogenic diabetes insipidus, to a minor subclinical concentrating defect, as in some patients with hypercalcemia.

The differential diagnosis of polyuria begins with characterization of the disorder as either an osmotic diuresis or a water diuresis as described above. Once it is ascertained that a polyuric patient is having a water diuresis, a water deprivation–Pitressin test is performed as described by Miller and co-workers. Briefly, water is withheld from 6 to 18 hours until either there is a plateau in hourly determinations of urine osmolality or there is a greater than 3–5 percent loss in body weight. Plasma osmolality and plasma AVP are then deter-

---

Table 1
Causes of Central Diabetes Insipidus

Trauma—postoperative, head trauma
Intracranial mass lesions—pituitary tumors, suprasellar tumors, granulomatous lesions, histiocytosis
Infectious—meningitis, encephalitis
Vascular—aneurysms
Familial
Idiopathic

Table 2
Causes of Impaired Renal Concentrating Ability

Osmotic diuresis per nephron
  Chronic renal failure (also disruption of countercurrent system and interference with
  adenylate cyclase–cAMP)
  Diuretic phase of acute tubular necrosis
  Postobstructive nephropathy (also interference with adenylate cyclase–cAMP)
  Salt-losing nephritis
  Glycosuria
Breakdown of renal medullary osmotic gradient
  Psychogenic polydipsia
  Low-protein diet
  Furosemide therapy
Disruption of the countercurrent system
  Sickle-cell nephropathy
  Medullary cystic disease
  Chronic pyelonephritis
  Sjögren's syndrome
  Light chain nephropathy
  Papillary necrosis
Interference with the adenylate cyclase–cyclic AMP system
  Lithium
  Demethychlortetracycline (Declomycin)
  Methoxyflurane

mined, and the patient is given 5 units of aqueous Pitressin subcutaneously. Urine samples for osmolality and volume are then obtained for two additional hours. The interpretation of the test is summarized in Table 3. Patients with either complete or partial central diabetes insipidus fail to concentrate maximally their urine after water deprivation and have subnormal plasma levels of AVP in association with elevated levels of plasma osmolality. After administration of exogenous AVP in the form of aqueous Pitressin they have a substantial increase in urine osmolality, although they usually do not achieve levels within the normal range. In contrast, patients with nephrogenic diabetes insipidus have less than maximally concentrated urine in association with elevated plasma concentrations of AVP. These patients are distinguished by the inability of their kidneys to respond to even pharmacologic doses of Pitressin. A special situation is the polyuria seen in patients having a primary disturbance in thirst regulation, i.e., psycho-

genic polydipsia. In these patients increased water intake leads to dilution of body fluids, physiologic suppression of AVP release, and polyuria. When this process is of long standing the renal medullary osmotic gradient is "washed out" and concentrating ability is impaired. The etiology can usually be suspected when plasma osmolality is slightly depressed or low normal in a patient with large urinary volumes and almost maximally dilute urine. After dehydration plasma AVP values may rise to the normal range but urine osmolality is subnormal and does not increase after Pitressin. These patients may present a special diagnostic problem because the intensity of their thirst drive is such that they go to great extremes to obtain water during a dehydration test, including drinking the water in flower vases and toilet bowls.

Central diabetes insipidus is best treated by replacement therapy with the deficient hormone or one of its analogues. A mixture of AVP and LVP (lysine

Table 3
Differential Diagnosis of Hypotonic Polyuria by Sequential Dehydration and Pitressin Administration

	P_{osm}	P_{AVP}	U_{osm}	
			After Dehydration	After Pitressin
Central diabetes insipidus	>N*	≪N†	≪N‡	↑ ↑
Partial central diabetes insipidus	sl.>N	<N	<N	↑ (>9%)
Psychogenic polydipsia	<N	<N	<N	No change
Nephrogenic diabetes insipidus	>N	>N	<or ≪N	No change

*The normal (N) range for plasma osmolality is approximately 280–290 mOsm/kg.
†Normal levels for plasma AVP range from 0.2 to 1.2 μU/ml but vary according to the method of assay.
‡Maximal U_{osm} after water deprivation is approximately 900–1200 mOsm/kg.

vasopressin, the antidiuretic principle of the order Suinae) can be given by slow intravenous infusion using aqueous Pitressin or subcutaneously using the long-acting preparation Pitressin Tannate in Oil. Synthetic lysine vasopressin is also available as a nasal spray (Diapid), which is administered every 4–6 hours. Recently, 1-desamino-8-D-arginine vasopressin (DdAVP), a form of AVP which has markedly less effect on smooth muscle contractility and considerably longer duration of action than AVP, has been introduced. The diminished effect on smooth muscle permits larger doses to be given without associated abdominal cramps or elevations of blood pressure, and the longer half-life in plasma permits good control of polyuria with only twice daily administration in many cases. The effectiveness of DdAVP is such that there should be little continued need for oral antidiuretic agents such as chlorpropamide, carbonmazepine, and clofibrate, which had been used earlier. All three of these agents produce decreased urine flow in patients with vasopressin-sensitive diabetes insipidus, particularly when there is only a partial defect. The basis for these beneficial effects is unclear and may be due to either enhanced sensitivity for AVP at the level of the collecting duct or increased AVP release. Plasma AVP levels have been found to be significantly less than control values after administration of carbamazepine in three out of four recent studies involving normal subjects. Also, there are conflicting data as to whether or not chlorpropamide stimulates AVP release. Furthermore, there is evidence that chlorpropamide stimulates renal medullary adenylate cyclase, inhibits renal prostaglandin synthetase, and inhibits renal phosphodiesterase, all of which would tend to augment the action of AVP at the level of the collecting duct. Given the effectiveness and lack of side effects of DdAVP, there is little need to utilize the oral agents, all of which have the potential for significant side effects.

In patients with nephrogenic diabetes insipidus, however, neither AVP nor any of the oral agents are effective. In this situation, a thiazide diuretic can, in a seemingly paradoxical way, be efficacious. The basis for the antidiuretic effect of the thiazide seems to relate to the depletion of extracellular volume which attends their administration. Volume depletion will increase proximal tubular reabsorption of salt and water, decrease the delivery of filtrate to the diluting segment, and thus diminish the diuresis.

Hypoosmolar Disorders

Dilution of extracellular fluid tonicity is a potential cause of significant central nervous system dysfunction. Acute decreases in ECF osmolality can produce cellular overhydration ultimately leading to cerebral edema, seizures, and coma. Frequently, hypoosmolality is detected as a significant fall in the serum sodium concentration on routine laboratory screening; however, not all instances of hyponatremia are associated with hypoosmolality. Important discrepancies between sodium concentration and osmolality exist whenever there is a substantial rise in the plasma concentration of osmotically active substances such as glucose or mannitol. Under these conditions one may see hyperosmolar hyponatremia (Table 4). The dissociation between sodium and osmolality under such circumstances is not due to a technical artifact in sodium measurement but rather is a reflection of the dilution of extracellular fluid constituents by water drawn out of cells down an osmotic gradient, i.e., extracellular fluid overhydration and cellular dehydration. The magnitude of the dilutional effect can be estimated for glucose as an observed fall of 1.6 mEq/liter in sodium concentration for each 100 mg/dl elevation of blood glucose above normal. The dilutional phenomenon can be reversed by insulin therapy, which facilitates the entry of glucose accompanied by water into the cells. Rarely, massive elevations of plasma lipids or total proteins will present with hyponatremia and normal plasma osmolality. In these situations the sodium concentration for each milliliter of plasma water is perfectly normal but the enormous elevations of fat or protein produce a proportionate decrease in the aqueous fraction of plasma which, in turn, results in a decreased measured sodium concentration expressed per unit volume of plasma. The extent of such changes in sodium concentration are relatively minor, such that plasma lipid concentrations in excess of 2500 mg/dl or plasma proteins of 15 g/dl produce a fall in sodium concentration of only a few milliequivalents per liter. In both circumstances the fall in measured sodium concentrations represent artifactual or pseudohyponatremia.

Hyponatremia is frequently found in association with diminished body fluid tonicity, i.e., hypoosmolar hyponatremia (Table 4). In this setting water enters the cells along an osmotic gradient, producing cellular overhydration and ultimately leading to central nervous system dysfunction (see above). The cellular overhydration occurs regardless of the volume of other body fluid compartments and may actually occur in the setting of severe contraction of the extracellular fluid compartment. Indeed, extracellular fluid volume depletion (hypovolemic hyponatremia) is a common cause of the hypoosmolar syndrome. In this syndrome there is a deficit in exchangeable sodium. Salt and water losses occur through the kidneys, as in salt-losing nephritis, or diuretic abuse, through extrarenal routes, as in losses to a third space (burns, pancreatitis, rhabdomyolysis), or through the gastrointestinal tract (emesis, diarrhea) and trigger several mechanisms which result in enhanced free water intake and impaired free water excretion. Hypovolemia activates both the renin–angiotensin system and the cardiac and carotid baroreceptors to stimulate thirst. At the same time enhanced secretion of AVP along with decreased renal blood flow and elevated proximal tubular reabsorption of glomerular filtrate combine to markedly limit renal water excretion. As a consequence, water balance becomes positive and dilution of body fluids ensues. This course of events can occur even in the absence of AVP; Brattleboro

Table 4
Hyponatremic States

Osmolality:	Hyperosmolar Hyponatremia, Cellular Dehydration	Euosmolar Hyponatremia, Artifactual Hyponatremia	Hypovolemic Hyponatremia	Hypoosmolar Hyponatremia, Hyponatremia With Minimal ECF Expansion	Hypervolemic Hyponatremia
ICF volume	↓	N	↑	↑	↑
ECF volume:	↑	N	↓	sl. ↑	↑
"Effective" blood volume	sl. ↑	N	↓	↑	↓
Urine sodium excretion	Variable	N	Renal ↑, extrarenal ↓	↑	↓
Etiology	↑$P_{glucose}$ ↑$P_{mannitol}$	↑$P_{protein}$ ↑P_{lipid}	Renal—diuretics, salt-losing nephritis Extrarenal–third space, nasogastric suction, vomiting	SIADH—malignancies, drugs, CNS, pulmonary disease, other Myxedema	Nephrosis Cirrhosis Congestive heart failure

Adapted from a figure by Schrier RW, Berl T: Disorders of water metabolism in Schrier RW (ed): Renal and Electrolyte Disorders. Boston, Little, Brown, 1976, p. 1.

rats, which have a hereditary absence of AVP, can be rendered hyponatremic after severe salt depletion. The diagnosis of hypovolemic hyponatremia is easily made by clinical evaluation of the state of hydration and by a few simple laboratory tests. The patients usually manifest dry mucous membranes, decreased skin turgor, and orthostatic tachycardia and hypotension. On laboratory evaluation they have hypoosmolar hyponatremia associated with mild azotemia. Urine sodium concentration can be used to differentiate extrarenal and renal etiologies; it is usually less than 20 mEq/liter in patients with extrarenal causes of volume depletion and greater than 40 mEq/liter in patients with renal salt wasting.

An important exception to the general principle that urinary sodium excretion is reduced in states of extrarenal sodium loss occurs during vomiting. In this situation the gastric losses of hydrochloric acid result in generation of a bicarbonate load and diuresis of alkaline urine. Since bicarbonate functions as a nonreabsorbable anion under these conditions, it fosters persistent renal losses of sodium in spite of hypovolemia. An important clue to the presence of this picture is a very low urinary chloride in association with high urinary sodium and alkaline urine.

Another potential exception occurs in some patients with diuretic induced sodium losses, who may have normal or low urinary sodium concentrations if they stopped their medication 1–2 days prior to the time of evaluation. The treatment in all instances is administration of adequate quantities of isotonic saline. This solution is, or course, slightly hypertonic to the extracellular fluid osmolality of the patients, but more importantly it restores the volume deficit, which permits renal excretion of the retained free water and normalization of plasma osmolality.

Hyponatremia is often found without any clinical evidence of either volume expansion or depletion (hy-

ponatremia with minimal ECF expansion; see Table 4). In these patients there is often subclinical evidence of slightly increased extracellular fluid volume in association with increases in intracellular fluid volume proportional to the decline in osmolality. Total body water is significantly increased, and exchangeable sodium is normal or perhaps slightly decreased. Blood urea nitrogen and uric acid concentrations are usually reduced, and the urine osmolality is less than maximally dilute (as would otherwise be expected under conditions of plasma hypoosmolality) and often is hypertonic to plasma. Urine sodium concentration is frequently elevated (greater than 40 mEq/liter), although it may be less than 40 mEq/liter if the patient is in negative salt and water balance at the time the urine sample is collected. If urine sodium concentrations are not clearly diagnostic of this syndrome, it may be useful to repeat the determination after saline loading, since patients with this syndrome have an exaggerated natriuresis after administration of isotonic saline or even after administration of a water load. Finally, plasma renin activity tends to be low and plasma aldosterone measurements normal or slightly reduced.

The clinical and laboratory picture described above is most commonly seen in association with the syndrome of inappropriate antidiuretic hormone (SIADH). This picture can also be seen in patients with hypothyroidism, although it is not clear that AVP is necessarily the major factor causing hyponatremia in that state.

To some extent the diagnosis of SIADH is one of exclusion, and efforts should be made to exclude the presence of other diseases that might impair water excretion independently of enhanced secretion of AVP. There are multiple causes for inappropriate AVP secretion. Malignant tumors, especially oat cell carcinomas, but also many other cell types, develop the capability to secrete large quantities of AVP sufficient to cause water retention. Severe hyponatremia is frequently the first manifestation of an underlying malignancy. Some authors have questioned the use of the term "inappropriate" in describing excessive secretion of AVP in circumstances other than those in which the AVP is produced by a malignant tumor. They have rightfully pointed out that there are multiple nonosmotic stimuli to AVP secretion and that signals from any one of them could produce a physiological or "appropriate" increase in plasma AVP that might be inappropriate for the level of osmolality. Since the precise cause for elevated AVP secretion and water retention is not always apparent in all instances, it is not unreasonable to continue using the same terminology (SIADH) in cases in which plasma AVP concentrations are inappropriate to known osmotic and nonosmotic stimuli.

Many pulmonary conditions other than malignancies have been found to produce SIADH, including tuberculosis, pneumonia, and lung abcesses. It has been postulated that some chest conditions might alter pulmonary compliance and in turn influence the firing rate of intrathoracic baroreceptors; however, AVP-like activity has been identified in one case of tuberculous abscess, suggesting local production of AVP by the diseased tissue. Central nervous system diseases such as encephalitis, meningitis, head trauma, and subarachnoid hemorrhage are also associated with SIADH. In some instances the enhanced secretion of AVP might be the consequence of increased intracranial pressure, since experimental elevations of intracranial pressure have been shown to stimulate secretion of AVP.

Drugs are an important cause of water retention and hyponatremia, although not all medications that impair water excretion necessarily do so by stimulation of AVP release. Some drugs such as chlorpropamide and indomethacin potentiate the action of AVP on the collecting duct. Other drugs, such as thiazide diuretics, also diminish water excretion but do so in part by a mechanism independent of AVP. The impaired water excretion in patients taking diuretics appears to be due to enchanced proximal reabsorption of filtrate such that there is reduced filtrate delivered to the loop of Henle. In addition, thiazides inhibit sodium transport in the cortical diluting segment. Furthermore, thiazides may produce potassium depletion and/or volume contraction, both of which may enhance AVP secretion and further impair water excretion. Many drugs, including clofibrate, chlorpropamide, opiate analgesics, nicotine, barbiturates, cyclophosphamide, and vincristine, are thought to cause hyponatremia by stimulating secretion of AVP. In some instances AVP release may not be the result of a direct effect on the hypothalamic–neurohypophyseal system but rather may be mediated by drug effects on other systems. For example, AVP release following systemic administration of nicotine can be substantially attenuated by either baroreceptor denervation or pretreatment with antihistamines, suggesting mediation by the vasomotor or emetic centers. Finally, some drugs, such as oxytocin, may bind to renal AVP receptors and initiate an antidiuretic response. This effect is clinically important, since sustained postpartum infusions of oxytocin along with dextrose in water frequently lead to substantial water retention and hyponatremia.

A picture of hypoosmolar hyponatremia consistent with the syndrome of inappropriate ADH secretion may also be seen in association with various forms of emotional stress. Psychosis is frequently associated with hyponatremia, and elevated plasma levels of AVP have been described in some psychotic patients. Major surgery, particularly after abdominal traction, can produce sustained elevations in plasma AVP that may, in part, contribute to postoperative fluid retention. Indeed, severe pain in the absence of surgery has been shown to elevate plasma AVP. It is not clear to what extent stress other than pain influences AVP secretion. Studies in rats have shown that many different stresses, such as high gravitational forces, ether, immersion, etc., do not stimulate AVP secretion, although they have substantial effects on ACTH release, as reflected by changes in plasma corticosterone levels. It is not always possible to attribute some cryptogenic cases of SIADH to stress, some cases have to be regarded as idiopathic, without any clearly defined etiology.

The treatment for SIADH has to be tailored to the underlying abnormality as well as the severity and chronicity of the observed fall in serum sodium concentration. Any obvious underlying cause such as ingestion of drugs potentially capable of causing water retention should be identified and the offending medication discontinued or the underlying illness treated. Rapid onset of hyponatremia frequently produces serious central nervous system complications, and patients having a 10 mEq/liter or greater fall in serum sodium concentration over 1–2 days and having evidence of diminished mental status may need to be treated on an urgent basis. Hantman and colleagues have proposed a treatment scheme in which hypertonic saline is infused along with furosemide. The furosemide serves to prevent excessive extracellular fluid volume expansion during saline infusion and also limits free water reabsorption by its effect on the renal countercurrent mechanism. Hypertonic saline infusion by itself has only short-lived beneficial effects since most of the sodium is rapidly excreted due to the exaggerated natriuresis seen in patients with SIADH. In many instances of SIADH, there is only mild hyponatremia of longstanding duration. In such cases it is sufficient merely to restrict water intake to a degree consistent with renal and insensible losses. In some patients with SIADH due to malignancy, such a treatment plan with drastic restriction of water intake may be difficult to tolerate on a chronic basis. In such patients oral administration of demeclocycline hydrochloride (Declomycin) can result in inhibition of the renal action of AVP and permit normal water intake. Lithium carbonate has also been used for this purpose but has been found to be less satisfactory.

The last major subgroup of hyponatremic disorders to be discussed is designated hypervolemic hyponatremia. The three main causes of this picture are hepatic cirrhosis, nephrotic syndrome, and congestive heart failure. The underlying pathophysiological disturbances vary in these conditions, but there is in common a strong tendency for salt and water retention. Exchangeable sodium is elevated in these conditions, and there is an even greater increase in total body water, producing dilution of body fluids. Water retention in these diseases is mediated by several different mechanisms. Alterations in systemic hemodynamics may result in enhanced proximal reabsorption of glomerular filtrate, which in turn diminishes distal delivery and limits free water formation independent of AVP. Reductions in "effective" or nonsplanchnic blood volume may result in stimulation of cardiopulmonary receptors and enhanced secretion of AVP. Finally, AVP clearance may be depressed in some instances of either renal or hepatic insufficiency. The diagnosis of hypervolemic hyponatremia can be established by the finding of hypoosmolar hyponatremia in an edematous patient in association with very low values (usually less than 20 mEq/liter) for urine sodium concentration. Plasma renin activity is typically elevated in these disorders, in contrast to SIADH. Treatment of the hyponatremia in such patients must be undertaken with considerable caution. Hypertonic saline infusion may aggravate the edema and produce only transient elevations in serum sodium concentration. Alternatively, severe water restriction or furosemide administration may produce acute circulatory embarrassment in some patients. It is important to realize that the hyponatremia is often relatively longstanding and is therefore unlikely to be associated with serious side effects. There is accumulating experimental evidence to suggest that the cellular overhydration and hypervolemia seen following acute reductions in plasma osmolality spontaneously resolve after 1–2 days when intracellular solute is lost and a new osmotic equilibrium is established. Moderate restriction of both salt and water usually suffices to minimize hyponatremia in such patients.

The diversity of treatment and the variable prognosis for the different hypoosmolar syndromes make it extremely important to determine the pathophysiologic basis for hyponatremia in individual patients. Careful clinical and laboratory evaluation should permit classification of most cases of hyponatremia (Table 4). Interestingly, plasma levels of AVP are generally of little value for differential diagnosis, since they are elevated (albeit to a variable degree) in all the major types of hypoosmolar hyponatremia. It is conceivable that in selected cases differential venous sampling for AVP may permit the distinction between pituitary and ectopic secretion. Plasma renin activity may be of significant diagnostic value in difficult cases. As noted above, plasma renin activity is significantly suppressed in SIADH, while it is elevated in sodium depletion and also in hepatic, renal, and cardiac disease associated with hyponatremia. Once the specific diagnosis is made, therapy can be initiated and tailored to the nature of the underlying disorder.

Hypernatremic Disorders

While hyponatremia is a rather common disorder, hypernatremia is a distinctly uncommon clinical problem. In all instances of hypernatremia there is accompanying hyperosmolality, although the converse is not always the case. The causes of hypernatremia, like those of hyponatremia, can be divided on the basis of the state of the extracellular fluid volume. Hypernatremia in association with expanded extracellular fluid volume (hypervolemic hypernatremia) can be seen in situations of iatrogenic administration of excessive quantities of sodium salts or in states of mineralocorticoid excess. The former condition can be seen shortly after a cardiac arrest when large quantities of intravenous sodium bicarbonate have been administered or following saline abortions. Primary hypersecretion of mineralocorticoids is also associated with modest increases in serum sodium concentration. It is likely that the minor degree of volume expansion seen with this state attenuates both AVP secretion and thirst such that there is a slight rise in serum sodium concentration. This phenomenon may be of clinical utility in distinguishing between primary and secondary hyperaldosteronism; in the former serum sodium is slightly elevated, and in the latter it is slightly decreased.

Occasionally, patients are seen who present with severe hypernatremia in the absence of any obvious disturbances in extracellular fluid volume (essential or normovolemic hypernatremia). The main defect in such patients appears to be in their sensation of thirst. Lacking a thirst drive, they have substantially reduced water intake and become hypernatremic. In most cases regulation of AVP secretion is also disturbed, although frank diabetes insipidus is not generally seen. In several well studied cases osmotic stimulation of AVP secretion seems to be selectively impaired with volume regulation remaining intact. As a consequence, whenever dehydration becomes sufficiently severe to activate the baroreceptors, the resultant rise in plasma AVP prevents further renal water losses. This phenomenon may have given rise to the impression that these patients had a "reset osmostat" for AVP secretion. This impression was based in part on the observation that dehydrated patients with this syndrome lowered their urine osmolality in response to water loading even though the plasma osmolality was still elevated above normal. Recently, careful determination of plasma levels of AVP and osmolality have been performed in patients with normovolemic hypernatremia under varying conditions of hydration. These studies showed that the hypernatremic patients have essentially the same "osmotic threshold" as normal subjects but they release substantially less AVP at any given level of osmolality. Polyuria is avoided, since the elevated levels of plasma osmolality result in sufficient osmotic stimulation to release AVP. In this setting renal concentrating ability is maintained at the expense of hyperosmolality. This could not occur in the usual patients with diabetes insipidus, since the elevated osmolality would stimulate thirst and the subsequent water ingestion would restore plasma osmolality to normal. The hypernatremic syndrome has been reproduced experimentally by lesions placed in the anteroventral third ventricular region in rats. This region appears to be of critical importance in integrating various stimuli for drinking behavior. Clinically, patients with this disorder may be asymptomatic or may present with episodic muscle weakness or paralysis. Chlorpropamide has been a uniquely effective therapy both by enhancing either the release or renal action of AVP and by an apparent direct effect on the hypothalamus to restore thirst and drinking behavior.

Hypernatremia can also be seen in the setting of severe volume depletion (hypovolemic hypernatremia). A relatively common cause of this picture is excessive nonrenal water loss under conditions of high ambient temperature. This syndrome may also be seen in elderly patients who become gradually dehydrated in a nursing home setting and are unable either to sense or to express their need for fluids.

Hypernatremia with volume depletion and adipsia may also have been seen as an acquired disorder in some patients with central nervous system disease. Serial observations of one such patient provide insight into the pathogenesis of this disorder. The patient initially presented with panhypopituitarism and central diabetes insipidus with polyuria but went on over a number of years to develop severe dehydration and oliguria associated with loss of the sensation of thirst. His urine osmolality measured during an episode of dehydration was hypertonic to plasma. It appeared that the patient had originally lost AVP secretion as the consequence of a pituitary tumor which had then extended to involve the thirst center, producing adipsia and hypernatremia. The absence of volume-stimulated AVP release probably contributed to the severity of his dehydration. The residual concentrating ability during dehydration may have been due to decreased renal blood flow with reduced distal delivery of filtrate or possibly to an effect of angiotensin on renal water handling. Although experience with this disorder is limited, some benefit has been obtained by treatment with exogenous AVP in the form of Pitressin and by forcing fluids.

REFERENCES

Andreoli TE, Grantham JJ, Rector F: Disturbances in Body Fluid Osmolality. Bethesda, American Physiological Society, 1977

Berl T, Anderson RJ, McDonald KM, et al: Clinical disorders of water metabolism. Kidney Int 10:117, 1976

Fichman MP, Michelakis AM, Horton R: Regulation of aldosterone in the syndrome of inappropriate antidiuretic hormone secretion (SIADH). J Clin Endocrinol Metab 39:136, 1974

Halter J, Goldberg AP, Robertson GL, et al: Selective osmoreceptor dysfunction in the syndrome of chronic hypernatremia. J Clin Endocrinol Metab 44:609, 1977

Hantman D, Rossier B, Zohlman R, et al: Rapid correction of hyponatremia in the syndrome of inappropriate secretion of antidiuretic hormone: An alternative treatment to hypertonic saline. Ann Intern Med 78:870, 1973

Miller M, Dalakos T, Moses AM, et al: Recognition of partial defects in antidiuretic hormone secretion. Ann Intern Med 73:721, 1970

Moses AM, Miller M: Drug induced dilutional hyponatremia. N Engl J Med 291:1234, 1974

Robertson G: The regulation of vasopressin function in health and disease. Recent Prog Horm Res 33:333, 1977

Robinson AG: Dd AVP in the treatment of central diabetes insipidus. N Engl J Med 294:507, 1976

Schrier RW, Berl T: Disorders of water metabolism, in Schrier RW (ed): Renal and Electrolyte Disorders. Boston, Little, Brown, 1976, p 1

Weitzman R: Current concepts on the factors regulating the secretion and metabolism of arginine vasopressin (antidiuretic hormone). Contemp Issues Nephrol (in press)

DISORDERS OF SODIUM METABOLISM

H. John Reineck

The maintenance of normal sodium balance is central to proper control of the extracellular fluid volume. Accordingly, disorders of sodium metabolism are manifested by alterations in volume homeostasis. Thus this chapter deals with those clinical conditions associated with abnormalities of volume regulation, i.e., edema formation and volume depletion. It should be pointed out that although these conditions may be accompanied by hypo- or hypernatremia, such disorders of tonicity are primarily due to abnormalities of the concentrating and diluting mechanisms, which are discussed in the preceding chapter.

EDEMATOUS STATES

Edema may be defined as the abnormal accumulation of fluid within the interstitial compartment. This phenomenon results from alterations of normal Starling's forces across capillary walls. Under normal circumstances mean capillary hydrostatic and oncotic pressure gradients along the length of the capillary circulation are in equilibrium and therefore no net interstitial accumulation of fluid occurs. In edematous states this equilibrium is upset, so that the mean oncotic pressure is insufficient to prevent the transcapillary movement of fluid caused by the hydrostatic pressure gradient between the intravascular and interstitial space. While edema may occur in anatomically localized areas, as occurs in lymphatic or venous obstruction or angioneurotic edema, this chapter deals only with generalized edema. This condition is associated with a variety of disorders which share a single common denominator, renal sodium retention.

CIRRHOSIS

Edema and ascites are prominent clinical findings in patients with hepatic cirrhosis, and by convention their presence defines "decompensated" cirrhosis. It should be pointed out, however, that a significant number of patients with so-called compensated cirrhosis, without edema or ascites, will exhibit impaired ability to excrete an administered salt load. Thus the terms compensated and decompensated, while abundant in the literature, are primarily descriptive and add little to our understanding of the pathogenesis of the salt retention which may accompany chronic liver disease.

Pathogenesis of Ascites Formation

Before discussing those factors which may be involved in mediating sodium retention in cirrhosis, it is appropriate to first confront the current controversy regarding the pathogenesis of ascites formation. As will be seen, this mechanism is central not only to understanding the etiology of sodium retention but also the formulation of a rational therapeutic approach to edema and ascites in cirrhotic patients.

Most authorities now agree that the basic pathophysiologic abnormality associated with ascites formation is an obstruction to hepatic venous outflow. Beyond this most fundamental understanding and despite decades of extensive research, controversy continues to surround our knowlege of the mechanism of ascites formation and its relationship to renal sodium retention. Fig. 1A schematically depicts the traditional theory of ascites accumulation. As hepatic parenchymal tissue is destroyed and replaced by fibrous scar, venous outflow becomes impaired and sinusoidal pressure increases. This process causes transudation of hepatic lymph into the peritoneal cavity. As portal hypertension develops, large collateral venous complexes form which "sequester" a large portion of the plasma volume. In addition, due to the high portal pressure, fluid transudation from splanchnic capillaries contributes further to ascites formation. These events lead to a reduction in "effective" or non splanchnic plasma volume which in turn causes renal salt retention. This traditional view is supported by several observations in cirrhotic patients. First, expansion of the extracellular or intravascular compartments by saline or dextran administration to patients with decompensated cirrhosis leads to increased sodium excretion. Second, neck-out water immersion, a maneuver known to increase central blood volume, leads to a natriuresis in cirrhotic patients which is quantitatively similar to that observed in normal subjects. Third, increased plasma renin activity is nearly universally observed in decompensated cirrhosis. If this parameter is a valid marker of "effective" plasma volume, this finding suggests that this elusive factor is decreased. In addition, the infusion of saralasin, a competetive inhibitor of angiotensin II, causes a marked fall in blood pressure in cirrhotics with ascites and edema, a finding similar to that seen in volume depleted normal subjects.

This traditional view of the pathogenesis of ascites formation has been recently challenged, however. Figure 1B depicts the "over-flow" theory, which may be summarized as follows. During the development of decompensated cirrhosis, renal sodium reabsorption is stimulated by mechanisms as yet unclear, resulting in expansion of the extracellular and intravascular fluid volumes. In the presence of increased hepatic sinusoidal pressure and obstructed hepatic venous outflow, this results in transudation of hepatic lymph and ascites formation. In the presence of portal hypertension the engorged splanchnic circulation also contributes to the ascites fluid.

Evidence favoring this "overflow" theory obtains from studies in cirrhotic patients and animal models of cirrhosis. First, measurements of plasma volume and cardiac output have consistently shown that these parameters are usually increased. Second, during spontaneous resolution of ascites, portal pressure does not fall. Third, the administration of mineralocorticoid to patients with portal hypertension and no ascites or

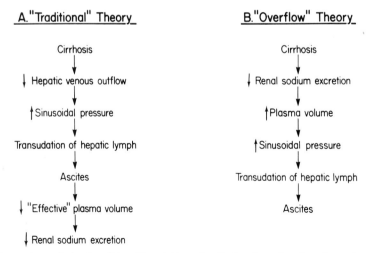

Fig 1. Comparison of the "traditional" and "overflow" theories of ascites formation in hepatic cirrhosis. [Adapted from Levinsky NG: Refractory ascites in cirrhosis. Kidney Int 14:93, 1978.]

edema fails to evoke the normal "escape" phenomenon (see the chapter on *Sodium Transport*) and results in edema and ascites. In dogs with chemically induced cirrhosis, Levy has demonstrated that renal sodium retention temporally precedes edema and acites formation. In addition, using radioisotope volume markers in conjunction with balance studies, Levy has found that in this model a significant portion of the retained salt and water remains in the nonsplanchnic circulation, indicating that "effective" or nonsplanchnic plasma volume is not diminished. Finally, Levy also has shown that after removal of ascitic fluid by paracentesis, reaccumulation of ascites is prevented by dietary sodium restriction.

Mechanism of Sodium Retention

Whether the afferent limb signaling sodium retention is a diminished "effective" plasma volume as is held by supporters of the traditional theory, or some as yet unidentified factor (or factors), as claimed by those favoring the overflow theory, has obvious importance to our understanding of the disordered sodium metabolism in cirrhosis. Of equal importance, however, is the nature of the efferent limb of this system, i.e., the mechanism by which the kidney retains sodium. While much progress has been made in this area, our knowlege remains incomplete.

Theoretically, sodium retention could result from either decreased glomerular filtration rate (GFR) or enhanced tubular reabsorption. Although most patients with decompensated cirrhosis have compromised GFR, it now seems clear that the most important abnormality is an increase in tubular reabsorption. The bulk of evidence, derived from clearance studies in cirrhotic patients, indicate that enhanced proximal reabsorption occurs. In addition, at least one study in man and micropuncture studies of animal models indicate that increased distal sodium reabsorption is also operative.

Hemodynamic Considerations

Total renal blood flow (RBF) is diminished in most patients with decompensated cirrhosis. Since GFR is usually similarly decreased, filtration fraction is often normal, yet since blood pressure is normal, the decrease in blood flow must represent increased renal resistance. If proximal reabsorption of sodium varies inversely with peritubular hydrostatic pressure (see the chapter on *Sodium Transport*) increase in vascular resistance would tend to enhance proximal reabsorption.

Although this explanation for salt retention in cirrhosis is highly speculative, current evidence suggests that renal vasoconstriction may be intimately involved in this phenomenon. Both systemic and intrarenal infusions of dopamine, a unique renal vasodilator substance, have been shown to result in a marked natriuresis in decompensated cirrhosis.

Redistribution of RBF to juxtamedullary structure has been reported in patients with cirrhosis. At the time of those studies, such a redistribution of RBF was thought to be associated with sodium retention. Sub-

sequently, the bulk of evidence tends to refute that hypothesis. Therefore it seems unlikely that these observations bear on the mechanism of increased sodium reabsorption.

Humoral Factors

Elevated plasma *aldosterone* levels have been repeatedly demonstrated in cirrhotic subjects with edema and ascites, and this increase is clearly due to increased adrenal secretion as well as decreased hepatic clearance. In addition, enhanced tubular sensitivity to the hormone has been reported. In view of its sodium retaining properties, an important role for aldosterone in the sodium retention of cirrhosis has been widely suggested. Multiple observations tend to refute this commonly accepted concept, however. First, the administration of spironolactone, a competitive inhibitor of aldosterone, produces at best a very mild natriuresis in these patients. Second, aminoglulethamide, which causes a marked fall in aldosterone levels, fails to increase urinary sodium excretion. Third, a recent report shows that in a significant number of cirrhotic patients ingestion of a high-salt diet resulted in suppression of aldosterone levels, but marked sodium retention still occurred. Fourth, water immersion stimulates sodium excretion despite the administration of exogenous DOCA. This last observation also indicates that if the stimulus to sodium retention is a diminished "effective" plasma volume, the sodium retention is not mediated by aldosterone. From these data it seems clear that this hormone is not the primary cause of salt retention in decompensated cirrhosis.

Estrogens have been demonstrated to exert significant sodium retention in normal man, and this effect is even greater in patients with cirrhosis, ascites, and edema. The finding that plasma estradiol and urinary estrogen excretion are elevated in cirrhotic individuals leads to speculation that this steroid hormone may mediate, at least in part, avid sodium reabsorption. Although to date no data refute this possibility, further study is required to confirm this relationship and define the relative importance, if any, of this mechanism.

The existence of a *"natriuretic hormone"* has been postulated by a large number of investigators to explain the natriuretic response to volume expansion in both man and animals. If such a substance indeed exists, the absence of this hormone could be, and has been, implicated in the salt retention of edematous states, including decompensated cirrhosis. To date, however, despite intensive efforts, isolation and identification of a "natriuretic hormone" have remained elusive. Since the very existence of this hormone remains in doubt, it seems premature at this time to attribute sodium retention to its absence.

Renal Nerves

Renal sympathetic nerve activaly has been implicated as playing a role in urinary sodium excretion (see the chapter on *Sodium Transport*). Further, renal nerve stimulation has been demonstrated to increase proximal sodium reabsorption, even in the absence of detectable hemodynamic alterations. It is therefore conceivable that enhanced adrenergic activity could mediate sodium retention in cirrhosis. At the present time, however, most evidence denies such a role.

Treatment of Decompensated Cirrhosis

As pointed out earlier in this chapter, the mechanism of ascites formation has important implications in its treatment. If the "over-flow" theory is correct, one might expect that early prevention of salt retention may also prevent the development of ascites. Likewise, reducing extracellular fluid volume should reduce its accumulation, and paracentesis should not result in volume depletion. On the other hand, if the more "traditional" theory is correct, diuretic therapy and/or paracentesis are fraught with hazard, since salt retention is a physiologic (and necessary) response to progressive liver disease which attempts to maintain a normal "effective" plasma volume. Thus until the issue of the mechanism of ascites formation is settled, therapeutic principals remain controversial and are currently based on empiric observations.

In this regard several principles should be kept in mind. First, the occurrence of ascites and edema in cirrhosis must be viewed as a sign of disease rather than a disease per se. Thus in the absence of respiratory embarassment from tense ascites and dermatologic complications of profound edema the stimulus to treat these signs is often primarily cosmetic. Second, the over zealous use of diuretics can precipitate a variety of complications. These include hyponatremia and hepatic encephalopathy, from hypokalemia and/or metabolic alkalosis, and, most significantly, "hepatorenal syndrome" (see the chapter on *Hepatorenal Syndrome*). Third, while peripheral edema may be mobilized from the interstitial to intravascular compartment at a virtually unlimited rate, the mobilization of ascites is quite finite. Studies addressing this point indicate that the maxium mobilization rate of ascites fluid is about 900 ml/day and in most patients is closer to 500 ml/day. Thus in cirrhotic patients with ascites and no peripheral edema, a weight loss of approximately 0.5–1 kg day is optimum.

Finally, some mention of the Le Veen shunt is in order. This unique device, which requires surgical intervention, removes ascitic fluid and returns it to the intravascular space via a peritoneal–jugular catheter. This procedure has been reported to result in resolution of ascites and in some cases improvement in GFR and normalization of renal sodium handling. While these reports are encouraging, experience with this intervention is still insufficient to allow its general recommendation.

HEART FAILURE

As in the case of cirrhosis, renal sodium retention often plays a prominent role in the clinical presentation of patients with heart failure. Historically, our understanding of the pathophysiology of edema formation is quite analogous to the current controversy surrounding ascites formation in cirrhosis. In the early 19th century, the "backward failure" theory was elaborated, stating that as a result of increased right atrial pressure, peripheral venous pressure also rose and resulted in transudation of fluid from the vascular to interstitial space. This loss of vascular volume triggered sodium retention in an attempt to restore vascular volume. In the first half of this century, the "forward failure" theory developed and held that as a result of some hemodynamic alterations renal sodium retention occurs, expanding the extracellular fluid volume. This expansion leads to change in Starling's forces across the microcirculation, resulting in edema. Measurements of plasma volume in patients with heart failure and edema indicate that this parameter is uniformly elevated. Thus although, as will be discussed below, elevated central venous pressure may be an important stimulus to renal sodium retention, it now seems clear that this enhanced sodium reabsorption is of primary importance in the pathogenesis of edema formation.

Before discussing the mechanisms of sodium retention in heart failure, it is appropriate to briefly address our current teleologic concept of this phenomenon. Figure 2 depicts the Frank-Starling relationship between cardiac output and left ventricular end-diastolic volume (LVEDV). Curve A represents this relationship in the normal heart and curve B that in the failing myocardium. It should be noted that in both situations a direct curvilinear relationship exists between cardiac output and LVEDV, but that at any given LVEDV the cardiac output is less in the failing than in the normal heart. Since LVEDV is largely determined by venous return and hence plasma volume, it is readily evident that one mechanism by which cardiac output can be "normalized" in the diseased heart is by increasing plasma volume and LVEDV. It is thus apparent that renal retention of sodium in heart failure is much more than an interesting and sometimes bothersome problem, rather representing a physiologic phenomenon by which the organism attempts to maintain cardiac output and thereby adequate tissue perfusion.

Mechanism of Sodium Retention

Afferent mechanism. The nature of afferent limb—i.e. sensing mechanism which signals the retention of sodium—is unclear, but several interesting observations shed some light on this issue.

Central venous pressure has been postulated as the afferent component of sodium retension in heart failure. This postulate is primarily based on observations published in 1956 by Hollander and Judson. These investigators compared two groups of patients with comparably severe heart disease, as judged by cardiac index, oxygen consumption, and pulmonary artery pressures; one group with peripheral edema demonstrated marked sodium retention, and the other, without edema, excreted administered sodium normally. The only parameter to differ significantly between these groups was the right ventricular end-diastolic pressure, which was greater in the former group of patients. The validity of the conclusion from this study is made somewhat suspect by the more recent finding that a significant number of patients with heart failure, normal venous pressure, and no edema or demonstrable sodium retention have an expanded plasma volume and increased total body sodium content, indicating that they have previously retained sodium and are now operating "normally" but with a "re-set volustat". In addition, normal individuals demonstrate an inverse relationship between central venous pressure and sodium excretion, as witnessed by the increase in urinary sodium excretion that accompanies the assumption of a supine position or during the maneuver of water immersion. Thus it seems possible the increase in right ventricular end-diastolic volume noted in salt-retaining edematous patients may have been a result of sodium retention rather than a cause.

Cardiac output was first proposed as an afferent mechanism for renal sodium retention along with the theory of "forward" heart failure. This mechanism may indeed be operative in many patients, but it certainly cannot account for edema formation in all instances, since a number of conditions (arteriovenous fistulae, thyrotoxicosis, anemia) are associated with heart failure, edema, and high cardiac output. In addition, as mentioned above, measurement of cardiac output fails to differentiate edematous patients with heart failure and those without evidence of sodium retention.

Volume receptors in the arterial side of the circulation have long been recognized as important determinants of antidiuretic hormone secretion. By analogy, it has been postulated that these same receptors (or some as yet unidentified receptor) may be functioning to signal renal sodium retention. Such a possibility gained support from elegant studies in patients with large arteriovenous fistulae. Acute closure of these fistulae results in a prompt increase in sodium excretion. Since AV fistulae result in an increased rate of arterial emptying into the venous circulation and thereby a low diastolic blood pressure, these observations were suggestive of an arterial baroreceptor. In thyrotoxicosis and anemia, a relative or absolute deficiency in tissue oxygen delivery is present. This finding is consistent with the existence of some chemoreceptor acting in the afferent system. Further, an enhanced AV oxygen difference is observed in virtually all cases of heart failure, regardless of high or low cardiac output. Unfortunately, efforts to locate and identify either a chemoreceptor or baroreceptor that functions in the afferent limb of sodium metabolism have been, to date, unsuccessful.

Efferent mechanisms. *Hemodynamic alterations* are currently thought to play an important role in the efferent limb of sodium retention in heart failure. Measurements of RBF and GFR in this condition consistently demonstrate that the former is reduced proportionately greater than the latter parameter, resulting in an increased filtration fraction (FF). As discussed in the chapter on *Sodium Transport,* this ratio of GFR:RBF

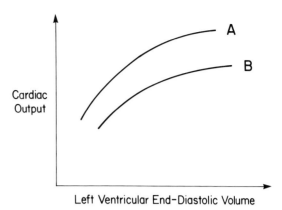

Fig 2. Frank-Starling relationship between cardiac output and left ventricular end-diastolic volume. A direct curvilinear relationship exists bwtween these parameters in both the normal (curve A) and failing myocardium (curve B). [Adapted from Humes HD, Gottlieb MN, Brenner BM: The kidney in congestive heart failure, in Brenner BM, Stein JH (eds): Sodium and Water Homeostasis. New York, Edinburgh, London, Churchill Livingstone, 1978.]

is thought to be an important determinant of proximal sodium reabsorption. Indeed, clearance studies in man and micropuncture data in animal models indicate that proximal reabsorption is enhanced in heart failure. These considerations lend support to the concept that an increase in FF and its attendant increase in peritubular capillary oncotic pressure and reduction in peritubular hydrostatic pressure mediate, at least in part, the sodium retention in heart failure.

In addition, however, it should be pointed out that studies in various models of this condition (i.e., AV fistulae, chronic thoracic vena cava obstruction, and pericarditis) indicate that loop of Henle sodium reabsorption is also increased. These findings are nor surprising in view of the inverse relationship observed between renal perfusion pressure and reabsorption along this segment (see the chapter on *Sodium Transport*).

The direct effector of the changes in renal hemodynamics in heart failure is not clear. Multiples studies indicate that *renin* release and *angiotensin II* formation are increased in this condition. Further, recent studies using an angiotensin antagonist, saralasin, and an angiotensin converting enzyme inhibitor indicate that the renin–angiotensin system may mediate the renal hemodynamic alterations and thereby the sodium retention in heart failure. At odds with this view is the observation in some patients with heart failure and sodium retention that a high-salt diet suppresses plasma renin activity while avid sodium reabsorption continues. Increased *renal nerve activity* has also been postulated to explain the hemodynamic abnormalities in heart failure. This postulate is largely based on the natriuretic response to alpha adrenergic blockage in patients with heart failure. On the other hand, high spinal anesthesia has failed to improve the decreased RBF in such patients. Thus while hemodynamic abnormalities probably are responsible for at least a portion of sodium retention in heart failure, the factors responsible for these changes remain controversial. In this regard, it should be pointed out that other vasoactive substances, including renal prostaglandins and the kinin system, may be involved, but further study will be required to define their role, if any.

Redistribution of renal blood flow to deep nephrons has been put forward as a possible determinant of sodium retention in heart failure, as in liver disease. Currently, the bulk of evidence denies that redistribution occurs in heart failure. Further, as pointed out in the chapter on *Sodium Transport,* whether this phenomonon has any role in determining urinary sodium excretion is now doubtful.

Aldosterone secretion rate is increased in most patients with heart failure; however, an important role of this hormone in sodium retention is suspect. This statement is based on the following observations: First, adrenalectomy and cortisone replacement fails to blunt the salt retention noted in dogs with pulmonic stenosis. Second, the administration of spironolactone to patients results in only a trivial increase in sodium excretion. Third, patients with heart failure fail to "escape" from exogenous mineralocorticoid administration, indicating that other factors must be operative. Fourth, plasma aldosterone levels may fall to normal levels in response to a high-salt diet, yet sodium retention persists.

Treatment of Heart Failure

In the preceding section on liver disease, it was pointed out that sodium retention in that condition demands treatment only rarely. In heart failure, however, a significant consequence of sodium retention is pulmonary congestion, which can result in life-threatening hypoxemia and which therefore constitutes a complication of major importance. As is the case with most medical problems, therapy should be aimed at correcting the underlying disease. Thus in heart failure improving myocardial contractility with digitalis remains the therapeutic cornerstone. In the past decade considerable data have accumulated indicating that reducing left ventricular afterload (systemic peripheral resistance) by administration of vasodilator drugs, such as nitroprusside, can also improve myocardial performance.

Diuretic therapy is, of course, also commonly employed. In patients with mild edema, thiazide diuretics are often sufficient. In patients with more severe salt retention, loop acting diuretics, i.e., furosemide or ethacrynic acid, are particularly effective. It should be pointed out that both of these agents are potent venodilators, a quality which facilitates their effectiveness in the treatment of pulmonary edema. Recent reports indicate that in patients with refractory failure, the diuretic response to loop diuretics can be markedly improved by the concomitant administration of vasodilators such as nitroprusside. Spironolactone and triamterene, potassium sparing diuretics, are of little efficacy alone, and their major role is in avoiding the hypokalemia which may accompany the thiazide and loop diuretics.

Finally, a word of caution regarding diuretic use in heart failure is appropriate. From Fig. 2, one will recall that a direct relationship exists between LVEDV and cardiac output. Thus excessive diuresis, while diminishing edema, may also decrease cardiac output and subsequently tissue perfusion and oxygenation.

NEPHROTIC SYNDROME

Edema is a cardinal feature of the nephrotic syndrome which results ultimately from the altered glomerular permeability to albumin. The pathogenesis of edema formation in this condition differs markedly from that described in decompensated cirrhosis and heart failure. This primary difference centers on the fact that in the previously discussed entities plasma volume is expanded and edema formation is generally held to result from renal sodium retention. In the nephrotic syndrome, our current understanding, based on measurements describing a contracted plasma volume, holds that renal sodium retention results from edema formation. According to this scheme hypoalbuminemia and its resultant diminished plasma oncotic pressure lead to transudation of fluid from the intravascular to the interstitial space, i.e., edema formation. This loss of plasma volume then constitutes the *afferent* signal for renal sodium retention, a phenomenon which can be viewed as a compensatory homeostatic mechanism to replenish plasma volume.

The *efferent* mechanism by which the kidney retains sodium is poorly understood. *GFR* is often reduced in nephrotic patients, particularly those with glomerulonephritis and diabetes, and may contribute to sodium retention in these entities. In patients with so-called lipoid nephrosis, however, GFR is often normal or even increased (presumably due to the decreased glomerular capillary oncotic pressure opposing filtration), and therefore enhanced tubular reabsorption of sodium must again be considered the primary cause of sodium retention.

The mechanism of increased tubular reabsorption apparently differs, at least in part, from those discussed in the preceding sections on cirrhosis and heart failure, conditions in which proximal reabsorption is increased. Clearance studies in man and micropuncture studies in animal models indicate that the proximal reabsorption is normal or even decreased. This observation is best explained by the hypoalbuminemia which despite an increased filtration fraction results in a normal or low peritubular oncotic pressure. Thus distal nephron sites must be responsible for the avid sodium retention in the nephrotic syndrome. The responsible mechanisms, however, are unclear. As mentioned earlier, *hemodynamic alterations* may affect loop of Henle reabsorption; however, a decrease in postglomerular perfusion pressure which might explain increased sodium reabsorption by this segment is, at present, conjectural.

Aldosterone, which clearly affects distal sodium reabsorption and is elevated in both plasma and urine in the nephrotic syndrome, may account, at least in part, for the enhanced distal reabsorption. Clinically, however, the use of spironolactone, an aldosterone antagonist, results in only a small increase in sodium excretion. In addition, sodium retention in the face of suppressed plasma aldosterone has recently been reported. The degree to which mineralocorticoids contribute to distal sodium retention in the nephrotic syndrome remains unknown. The possibility that some as yet unidentified *"natriuretic hormone"* may be decreased or ineffective in the nephrotic syndrome remains an unproven but possible explanation. In this regard the extensive work by Bricker and his colleagues postulating a distally acting hormone may be pertinent (see the chapter on *Chronic Renal Failure— Pathophysiology*). Finally, no data examining the possible role of other factors postulated to affect distal sodium transport (e.g., prostaglandins, medullary blood flow) are available.

Treatment

From the above discussion it is apparent that the accumulation of edema is a secondary phenomenon in the nephrotic syndrome resulting from the altered glomerular permeability to albumin and the subsequent hypoalbuminemia. Thus the ideal treatment of this syndrome would be correction of the urinary albumin excretion. Unfortunately, only in lipoid nephrosis is such treatment consistently effective. Further, since administered albumin is rapidly excreted, this mode of therapy is ineffective. Therefore dietary sodium restriction and diuretic therapy provide our only useful therapeutic modalities in most patients with this disorder.

For dietary sodium restriction alone to be effective requires that sodium intake be less than urinary sodium excretion, a very low figure indeed. Such a diet is difficult to prepare and quite unpalatable. Therefore diuretics,which increase sodium excretion are often employed. It cannot be overemphasized that edema per se is generally not harmful; therefore the benefits of diuretic use must be weighed against potential complications. In that regard, one must recall that renal sodium retention in the nephrotic syndrome represents a compensatory mechanism which restores plasma volume. Therefore rapid and massive diuresis may result in hypovolemia, hypotension, and pre-renal azotemia. When superimposed on an already compromised GFR (as in patients with glomerulonephritis or diabetic nephropathy) these complications may be disastrous. On the other hand, it should be pointed out that when diuretics are judiciously and cautiously used, the loss of salt and water transiently concentrates plasma proteins, mobilizes fluid from the interstitial to the intravascular space, and maintains plasma volume.

The choice of diuretic agents is largely empiric. In general, thiazide diuretics are tried initially, if ineffective, more potent loop acting agents—furosemide or ethacrynic acid—may be tried. Spironolactone or triam-terene alone are usually not effective and their use is primarily adjunctive, potentiating the diuretic effect of more proximally acting agents or avoiding the potassium depletion which may occur with loop acting or thiazide preparations. This latter phenomenon may be particularly prominent in patients receiving high-dose steroids. Finally, it should be cautioned that the potassium sparing agents should be avoided in patients with significant renal insufficiency, since sudden and life-threatening hyperkalemia may develop.

IDIOPATHIC EDEMA

Idiopathic edema is a disease occurring exclusively in women characterized by renal sodium retention and edema formation in the absence of cardiac, hepatic, or renal disease. Although the disease may be cyclic, with edema-free periods of normal sodium balance, many women with this condition chronically retain sodium, requiring constant dietary sodium restriction and/or diuretic therapy. The pathophysiology of idiopathic edema, as its name implies, is unknown. Because no animal model of the disease is available, thorough investigation of the problem is difficult. Nevertheless, several interesting observations have recently been made and deserve consideration here.

Afferent Mechanisms

Several groups of investigators have described possible afferent mechanisms which signal the need for renal sodium retention. In virtually all of these proposals, an absolute or relative decrease in plasma volume is postulated. *Hypoalbuminemia,* possibly due to altered peripheral capillary permeability to protein, has been reported in these patients. The bulk of data, however, suggests that hypoalbuminemia is quite rare in this condition. Because the disease occurs exclusively in females and generally in premenopausal women, *estrogen* has been postulated to play an important role in the sodium retention. Since the hormone is capable of causing vasodilatation, the vascular holding capacity could conceivably be increased out of proportion to plasma volume. Such circumstances would result in an ''ineffective'' plasma volume, and sodium retention would result in an effort to ''refill'' the intravascular space. Indeed, elevated estrogen levels have been reported in women with idiopathic edema, but normal values have also been cited. It is possible, of course, that increased vascular sensitivity to estrogen exists, explaining the observed normal values reported. *Excessive orthostatic pooling* of blood during upright posture has been described in some women with idiopathic edema, yet since sodium retention is noted in other patients remaining supine, this explanation probably cannot explain the syndrome in all patients. It is possible also that more than one afferent mechanism exists and that we are dealing with more than a single entity.

As attractive as these postulates appear, a recent study casts grave doubt on a role for any of these mechanisms in the afferent limb in idiopathic edema. In that study, plasma renin and aldosterone levels were observed to be normal prior to salt loading and to suppress normally in response to a high-sodium diet. If plasma renin is accepted as a marker of "effective" plasma volume, it appears unlikely that alterations in this rather nebulous factor is involved.

Efferent Mechanisms

Since GFR is normal in idiopathic edema, enhanced tubular reabsorption must be the cause of sodium retention. Measurements of RBF have shown this parameter to also be normal. In view of the normal systemic blood pressure in these patients, it follows that renal resistance must also be normal. These observations therefore make it unlikely that *hemodynamic factors* play an important efferent role in renal sodium retention. It should be pointed out, however, that these findings do not preclude distributional changes in GFR or RBF from contributing to the abnormality. As in other edematous states, *aldosterone* has received considerable attention as the mediator of renal sodium retention. Conflicting data exist regarding its role in idiopathic edema, levels being reported as elevated in some studies and normal to low in others. The lack of hypokalemia, hypertension, and the poor therapeutic response to the aldosterone antagonist spironolactone make a primary role of this hormone unlikely. *Estrogen* has been shown to elicit renal sodium retention by a direct effect at the level of the renal tubule. As noted above, however, data concerning estrogen levels in this disease are also conflicting. Finally, it is possible that *renal sympathetic nerve activity* is increased in idiopathic edema. No available data shed light on this possibility, however.

Treatment

Dietary sodium restriction and diuretic therapy usually are effective in controlling symptomatic edema in this disease. Low to moderate doses of thiazide diuretics are generally sufficient.

SODIUM DEPLETED STATES

Sodium depletion represents the antithesis of edematous states and by virtue of sodium's central role in determining extracellular volume is invariably associated with contraction of this fluid compartment. The clinical findings in this condition are often dramatic and consist of orthostatic hypotension and tachycardia, decreased jugular venous pressure, dry mucous membranes, poor skin turgor, and in severe cases sunken eyes and intense vasoconstriction. Patient's symptoms are often less specific and include enhanced thirst, muscle cramps and weakness, headache, and lassitude. Because plasma volume is a vital component of the extracellular fluid volume, profound sodium depletion may lead to vascular collapse and shock. In addition, it should be stressed that in patients with underlying renal insufficiency, sodium depletion may lead to dramatic worsening of renal function and precipitate frank uremia.

Laboratory findings, while not pathognomic, often aid in detecting less dramatic degrees of volume deple-

tion. An elevation in hemoglobin concentration (hemoconcentration), a disproportionate increase in blood urea nitrogen compared to serum creatinine, and elevated plasma renin activity are common findings. It should be stressed that serum sodium concentration bears no relationship to extracellular fluid volume and may be high, low, or normal depending on concomitant water balance (see the chapter on *Aldosterone*).

The causes of sodium depletion are extensive and may be divided into those due to extrarenal sodium loss and those due to excessive urinary excretion of sodium. In general, these two catagories may be readily differentiated by urinary sodium determination. When sodium depletion occurs from extrarenal losses, renal sodium retention occurs and urine sodium concentration is usually less than 10 mEq/liter. Values greater than 20 mEq/liter are indicative of renal causes. The clinician should be aware of one very important exception to this rule. In cases of metabolic alkalosis of nonrenal cause, particularly when severe or during its generation, urinary sodium concentrations may be quite high. In this setting urinary chloride concentrations will accurately separate renal and extrarenal causes of volume depletion (see the chapter on *Disorders of Acid–Base Metabolism*).

Causes of Sodium Depletion

Since this chapter deals with "disorders of sodium metabolism," nonrenal causes of sodium depletion will not be discussed. Renal causes of excessive sodium losses are listed in Table 1.

Causes extrinsic to the kidney. Solute diuresis. Endogenous substances such as urea and glucose are capable of causing an osmotic diuresis and natriuresis when large loads of these substances are filtered. Since endogenous urea accumulates as a result of renal insufficiency, this phenomenon probably seldom causes significant sodium depletion except, as discussed below, as a component of the diuretic phase of acute renal failure and post-obstructive diuresis. Glucose induced osmotic diuresis, on the other hand, is a common cause of the profound volume deficits which may accompany diabetic ketoacidosis or hyperglycemic nonketotic coma.

A variety of exogenously administered substances,

Table 1
Renal Causes of Sodium Depletion

Causes due to factors extrinsic to the kidney
    Solute diuresis —endogenous, exogenous
    Diuretics
    Mineralocorticoid deficiency

Causes due to factors intrinsic to the kidney
    Chronic renal failure
    Salt-wasting renal diseases
    Postobstructive renal disease
    Nonoliguric acute renal failure
    Diuretic phase of acute renal failure

including urea, mannitol, and x-ray contrast media, may cause significant increases in urinary sodium excretion by their action as osmotic diuretics. Additionally, administration of salts of poorly reabsorbable anions may increase sodium excretion. Bicarbonate and sulfate salts are common examples of such substances.

Diuretics. Virtually all diuretic agents increase urinary sodium excretion by varying degrees, and excessive use of these drugs, particularly potent loop acting diuretics, may result in significant sodium depletion. It should be pointed out that the use of urinary sodium concentration to distinguish renal and nonrenal causes of sodium depletion may be difficult to interpret under these circumstances. In that regard, knowledge of the duration of action of commonly employed diuretics is helpful (Table 2).

Aldosterone deficiency. Although the relative importance of aldosterone in edematous states and its role in normal sodium metabolism are unclear, it is well established that the absence of this hormone results in renal sodium wasting. Three general categories of aldosterone deficiency have been documented. First, primary adrenal insufficiency (Addison's disease) is associated with a variety of diseases, including pernicious anemia, thyroiditis, diabetes mellitus, and granulomatous processes. Because glucocorticoid deficiency also exists with this entity, hyperpigmentation and hypoglycemia are often prominent findings. Second, hypoaldosteronism due to enzyme deficiencies is now well characterized. Virilizing congenital adrenogenital syndrome, a deficiency in 21-hydroxylase, results in a shunting of steroid precursors from the mineralocorticoid pathway to androgen production. In addition, other sporadic and rare enzyme deficiencies have also been reported. Chronic heparin therapy has also been reported to result in isolated hypoaldosteronism. The third category of aldosterone deficiency is termed "hyporeninemic hypoaldosteronism" (see the following chapter). Although the exact nature of this entity is not well established, it is hypothesized to result from a deficiency in renin production. It should be pointed out that this phenomenon occurs almost exclusively in patients with moderate renal insufficiency, and volume depletion is rarely a prominent manifestation. Rather, hyperkalemia and hyperchloremic acidosis usually bring this entity to the physician's attention.

Causes intrinsic to the kidney. If dietary sodium is abruptly decreased in patients with *chronic renal insufficiency* of virtually any cause, urinary sodium excretion does not similarly decrease. Thus chronic renal failure, strictly speaking, is associated with salt wasting. It should be stressed that this phenomenon is rarely of clinical importance, possibly because, as recently observed, in the face of prolonged salt restriction sodium balance is restored.

This phenomenon of "salt wasting" with chronic renal failure should be distinguished from that observed in some patients with *interstitial renal disease.* Such

Table 2
Duration of Action of Commonly Used Diuretics

Diuretic		Duration
Acetazolamide		6–8 hours
Furosemide	Oral:	6 hours
	i.v.:	2 hours
Ethacrynic acid	Oral:	6–8 hours
	i.v.	3 hours
Thiazides		
Chlorothiazide		6–12 hours
Hydrochlorothiazide		12–18 hours
Chlorthalidone		24 hours
Trichlormethiazide		24 hours
Triamterene		12–16 hours
Spironolactone		2–3 days

patients, particularly those with medullary cystic disease, may demonstrate negative sodium balance in the presence of normal dietary sodium intake. As a result, volume depletion may be a prominent clinical problem in such patients. Renal salt wasting may also occur following relief of urinary tract obstruction (*postobstructive diuresis*), during the *diuretic phase of acute renal failure,* and occasionally during the course of *nonoliguric acute renal failure.* It should be stressed that while true salt wasting may occur in these settings, the liberal administration of sodium may result in increased urinary sodium excretion. Hence it is important to determine that the "salt wasting" is not, in fact, an appropriate renal response to sodium administration.

Treatment

The treatment of sodium depletion obviously requires restoration of the extracellular fluid volume. Such restoration is best accomplished by sodium chloride administration, since anions other than chloride are less well reabsorbed by the renal tubule. The amount of sodium chloride to be administered depends upon the degree of volume depletion. If weight before volume depletion is known, this parameter provides a valid index of fluid needs (1 liter/kg weight loss). In the absence of hemorrhage or hemolysis, the degree of hemoconcentration (i.e., percentage rise in hemoglobin concentration) should proportionately reflect the percentage loss of extracellular fluid volume. Finally, the tonicity of the fluid replacement will be largely dependent on the serum sodium concentrations prior to initiating therapy. In the presence of severe volume depletion, however, isotonic saline is preferable, even in the presence of hypertonic body fluids, since correction of tonicity is less important in this setting.

REFERENCES

Anderson RJ, Linas SL: Sodium depletion states, in Brenner BM, Stein JH (eds): Sodium and Water Hemeostasis. New York, Edinburgh, London, Churchill Livingstone, 1978, p 154

Chonko AM, Bay WH, Stein JH, et al: The role of renin and

aldosterone in the salt retention of edema. Am J Med 63:881, 1977

Epstein FH, Post RS, McDowell M: Effects of an arteriovenous fistula on renal hemodynamics and electrolyte excretion. J Clin Invest 32:233, 1953

Epstein M: Renal sodium handling in cirrhosis, Epstein M (ed): in The Kidney in Liver Disease. New York, Elsevier North-Holland, 1978, p 35

Ferris TF, Bay WH: Idiopathic edema, in Brenner BM, Stein JH (eds): Sodium and Water Hemeostasis. New York, Edinburgh, London, Churchill Livingstone, 1978, p 131

Hollenberg W, Judson WE: The relationship of cardiovascular and renal hemodynamic function to sodium excretion in patients with severe heart disease but without edema. J Clin Invest 35:970, 1956

Humes HD, Gottlieb MN, Brenner BM: The kidney in congestive heart failure, in Brenner BM, Stein JH (eds): Sodium and Water Homeostatis. New York, Edinburgh, London, Churchill Livingstone, 1978 p 51

Levinsky NG: Refractory ascites in cirrhosis. Kidney Int 14:93, 1978

Levy M: The kidney in liver disease, in Brenner BM, Stein JH(eds): Sodium and Water Homeostasis. New York, Edinburgh, London, Churchill Livingstone, 1978, p 73

Lieberman FL, Dennison EK, Reynolds TB: The relationship of plasma volume, portal hypertension, ascites and renal sodium retention in cirrhosis; The overflow theory of ascites formation. Ann NY Acad Sci 170:202, 1970

CLINICAL DISORDERS OF POTASSIUM METABOLISM

Robert T. Kunau, Jr., and Jay H. Stein

HYPOKALEMIA

Table 1 lists those disorders which can be associated with hypokalemia. These disorders are generally divided into categories wherein hypokalemia results from inadequate intake, excessive losses either through the gastrointestinal tract or the kidneys, or through a shift of potassium from the extracellular to the intracellular compartment. It should also be recognized that more than one mechanism may be involved in a number of the disorders.

Inadequate Potassium Intake

A poor dietary intake is rarely, if ever, the only cause for potassium depletion, but it may be a contributing factor in those patients who are experiencing potassium loss for other reasons.

Gastrointestinal Loss of Potassium

Vomiting. Vomiting not infrequently results in hypokalemia; however, it is not the loss of potassium in the vomitus which is responsible, since the potassium concentration in gastric juice rarely exceeds 10 mEq/liter; rather, the major cause of hypokalemia in this setting appears to result from the associated metabolic alkalosis increasing renal potassium excretion and shifting potassium.

Diarrhea. In the colon, water and sodium are reabsorbed and potassium is secreted. As a result, the potassium concentration in the stool water is usually higher than that of sodium. Although the potassium concentration decreases as the stool volume increases during diarrhea, the potassium loss in the stool in diarrheal states is roughly proportional to the stool volume.

A villous adenoma of the colon can induce profound potassium depletion, perhaps, in part, because of an alteration in colonic permeability by some substance produced by the adenoma.

Chronic laxative abuse is known to cause hypokalemia. These patients may have a number of psychological problems and may deny laxative use.

Renal Loss of Potassium

Diuretics. Hypokalemia is not infrequently cited as a complication of diuretic therapy. Several mechanisms seem to be involved—(1) an increase in distal tubular flow rate; (2) impairment of potassium reabsorption in the thick ascending limb in the case of ethacrynic acid and furosemide; and (3) an increase in bicarbonate delivery to the distal nephron, thereby altering the intraluminal pH or the transepithelial potential difference.

Despite what appears to be a favorable environment for the development of hypokalemia, frequently the degree of potassium deficiency seen in patients on diuretic therapy is very modest. Presumably, this can be attributed to a diuretic-induced decrease in the extracellular fluid volume which may result in a diminution in filtrate delivery to distal potassium secretory sites. Further, any fall in the serum potassium would tend to counterbalance any effect of volume depletion to enhance aldosterone production. Finally, the diuretic-induced volume depletion may enhance potassium reabsorption in the collecting duct.

Because the need for potassium supplementation may be extremely variable, it seems inappropriate to arbitrarily provide all patients on diuretic therapy with potassium supplements; however, in the digitalized patient or those patients with decreased intake, with primary or secondary aldosteronism, or undergoing a profound diuresis, potassium supplementation may be appropriate.

Mineralocorticoid excess. Primary aldosteronism. The clinical syndrome seen with increased production of aldosterone, i.e., hypertension, suppression of plasma renin activity, hypokalemia, and metabolic alkalosis, is frequently the result of an isolated adrenal adenoma, the removal of which usually reverses these abnormalities. In those patients in whom bilateral adrenal hyperplasia rather than an adenoma is the cause of the increase in aldosterone production, the patients tend to have lower aldosterone levels, higher peripheral vein renin activity, and less alteration of the serum bicarbonate and potassium values. As surgery in these latter patients may not be beneficial in relieving the hypertension, differentiation of this condition from that due to an adenoma is critical.

Hyperaldosteronism may also be seen in two other conditions. A group of patients has been described with increased aldosterone excretion but without a consistent suppression of the plasma renin in whom desoxycorticosterone readily decreased the level of aldosterone excretion. Hypokalemia was infrequent in these patients. Second, two patients with hypertension, hypokalemia, intermittent elevations in urinary 17-keto- and hydroxysteroids, and increased secretion of 18-hydroxycorticosterone have been reported. These abnormalities disappeared with glucocorticoid administration.

Cushing's syndrome. Cushing's syndrome is not infrequently the cause of hypokalemia, although the cause is not readily apparent. Aldosterone secretory rates may be normal; however, the hypokalemia may be related, in part, to the mineralocorticoid effect of cortisol or possibly to an increase in the secretion of other mineralocorticoids.

Numerous neoplasms produce an ACTH-like substance which may lead to excessive production of cortisone, desoxycorticosterone, and corticosterone and a clinical picture of Cushing's syndrome. The hypokalemia in these patients may be quite severe. Diagnosis depends upon demonstration of the primary tumor.

Accelerated hypertension and renal artery stenosis. Hypokalemia may be seen in patients with accelerated hypertension even in the presence of significant renal functional impairment and has been reported in approximately 15 percent of patients with renal artery stenosis. Hyperaldosteronism and an increase in filtrate delivery to distal parts of the nephron as a consequence of the hypertension are possible contributing factors to the development of the hypokalemia.

Renin producing tumors. Renin producing tumors of the kidney, the so-called Robertson-Kihara syndrome, have been associated with hypertension, hypokalemia, hyperaldosteronism, and unilateral elevations of the renal venous renin activity without angiographic evidence of renal arterial disease. The tumors, which are usually hemangiopericytomas, are frequently quite small but may be seen on arteriography. A Wilms' tumor may be associated with a similar syndrome.

Adrenogenital syndrome. A deficiency of either of two enzymes, 11-hydroxylase or 17-hydroxylase, in the adrenal gland may cause hypertension and hypokalemia. These findings occur because the associated decrease in plasma cortisol results in an increase in ACTH production. The increased output of ACTH stimulates the formation of the mineralocorticoid desoxycorticosterone, and hypertension and hypokalemia occur.

Licorice administration. The active principle of licorice extract is similar in action to desoxycorticosterone. Thus ingestion of large amounts of licorice for prolonged periods of time will cause a clinical syndrome similar to hyperaldosteronism except that endogenous aldosterone production is reduced.

Bartter's syndrome. In 1962, two patients were described who manifested the following findings: growth retardation, impaired urinary concentrating ability, hyperaldosteronism, hyperreninemia, normotension, insensitivity to exogenous angiotensin II, and

Table 1
Classification of Hypokalemic Disorders

Inadequate dietary intake

Gastrointestinal losses
Vomiting
Diarrhea of various causes
Chronic laxative abuse

Renal losses
Diuretics
Mineralocorticoid excess
Primary aldosteronism—adenoma, bilateral hyperplasia
Cushing's syndrome
Accelerated hypertension
Renal vascular hypertension
Renin producing tumor
Adrenogenital syndrome
Licorice excess
Bartter's syndrome
Liddle's syndrome
Renal tubular acidosis
Metabolic alkalosis
Acute hyperventilation
Starvation
Ureterosigmoidostomy
Antibiotics—carbenicillin, amphotericin, gentamicin
Diabetic ketoacidosis
Acute leukemia

Cellular shift
Alkalosis
Periodic paralysis
Barium poisoning
Insulin administration

hypertrophy and hyperplasia of the juxtaglomerular apparatus.

The syndrome appears to be more common in blacks, may show a familial incidence, and may be associated with an increased incidence of mental retardation.

The laboratory findings include modest to marked hypokalemia (e.g., 1.5–2.5 mEq/liter), an elevated plasma bicarbonate concentration, and an alkaline arterial pH. The creatinine clearance is usually normal. Magnesium depletion, hyperuricemia, and polycythemia have all been described. A urinary concentrating defect, resistant to vasopressin, is also present. Inappropriately elevated levels of potassium and increased quantities of prostaglandin E (PGE) are found in the urine.

Although the plasma renin is high, it does fall after appropriate intervention. The aldosterone production may be elevated, normal, or reduced, the last likely due to the inhibitory effect of hypokalemia. The pressor response to exogenous angiotensin II may be blunted but can be enhanced with expansion of the extracellular fluid volume.

The renal biopsy invariably reveals hypertrophy and hyperplasia of the cells of the juxtaglomerular apparatus. In addition, hyperplasia of the medullary interstitial cells has been reported. The latter finding is of particular interest in that the renal medullary interstitial cells are the probable site of production of renal prostaglandins and other vasoactive lipids.

The pathogenesis of Bartter's syndrome is unknown. The original suggestion that the condition represented a resistance to the vasoconstrictor effect of angiotensin II does not seem to be the case. Another proposal, that renal salt wasting is the basic defect, with hyperreninemia and hyperaldosteronism occurring secondarily, also has failed to be consistently documented. The renal potassium loss in Bartter's syndrome is not due only to excess aldosterone secretion, since the hormone may be normal or even reduced in certain patients with Bartter's syndrome. In addition, neither spironolactone nor aminogluthemide, an inhibitor of aldosterone synthesis, will completely correct the potassium deficit. Bilateral adrenalectomy may attenuate the hypokalemia but does not result in restoration of the plasma potassium.

A recent theory has been proposed to account for many of the features of Bartter's syndrome. This proposal is presented in Fig. 1. It is possible that the marked increase in urinary PGE excretion in patients with Bartter's syndrome is secondary to the renal potassium loss. In support of this is the observation that potassium deficiency in the dog can result in a marked increase in urinary PGE excretion. Systemic infusions of prostaglandins may alter the circulation and lead to renin release. To the extent that prostaglandins produced in the kidney escape degradation in the lung, the systemic effect of the prostaglandins may directly or indirectly stimulate renin release and subsequently, through angiotensin II release, enhance production of aldosterone. The resistance to exogenous angiotensin II would then be due to the high endogenous levels of angiotensin II. This sequence of events would

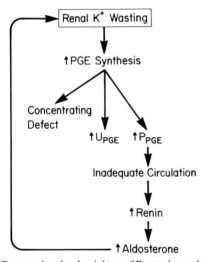

Fig. 1. Proposed pathophysiology of Bartter's syndrome. The relationship of urinary potassium wasting to the other metabolic derangements is emphasized. [Reprinted with permission from Bardgette JJ, Stein JH: Pathophysiology of Bartter's syndrome, in Brenner BM, Stein JH (eds): Acid-Base and Potassium Homeostasis. New York, Churchill Livingstone Inc and Longman Inc, 1978, p 282.]

also explain the reversal of angiotensin insensitivity with indomethacin, an inhibitor of prostaglandin synthesis.

The excessive PGE production may also explain the concentrating defect found in this disorder since there is sufficient evidence from both in vivo and in vitro studies that PGE may antagonize the hydroosmotic effection of vasopressin.

The therapy of Bartter's syndrome should include potassium chloride, which may be required in large quantities, and agents which minimize potassium secretion in the distal nephron. Propranolol has been used with varying success. Finally, indomethacin has been demonstrated to correct or ameliorate some of the metabolic abnormalities of the syndrome, at least for a short period of time. This effect is presumably due to the inhibitory effect of indomethacin on renal prostaglandin production and the secondary events which follow. It should be noted, however, that indomethacin may reduce the severity of the hypokalemia seen to the extent that the latter is aldosterone dependent but that the drug does not correct the potassium wasting state.

Liddle's syndrome. In 1963, a 16 year old girl was described with the clinical findings of hypokalemic metabolic alkalosis, hypertension, and a reduction in aldosterone secretion rate on either a normal or low-sodium diet. Neither inhibition of aldosterone synthesis nor an aldosterone antagonist affected the state of sodium retention or the kaliuresis; however, triamterene, an agent which inhibits distal ion transport independent of aldosterone, resulted in a natriuresis and potassium retention. Enhanced sodium reabsorption and potassium secretion in some portion of the distal nephron has been proposed as the cause of this condition. Further, abnormalities observed in red cell sodium flux suggested that the disorder may not be limited only to the kidney.

Renal tubular acidosis (RTA). Hypokalemia is common in both the distal (type I) and proximal (type II) forms of RTA (see also the following chapter and the chapter on *Transport Disorders*), but the etiology is quite different. In the former, the distal tubular permeability to potassium would appear to be altered, permitting enhanced diffusion of potassium into the lumen from the cell. In the latter (type II), the reduction in the reabsorptive capacity of the proximal nephron for bicarbonate floods the distal nephron with an anion which is poorly reabsorbed; as a result, the intraluminal negativity may increase, resulting in a more favorable gradient for potassium entry into the lumen.

Although elevated aldosterone levels have been reported in both types of RTA, the role this plays in the kaliuresis is unclear.

Starvation. Although the serum potassium may not fall significantly, perhaps because of the attendant acidosis, potassium excretion may increase during the induction of starvation. It is possible that this kaliuresis is due to the increased delivery of organic anions to the distal nephron resulting in a more favorable electrical gradient for potassium entry into the lumen.

Ureterosigmoidostomy. In addition to the well known development of metabolic acidosis which can be seen in patients with surgical implantation of the ureters, hypokalemia may result in this condition because of the secretion of bicarbonate and potassium in exchange for sodium chloride in the colon.

Antibiotics. Several antibiotics may cause hypokalemia. Amphotericin B may alter the membrane permeability leading to an increase in potassium entry into the tubular lumen. Carbenicillin increases potassium excretion presumably by behaving as a nonreabsorbable anion in the distal tubule. Gentamicin also increases the urinary loss of potassium, although the mechanism is unclear.

Diabetic ketoacidosis. Because of the concomitant acidosis, hypokalemia is infrequent in patients with diabetic ketoacidosis, yet total body potassium depletion is common, undoubtedly due to the renal potassium loss which occurs as a result of the osmotic diuresis of ketosis as well as to other related factors. Replacement therapy becomes essential as insulin is given and the blood pH returns toward normal.

Acute leukemia. Although controversial, it has been proposed that chronic lysozymuria in patients with acute myeloid, myelomonocytic, or monocytic leukemia may induce renal potassium wastage.

Transcellular Shifts of Potassium

Alkalosis. Acute variations in the systemic acid–base balance may have profound effects on the transcellular distribution of potassium. Alkalosis, either of metabolic or respiratory origin, can result in a movement of potassium into cells, whereas acidosis has the opposite effect. These shifts have been felt to occur in response to hydrogen ion movement in the opposite direction. In addition, however, recent evidence indicates that transcellular potassium shifts may occur in response to bicarbonate gradients between the intra- and extracellular compartments in the absence of a change in extracellular pH.

It should be appreciated, however, that the magnitude of the fall of the serum potassium in alkalotic states is also dependent upon the renal losses which occur. Although acute alkalosis of either respiratory or metabolic origin can increase potassium excretion, persistent urinary losses occur only in metabolic alkalosis. The reason for this is unclear but may be related to a persistently elevated intracellular pool of potassium in the distal nephron during chronic steady-state metabolic alkalosis.

Periodic paralysis. In the hypokalemic form of this disorder, intermittent attacks are characterized by muscle weakness, including paralysis, and a decrease in the serum potassium level.

The attacks are precipitated by a number of factors, including an interval of rest after exercise, ingestion of a high carbohydrate load, infections, trauma, tension, and alcohol. These attacks may last for 24 hours.

The etiology of the attacks is unclear. The observed fall in the serum potassium is associated with a decrease in urinary potassium excretion, suggesting that potassium must be moving from the extracellular to the intracellular compartment. A period of sodium retention usually precedes an attack, with a natriuresis and diuresis commonly occurring after it.

A number of theories have also been proposed to account for this disorder, although at the present time there are insufficient data to conclude that one is more attractive than the others.

Acetazolamide, a carbonic anhydrase inhibitor, in doses of 375–500 mg has been reported to be a more effective therapeutic agent than either potassium administration or spironolactone. The clinical improvement seen with this agent may be due to the effects of the metabolic acidosis which follows acetazolamide administration, the acidosis decreasing the rate of potassium entry into cells.

Barium poisoning. Rarely, soluble barium salts may be extremely toxic, resulting in death within hours after ingestion. A rapid and profound decrease in serum potassium may occur in this condition, presumably as the result of a shift of potassium into cells.

Insulin. Insulin is known to have a potent influence on the cellular uptake of potassium. This not only is a pharamacological effect of this hormone but also may be an important part of its physiological role. Further, it is conceivable that insulin administration may transiently decrease the serum potassium, although this effect is usually not recognized clinically.

Therapy of Potassium Depletion

General guidelines have been proposed in an attempt to correlate the degree of hypokalemia with the magnitude of the total body potassium deficit; however, this type of analysis must be done with caution, since the patient with acidosis and hypokalemia will have a much greater total body deficit than an alkalotic patient with a similar degree of hypokalemia.

Modest potassium depletion can be remedied with oral potassium chloride, either as an elixir or as Slow-K. The latter is a sugar coated tablet in which the potassium chloride crystals are imbedded in an inert, insoluble wax. This product does not have a repugnant taste, as is the case with liquid potassium chloride, and rarely, if ever, results in the small bowel ulcerations seen previously with enteric coated potassium chloride tablets.

Parenteral therapy should be used in those patients who demonstate altered neuromuscular or myocardial function on the basis of potassium depletion or in those patients who cannot take potassium orally. Intravenous potassium chloride can be given at the rate of 10 mEq/hour. If more rapid replacement is deemed necessary, it should be performed only with adequate monitoring. Finally, although perhaps obvious, the importance of knowing the status of renal function prior to potassium administration cannot be overemphasized.

HYPERKALEMIC DISORDERS

The conditions associated with hyperkalemia are listed in Table 2. This list is divided into categories which delineate the various mechanisms by which hyperkalemia may be generated. These categories include

Table 2
Classification of Hyperkalemia

Pseudohyperkalemia
  Improper collection of blood
  Hematologic disorders with white blood cell or platelet count
Exogenous potassium load
  Oral or intravenous KCl
  Potassium-containing drugs
  Transfusion
  Geophagia

Cellular shift in potassium
  Tissue damage—trauma, burns, rhabdomyolysis
  Destruction of tumor tissue
  Digitalis overdose
  Acidosis
  Hyperkalemic periodic paralysis
  Hyperosmolality
  Succinylcholine
  Arginine infusion

Decreased renal potassium excretion
  Acute renal failure
  Chronic renal failure
  Potassium sparing diuretics
  Mineralocorticoid deficiency
    Addison's disease
    Bilateral adrenalectomy
    Hypoaldosteronism—hyporeninemic hypoaldosteronism, heparin therapy, specific
      enzymatic defect, tubular unresponsiveness
  Congenital adrenal hyperplasia
  Primary defect in potassium transport

exogenous potassium loads, transcellular shifts of potassium, and impaired renal excretion.

Pseudohyperkalemia

There are a number of causes of a false elevation of the potassium concentration of the blood. The serum concentration is normally 0.5 mEq/liter higher than plasma because of the release of potassium from platelets and other cells during clotting. Further, exercise of the forearm to better delineate a vein for venipuncture can result in a release of potassium from muscle and local hyperkalemia. Other problems include hemolysis and the passage of potassium from cells to plasma upon standing. All can be easily remedied.

In patients with hematologic disorders characterized by increased platelet or leukocyte counts, pseudohyperkalemia may be noted if the cellular elements are not rapidly separated from the plasma. The hyperkalemia in this instance results from leakage of potassium from the cells in vitro.

Exogenous Potassium Load

Although in patients with normal function substantial amounts of potassium can be administered with safety, this is not the case in the patient with renal functional impairment. This is particularly true when the urinary flow rate is low because of the flow-dependent nature of potassium excretion. Hyperkalemia can also be induced by the administration of stored blood, by large amounts of potassium penicillin, or by the administration of potassium in non-rigid parenteral fluid containers.

Another instance of hyperkalemia being induced in the presence of renal insufficiency was reported in five patients who ingested riverbed clay which contained large quantities of potassium.

Cellular Shifts of Potassium

Tissue damage. Cellular damage from a number of causes, including rhabdomyolysis, burns, etc., may release large quantities of potassium into the extracellular space. In the presence of normal renal function, most of the potassium might be expected to be excreted. Not infrequently, however, renal functional impairment is also present.

Recently, a comparable syndrome has been described in patients with Burkitt's lymphoma and in patients with lymphocytic leukemia. In the period immediately after the initiation of chemotherapy, there is marked cellular destruction with the release of potassium.

Marked hyperkalemia may also be seen in patients who take an overdose of digitalis. The hyperkalemia in this situation presumably results from a digitalis-induced decrease in the activity of the cation pump in the cell membrane, thereby inhibiting potassium uptake into the cell.

Hyperkalemic periodic paralysis. In 1956, a family was described in which several members had episodic paralysis. Several features, however, differentiated this entity from hypokalemic periodic paralysis. First, hyperkalemia rather than hypokalemia was present during the attacks. Moreover, the attacks began at a younger age, were of shorter duration, and occurred more frequently than in the hypokalemic form of periodic paralysis.

The paralytic attacks characteristically occur when the patient is resting following vigorous exercise, the weakness involving multiple muscle groups. Coughing and swallowing may also be affected. The onset of the paralysis is quite rapid, the peak being reached in 30 min or less.

In addition to the hyperkalemia seen during the attacks, a fall in the serum sodium and chloride and a rise in the serum bicarbonate can be noted. Further, the paralytic attacks can be associated with an increase in urinary potassium excretion and a decrease in sodium excretion.

As with the hypokalemic variety of periodic paralysis, the etiology of this disorders is unclear. Thiazide diuretics, carbonic anhydrase inhibitors, and mineralocorticoids have all been shown to be effective prophylactic agents.

Hyperosmolality. Hyperosmotic infusions of mannitol or saline can lead to hyperkalemia. This effect presumably is due to an alteration in the permeability of the cellular membrane permitting potassium to "leak" from the intracellular to the extracellular compartment.

Succinylcholine administration. Due to a release of potassium from muscle during cellular depolarization, depolarizing muscle relaxants such as succinylcholine may result in hyperkalemia. Patients with trauma, burns, tetanus, renal failure, and various neuromuscular diseases seem to have an exaggerated response to the drug. Tubocurarine will attenuate the succinylcholine-induced muscle release of potassium.

Arginine. Arginine hydrochloride is used primarily for the treatment of metabolic alkalosis and as a test of pituitary function; however, since this amino acid may enter cells in exchange for potassium, its administration may lead to hyperkalemia.

Decreased Renal Excretion of Potassium

Acute renal failure. Hyperkalemia is a well known complication of acute renal failure. In a recent extensive series of patients having multiple traumatic injuries and acute renal failure, the serum potassium concentration was found to be above 7.0 mEq/liter at least once in half of the subjects.

The hyperkalemia seen in the patient with acute renal failure is likely attributable to a number of factors. In those patients with oliguria, the decrease in the flow rate of tubular fluid in both the distal convoluted tubule and the collecting duct would severely limit potassium excretion. Further, in many of the patients, tissue breakdown and acidosis contribute to the hyperkalemia.

Chronic renal failure. In the patient with chronic renal failure, the serum potassium may be decreased, normal, or elevated depending upon the potassium intake, urine volume, and the adequacy of both the renal and extrarenal mechanisms to compensate for the reduction in the renal mass.

Although the ability to excrete a potassium load is impaired in chronic renal disease, important but poorly understood compensatory mechanisms come in to play to increase potassium excretion per nephron. In fact, potassium excretion may exceed the filtered load in patients or experimental animals with a reduction in functional renal mass.

The factors responsible for the adaptive increase in potassium excretion per nephron when the renal mass is reduced have yet to be clarified. In dogs in which the renal mass was reduced by ligating a major portion of the arterial supply to one kidney and contralateral nephrectomy, potassium excretion increases in hours and within days returns to control levels. This adaptive response is not altered by maintaining mineralocorticoid activity at a high or low level, by altering sodium balance, or by aortic constriction.

Recent micropuncture studies of remnant kidneys in the rat have shown that the adaptive increase in potassium excretion as renal mass is reduced is associated with a number of changes in intrarenal potassium transport. First, a high single nephron glomerular filtration rate increases the absolute quantity of potassium delivered to the distal nephron. Second, distal tubular potassium secretion is enhanced, presumably, in part, as a result of the increase in the flow rate of tubular fluid. Lastly, on occasion, nephron sites beyond the superficial distal tubule contribute meaningfully to the amount of potassium found in the final urine.

There are also two extrarenal mechanisms for maintaining a normal serum potassium concentration in patients with renal failure. First, it is well known that an animal on a high-potassium diet for a prolonged period of time is better able to maintain the serum potassium concentration in a relatively normal range than in an unadapted animal even in the absence of kidneys. Prior adrenalectomy abolishes this adaptive mechanism. Presumably administered potassium moves more readily into muscle and possibly bone in the adapted animal by an aldosterone dependent mechanism. Thus if the patient with chronic renal failure is analogous to the potassium adapted subject, this mechanism will play a role in the regulation of the serum potassium concentration independent of renal function.

Second, patients on hemodialysis with a normal intake of potassium but with essentially no renal excretion of potassium, diarrhea, or significant potassium loss in the dialysate may not be hyperkalemia. Metabolic studies have revealed that 25–75 percent of their daily dietary potassium was excreted in the stool. In further studies in a larger series of patients with a creatinine clearance less than 5 ml/min, the magnitude of the potassium loss was proportional to the net weight of the stool and the potassium intake. The increased stool potassium excretion was not reversed by variations in sodium intake or by diuretics. It may also be of interest that colonic mucosal $Na^+ K^+$ ATPase increases during potassium adaptation in the rat and that this response is abolished by adrenalectomy. In any case, it seems likely that increased intestinal excretion of potassium may play a role in maintaining the serum potassium concentration in some patients with far advanced renal disease.

In spite of these multiple adaptive mechanisms for regulating the serum potassium concentration, there are numerous reports of patients with varying degrees of renal insufficiency who have persistent hyperkalemia. This abnormality has been reported in a patient with resolving acute glomerulonephritis, subjects diagnosed as having chronic pyelonephritis, and patients with renal failure and marked salt wasting. Although it is not possible retrospectively to define the specific mechanisms involved in these earlier reports, it seems possible that at least some of these patients did in fact have hyporeninemic hypoaldosteronism (see below).

By the time the patient with renal disease develops endstage renal insufficiency requiring dialysis, there is frequently depletion of total body potassium stores. This may be due to the associated vomiting, diarrhea, and anorexia seen with uremia.

Potassium sparing agents. The aldosterone antagonist aldactone, and amiloride and triamterene, which are not aldosterone dependent, decrease distal tubular potassium secretion.

The administration of these agents may result in hyperkalemia, particularly in those patients with renal insufficiency in whom enhanced potassium secretion is necessary to maintain potassium balance. In addition, death due to hyperkalemia has occurred in diabetic patients with normal renal function taking these drugs, perhaps, in part, due to an attenuated insulin response to hyperkalemia in this situation.

Addison's disease. It has been recognized for some time that the serum potassium increases after adrena-lectomy. Although unusual, the signs and symptoms of hyperkalemia may be a prominent feature of Addison's disease. The hyperkalemia, in large part, is likely due to the absence of a mineralocorticoid effect on potassium excretion in the distal nephron. Interestingly, hyperkalemia is unusual in the Addisonian patient who receives cortisone replacement alone, presumably due to the mineralocorticoid effect of this agent.

Hypoaldosteronism. This entity is defined as a selective deficiency of aldosterone in the absence of abnormalities of glucocorticoid secretion.

Most adult cases of hypoaldosteronism fit into the category known as hyporeninemic hypoaldosteronism. The first report of isolated hypoaldosteronism involved an elderly patient with mild renal insufficiency, hyperkalemia, renal salt wasting, and cardiac conductive defects. Since this patient with hypoaldosteronism had normal cortisol secretion, it seemed surprising that hyperkalemia was present. The major clinical manifestations in patients with this disorder are the hyperkalemia and a metabolic acidosis. Both of these effects are presumably directly related to the impaired production of aldosterone.

That preexisting renal disease is an important factor in clinically recognizable selective hypoaldosteronism is now clear. In fact, it may be that the renal disease is responsible, in part, for the hypoaldosteronism. Plasma renin activity and aldosterone production are decreased in these patients and do not rise appropriately after various stimuli (Fig. 2 and 3). Associated diseases in these patients include diabetes, gout, pseudogout, and

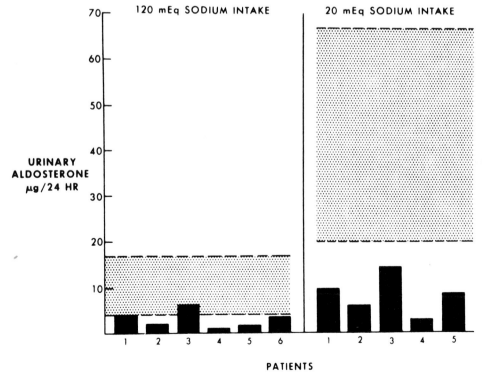

Fig. 2. Urinary aldosterone excretion during normal sodium (120 mEq per day) and low sodium (20 mEq per day) intakes in patients with hyporeninemic hypoaldosteronism. The stippled areas indicate the ranges for normal subjects. [Reprinted by permission from Schambelan M, Stockigt JR, Biglieri EG: Isolated hypoaldosteronism in adults. N Engl J Med 287:809, 1972.]

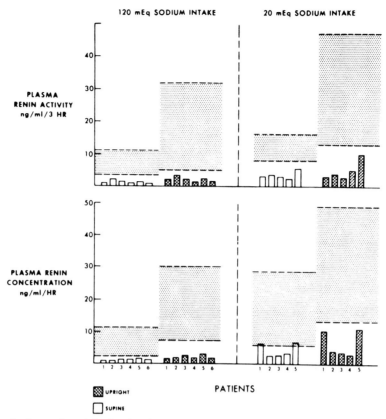

Fig. 3. Supine and upright levels of plasma renin activity and concentration in patients with hyporeninemic hypoaldosteronism on normal and low sodium intakes. The stippled areas indicate the ranges for normal subjects. [Reprinted by permission from Schambelan M, Stockigt JR, Biglieri EG: Isolated hypoaldosteronism in adults. N Engl J Med 287:809, 1972.]

primary hyperparathyroidism. Perhaps in some way the renal disease results in an acquired abnormality of the juxtaglomerular apparatus such that renin is decreased and that angiotensin II and aldosterone formation are subsequently diminished. Why the resultant hyperkalemia, in and of itself, does not increase aldosterone production and restore potassium balance is unclear. Patients with this syndrome have been treated with mineralocorticoid therapy, e.g., fludrocortisone, with amelioration of the hyperkalemia and acidosis (Fig. 4). In those patients with this syndrome who are hypertensive, furosemide rather than a mineralocorticoid is an appropriate form of therapy.

Heparin and related compounds have been shown to cause a natriuresis and a decrease in potassium excretion. This effect has been shown to be due to a decrease in secretion and excretion of aldosterone.

Hypoaldosteronism may also be due to a specific enzymatic defect (see below). In addition, there are scattered reports of patients with tubular insensitivity to aldosterone.

Congenital enzymatic defects in mineralocorticoid production. In the previous section on hypokalemic disorders, it was pointed out that certain forms of the adrenogenital syndrome may be associated with a reduction in the serum potassium concentration. There are also other enzymatic disorders in which aldosterone production is markedly depressed and the secretion of

other mineralocorticoids is not increased. The most common cause of hyperkalemia in these disorders is a 21-hydroxylase defect where salt wasting and virilization are usually also present. A selective defect in aldosterone secretion has been described in two infants with a familial deficiency of the enzyme 18-hydroxydehydrogenase. These patients clinically presented with growth failure, hyperkalemia, and acidosis, which were corrected by salt and mineralocorticoid deficiency.

Primary defect in potassium excretion. Hyperkalemia due to a defect in the renal handling of potassium has been described. These patients have normal renal and adrenal function but may have a number of associated clinical findings including metabolic acidosis, short stature, hypertension, and a modest acidifying defect. It has been suggested that an abnormality in distal tubule potassium secretion is responsible for the hyperkalemia. Chlorthiazide appears to be an effective therapeutic agent.

Treatment of Hyperkalemia

The severity of hyperkalemia as judged by electrocardiographic (ECG) changes and other criteria does not always correlate with the level of serum potassium. In most patients, ECG changes will be present by the time the serum potassium reaches 7 mEq/liter. In patients with somewhat lower levels of serum potassium and with no abnormalities in ECG, potassium restriction and liberalization of sodium intake may be adequate

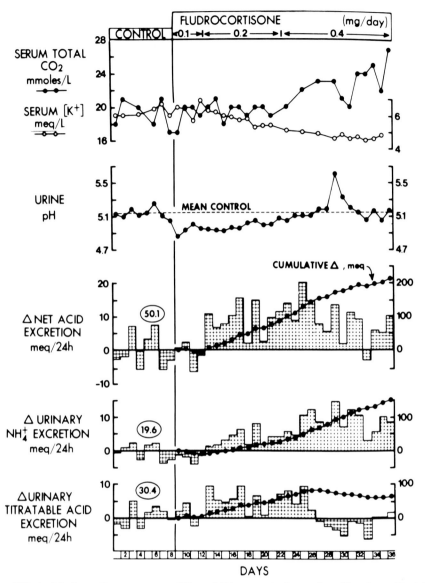

Fig. 4. Effect of fludrocortisone on serum CO_2 and K^+ concentration, urine pH, urinary titratable acid, ammonium, and net acid excretion in a patient with hyporeninemic hypoaldosteronism and chronic renal insufficiency (creatinine clearance 35 ml/min/1.73 m^2). In the three bottom panels, the hatched bars represent the differences between the measured value of acid excretion and the mean value before therapy; the magnitude of these differences is indicated by the scale on the left-hand side of the panel. For reference, the mean control values are designated by the numerals within the ellipses. The accumulated values of the daily differences are shown by the solid circles and are indicated by the scale on the right-hand side of the panel. [Reprinted by permission from Sebastian A, Schambelan M, Lindenfield S, et al: Amelioration of metabolic acidosis with fludrocortisone therapy in hyporeninemic hypoaldosteronism. N Engl J Med 297:576, 1977.]

therapy. If, however, there are significant electrocardiographic changes (widened QRS, heart block, ventricular arrhythmias), the situation should be considered a medical emergency. First, a calcium infusion should be given to reverse the cardiotoxic effects of hyperkalemia. One to three ampoules of 10 percent calcium gluconate are infused intravenously over 3–5 min during ECG monitoring. The onset of action of calcium is within 1–5 min but is relatively transient, and other, more long lasting agents must be used. These would include the

administration of glucose and insulin and/or alkali therapy. A solution of 500 ml of 10 percent glucose with 10 units of regular insulin may be given over 30 min and then administered at a reduced rate if necessary. The onset of action of glucose and insulin is within 30 min and the effect may last for several hours.

Alternatively, two or three ampoules of sodium bicarbonate (each ampoule provides 44 mEq of sodium bicarbonate) is added to 1 liter of glucose and infused over 1–2 hours. With the rise in blood pH, potassium moves into cells decreasing the hyperkalemia within 1 hour. This effect may persist for several hours if the blood pH is maintained and endogenous potassium release is not large.

The effect of this form of therapy is to drive potassium into cells and to not remove the potassium from the body. Cation exchanges resins of the sodium cycle such as sodium polystyrene sulfonate (Kayexalate) are quite useful in achieving this latter goal. They can be given orally or per rectum as an enema. It has been estimated that approximately 1 mEq of potassium is exchanged for each gram of resin administered. Sixty to eighty grams are given orally per day in combination with varying amounts of 70 percent sorbitol, which prevents the constipation otherwise frequently seen with the resin. In addition, in the presence of adequate renal function, diuretics such as the thiazides may be of benefit by enhancing urinary potassium excretion.

Either peritoneal dialysis or hemodialysis has been used to treat hyperkalemia, yet the other therapeutic modalities mentioned will usually satisfactorily control the hyperkalemia, while dialysis may be necessary to control the other abnormalities associated with renal failure.

REFERENCES

Bardgette JJ, Stein JH: Pathophysiology of Bartter's syndrome, in Brenner BM, Stein JH (eds): Acid-Base and Potassium Homeostasis. New York, Churchill Livingstone Inc and Longman Inc, 1978, p 282

Bartter FC, Gill JR, Frolich JC, et al: Prostaglandins are overproduced by the kidneys and mediate hyperreninemia in Bartter's syndrome. Clin Res 24:490A, 1976 (Abstr)

Burnell JM, Villamil MF, Uyeno D, et al: The effect in humans of extracellular pH change on the relationship between serum potassium concentration and intracellular potassium. J Clin Invest 35:935, 1956

Conn JW: Primary aldosteronism: A new clinical syndrome. J Lab Clin Med 45:6, 1955

Giebisch G: Renal potassium excretion, in Rouiller CT, Muller AF, (eds): The Kidney, New York and London, Academic Press, Vol 3, 1971, p 329

Schambelan M, Stockigt JR, Biglieri EG: Isolated hypoaldosteronism in adults. N Engl J Med 287:809, 1972

Sebastian A, Schambelan M, Lindenfield S, et al: Amelioration of metabolic acidosis with fludrocortisone therapy in hyporeninemic hydoaldosteronism. N Engl J Med 297:576, 1977

Spitzer A, Edelman CM, Goldberg LD, et al: Short stature, hyperkalemia, and acidosis; A defect in renal transport of potassium. Kidney Int 3:251, 1973

DISORDERS OF ACID–BASE METABOLISM

Jose A.L. Arruda and Neil A. Kurtzman

METABOLIC ALKALOSIS
Definition

Metabolic alkalosis is a primary pathophysiologic state characterized by a gain of bicarbonate or loss of nonvolatile acid from extracellular fluid.

Generation

In order to generate metabolic alkalosis one must have a gain of base or a loss of acid. The gain of base usually results from the administration of alkaline solutions. The loss of acid may be via the gastrointestinal tract or from the kidney. Depletion of hydrochloric acid from the stomach as the consequence of vomiting or nasogastric suction leaves behind large amounts of bicarbonate.

The body produces 60–100 mEq of acid daily as the consequence of normal metabolism. The kidney is thus required to excrete 60–100 mEq of acid daily. For each mEq of acid excreted in the urine 1 mEq of new bicarbonate will be generated and added to the blood, maintaining normal acid–base homeostasis. In order for the kidney to generate metabolic alkalosis net acid excretion must increase at least transiently, resulting in the addition of excess amounts of bicarbonate to the blood.

The fact that new bicarbonate is added to the blood (regardless of the mechanism) does not necessarily mean that metabolic alkalosis will ensue. The new bicarbonate may be excreted by the kidney, thus preventing metabolic alkalosis. It is clear that in order for sustained metabolic alkalosis to be present, the excess bicarbonate generated or administered must not be excreted, i.e., the high bicarbonate present in the filtrate must be reclaimed by the kidney in order to maintain the metabolic alkalosis. An increase in bicarbonate reabsorption unaccompanied by the gain of bicarbonate or loss of acid cannot generate metabolic alkalosis.

Two mechanisms are then extremely important in metabolic alkalosis—(1) the generation of new bicarbonate and (2) the maintenance of a high plasma bicarbonate concentration, which is accomplished by increased tubular reabsorption of bicarbonate.

Role of Potassium and Aldosterone in the Generation of Metabolic Alkalosis

The kidney can generate metabolic alkalosis if there is an increased capacity of the distal nephron to secrete hydrogen ion at a time when there is adequate distal sodium delivery. Aldosterone excess increases sodium reabsorption in the distal nephron and enhances potassium excretion. The sodium retained results in extracellular volume expansion, which in turn depresses proximal reabsorption increasing distal sodium delivery. Patients with aldosterone excess commonly have metabolic alkalosis. The generation and the maintenance of metabolic alkalosis in patients with primary mineralocorticoid excess is likely the consequence of accelerated distal hydrogen ion secretion, which is driven by both steroid excess and potassium depletion.

Maintenance and Correction

The following factors seem to be important in the maintenance of metabolic alkalosis:

ECV contraction. The degree of metabolic alkalosis generated by potassium depletion and mineralocorticoid excess can be significantly altered by variations in the salt intake. Volume contraction enhances bicarbonate reabsorption and thus maintains a higher plasma bicarbonate concentration. Expansion of the extracellular volume with saline should then correct metabolic alkalosis. Correction of metabolic alkalosis can be achieved by expansion of the extracellular fluid volume with a solution that contained the same concentration of sodium chloride and bicarbonate as the plasma of the alkalotic subject. Expansion of extracellular fluid volume with this solution leads to the excretion of bicarbonate and retention of chloride resulting in correction of the metabolic alkalosis. This correction is not caused by an increase in glomerular filtration rate or a decrease in mineralocorticoid activity. Rather, the correction seemed to be caused by expansion of extracellular volume.

Potassium depletion. Potassium depletion enhances bicarbonate reabsorption and thus can maintain metabolic alkalosis. Most cases of metabolic alkalosis can be corrected by volume expansion alone without repletion of potassium deficits. There are a few cases, however, of metabolic alkalosis associated with severe potassium depletion that are not corrected by saline alone ("saline resistant metabolic alkalosis"). These causes are usually secondary to primary aldosteronism or Cushing's syndrome but can also be found in other diseases associated with severe potassium depletion. In patients with primary aldosteronism metabolic alkalosis is maintained by a distal mechanism. Although these patients are potassium depleted they are also volume expanded. Potassium depletion enhances proximal bicarbonate reabsorption, whereas volume expansion depresses it. These two mechanisms tend to counterbalance each other; therefore enhanced proximal reabsorption does not play a major role in the maintenance of this type of metabolic alkalosis. This explains why saline alone does not correct the metabolic alkalosis.

There is no question that potassium depletion alone may maintain metabolic alkalosis regardless of the mechanism responsible for its generation if the degree of potassium depletion is extreme. Severe potassium depletion may increase proximal bicarbonate reabsorption to such a marked extent that volume expansion cannot lower it to the "normal" range. For example, a patient with severe hypokalemia may be volume contracted and have a plasma bicarbonate concentration of 50 mEq/liter. Volume expansion without replacing the potassium deficit may lower bicarbonate concentration to 40 mEq/liter. Full correction of the alkalosis requires potassium administration.

Patients whose effective arterial blood is contracted, who have metabolic alkalosis, and whose volume cannot be expanded by saline administration (e.g., congestive heart failure, cirrhosis) will have a type of alkalosis that may be both saline and potassium resistant. For it to be corrected, effective arterial blood volume must be restored to normal; in the case of the patient with congestive heart failure, cardiac performance must improve. The key for the understanding of metabolic alkalosis is the accurate assessment of effective volume.

Causes

Table 1 shows the causes of metabolic alkalosis and the factors responsible for its maintenance. It is important to realize that the factors responsible for the generation of metabolic alkalosis need to be present only transiently; it is necessary to look for the factors responsible for the maintenance of the metabolic alkalosis as well as for the initial cause.

Gastric Alkalosis

The hydrochloric acid concentration of gastric juice may be as high as 160 mEq/liter. The concentrations of sodium and potassium in this fluid are about 10–20 mEq/liter. Thus a patient who is vomiting or who undergoes gastric suction sufficient to result in a loss of 250 ml/hr of gastric juice might lose 40 mEq of hydrochloric acid per hour. Each mEq of hydrochloric acid lost from the body represents 1 mEq of sodium bicarbonate added to extracellular fluid. Thus severe protracted vomiting or prolonged gastric aspiration can result in the addition of as much as 1000 mEq of bicarbonate to the extracellular fluid per day. Such an extreme degree of gastric hypersecretion is likely to be seen only in patients with Zollinger-Ellison syndrome.

With vomiting or gastric drainage the following sequence of events takes place (Fig. 1): The loss of hydrochloric acid in vomitus results in a rise in the plasma bicarbonate concentration with little change in plasma sodium or potassium concentration. The concentration of sodium and potassium in gastric juice is relatively low. When the plasma bicarbonate concentration rises to a level which exceeds the reabsorptive capacity for bicarbonate of the proximal tubule, increased amounts of bicarbonate are delivered to the distal nephron. Some of the sodium is exchanged for potassium, while most escapes in the urine with the bicarbonate. Thus, initially there is an increase in the excretion of sodium bicarbonate in the urine. This results in an increase in the urine pH. Owing to the loss of chloride in the vomitus there is an immediate decline in chloride concentration. To the extent that sodium bicarbonate is lost in the urine there is an equivalent loss of salt and water from the extracellular fluid. This is because the loss of sodium bicarbonate is coupled to the loss of hydrochloric acid. The loss of salt and water results in contraction of the effective arterial blood volume. This in turn results in a number of physiologic alterations.

As volume becomes contracted there is an increased stimulus to proximal bicarbonate reabsorption. Thus, a greater fraction of the filtered bicarbonate is reabsorbed and returned to the extracellular fluid. This event tends to perpetuate the metabolic alakalosis which was generated initially by the loss of gastric acid. Decreased amounts of sodium bicarbonate are delivered to the distal nephron. Owing to the development of volume contraction, increased amounts of aldosterone are secreted. Thus aldosterone enhances the exchange of sodium for potassium in the distal nephron and results in an increase in urinary potassium. It is this loss of urinary potassium which results in the hypoka-

Table 1
Generation and Maintenance of Metabolic Alkalosis

Generation	Example	Maintenance
Loss of acid from extracellular space		
Loss of gastric fluid	Vomiting	↓ Effective arterial volume, (EAV)
Loss of acid into urine—increased distal Na delivery in presence of hyperaldosteronism	Primary aldosteronism Diuretic administration	K depletion and aldosterone excess ↓ EAV and K depletion
Loss of acid into cells—K deficiency	Contributing factor	K deficiency
Loss of acid into stool	Congenital chloride-losing diarrhea	K deficiency and ↓ EAV
Excessive HCO_3 loads		
Absolute		
Oral or parenteral loads of HCO_3 alkalinizing salts	$NaHCO_3$ administration, milk alkali syndrome	↓EAV or continuous administration, K deficiency
Metabolic conversion of salts of organic acids (e.g. ketones, lactate) to HCO_3	Lactate, acetate, citrate administration	↓EAV, K deficiency, or continuous administration
Relative—alkaline loads in renal failure	Alkali administration to patients with renal failure	Renal failure
Posthypercapnic state	Correction of chronic hypercapnia in presence of a low salt diet	↓EAV

263

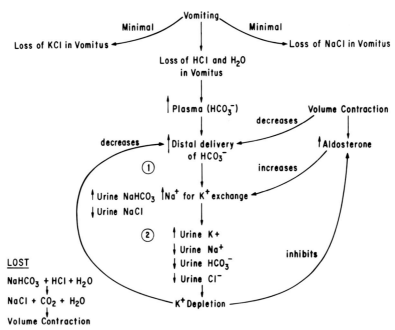

Fig. 1.   A schema of alkagastric alkalosis.

lemia of vomiting, not the loss of potassium in gastric juice. Since smaller and smaller amounts of bicarbonate are being delivered to the distal nephron because of enhanced proximal bicarbonate reabsorption, urinary sodium and bicarbonate concentrations decrease. This results in a fall in urine sodium concentration as well as a fall in urine pH.

The development of potassium depletion inhibits the adrenal synthesis of aldosterone and plasma aldosterone concentration now falls. Proximal bicarbonate concentration is further stimulated by the development of hypokalemia. These events, as outlined in Fig. 1, result in the characteristic findings of protracted vomiting. The plasma bicarbonate concentration and pH are high. Urine sodium, chloride, and bicarbonate are low. Urine potassium tends to be higher than sodium. Plasma aldosterone concentration is "normal." When plasma aldosterone concentration is corrected for the degree of hypokalemia present it may be considered to be "elevated."

Several practical points deserve emphasis from the above formulation. If the patient is seen early in the course of vomiting, measurement of the urine sodium as an index of effective arterial blood volume may yield results which are difficult to interpret. Since sodium bicarbonate is lost in the urine in large amounts early in vomiting, urine sodium may be high even though volume is contracted. In patients with gastric alkalosis the urine chloride, not sodium, should be used as a marker of volume. Since the loss of salt and water sets into play the entire array of pathophysiologic events just described, the cornerstone of the treatment of gastric alkalosis is the replacement of salt and water. It goes without saying that potassium deficits should likewise be replaced. In patients without serious circu-

latory or renal disease the urine chloride concentration may be used as an index of effective salt replacement. Adequate amounts of salt will not have been given until such time as the urine chloride concentration starts to rise.

The Kidney and Generation of Metabolic Alkalosis

As discussed previously, the kidney can produce metabolic alkalosis by enhancing distal hydrogen ion excretion, thus adding new bicarbonate to the extracellular fluid. Required for the renal generation of metabolic alkalosis are (1) enhanced capacity to secrete hydrogen ions and (2) adequate delivery of sodium salts to the distal nephron when increased avidity for sodium is present. This will allow reabsorption of sodium and secretion of hydrogen ions. Increased delivery of sodium to the distal nephron may result from the following sources: (1) dietary sodium chloride, (2) depressed sodium reabsorption by diuretics, and (3) administration of sodium salts or poorly reabsorbable anions. If there is a strong stimulus for sodium retention in the distal tubule (i.e., hyperaldosteronism), sodium will be retained and hydrogen will be secreted.

Steroids. Clinical conditions associated with excessive mineralocorticoid activity are almost invariably associated with metabolic alkalosis. Examples of these include Cushing's disease, adrenal adenoma, malignant hypertension, renal artery stenosis, adrenogenital syndrome, and other related syndromes. Administration of mineralocorticoids is commonly associated with metabolic alkalosis. After administration of these hormones the following events take place:

1. Increased sodium reabsorption in the distal nephron, with enhanced potassium excretion.
2. Retention of sodium expands extracellular volume

and depresses proximal reabsorption, which leads to increased distal delivery of sodium which is exchanged for potassium and hydrogen. Acid excretion, as well as potassium excretion, is therefore increased.

3. Metabolic alkalosis ensues because acid excretion is enhanced as the consequence of two different mechanisms—potassium depletion, in the presence of aldosterone, enhances acid excretion, and increased levels of aldosterone further enhance acidification of the urine when the subject is potassium deleted.

Experimental studies in animals have shown that if expansion of extracellular volume is prevented by giving steroid treated animals a sodium-free diet, metabolic alkalosis does not develop. A low-salt diet enhances proximal reabsorption, curtailing the amount of sodium delivered to the distal tubule and preventing an increase in acid excretion.

The maintenance of steroid induced metabolic alkalosis results from two mechanisms. First, potassium depletion enhances proximal bicarbonate reabsorption. Second, in the presence of excessive amounts of aldosterone, distal bicarbonate reabsorption is also enhanced. It is likely that this type of metabolic alkalosis is maintained mainly by a distal mechanism.

The effects of potassium depletion and extracellular volume expansion on proximal bicarbonate reabsorption tend to counterbalance each other. Therefore increased proximal reabsorption does not seem to play a major role in the maintenance of this metabolic alkalosis.

Bartter's syndrome. This syndrome is associated with metabolic alkalosis; it may represent a form of salt wastage due to the defective reabsorption of chloride in the loop of Henle. This salt wastage leads to a contracted plasma volume which stimulates renin and aldosterone production. Potassium reabsorption also seems to be impaired, since adrenalectomy does not correct the severe hypokalemia found in these patients. This form of metabolic alkalosis seems to be generated by the severe potassium depletion and mineralocorticoid excess; it is maintained by enhanced proximal reabsorption secondary to contracted plasma volume as well as by an enhanced distal mechanism.

Hypercapnia. Chronic hypercapnia enhances acid and chloride excretion. At the same time it stimulates bicarbonate reabsorption, causing an increased concentration of plasma bicarbonate. Following the return of the pCO_2 to normal there usually is retention of chloride and excretion of bicarbonate in the urine. If patients with hypercapnia are on a low-salt diet or are treated with diuretics, proximal reabsorption will be enhanced and bicarbonate reabsorption will remain elevated following the return of the pCO_2 to normal, resulting in posthypercapnic metabolic alkalosis. Correction of this type of metabolic alkalosis can be accomplished by salt administration. This syndrome may result if effective

arterial volume is contracted for any reason, such as congestive heart failure. In this latter instance, successful treatment of the heart failure is required to correct the alkalosis; salt administration here is contraindicated.

"Contraction" alkalosis. Administration of diuretics such as thiazides, ethacrynic acid, and furosemide is commonly associated with metabolic alkalosis. The generation of this type of metabolic alkalosis is due to enhanced acid excretion brought on by potassium depletion and secondary hyperaldosteronism. Once generated, diuretic induced metabolic alkalosis is maintained by volume contraction and potassium depletion. It has been suggested that ethacrynic acid and furosemide, which have their diuretic site of action in the loop of Henle, may induce metabolic alkalosis without loss of acid. This alkalosis has been called "contraction" alkalosis; it is thought to be due to enhanced excretion of sodium and chloride without proportional losses of bicarbonate (bicarbonate reabsorption in the loop of Henle is small or absent). It should be pointed out, however, that adrenalectomized dogs given maintenance doses of dexamethasone and DOCA and treated with furosemide failed to develop metabolic alkalosis. When the dogs were volume contracted at a time when large amounts of DOCA were given, metabolic alkalosis developed. Contraction per se seems a simplistic explanation for this type of metabolic alkalosis. It seems likely that excess renal acid excretion must occur for it to develop.

Postfasting metabolic alkalosis. Metabolic alkalosis is known to occur in fasting patients when they return to a normal diet with a high glucose content. Bicarbonate reabsorption measured in these patients correlates with sodium balance. Bicarbonate reabsorption is low in the first week of fasting when the sodium balance becomes positive but metabolic alkalosis is not present. Glucose administration leads to a further increase in bicarbonate reabsorption and metabolic alkalosis. The maintenance of this type of metabolic alkalosis seems to be caused by contracted extracellular volume and the enhancing effect of glucose on bicarbonate reabsorption. The mechanism responsible for the generation of this type of metabolic alkalosis is not clear at the present time, although it may be secondary to increased acid excretion.

Metabolic alkalosis secondary to hypercalcemia and hypoparathyroidism. A few cases of metabolic alkalosis have been reported in association with hypoparathyroidism. Hypercalcemia is more commonly associated with metabolic alkalosis. It is likely that parathyroid hormone depresses bicarbonate reabsorption and its absence enhances it. Hypercalcemia, by suppressing parathyroid hormone secretion or by a direct effect, may also increase bicarbonate reabsorption. Although these observations could explain the maintenance of metabolic alkalosis in these conditions, they leave unresolved the question of how the metabolic alkalosis is generated. Parathyroid hormone has been shown to have an inhibitory effect on acid excretion, and, theoretically, lack of parathyroid hormone could lead to enhanced acid excretion; this, however, has yet to be proven. The generation of metabolic alkalosis secondary to hypercalcemia has been attributed to a greater availability of the buffering capacity of the skeleton secondary either to bone destruction or increased bone turnover.

Metabolic alkalosis secondary to excessive bicarbonate loads. Administration of sodium bicarbonate in doses up to 140 g/day for periods extending to 3 weeks has been shown to produce metabolic alkalosis with plasma bicarbonate levels of 33–36 mEq/liter. There was a linear relationship between the doses of sodium bicarbonate administered and the rise in serum bicarbonate. Note that the dose of bicarbonate used was very high. If volume contraction or potassium depletion does not develop, this type of metabolic alkalosis will correct as soon as bicarbonate administration ceases because of the kidney's intrinsic capacity to excrete enormous amounts of bicarbonate. In renal failure, however, a smaller dose of sodium bicarbonate may produce metabolic alkalosis because of the limited capacity of the severely diseased kidney to excrete a sodium load.

Congenital alkalosis with diarrhea. This is a rare form of metabolic alkalosis. Patients with this disease have hypochloremia, a high stool chloride concentration, and an absence of chloride in the urine. The stool chloride concentration is higher than the sum of sodium and potassium concentrations. This is in contrast with all other diarrheal states, in which the sum of sodium and potassium concentrations in the stool is higher than the chloride concentration. These patients have a defect in the chloride–bicarbonate pump in the ileum. They are unable to transport chloride against an electrochemical gradient; this defect results in a loss of chloride and acid in the stool, which in turn causes metabolic alkalosis.

Respiratory adjustment. Metabolic alkalosis may lead to compensatory hypoventilation and consequent carbon dioxide retention. Uncomplicated metabolic alkalosis is not always associated with alveolar hypoventilation. The magnitude of the hypoventilation in metabolic alkalosis is not great; the pCO_2 is usually not higher than 55 mm Hg. This is in contrast to metabolic acidosis, where a reduction in plasma bicarbonate is always associated with a marked reduction in PCO_2.

Treatment

Once the pathophysiology of the type of metabolic alkalosis has been delineated, treatment is usually simple. If volume contraction is the perpetrating mechanism it should be restored to normal. Potassium deficits should be corrected. If primary mineralocorticoid excess is present it may be antagonized by the administration of spironolactone prior to definitive therapy.

In patients with metabolic alkalosis and contraction of effective arterial volume due to severe cardiac or liver disease the infusion of large volumes of sodium chloride will not only fail to correct the metabolic alkalosis but may cause further clinical deterioration. Acidifying agents such as ammonium chloride and arginine hydrochloride can be used to correct metabolic alkalosis in these situations but also may prove hazardous. If effective arterial volume cannot be restored toward normal, hydrochloric acid can be infused through a central venous catheter. Over a 12–24 hour period 150 ml of 1 N hydrochloric acid may be administered; this procedure is also, however, not without hazard, since leakage of the acid into the mediastinum has been reported. This technique can also be applied to patients with severe renal failure. Carbonic anhydrase inhibition and hemodialysis are special techniques which may be indicated for treatment of metabolic alkalosis on rare occasions.

METABOLIC ACIDOSIS
Definition and Generation

Metabolic acidosis is a primary pathophysiologic state characterized by a gain of strong acid or a loss of bicarbonate from the extracellular fluid. The loss or gain of acid may occur through either renal or extrarenal mechanisms. It is easy to distinguish if the acidosis is caused by a gain of acid or a loss of base by calculating the anion gap. The anion gap is calculated by subtracting the sum of sodium and potassium from the sum of chloride and bicarbonate. This difference between the cations and anions represents the anions normally present in the blood which are not measured routinely (phosphate, sulfate, organic acids, etc.). The normal anion gap is 12–16 mEq/liter. Metabolic acidosis secondary to a gain of acid will be associated with an increased anion gap except when the acid gained is hydrochloric acid. Metabolic acidosis caused by a loss of base will be associated with a normal anion gap. The causes of metabolic acidosis are shown in Table 2.

Either the loss of bicarbonate from extracellular fluid or the addition of nonvolatile acid to this compartment will result in metabolic acidosis. The simplest form of metabolic acidosis resulting from the gain of acid is the administration of endogenous acids such as ammonium chloride. Disease states associated with the incomplete oxidation of lipids results in ketoacidosis, diabetes mellitus being the most common example of this form of metabolic acidosis. Similarly, incomplete oxidation of carbohydrates will result in the generation of lactic acid. Normal protein metabolism results in the formation of sulfuric and phosphoric acid which is normally excreted in the urine. The presence of renal failure will result in metabolic acidosis, which is the consequence of the failure to excrete these acids resulting from normal protein metabolism.

Both the GI tract and the kidney have the capacity to excrete bicarbonate. Thus metabolic acidosis may result from excessive loss of bicarbonate in the stool; diarrheal acidosis is the most prominent example of this type of metabolic acidosis. Disorders of renal tubular transport likewise may result in bicarbonate wastage or

Table 2
Causes of Metabolic Acidosis

General Mechanism	Specific Mechanism	Examples
Gain of Acid	Gain of exogenous acid	HCl = NH_4Cl, arginine chloride, lysine chloride, intravenous hyperalimentation; sulfuric acid—methionine
	Incomplete oxidation of fat (ketoacids)	Diabetes; starvation; alcohol
	Incomplete oxidation of carbohydrate (lactic acid)	Shock; phenformin therapy; diabetes; cirrhosis; leukemia
	Other organic acids	Methanol; paraldehyde*; ethylene glycol*
	Normal protein metabolism	Renal failure
Loss of HCO_3	Gastrointestinal loss of HCO_3	Diarrhea; loss of pancreatic, biliary or intestinal secretions; ureterosigmoidostomy; ingestion of calcium chloride; cholestyramine; or magnesium sulfate
	Renal loss of HCO_3	Distal renal tubular acidosis; proximal renal tubular acidosis

*May be due to lactic acid generation consequent to increased (NADH/NAD).

acid retention and metabolic acidosis. Both proximal and distal tubular acidosis are examples of these mechanisms.

Acidosis of renal origin can ensue through five different mechanisms: (1) impaired hydrogen ion secretion, (2) normal hydrogen ion secretion with increased acid back diffusion, (3) impaired ammonium production, (4) decreased absolute acid excretion due to reduced renal mass, and (5) loss of bicarbonate in the urine.

The first two mechanisms are involved in the pathogenesis of the distal renal tubular acidosis. Impaired ammonium production may account in part for the metabolic acidosis of hypoaldosteronism and of hyperkalemia. Loss of significant amounts of bicarbonate in the urine is the mechanism responsible for the proximal renal tubular acidosis. Reduced renal mass will result in an absolute decrease in acid excretion and metabolic acidosis.

Mechanisms for the Generation of Renal Acidosis

There are at least five types of metabolic acidosis resulting from impaired distal acidification which seem possible. As discussed below, the absence of aldosterone will impair the capacity of the distal nephron to excrete acid and will result in metabolic acidosis. The classical form of distal RTA, which may occur spontaneously or as the result of drug toxicity or systemic disease, is a form of metabolic acidosis associated with hypokalemia. Theoretically this type of defect is limited to acidification. The capacity to secrete potassium is intact; potassium wastage, which is the consequence of volume contraction, hyperaldosteronism, and an inability to exchange sodium for hydrogen, results in hypokalemia. This type of metabolic acidosis may be the result of either impaired hydrogen ion secretory capacity or an inability to maintain a normal hydrogen ion gradient between the lumen of the distal nephron and the peritubular environment (Table 3).

Recently it has become clear that some patients with distal RTA have impaired potassium secretion which accompanies their impaired acidification. This inability to secrete potassium is not the result of aldosterone deficiency. Unpublished observations made by us suggest that the inability to secrete potassium may be the result either of impaired secretory capacity for potassium or of a gradient-type defect. This gradient-type defect is, we think, the result of an inability to maintain the expected negative intratubular potential difference characteristic of the distal nephron. Thus while the capacity to secrete potassium may be intact, potassium excretion will be diminished.

Table 3
Distinction Between a Gradient RTA and Secretory RTA

	Secretory Defect	Gradient Defect
Minimal urine pH during acidosis or with NH_4Cl	> 5.5	> 5.5
Urine–blood pCO_2 gradient in maximally alkaline urine (urine pH > 7.8)	< 10 mm Hg	< 10 mm Hg
Urine pH following Na_2SO_4 infusion	> 5.5	< 5.5
Urine–blood pCO_2 gradient during neutral phosphate infusion (urine pH 6.8–7.4) or Tris administration (urine pH 6.8–8.0)	< 10 mm Hg	30 mm Hg

If the mechanisms responsible for the generation of distal RTA are not clear, the clinical consequences are. The invariable occurrence of hyperchloremia and altered potassium concentration is also accompanied with a severe form of metabolic bone disease. Because of persistent acidemia extracellular buffers are completely exhausted. Further buffering requires the titration of bone buffers, which results in osteomalacia and release of large amounts of calcium into the extracellular fluid compartment. This calcium which is lost in the urine in turn predisposes the patient with this disorder to the development of nephrocalcinosis and nephrolithiasis. All the features of the hypokalemic variety of this disorder are reversed by alkali administration.

Renal acidification defect due to decreased ammonium production. In this type of acidification defect the ability to lower urine pH should be normal, since the hydrogen ion secretory mechanism is intact; for any given urine pH ammonium excretion would be decreased in comparison to normal animals. Since the capacity to raise urinary pCO_2 (see below) in maximally alkaline urine is not dependent on ammonia production, it would be expected that urinary pCO_2 would be normal in the presence of this defect. Impaired ammonia production may account for the acidification defect due to selective aldosterone deficiency and hyperkalemia. We have demonstrated that in both conditions urinary pCO_2 in maximally alkaline urine is normal.

Recent studies from our laboratory have demonstrated that decreased distal delivery of sodium plays an important role in this form of metabolic acidosis. Patients with aldosterone deficiency are likely to waste sodium and become volume contracted. Volume contraction, by reducing glomerular filtration rate and enhancing proximal sodium reabsorption, decreases distal delivery of sodium. Without adequate amounts of sodium to be exchanged for hydrogen ion in the collecting duct, acid will be retained, ammonium excretion will be curtailed, and metabolic acidosis will result. The importance of decreased distal delivery as a pathogenetic factor in the metabolic acidosis of selective aldosterone deficiency is underscored by the fact that rats with this disorder undergo complete correction of metabolic acidosis following administration of a high sodium chloride diet.

Renal acidosis due to a reduction in nephron mass. Chronic renal failure is almost invariably associated with metabolic acidosis once the GFR falls to 25 percent of normal. The most common form of metabolic acidosis in chronic renal failure is that associated with an increased anion gap. The mechanism whereby chronic renal failure leads to metabolic acidosis seems to result from decreased excretion of ammonium. Absolute excretion of ammonium is decreased not because of any specific defect in ammonia production but simply because the number of nephrons is reduced; indeed ammonium excretion per nephron (calculated by dividing ammonium excretion per GFR) is higher than normal. Titratable acid excretion is normal or slightly decreased in renal failure, since absolute phosphate excretion is normal due to high plasma phosphate and increased parathyroid hormone levels. Bicarbonate wastage is rare in renal failure. We have recently demonstrated that bicarbonate reabsorption in patients with chronic renal failure is higher than when renal function is normal if the effect of volume expansion on bicarbonate reabsorption is taken into account. This study suggests that total hydrogen ion secretion per nephron (measured as bicarbonate reabsorption in renal failure) increases, as does ammonium excretion per nephron.

The other form of metabolic acidosis occasionally seen in patients with renal failure is associated with a normal anion gap. This form of hyperchloremic acidosis is more frequent in patients with interstitial nephritis and salt losing nephritis. It has been suggested that these patients lose the capacity to form ammonia due to the more severe involvement of the medulla. Consequently the loss of sodium with anions of endogenous metabolism leads to sodium depletion and volume contraction, which in turn leads to enhanced proximal reabsorption of sodium chloride. In the extracellular fluid the ratio of sodium in chloride is 1.4:1; reexpansion of the extracellular fluid with sodium chloride in a ratio of 1:1 will lead to hypercloremic acidosis.

This form of hyperchloremic acidosis is by no means seen exclusively in patients with interstitial nephritis. It can be present in patients with moderate chronic renal failure of any etiology. The pathogenesis of this form of acidosis seems to result from volume contraction. If a patient with moderate chronic renal failure is salt restricted, he will continue to lose sodium with anions from endogenous acid produced by metabolism. Volume contraction will enhance reabsorption of sodium chloride in a ratio of 1:1, and consequently hypercloremic acidosis almost invariably indicates contraction of effective arterial blood volume; the finding of hyperchloremic acidosis should alert the physician to look for the cause of volume contraction.

Assessment of Urinary Acidification

In the presence of metabolic acidosis, the kidney normally enhances acid excretion and lowers urine pH. The finding of a urine pH inappropriately high for the degree of metabolic acidosis indicates that impaired renal acid excretion is at least in part responsible for the metabolic acidosis. In the presence of marked metabolic acidosis the urine pH should be lower than 5.5. The finding of a urine pH higher than 5.5 indicates impaired renal acidification. Urine pH is influenced by the urine flow. In subjects excreting an acid urine, water diuresis results in an increase in urine pH (a mean increase of 0.35 pH units). Net acid excretion has been reported to be unchanged, increased, or decreased. If the urine flow is increased by osmotic diuresis, the urine pH decreases and net acid excretion increases. If there is any doubt regarding the diagnosis of renal tubular acidosis, one may assess the acidification mechanism by one of the following tests:

Ammonium chloride loading test. Ammonium chloride is administered orally in a dose of 0.1 g/kg body weight daily for 3 days. On the third day urine is collected; the urine pH then should be lower than 5.5. Wrong and Davies have used a single dose of ammonium chloride (1.9 mEq = 0.1 g/kg), and urine samples were collected hourly from 2 to 8 hours after the ammonium chloride ingestion. All urine samples after 2 hours of ingestion of ammonium chloride had urine pH levels of 5.3 or less. Ammonium and titratable acid excretion also increased normally.

Ammonium chloride is irritating to the stomach and may cause vomiting; to avoid vomiting one should use gelatin capsules of ammonium chloride. The total dose of ammonium chloride should be ingested in a period of 1 hour.

Another substance used to test acidification is calcium chloride at a dose of 2 mEq/kg body weight (calcium chloride should be dissolved in water). In the small bowel the following reaction takes place:

$$CaCl_2 + 2NaHCO_3 \rightleftharpoons CaCO_3 + 2NaCl + CO_2 + H_2O$$

Oral administration of $CaCl_2$ thus causes a loss of bicarbonate from the gastrointestinal tract and thus can result in metabolic acidosis. Ammonium chloride and calcium chloride have been shown to give the same results when used to assess urinary acidification. Calcium chloride should be used in patients who cannot tolerate ammonium chloride or in patients who have a contraindication to ammonium chloride ingestion (e.g., cirrhosis).

Sodium sulfate infusion. Administration of sodium sulfate to normal subjects who are avidly retaining sodium results in a decrease in the urine pH and increased ammonium excretion. If the subject is not reabsorbing sodium avidly, sodium sulfate increases the urine pH apparently by acting as an osmotic diuretic and increasing bicarbonate excretion. Patients to be tested with sodium sulfate must receive a salt retaining hormone (9α-fluorohydrocorticosterone, 1 mg orally over a period of 12 hours, or deoxycorticosterone acetate, 5 mg intramuscularly 12 hours and 2–4 hours before the study). If the subjects are put on a low-salt diet the test will give more reliable results. One liter of 4 percent sodium sulfate is infused over 40–60 min. Sodium bicarbonate is added to the sodium sulfate infusion in order to avoid acidosis secondary to rapid sodium sulfate infusion (30 mEq sodium bicarbonate per liter of sodium sulfate). Urine collections should continue for 2–3 hours after sodium sulfate infusion is discontinued. Normal individuals lower urine pH below 5.5, and in most of them urine pH falls below 5.

In the presence of a stimulus for sodium retention, sodium sulfate increases the negative intratubular po-

tential (sulfate is a nonreabsorbable anion). Since net hydrogen ion excretion is apparently the result of active hydrogen ion secretion minus passive hydrogen ion back diffusion, sodium sulfate likely increases net hydrogen ion excretion by increasing the negative intratubular potential and thereby restricts passive back diffusion of hydrogen ion.

The major disadvantage of sodium sulfate is that it does not lower the urine pH if the subject is not reabsorbing sodium avidly. Urinary sodium concentration before sodium sulfate infusion should be low in order to facilitate an adequate assessment of the response to sodium sulfate. The lack of acidification with sodium sulfate can either indicate that there is an acidification defect or that the individual was not reabsorbing sodium avidly.

Hydrogen ion secretion in the distal nephron is dependent on the sodium for hydrogen ion exchange. If there is inadequate delivery of sodium to the distal nephron due to enhanced sodium reabsorption in the more proximal parts of the nephron, hydrogen ion secretion may be impaired. Sodium sulfate infusion increases distal delivery of sodium and enhances acid excretion. It has been suggested that patients with cirrhosis have a distal acidification defect when tested with calcium chloride administration. Another study, however, demonstrated that patients with cirrhosis showed a normal response to sodium sulfate infusion. It is possible that the lack of acidification with calcium chloride was due to inadequate distal delivery of sodium; sodium sulfate infusion, by increasing distal delivery of sodium, promoted hydrogen ion secretion. Alternatively, the failure to enhance hydrogen ion secretion with calcium chloride and the normal response to sodium sulfate could mean that increased acid back diffusion may account for the acidosis of some patients with cirrhosis.

Sodium sulfate infusion apparently stimulates hydrogen ion secretion by restricting back diffusion of hydrogen ion. One would expect sodium sulfate infusion to result in a normal acidification if the mechanism of the acidification defect is increased acid back diffusion; on the other hand, if the acidification defect is due to impaired hydrogen ion secretion, one would expect no response to sodium sulfate infusion (Table 3).

Urinary carbon dioxide tension. Alkalinization of the urine (pH > 7.8) results in an increase in urinary pCO_2 to a value considerably above that of plasma. The high urinary pCO_2 of alkaline urine has been attributed to delayed dehydration of carbonic acid. Carbonic anhydrase is not present on the luminal epithelial cell surface of the distal nephron. Therefore the dehydration of carbonic acid proceeds slowly such that it occurs to a large extent after the urine has left the nephron and is in the "lower" urinary tract, where the suface to volume relationship is such that the diffusion of carbon dioxide from urine to blood is not favored.

When the urine pH is less alkaline, about 7, the urinary pCO_2 also may be considerably higher than that of plasma provided that sufficient amounts of phosphate are present in the urine. In this instance hydrogen ion secreted from the distal nephron is partitioned between HCO_3^- and HPO_4^{2-}; $H_2PO_4^{2-}$ serving as buffer in turn may donate a hydrogen ion which will titrate HCO_3^- in the "lower" urinary tract to H_2CO_3, resulting in a high urinary CO_2 tension. Note that in both these instances, urinary pH 7 or urinary pH 8, the high urinary pCO_2 has been attributed to hydrogen ion secretion by the distal nephron.

Another mechanism for the formation of a high urinary pCO_2 which does not require the secretion of hydrogen ion by the distal nephron is the reaction of HCO_3^- with HCO_3^-, which forms H_2CO_3 and CO_3^{2-}. The H_2CO_3 formed in turn will break down and form CO_2. Thus the concentration of the urine in the collecting duct under conditions of alkaline diuresis results in an increase in the concentration of urinary $HCO_3\cap-$. This increase in urinary HCO_3^- in and of itself will raise urinary pCO_2. As can be seen,

$$\text{Acidification } H^+ \searrow$$
$$+ HCO_3^- \rightleftarrows H_2CO_3 \rightleftarrows CO_2 + H_2O$$
$$\text{Concentration } HCO_3^- \nearrow$$

The high urinary pCO_2 of an alkaline urine is the sum of the H_2CO_3 formed as a result of H^+ secretion and the result of urinary concentration which increases urinary HCO_3^- concentration. Thus, states associated with marked impairment of urinary concentrating ability, e.g., chronic renal failure, will be associated with a diminished urinary pCO_2 even in the face of normal or accelerated H^+ secretion when the urine is highly alkaline. There is no question, however, that the elevated pCO_2 observed in less alkaline urine is solely the result of H^+ secretion, provided that adequate amounts of phosphate buffer are present.

Bicarbonate titration. Another method to assess proximal and distal acidification defects is to measure bicarbonate reabsorption at different plasma bicarbonate levels. This can be done by infusing sodium bicarbonate in order to produce stepwise increments in plasma bicarbonate. For each increase in plasma bicarbonate (e.g. 4 mEq/liter), bicarbonate concentrations in the blood and urine and glomerular filtration rate are determined. Bicarbonate reabsorption can be calculated and plotted against plasma bicarbonate. At low plasma levels normal individuals reabsorb 100 percent of the filtered bicarbonate, and as the plasma level increases reabsorption increases until the plasma level reaches 24–26 mEq/liter. Bicarbonate then starts to appear in the urine (renal bicarbonate threshold). At a plasma level of about 28 mEq/liter bicarbonate reabsorption is maximal [tubular maximum (T_m) for bicarbonate].

In patients with distal renal tubular acidosis bicarbonate reabsorption is incomplete at low plasma levels of bicarbonate. At normal plasma bicarbonate levels the fraction of filtered bicarbonate excreted in the urine is around 3 percent (calculated by dividing bicarbonate excreted by filtered bicarbonate). Bicarbonate T_m thus is normal or slightly increased. In proximal renal tubular acidosis there is a defect in the proximal tubule with a decrease in the bicarbonate T_m, or, alternatively, bicarbonate T_m is normal but there is increased splay of the bicarbonate titration curve. In both situations large amounts of bicarbonate are spilled in the urine; the fraction of filtered bicarbonate excreted in the urine at normal plasma bicarbonate levels is greater than 15 percent. At low plasma bicarbonate levels bicarbonate reabsorption is complete and the urine pH may be appropriately acid. Thus, it is important to realize that one may have proximal renal tubular acidosis with an acid urine pH. The urine becomes alkaline when the plasma is increased to normal levels.

Diagnosis

The diagnosis of metabolic acidosis can be made by identifying a clinical cause known to produce metabolic acidosis accompanied by laboratory values (low pH, low bicarbonate, etc.) associated with metabolic acidosis. It cannot be overemphasized that this diagnosis, or that of any acid–base disturbance, cannot be made on the basis of laboratory values alone. Both history and appropriate laboratory values are required for a diagnosis to be made.

Once the diagnosis has been established, the kind of metabolic acidosis present can be determined without much difficulty. The presence of an anion gap steers the clinician to a consideration of one of the seven types of metabolic acidosis listed in Table 4. History, physical, and laboratory data should point to the final diagnosis without difficulty.

If the metabolic acidosis is not associated with an anion gap it will be associated with hyperchloremia. Only three events result in hyperchloremia—hyperchloremia will be manifested in patients with hyperchloremic metabolic acidosis, with respiratory alkalosis, and with dehydration. The effects of dehydration can be assessed by examining the serum sodium concentration. If the serum sodium is not elevated, then the hyperchloremia is not the result of dehydration and must be the result of either metabolic acidosis or respiratory alkalosis. If hypernatremia is present, one can correct the chloride concentration for the degree of dehydration; if the chloride concentration after this correction is still elevated, then dehydration is accompanied by an acid–base disturbance. Evaluation of the patient's history and laboratory values are then necessary to distinguish hyperchloremic metabolic acidosis from respiratory alkalosis.

Hyperchloremic metabolic acidosis may be the result of ammonium chloride administration, loss of sodium bicarbonate from diarrhea, or loss of bicarbonate and retention of acid by the kidney. Patients ingesting ammonium chloride should have a history of doing so and should have a maximally acid urine pH and high values of urinary ammonium. Patients with diarrhea will likewise have a very low urine pH (less than 5.5) and high urinary ammonium excretion.

Patients with proximal renal tubular acidosis may have evidence of other defects in proximal tubular transport, i.e., phosphaturia, glycosuria, uricosuria, and amino aciduria (Table 5). Bicarbonate reabsorption, as assessed by bicarbonate loading studies, will be depressed, but these patients will acidify their urine normally if they are allowed to develop severe degrees of acidemia. Patients with distal renal tubular acidosis will not acidify the urine maximally (pH > 5.5, usually > 6.0) despite the presence of severe acidemia. Patients with aldosterone deficiency will lower the urine pH to levels seen in normal subjects with severe acidemia; ammonium excretion, however, will be low and plasma and urinary aldosterone levels will also likely be low. This form of metabolic acidosis is also associated with hyperchloremia.

Respiratory Compensation to Metabolic Acidosis

The first line of defense against metabolic acidosis is titration of the hydrogen ion by the body buffers. In addition there is a prompt increase in alveolar ventilation with increased elimination of carbon dioxide. It has been suggested that the hyperventilation of metabolic acidosis is mediated by the stimulation of chemoreceptors in the carotid and aortic bodies. The maximum respiratory compensation in metabolic acidosis is achieved in 24 hours. For each mEq decrease in bicarbonate one would expect a decrease in plasma pCO_2 of 1.3 mm Hg. The finding of plasma pCO_2 lower than the expected value indicates the presence of an associated primary respiratory alkalosis; if the pCO_2 is higher than the expected value there is either an associated respiratory acidosis or not enough time has elapsed for maximum compensation. Respiratory compensation minimizes the changes in blood pH, but it is usually not sufficient to keep the blood pH within normal limits. It is also important to realize that it is physiologically impossible to lower plasma pCO_2 below 10 mm Hg, and thus if respiratory compensation is at maximum level further deterioration of the acidosis will not be accompanied by additional respiratory compensation.

Table 4
Causes of Increases in Anion Gap

Metabolic acidosis
Lactic acidosis
Ketoacidosis
Renal failure
Paraldehyde
Salicylate
Methanol
Ethylene glycol
Metabolic alkalosis

Physiological Consequences of Metabolic Acidosis

Acidosis causes a depression of myocardial contractility and thus can impair cardiac function. Acidosis also increases the release of catecholamines; the effect of these substances on myocardial contractility may counteract the effect of acidosis, and cardiac function may thus remain normal. In peripheral vessels similar to the heart, acidosis tends to decrease peripheral resistance whereas catecholamines tend to increase it; the net result may be an increase or decrease in peripheral resistance depending on which factor predominates. Pulmonary artery and peripheral veins respond to acidosis with increased vasoconstriction.

Acidosis shifts the oxyhemoglobin dissociation curve to the right, and this increases the availability of oxygen to the tissues. On the other hand, acidosis may decrease 2,3-diphosphoglycerate (2,3-DPG) in the red blood cell; a decrease in 2,3-DPG may shift the oxyhemoglobin dissociation curve to the left and thus may neutralize the effect of acidosis per se on the dissociation of this curve.

Treatment

It is important to determine the cause of metabolic acidosis and remove or control it. For example, in most patients with diabetic ketoacidosis control of diabetes alone will be sufficient to correct the metabolic acidosis. If the metabolic acidosis is severe and symptomatic it should be treated with sodium bicarbonate. Plasma bicarbonate should not be returned to normal because

Table 5
Classification and Types of Renal Tubular Acidosis

Mechanism	Example
Impaired proximal H$^+$	
Secretion (proximal RTA)	Proximal RTA
	Franconi's syndrome
	Tetracycline
	Acetazolamide
Impaired distal acidification	
Impaired H$^+$ secretion	Classical distal RTA (?)
	Hyperglobulinemic states (?)
Increased acid back diffusion	Amphotericin (?)
	Classical distal RTA (?)
	Hyperglobulinemic states (?)
Mineralocorticoid deficiency	Addison's disease
	Selective hypoaldosteronism

the patient is hyperventilating and hyperventilation will continue after the acidosis is corrected; this return of plasma bicarbonate to normal will result in overcompensated metabolic alkalosis. The amount of sodium bicarbonate used to raise the plasma bicarbonate can be calculated in the following way: Normally the ratio of plasma bicarbonate concentration to carbonic acid (arterial $pCO_2 \times 0.03$) is 20. A ratio of 20, when fitted to the Henderson-Hasselbalch equation [$pH = 6.1 + \log(HCO_3/H_2CO_3)$] gives a pH of 7.4 (the log of 20 is 1.3). Thus, the amount of bicarbonate to be infused should not raise this ratio above 20. For example, a patient with a bicarbonate concentration of 6 mEq/liter and plasma pCO_2 of 20 mm Hg should not have plasma bicarbonate raised above 12 mEq/liter [$6/(0.03 \times 20) = 10$; $12/(0.03 \times 20) = 20$].

Desired plasma bicarbonate minus actual plasma bicarbonate equals deficit of bicarbonate per liter; total body water equals 60 percent of body weight; total bicarbonate deficit equals total body water times deficit of bicarbonate per liter. For example, a patient weighing 50 kg has metabolic acidosis with a plasma bicarbonate of 12 mEq/liter and one wants to raise his plasma bicarbonate to 18 mEq/liter. Bicarbonate deficit is $18 - 12 = 6$ mEq/liter; total body water is $0.6 \times 50 = 30$; total bicarbonate deficit is $30 \times 6 = 180$ mEq. It is important to realize that the volume of distribution of bicarbonate approximates total body water and not extracellular water. In some patients with metabolic acidosis the amount of bicarbonate required to raise the plasma bicarbonate may be higher than the amount calculated by the method described above. There are a few conditions in which this situation may happen: (1) when there is continuous external loss of bicarbonate; (2) when there is continuous production of acid, e.g., lactic acid, which consumes the bicarbonate which is being infused, and (3) in some patients with severe metabolic acidosis the amount of sodium bicarbonate required to raise the plasma bicarbonate to the desired level may be four or five times greater than the calculated value. It has been recently demonstrated that in patients with severe metabolic acidosis the amount of bicarbonate remaining in the extracellular fluid is much less than in patients with moderate metabolic acidosis or in patients with normal plasma bicarbonate. In severe metabolic acidosis there is considerable intracellular hydrogen ion buffering. Hydrogen ions move in and potassium leaves the cell. During correction of this form of metabolic acidosis the reverse sequence of events occurs: hydrogen ions leave the cell and potassium enters the cell (it is also possible that bicarbonate enters the cell). This explains why the amount of sodium bicarbonate may be greater than the calculated value.

There are other alkalinizing agents, such as Tris, sodium lactate, and sodium acetate. Sodium bicarbonate is clearly better than these agents, and there is probably no indication for their use.

ACUTE AND CHRONIC RESPIRATORY ALKALOSIS
Definition

Respiratory alkalosis is a primary pathophysiologic state characterized by an increase in alveolar ventilation (CO_2 excretion) relative to CO_2 production. A primary reduction in pCO_2 will lead to an increased pH. It will also be associated with a slight decrease in bicarbonate concentration. This reduction in bicarbonate concentration occurs immediately upon reduction in pCO_2 and slightly minimizes the increase in pH. With maximal hyperventilation the plasma bicarbonate may decrease to values as low as 15 mEq/liter. This effect is due to tissue buffering and does not represent any renal compensatory mechanism. It is reversible immediately upon return of the pCO_2 to normal.

Causes

Table 6 shows a list of clinical conditions associated with respiratory alkalosis. To produce respiratory alkalosis, hyperventilation must be present. Hypoxia, however, may or may not be present. In pulmonary diseases, for example, the stimulus for hyperventilation is hypoxia, and this will lead to hyperventilation. Since CO_2 is 20 times more diffusable than O_2, hypoxia will be associated with hypocapnia. On the other hand, if the stimulus for hyperventilation is in the central nervous system, such as in salicylate intoxication, hypoxia will not be present.

Ionic Transfers Between Intracellular and Extracellular Fluid

In acute respiratory alkalosis plasma bicarbonate falls and pH and plasma chloride increase. There is also a significant decrease in plasma phosphate concentration. Intracellular hydrogen ion concentration decreases; this is due to a movement of hydrogen ion out of the cell to the extracellular fluid to minimize changes in blood pH. The hydrogen ion that leaves the cell is replaced by the movement of sodium and potassium into the cell. There is an exchange between chloride and bicarbonate as chloride leaves the cell and is replaced by bicarbonate. Only about half of the decrement in plasma bicarbonate can be accounted for by the observed concomitant changes in sodium, potassium, and chloride. Lactic acid generation is increased and is responsible for about 35 percent of the reduction in plasma bicarbonate concentration.

Thus, the acute defense of respiratory acidosis is due to a combination of renal (see below) and extrarenal mechanisms. Bicarbonate is lost in the urine and acid is retained. Hydrogen ion leaves the cell; lactic acid is generated at an increased rate. All of these events serve to return the plasma pH toward normal.

Chronic Respiratory Alkalosis

The mechanism by which adaption to chronic hypocapnia takes places works via a marked decrease in net acid excretion. This decrease in net acid excretion is achieved mainly through a decrease in ammonium excretion. The remainder of the fall in net acid excretion

Table 6
Causes of Respiratory Alkalosis and Acidosis

Location	Mechanism	Examples
Respiratory alkalosis		
Central nervous system	Direct stimulation of the respiratory center	Emotion Acetylsalicylic acid Organic disease Progesterone
Peripheral chemoreceptors	Reflex stimulation of the respiratory center	Hypoxemia
Intrathoracic receptors	Reflex stimulation of the respiratory center	Localized pulmonary disease
Respiratory acidosis		
Central nervous system	Inhibition of respiratory center	Drugs (opiates, anesthetics, sedatives), brain lesion
Nerves, muscles, chest well	Impaired function of nerves, muscles, or the chest wall	Nerves —poliomyelitis Muscle —miasthenia gravis Chest wall—trauma
Alveolar capillary	Impaired gas exhange	Emphysema Pulmonary edema

is due to a decrease in titratable acid excretion; no significant loss of bicarbonate occurs in the urine. This suppression of acid excretion in patients on a normal salt diet is mediated by a decrease in sodium reabsorption. When sodium is not available the adaptation is mediated through enhanced potassium excretion. The suppression of acid excretion during chronic hypocapnia is quite marked and is sufficient to prevent a major decrease in plasma hydrogen ion concentration. For example, after pCO_2 reduction to 15–20 mm Hg, plasma hydrogen ion concentration decreases by only 2–5 nm/liter. It therefore follows that adaptation to chronic hypocapnia is almost 100 percent complete.

It should be emphasized that the defense of pH is significantly more effective in chronic hypocapnia than in chronic hypercapnia. In chronic hypercapnia, the plasma hydrogen ion concentration increases 0.33 nm/liter with each mm Hg increase in pCO_2; in chronic hypocapnia plasma hydrogen ion concentration decreases only 0.17 nm/liter with each mm Hg decrease in pCO_2.

Treatment

There is no specific treatment for respiratory alkalosis except eliminating the underlying cause.

RESPIRATORY ACIDOSIS

Definition

Respiratory acidosis is a primary pathophysiologic state characterized by a decrease in alveolar ventilation (CO_2 excretion) relative to CO_2 production. A primary increase in plasma pCO_2 will result in a decrease in blood pH. During acute respiratory acidosis the plasma bicarbonate increases slightly, approximately 1 mEq per each 10 mm Hg increase in pCO_2. This increase in plasma bicarbonate occurs within minutes and is secondary to the titration of body buffer. As a consequence of the increase in pCO_2 there is a shift of the equilibrium of the following reaction to the left,

$$H + HCO_3 \rightleftharpoons H_2CO_3 \rightleftharpoons CO_2 + H_2O$$

with a consequent increase in plasma HCO_3. Inasmuch as the increase in plasma bicarbonate is of small magnitude, this mechanism of tissue buffering is not very effective in minimizing the effect of hypercapnia on the blood pH. In acute respiratory acidosis there are ionic exchanges between extracellular and intracellular fluid. Potassium and bicarbonate leave the cell in exchange for hydrogen ion and chloride (red cell), hence the development of hyperkalemia and hypochloremia during acute respiratory acidosis.

Causes

The causes of respiratory acidosis are shown in Table 6.

Chronic Hypercapnia

The mechanism responsible for the adaptation to chronic hypercapnia has been well studied in dogs. Plasma bicarbonate concentration rises during the first day of exposure to a high carbon dioxide environment and continues to rise slowly over the next 5–6 days to a final concentration of 35–38 mEq/liter. The rise in plasma bicarbonate concentration during the first day is mainly due to tissue buffering because acid excretion is practically unchanged. Over the following days net acid excretion is markedly enhanced, accounting for the estimated increase in the extracellular bicarbonate concentration. Plasma chloride concentration decreases in an inverse fashion with bicarbonate, and chloride excretion is enhanced.

Recovery from hypercapnia was studied in dogs with normal and low-salt diets. The animals on a normal salt diet showed a prompt reduction in plasma bicarbonate concentration to normal, and plasma chloride rose simultaneously to normal. By contrast, in the animals on a low-salt diet bicarbonate concentration did not return to normal levels and the animals became mildly alkalotic. When the animals on a low-salt diet were put on a normal salt diet, the plasma bicarbonate concentration returned to normal and the alkalosis was corrected. These results indicate that volume contracted subjects with respiratory acidosis reclaim the bicarbonate generated by chronic hypercapnia because of enhanced proximal reabsorption and thus maintain a high plasma bicarbonate concentration.

The pattern of adaptation to chronic respiratory acidosis in man has been derived by studying patients with chronic lung disease. In patients with uncomplicated respiratory acidosis the plasma bicarbonate is usually less than 45 mEq/liter even when the plasma pCO_2 is as high as 100 mm Hg. The relationship between hydrogen ion concentration and pCO_2 is linear in both acute and chronic respiratory acidosis, but the slope of H^+/pCO_2 is strikingly different between acute and chronic hypercapnia; for each 1 mm increase in pCO_2 hydrogen ion concentration increases 0.77 nmol/liter in acute hypercapnia but only 0.32 nmol/liter in chronic hypercapnia. Values of hydrogen ion concentration and plasma bicarbonate outside the expected range should alert the clinician for the presence of mixed acid–base disturbances. History and careful clinical evaluation of the patient are the essential requirements in order to make the accurate diagnosis of mixed acid–base disturbances.

The symptoms of acute respiratory acidosis are those of carbon dioxide narcosis; headache, confusion, blurred vision, tremor, asterixis, delerium, and coma. In chronic hypercapnia the patient may be asymptomatic.

Treatment

The treatment of acute respiratory acidosis is aimed at restoring normal ventilation by treating the underlying disease and appropriate supportive measures (such as bronchodilators, use of artificial respirators, etc.). There is no indication for the use of sodium bicarbonate in acute hypercapnia except in the presence of life-threatening acidosis (blood pH < 7.0). In chronic respiratory acidosis the treatment is again directed towards improving the alveolar ventilation. Sudden normalization of plasma pCO_2 in patients with chronic respiratory acidosis through the use of artificial ventilation may lead to a marked rise in blood pH because the renal excretion of bicarbonate lags behind (usually 24–48 hours) the rapid respiratory correction of the pCO_2. This sudden rise in blood pH may cause dizziness, coma, and death. This problem can be avoided if the pCO_2 is decreased slowly and time is allowed for the kidney to excrete the excess bicarbonate. In the presence of volume contraction the kidneys will not be able to excrete the excess bicarbonate owing to the enhanced proximal reabsorption, and the state of posthypercapnic metabolic alkalosis will ensue.

REFERENCES

Arruda JAL, Kurtzman NA: Metabolic acidosis and alkalosis. Clin Nephrol 5:215, 1977

Arruda JAL, Kurtzman NA: Metabolic and respiratory alkalosis, in Kurtzman NA, Martinez-Maldonado M (eds): Pathophysiology of the Kidney. Springfield, Ill., Charles C. Thomas, 1977, p 354

Kurtzman NA, White MG, Rogers PW: Pathophysiology of metabolic alkalosis. Arch Intern Med 131:702, 1973

Rector RC Jr: Acidification of the urine, in Orloff S, Berliner RW (eds): Handbook of Physiology, Baltimore, Williams & Wilkins, 1973, p 431

Sebastian A, McSherry E, Morris RC Jr: Metabolic acidosis with special reference to renal acidosis, in Brenner B, Rector FC Jr (eds): The Kidney, vol. 2. Philadelphia, W.B. Saunders, 1976, p 615

Seldin DW, Rector FC Jr: The generation and maintenance of metabolic alkalosis. Kidney Int 1:306, 1972

Thier SO, McCurdy DK, Rastegar A: Metabolic and Respiratory Acidosis, in Kurtzman NA, Martinez-Maldonado M (eds): Pathophysiology of the Kidney. Springfield, Ill., Charles C. Thomas, 1957, p 335

Specific Renal Diseases

IMMUNOLOGIC CONSIDERATIONS*

Curtis B. Wilson

Two well defined humoral immune mechanisms appear to be responsible for most glomerulonephritis and an undetermined amount of tubulointerstitial nephritis in man. The most frequently found mechanism involves the formation of circulating antigen–antibody complexes (with exogenous or endogenous antigens) as part of the body's normal immunologic surveillance or in association with autoimmune responses. These immune complexes have no specificity for the kidney but become trapped within the glomerulus, where they can cause an inflammatory reaction. The less frequent of these mechanisms of immunologic renal injury involves the formation of antibodies specific for antigens in or of the kidney. In man, the only nephritogenic immune response of this type found to date is that of antibodies reactive with antigens present in the glomerular basement membrane (GBM) or occasionally within the tubular basement membrane (TBM). Other antigenic systems in the glomeruli are currently being identified in experimental models and may someday become important in human disease.

These two mechanisms of immunologic injury can be differentiated by their distinctive patterns of immunoglobulin deposition (Fig. 1). Anti–basement membrane antibodies react in a smooth linear pattern along the GBM or TBM; immune complexes that settle randomly out of circulating blood appear as irregular granular deposits on the membranes when viewed by the immunofluorescent technique (see the chapter on *Immunofluorescence*).

Immunologic reactions induced nonspecifically (by the deposition of circulating immune complexes) or specifically (by anti–basement membrane antibodies) activate mediators of immunologic injury. For example,

*This is publication 1615 from the Department of Immunopathology, Research Institute of Scripps Clinic, 10666 N. Torrey Pines Rd., La Jolla, Calif. This work was supported in part by USPHS Grants AM-20043, AM-18626, and AI-07007 and BRS Grant RRO-5514.

in experimentally produced glomerulonephritis, glomerular fixation of anti-GBM antibodies usually leads to the rapid fixation of complement, the products of which attract and trap polymorphonuclear leukocytes through chemotaxis and immune adherence. The polymorphonuclear leukocytes contain many materials that are phlogogenic, including lysozymal enzymes that can fragment and solubilize the GBM.

Complement components almost always accompany presumed immune complex deposition in human glomeruli but, curiously, are found less frequently in patients with anti-GBM antibody-induced nephritis. In addition to mediating injury by activating complement proteins, immune reactions also result in release of vasoactive substances and activation of the kinin and coagulation systems. Possible contributions from the latter three mediators to immunologic renal injury in man has not yet been clearly defined.

Interest has focused recently on possible "nonimmunologic" activation of mediators, such as complement, that could initiate or perpetuate renal injury. Complement components can be identified in glomeruli and tubulointerstitial tissue of kidneys in the absence of detectable immunoglobulin deposits, therefore possibly accumulating from a nonimmunologic cause. Proteins of the coagulation system are also found in kidneys, perhaps as "nonimmune" mediators of renal injury in conditions such as systemic coagulopathies, hemolytic uremic syndrome, or eclampsia.

The major immunologic processes that lead to glomerular injury center around humoral immune responses; cellular mechanisms appear to play only minor roles. In contrast, cellular infiltration is often a prominent feature of tubulointerstitial nephritis, although the exact contribution of cellular immunity to this condition is not clear.

RENAL DISEASES CAUSED BY DEPOSITION OF CIRCULATING IMMUNE COMPLEXES

Experimental Models of Immune Complex Induced Renal Injury

Experimental immune complex glomerulonephritis. Experimental serum sickness glomerulonephritis. The principles by which deposition of

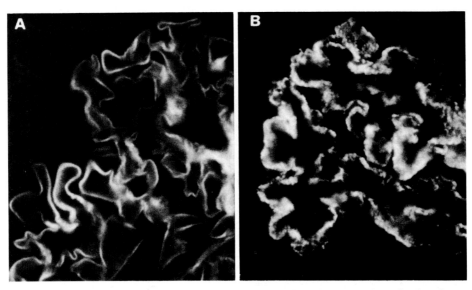

Fig. 1. (A) Linear deposits of IgG are seen outlining the GBM of a glomerular tuft taken from a patient with anti-GBM antibody-induced glomerulonephritis. (B) Irregular granular deposits of IgG, typical of those seen in patients with immune complex forms of glomerulonephritis, can be contrasted with the smooth, continuous deposits of anti-GBM antibodies shown in part A.

circulating immune complexes in the glomeruli leads to renal injury are best understood by considering experimental esrum sickness. After one injects large amounts of foreign serum proteins such as bovine serum albumin (BSA) into rabbits, the BSA equilibrates in the intra- and extravascular fluids and then disappears from the circulation at a rate determined by its nonimmune catabolism. Four to five days after infection, antibody forms and begins to combine with the circulating antigen. Initially, small immune complexes form because of the excess circulating antigen; however, as antibody production increases, the immune complexes enlarge sufficiently to be removed by the reticuloendothelial system. During this phase of immune elimination, immune complexes become trapped in the vascular beds including the glomerulus, and glomerulonephritis thus results. Quantitative studies have shown that about 18 μg of immune complexed antigen, or 4.4×10^8 molecules of antigen per glomerulus, deposit in the kidneys of each rabbit, where they incite a severe but transient inflammatory response. Once deposited, the complexes are in equilibrium with antigen or antibody from the circulation, so that their final composition may be continuously modified.

Rabbits can also be given BSA daily in amounts (10–200 mg) calculated to balance their antibody production, which causes chronic serum sickness and nephritis over an immunization period of 6–8 weeks (Fig. 2A). The types of nephritis that develop in this manner resemble the entire spectrum of glomerulonephritis lesions identified in man. Approximately 0.5 percent of the daily dose of antigen deposits by the time proteinuric glomerulonephritis is overt in this model. The half-disappearance rate of the antigen from the glomeruli is on the order of 5 days. Circulating antigen

and antibody continue to interact with the glomerular immune complex deposits. The most convincing evidence of the ongoing interaction is that the glomerular-bound complexes can be removed from the glomeruli by injecting the animals with a huge excess of antigen, which is known to dissociate antigen–antibody complexes. If rabbits are so treated before irreversible renal damage occurs, the antigen excess therapy can reverse the process.

Glomerular histologic responses in this model vary; early mesangial changes are followed by diffuse proliferative, proliferative and crescent-forming, or predominantly membranous forms of glomerulonephritis. The histologic manifestations seem to relate to the intensity and tempo with which the immune complex deposits within the mesangium and/or glomerular capillary wall. These varied histologic responses to a single immunogenic stimulus indicate that the form that glomerulonephritis assumes in large part reflects the host's response rather than the inciting mechanism. Routine histologic examination of the kidney, then, is of little use in identifying the immunopathogenic mechanism that is responsible; instead, detailed immunopathologic study is needed. Studies in the serum sickness model suggest that several interrelated events influence the glomerular deposition of immune complexes from the circulation. The size of the complex, determined largely by the relative antigen–antibody ratio, is of great importance. The avidity of the antibody may also affect the size and stability of the complex. Very large complexes tend to localize in the glomerular mesangium, and smaller complexes seem to deposit in the glomerular capillary wall. Vasoactive amines released during the antigen–antibody reactions that end in immune complex formation appear to be important in altering

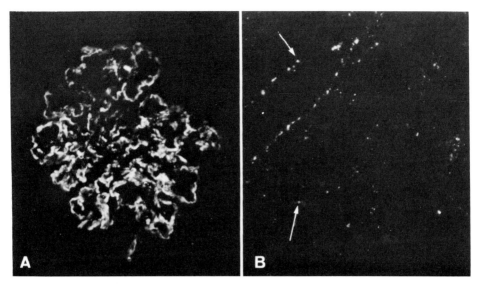

Fig. 2. (A) Typical diffuse granular deposits of BSA are observed in glomerular immune complex deposits in a rabbit with chronic serum sickness glomerulonephritis. (B) Extraglomerular deposits of BSA are observed in immune complexes deposited along the tubular basement membranes and peritubular capillaries of a rabbit with chronic serum sickness nephritis.

vascular and perhaps glomerular permeability and so enhance the deposition of the complexes, particularly in acute forms of serum sickness. The efficiency of handling of immune complexes by the reticuloendothelial system also influences the persistence of immune complexes in the ciruclation, thereby having an impact on the deposition of complexes in the vascular tissue. The mesangial area of the kidney seems to process aggregated or immune complexed proteins and could influence their glomerular pathogenicity. Hemodynamic factors are also of considerable importance, with alterations in blood flow, hypertension, and interruptions in the continuity of flow by bifurcations or constrictions all elements that participate in immune complex deposition.

In man, the glomerular capillary bed appears to be more susceptible to immune complex deposition than other capillary beds; in fact, the deposition may be confined to this locale in many primary immune complex glomerulonephritides. In systemic immune complex disorders, particularly when the load of circulating immune complexes is overwhelming, these complexes localize in many vascular beds, leading to the manifestations of diffuse vasculitis. All circulating complexes in man, however, do not settle within the glomerular capillary bed. Generally little glomerular deposition occurs in patients with rheumatoid arthritis, in spite of continued and significant amounts of immune complex material in their circulation.

Other experimental models of immune complex glomerulonephritis. A rather large array of experimental immune complex glomerulonephritides is available for study. Several experimental viral infections, particularly those of a chronic nature, produce immune complex glomerulonephritis in a number of experimental laboratory animals. Antigens derived from the hosts of experimental bacterial or protozoan infections can also cause glomerulonephritis in animals. Endogenous antigens are also identifiable in experimental immune complex nephritis, with DNA and other nuclear materials as well as murine retroviral antigens found in several strains of mice that spontaneously develop an autoimmune disease similar to systemic lupus erythematosus in man. Other endogenous antigens, such as thyroglobulin, erythrocyte antigens, histocompatibility antigens, and renal tubular epithelial antigens, have also been implicated in spontaneous or experimental immune complex nephritis in animals. Experimental thyroiditis, for example, can be induced in rabbits immunized with thyroglobulin, which leads to the formation of circulating antithyroglobulin antibody. Purposeful liberation of large amounts of thyroglobulin through radiation induced thyroid injury can shift the ratio of antigen and antibody, favoring the formation of nephritogenic circulating immune complexes.

Experimental immune complex induced tubulointerstitial nephritis. An experimental situation in which the amount of immune complex formed is large allows complexes to deposit within the extraglomerular renal tissue, including the TBM, peritubular capillaries, and interstitium (Fig. 2B). Rabbits with chronic serum sicknesses that form large amounts of immune complexes contain these extraglomerular deposits in addition to rather widespread systemic vascular deposits of immune complexes. Similar extraglomerular deposits are identifiable in some mice from the strains that are susceptible to systemic lupus erythematosus–like immune complex disease; however, since the quantity of immune complexes does not seem to be the sole determinant governing the deposition in extraglomerular sites, the nature of the complexes or other factors must be considered. For example, immune complexes formed during acute serum sickness more often deposit in extraglomerular vascular sites than complexes formed during chronic serum sickness, even though the overall quantities of immune complexes may be much greater in the latter model.

Immune complexes can also form directly within the renal tissue of rabbits immunized against renal tubular antigens. These rabbits develop tubulointerstitial nephritis without glomerular deposits of immune complexes. Complexes apparently form when antigen diffusing from the tubular cells interacts with antibody in the extravascular fluids. This type of in situ immune complex formation also occurs in the thyroid glands of mice with experimentally induced thyroiditis and in

rabbits that develop orchitis subsequent to vasectomy, but it is unknown so far in humans with nephritis.

Immune Complex Induced Renal Disease in Man

Immune complex glomerulonephritis in man. Clinical–pathologic features. When examined with immunofluorescence, approximately 80 percent of renal biopsies from patients with glomerulonephritis contain granular immunoglobulin and complement deposits (Figs. 3A–3C). Since the antigen(s) in these granular deposits usually is not known, one can only assume that the complexes are of immunologic origin and that the patients have immune complex induced glomerulonephritis. The assumption seems justifiable in view of the available clinical and experimental data. The glo-

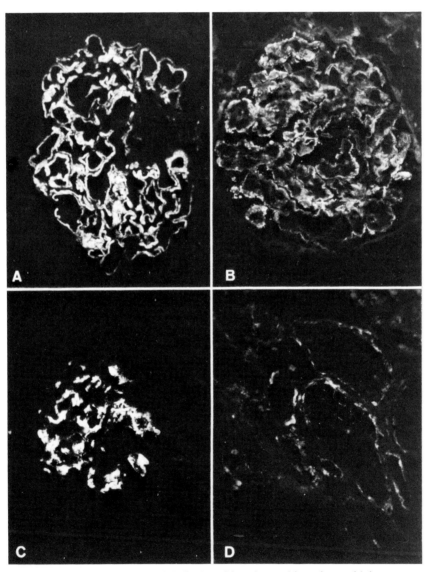

Fig. 3. Differing patterns of immunoglobulin deposition observed in patients with immune complex induced renal disease. (A) Diffuse granular deposits of IgG are seen outlining the GBM from a patient with membranous glomerulonephritis. (B) Diffuse granular deposits of IgG are seen in the GBM and mesangium from a patient with proliferative glomerulonephritis. (C) Granular deposits of IgA confined largely to the mesangium are observed in a patient with mesangial proliferation and recurrent bouts of gross hematuria. (D) Granular deposits of IgG are observed within the TBMs and peritubular capillaries of a patient with systemic lupus erythematosus.

merular and sometimes tubulointerstitial deposits of these patients may be part of a systemic immune complex disorder such as systemic lupus erythematosus or may be confined to the kidney in primary immune complex nephritis. Immune complexes also deposit occasionally within the lung, leading to pulmonary hemorrhage and nephritis and a presentation of Goodpasture's syndrome. The buildup of immune complexes in glomeruli can cause the entire spectrum of clinical–pathologic forms of glomerulonephritis known in man. Focal and mesangial forms of nephritis appear to be caused by the segmental or mesangial localization of immune complexes, which produce local and focal proliferation manifested clinically largely by proteinuria and/or hematuria. In some patients, this type of deposit is the forerunner of more severe histologic involvement and in others is the sole signal of immune complex disease. Patients with Henoch-Schönlein purpura often have local proliferation and corresponding local immune complex deposition. Some patients with systemic lupus erythematosus may present with and retain a mild focal nephritis with segmental immune complex deposits. Granular deposits of IgG, often with prominent IgA, are found in the mesangial areas and in segments of the GBM in some patients with focal proliferative nephritis and recurrent bouts of gross hematuria. The findings have been consistent enough in these patients so that their disease has been termed IgG–IgA nephropathy. The clinical symptomatology of these patients may exacerbate rapidly following a respiratory infection. The mesangial localization of the deposits suggests that the "complexes" may be large and have formed from preexisting antibody in a state of relative antibody excess.

In more diffuse proliferative forms of nephritis, the immune complex deposition tends to be widespread within the glomerular capillary wall. Patients with poststreptococcal glomerulonephritis, for example, generally have diffuse deposits of immunoglobulin and complement that appear on electron microscopic examination as subepithelial deposits or "humps." In some patients with poststreptococcal nephritis, particularly those examined late in the course of the disease, complement deposits tend to overshadow those of immunoglobulin. Patients with diffuse proliferative forms of nephritis, including those with systemic lupus erythematosus, characteristically develop nephritis with hematuria, proteinuria, and often impaired renal function. Nephrotic syndrome and hypertension of varying severity may complicate their disease. Immune complex deposition can also induce rapidly progressive forms of proliferative glomerulonephritis that are complicated by extensive epithelial crescent formation. Histologically, these lesions are indistinguishable from those caused by anti-GBM antibodies. In these diffuse proliferative forms of glomerulonephritis, with or without crescent formation, granular IgG, often with IgA, IgM, and C3, is present diffusely in the GBM along with electron-dense deposits in a conforming pattern. In some patients with rapidly progressive courses and diffuse prolifera-

tive, crescent-forming glomerulonephritis, little or no immunoglobulin or complement are evident in the glomeruli. Whether the latter patients' diseases have an immune etiology or not is unknown. Perhaps some patients' immune deposits are removed rapidly by the intensity of the inflammatory response and are thereby unavailable for identification.

Patients with membranous glomerulonephritis have typically thickened GBMs with little proliferative change and granular accumulations of immunoglobulin and complement diffusely along the GBMs. As a rule, these patients also have striking subepithelial electron-dense deposits, and as the disease progresses basement membrane material extends subepithelially and eventually engulfs the immune complex deposits. IgG, and less frequently IgA or IgM, usually with heavy C3 deposits, is observed by immunofluorescence in these patients. In general, individuals with this lesion have severe proteinuria, resulting in sufficient protein loss to cause nephrotic syndrome. Progression to renal failure is usually slow, and remission can occur.

Membranoproliferative glomerulonephritis, characterized by thickening of the glomerular capillary wall, mesangial proliferation, and lobular appearance of the glomeruli, is another histologic form of nephritis linked with immune complex deposition. Many of these patients have hypocomplementemia and heavy complement deposition, which often overshadows any immunoglobulin deposits that are present. Complement deposits are frequently very coarse and beaded in appearance. Serologic studies have detected abnormalities in complement concentrations suggestive of alternative complement pathway activation in these patients. The forms of this disease can be subdivided on the basis of the renal tissue's appearance in the electron microscope. Biopsies from patients with a subendothelial dense deposit form of the disease have many manifestations suggesting immune complex induced nephritis, whereas tissues from patients with the diffuse intramembranous dense deposit type have signs more indicative of primary complement activation. Many of these patients have circulating materials termed "nephritic factors" that actually activate the complement sequence via its alternative pathway. These factors are now known to be immunoglobulins reactive with specific combinations of complement components, and as such are immunoconglutinins. There is little evidence that they are nephritogenic per se. Interestingly, similar factors have been identified in patients with partial lipodystrophy, and these patients occasionally develop glomerulonephritis. Chronic complement activation conceivably could predispose an individual to the development of immune complex glomerulonephritis by influencing the body's ability to control infectious agents and process immune complexes. Patients with certain congenital complement deficiencies have an unusually high frequency of immune complex disease of the systemic lupus erythematosus variety.

Patients with focal and segmental glomerulosclerosis, a condition often responsible for steroid-resistant nephrotic syndrome in children, also have signs of segmental immunoglobulin and complement deposition in their glomeruli, often with striking amounts of IgM in the areas of sclerosis. The immunofluorescent findings in focal glomerulosclerosis differentiate it from the so-called minimal change disease, another common cause of nephrotic syndrome in childhood. Minimal change disease has no clearcut immunologic basis, although it does respond dramatically to steroid therapy and is sometimes aggravated by atopy. Elevation in serum IgM levels and suggestions of thymus cell dysfunction or release of lymphocyte factor(s) continue to stimulate interest in identifying its possible immune pathogenesis.

Like minimal change disease, conditions such as diabetes mellitus, hereditary renal disease, and systemic coagulopathies have no clearcut immune pathogenesis; however, certain features have triggered the interest of the immunopathologist. In patients with diabetes mellitus, the thickened GBM and TBM of the kidney contain unusually large amounts of IgG and albumin, apparently trapped there nonspecifically. In experimentally induced diabetes mellitus, mesangial deposits of IgG and C3 develop that are suggestive of immune complex deposits; moreover, the deposition is reversed by the correction of the diabetic environment. Familial renal disease, characterized by glomerulonephritis and nerve deafness (Alport's syndrome), is not generally classed with the immune disorders. In fact, electron microscopic observations have suggested that defects in basement membrane structure are present. Interestingly, some individuals with this condition appear to lack the usual nephritogenic GBM antigens and can develop anti–basement membrane disease when transplanted with normal human kidneys containing these antigens. Coagulopathies, including the thrombotic microangiopathies, are often associated with glomerular and vascular disease, of which hemolytic uremic syndrome, disseminated intravascular coagulation, thrombotic thrombocytopenic purpura, and preeclampsia/eclampsia are examples. The relationship between these rather varied entities is vague, and whether a clearcut immune mechanism responsible for activation of the intravascular coagulation will emerge is unknown.

Nature of antigen–antibody systems. Human immune complex glomerulonephritis can be caused by both endogenous and exogenous antigens. There is little reason to assume that a single antigen–antibody system is involved in each patient's disease; indeed, multiple antigen–antibody systems contribute to the immune complexes deposited in individuals with systemic lupus erythematosus. Actually, several immune complex systems could participate, either sequentially or simultaneously. No one really knows whether immune complex nephritis always results from unusual quantities or types of immune complexes or sometimes relates to the abnormal handling of small and more or less physiologic quantities of complexes that constitute every normal individual's immunologic apparatus. Almost any exogenous (or endogenous) antigen capable of remaining in

the circulation long enough to interact with antibody could conceivably participate in immune complex formation and subsequent renal deposition.

Exogenous antigens. Foreign serum proteins, toxoids, or drugs, whether used therapeutically or taken illicitly, carry with them the potential for forming immune complexes. Renal disease that includes immunofluorescent and electron microscopic findings typical of immune complex deposits have been associated with drug administration including penicillamine, sulfa compounds, trimethadone, mercury, gold, and illicit drugs such as heroin. The drug itself, some contaminant of the drug, or even some immunogenic tissue interaction with the drug could lead to the immune complex formation and deposition.

Bacterial, parasitic, and viral infections, particularly when persistent, are often associated with immune complex nephritis, and the antigens of the infecting organism are identifiable in the glomerular deposits. Nephritogenic streptococcal infection has long been linked with glomerulonephritis, with immunopathologic studies including electron microscopy indicating that immune complexes are deposited on tissues and circulate in blood. Streptococcal antigens have been identified in the glomeruli of such patients, particularly when biopsies are obtained early in the course of nephritis. The composition of these glomerular deposits may include cryoglobulins as well. Of particular interest to this subject are experimental studies showing that streptococci can alter autologous immunoglobulin and induce cryoglobulins in rabbits. The prominence of complement deposits in the glomeruli of some patients with poststreptococcal glomerulonephritis also suggests that this mediator sytem may help to initiate or perpetuate their renal lesions. The pathogenesis of poststreptococcal nephritis, then, seems to be extremely complicated, with immune complexes presumably containing antigens from the streptococcal infection, cryoglobulins, and complement abnormalities all possible participants.

Nephritogenic immune complexes containing antigens from infectious organisms may cause glomerulonephritis in patients with infected ventricular atrial shunts, endocarditis, pneumonia, typhoid, and syphilis. Immune complex nephritis also sometimes complicates leprosy and fungal infection. Parasitic infection is another frequent source of antigens for nephritogenic immune complex formation, as exemplified by the granular glomerular deposits containing antigens from *Plasmodium malariae* or *P. falciparum* infections in patients with malaria and schistosomal or toxoplasma antigens in patients with corresponding infections.

Viral infections can provide antigens for nephritogenic immune complex formation. For instance, hepatitis B antigen has been implicated in both immune complex nephritis and vasculitis in patients with this infection. Measles antigens have been found in the glomerular deposits of patients with subacute sclerosing panencephalitis, and Epstein-Barr viral antigens have been identified in glomerular deposits of patients with Burkitt's lymphoma. Glomerular injury clearly accompanies other viral infections, and the corresponding antigens almost surely contribute to nephritogenic immune complex formation in some of these patients, as future research should show.

Endogenous antigens. Participation of endogenous antigens in the formation of circulating nephritogenic immune complexes is best exemplified in systemic lupus erythematosus. The nuclear antigens that characterize this autoimmune disease appear in glomerular immune complex deposits, and antibodies recovered from these deposits react with a variety of nuclear components. The disease activity seems to correlate most closely with the presence of antibodies to DNA and presumably their corresponding immune complexes. Circulating immune complexes are easily identifiable in patients with systemic lupus erythematosus, who often have evidence of widespread immune complex deposition involving extraglomerular renal tissue and other vascular beds throughout the body. Some investigators have recently postulated a role for the yet to be identified human retroviral (C-type oncornaviral) infections in the induction of systemic lupus erythematosus. Although intriguing, this speculation is based largely on virologic studies in certain mouse strains with spontaneous lupus-like disease, and no convincing evidence of such an association in man is now at hand.

Other endogenous antigens have been identified in patients with glomerulonephritis. One of this antigenic group is thyroglobulin that complexes with antithyroglobulin antibody and occasionally causes nephritis in patients with thyroiditis. In one such patient, renal injury occurred in association with thyroid-induced radiation injury, perhaps through the release of antigens, increasing the amount and nephritogenicity of circulating complexes. Renal tubular antigens seemed to be part of immune complex deposits of membranous glomerulonephritic patients in Japan and of a few patients with sickle-cell anemia or renal carcinoma in this country. This mechanism does not appear to be common, however. Endogenous antigens from neoplastic tissues can also form into nephritogenic immune complexes. Cryoglobulins containing immunoglobulin, which may itself serve as an "antigen," can cause vascular and glomerular deposition and injury as well.

Presumed immune complex glomerulonephritis with unidentified antigens. Although a large number of antigens have now been identified in nephritogenic immune complexes, the exact nature of the antigen–antibody system has eluded detection in most instances. The nature of the immune complex is as yet unidentified in patients with Henoch–Schönlein purpura, whose renal tissue provides abundant immunofluorescent evidence to suggest an immune complex etiology. Immunofluorescent deposits suggestive of immune complex deposition are found in patients with vasculitis, patients with neoplasia, sarcoidosis, Landry-Guillain-Barré-Strohl syndrome, amyotrophic lateral sclerosis, multiple sclerosis, etc. Identification of the antigen involved in each of these circumstances could, in turn, help to establish the etiology of the primary disease.

Immune complex deposits are also prominent in patients with renal vein thrombosis. In most instances, the renal vein thrombosis appears to be a complication of hypercoagulability in persons whose nephrotic syndrome was induced by a preceding immune complex induced nephritis. Renal vein thrombosis has been questioned as the trigger that releases renal antigens, stimulating immune complex formation and subsequent glomerular deposition. Renal tubular antigens were identified tentatively in the glomerular deposits of one such patient.

Diagnostic features. Immunofluorescence used to detect typical granular deposits of immunoglobulin and complement is currently the key to diagnosing immune complex disease (see the chapter on *Immunofluorescence*). Confirmation that the deposit actually is an immune complex requires identification of the specific antigen–antibody system in question. Since, as already noted, the number of antigens involved is potentially very large, the patient's physician must serve as a detective to narrow the field of possible antigens to a number that can be tested by direct immunofluorescence study with specific antisera or by elution studies to recover antibodies from the glomerular deposits for subsequent identification of antibody reactivity.

Detection of circulating immune complexes. Recently, techniques have become available for screening sera of patients with immune complex glomerulonephritis for the presence of circulating immune complexes. At first, techniques were based on measuring physical-chemical changes in immunoglobulin by ultracentrifugation or chromatography studies or by precipitation in polyethylene glycol. More recently, the interaction of immune complexes with rheumatoid factor, complement components, or cellular receptors has gained the attention of immunopathologists, and radioimmunoassays developed for this purpose are now capable of detecting immune complexes in quantities approximating 10 μg/ml. Methods such as the Raji cell assay, based on the interaction of immune complexes with cell surface complement receptors and subsequent radioimmunoassay quantitation of bound immunoglobulin, or techniques employing the interaction of immune complexes with C1q, have been applied to the study of patients with immune complex disease. The use of these assays, particularly when several are combined, has shown that patients with acute forms of nephritis more frequently have circulating immune complexes than patients with indolent forms. Just why circulating immune complexes are not found in all patients with immunofluorescent evidence of glomerular immune complex localization is unknown. Perhaps the immune complex assays are not yet sensitive enough or specific enough to reveal the particular nephritogenic complexes of interest. The amount of immune complexes in circulating blood may well fluctuate or may be insufficient for detection after the early stage of disease has passed. One could also speculate that patients with rather indolent forms of immune complex disease and little alteration in the amount of circulating immune complexes may develop nephritis because they are abnormal in respect to the processing of more or less normal amounts of complexes produced during day-to-day immune responses. In such patients, the immune complex disease may develop not so much as the result of an unusual amount of complex material but due to alterations in immune complex clearing or handling.

Therapeutic considerations. Treatment of immune complex nephritis currently relies heavily on nonspecific antiphlogogistic or immunosuppressive regimens that include drugs such as corticosteroids, cyclophosphamide, azathioprine, etc., either used alone or combined. Theoretically, immune complex nephritis could best be treated by identifying and eradicating the antigenic source in the case of exogenous antigens or developing maneuvers to terminate the autoimmune response in the case of endogenous antigens. Elimination of circulating immune complexes might also be possible through extracorporeal procedures employing materials capable of binding complexes. Relatively specific immunoabsorbants to remove an antigen–antibody system whose identity is known could also be useful therapeutically. Now, less specific plasma exchange therapy is being evaluated as a means of altering levels of immune complexes, or perhaps of mediators of inflammation (complement, etc.), even when the antigen–antibody system is not identified.

Immune complex glomerulonephritis often progresses to renal failure, so that the physician may need to consider renal transplantation. Unfortunately, immune complex deposits can develop in a transplanted kidney either as the original immune complex disease recurs or as immune complexes form during the numerous antigenic challenges of the posttransplant course, including those by histoincompatibility antigens and antigens from infections in the immunosuppressed recipient.

Immune complex induced tubulointerstitial nephritis in man. Systemic lupus erythematosus is currently the clearest example of a disease in which extraglomerular immune complex deposits can lead to tubulointerstitial injury (Fig. 3D). About 70 percent of kidneys from patients with systemic lupus erythematosus have evidence of immune complex deposition in arteries, peritubular capillaries, interstitial tissue, and TBMs. Immune complex deposits contain immunoglobulin, complement, and nuclear antigens similar to the deposits located in glomeruli. This observation suggests that the extraglomerular deposits forming in the circulation are subsequently depositing in extraglomerular tissues. These extraglomerular deposits in kidneys from patients with systemic lupus erythematosus correlate well with histologic interstitial damage; however, it is unknown if immune complexes contribute to the development of primary tubulointerstitial nephritis, either by depositing from the circulation or by forming in situ. Renal tubular dysfunction, particularly renal tubular acidosis, which complicates autoimmune diseases such as Sjögren's

syndrome and other conditions of hypergammaglobulinemia, is an indicator but not proof that immune processes may be involved.

RENAL DISEASE CAUSED BY SPECIFIC IMMUNE REACTIONS TO ANTIGENS IN OR OF THE KIDNEY

Experimental Models of Specific Immune Reactions

The most common example of nephritis related to antibodies specific for antigens in the kidney, and the only example as yet identified in man, involves immune responses directed toward antigens in the GBM or TBM. The nephrotoxicity of anti-GBM antibodies has been recognized for many years, but only recently have similar reactions been attributed to anti-TBM antibodies. Recent observations in experimental animals have suggested that non-basement membrane glomerular and tubular antigens are also involved in immunologic tubular injury through their direct and specific interactions with antibodies. In other experimental studies, antigens clearly became trapped within the kidney, particularly the glomerulus, subsequently reacted in situ with their corresponding antibodies, and instigated renal injury and damage.

Experimental anti-GBM antibody-induced glomerulonephritis. Heterologous anti-GBM antibodies. The nephrotoxic effects of antikidney antibody were first demonstrated in 1900. During the 1930s Masugi thoroughly studied the model of nephrotoxic nephritis, and the disease is still sometimes referred to as Masugi nephritis, although in the 1950s the disease's cause was convincingly shown to be antibodies reactive with the GBM. Subsequently, the term nephrotoxic nephritis was largely discarded. Experimentally, one produces this disease by immunizing animals with basement membrane preparations in adjuvant, then removing the anti–basement membrane antibodies they form in response. These anti–basement membrane antibodies passively administered intravenously cause acute nephritis that occurs in two phases. The first, or heterologous, phase reflects the direct toxic effects of the antibody. The second, the delayed, or autologous, phase, occurs some days later when the recipient produces antibody reactive with the foreign immunoglobulin bound to the basement membrane. The occurrence and severity of the heterologous phase depends upon the quantity of antibody administered and varies with the species tested. Approximately 75 μg of antibody are required per gram of rat kidney to induce clinically apparent nephritis, but only 5 and 15 μg/g are required to induce acute injury in the sheep and rabbit, respectively. By making some assumptions, one can calculate that rats sustain immediate glomerular injury after about 1.2×10^{10} molecules of antibody bind per glomerulus, or 1 antibody molecule for every 20 nm^2 of glomerular capillary filtering surface. Depending on the steric factors involved, perhaps half of the filtering surface would then be covered by antibody.

The delayed, or autologous, phase of injury ensues 7–10 days after the administration of antibody, when the recipient forms antibody reactive with the heterologous immunoglobulin bound in his glomeruli. As little as 2 μg of antibody bound to the GBM is sufficient to cause glomerular injury during the autologous phase. The injury can be augmented by actively or passively immunizing the experimental animal against the autologous immunoglobulin. This phase of injury is the classic example of a foreign antigen planted in the glomerulus for subsequent interaction with host antibody. More will be said in a moment about other planted antigens in the induction of nephritis.

Nephritogenic anti-GBM antibodies are generally produced for experimental purposes by immunizing animals with basement membrane rich fractions of kidney; however, other organs rich in vascular basement membranes can be used to induce nephritogenic cross-reactive antibodies. Lung, placenta, and lymphoid connective tissue, for example, are all good sources of antigen. Even though nonrenal tissues are used to induce antibodies, the related injury is usually confined to the kidney, although on occasion pulmonary injury can be induced as well.

Nephritis induced by administering heterologous anti–basement membrane antibodies is generally of an acute proliferative type, often complicated by crescent formation. These antibodies are seen along the GBM as linear deposits when one uses immunofluorescent techniques (Fig. 4A). Experimental anti–basement membrane antibody-induced injury can be induced in any of several species, each of which varies in the severity and chronicity with which the lesion evolves.

Within minutes after the administration of complement-fixing anti-GBM antibodies, polymorphonuclear leukocytes accumulate within the glomerular capillary loops, where they displace the endothelium and approximate themselves along the basement membrane, producing lysozymal enzyme injury. Polymorphonuclear leukocyte infiltration is transient, lasting only a few hours, and may be replaced by an infiltrate of more mononuclear nature. Avian and certain mammalian anti-GBM antibodies can induce immediate glomerular injury in the absence of complement and polymorphonuclear leukocyte participation, indicating that other as yet unidentified mediation pathways of injury must be involved.

Alterations in physiologic function of the glomerulus occur within minutes after the administration of the antibody. A decrease in glomerular filtration is observed, caused by a complement-dependent vasoconstrictive element and a complement-independent decrease in the permeability of the GBM to water. Proteinuria rapidly ensues, after which the disease may progress to irreversible renal failure or slowly resolve over a period of weeks or months.

Autoimmune anti-GBM responses. It has been possible to induce an autoimmune response to an animal's own GBM antigens by immunization with homologous or heterologous basement membrane preparations suspended in adjuvant. Sheep appear to be particularly susceptible, and they develop fulminant anti-GBM nephritis after immunization with any of a variety of basement membranes in Freund's adjuvant.

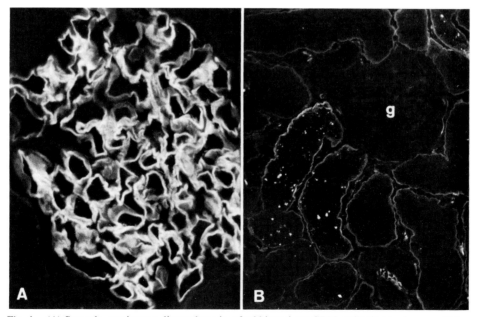

Fig. 4. (A) Smooth, continuous, linear deposits of rabbit anti–rat GBM antibody are shown outlining the GBM of a rat 1 hour after passive intravenous administration of the heterologous anti-GBM antibody. (B) Continuous, circumferential, linear deposits of IgG are seen outlining the TBMs of a Brown Norway rat 10 days after immunization with bovine TBM incorporated in complete Freund's adjuvant with pertussis vaccine. The antibodies produced do not react with the GBM of the glomerulus (g).

The immunized sheep characteristically have an intense linear accumulation of anti-GBM antibodies along their GBMs and circulating anti-GBM antibodies that are capable of transferring the nephritis to healthy sheep.

Autologous basement membrane antigens present in the urine have also been used to induce anti-GBM antibody responses. Indeed, rabbits can be caused to develop anti-GBM antibodies and nephritis upon immunization with basement membrane antigen rich fractions from their own urine. Similar antigenic materials have been identified in the circulation and have been noted to increase in concentration after nephrectomy. This suggests that these materials may be part of a pool derived from basement membrane metabolism and normally excreted into the urine. Reintroduction of these materials in an immunogenic way could perhaps explain the spontaneous induction of autologous anti-basement membrane responses in some individuals.

Experimental anti-TBM antibody-induced tubulointerstitial nephritis. Heterologous anti-GBM antibodies generally contain antibodies reactive with the TBM as well; however, in vivo binding of such antibodies is usually confined largely to the GBM. Publications of the last few years have described several models of autologous anti-TBM antibody formation and subsequent tubulointerstitial nephritis. Guinea pigs immunized with rabbit cortical basement membrane in adjuvant develop antibodies reactive with both GBM and TBM. Histologically, the injury is confined largely to the tubulointerstitial tissue and is associated with the development of severe tubulointerstitial nephritis. Passive transfer of these antibodies induces tubulointerstitial nephritis in normal guinea pigs. Studies to characterize the nature of the anti-GBM and anti-TBM antibody responses suggest that reactivity with the GBM is directed largely toward its collagen elements and is not particularly nephrotoxic, while the anti-TBM response is directed predominantly to its noncollagenous portions and is nephrotoxic.

Rats immunized with homologous kidney in complete adjuvant develop anti-TBM antibodies and tubulointerstitial nephritis. Brown Norway rats can be induced to form anti-TBM antibodies in the absence of anti-GBM antibodies by immunization with homologous kidney or bovine renal basement membrane. Immunization with bovine renal basement membrane causes anti-TBM antibodies to form and bind to the TBM beginning about 6 days after immunization (Fig. 4B). By 10 days, complement is also bound, and an intense polymorphonuclear leukocyte interstitial infiltrate follows. The polymorphonuclear leukocytes are subsequently replaced by infiltrating mononuclear cells, producing a conspicuous mononuclear interstitial infiltrate containing giant cells. The Brown Norway is the only strain of rat known to have sufficient antigen and to respond immunologically in such a way that severe tubulointerstitial nephritis develops. Lewis rats, for example, can form anti-TBM antibodies but lack the relevant antigen in their TBMs and therefore do not develop injury. If a Lewis rat is transplanted with an antigen-positive kidney taken from a Brown Norway/Lewis cross, the Lewis rat forms antibodies capable of reacting with the TBM of the transplant but not of its native kidney. These observations are relevant to transplantation in humans, for whom kidneys of somewhat differing TBM antigenicity may be used.

Nephritogenic immune responses involving other antigens in or of the kidney. Antigens derived from non-basement membrane structural components of the kidney or extrarenal antigens that are fortuitously trapped within the kidney might be involved in nephritogenic immune responses. For example, a spontaneously occurring glomerulonephritis in rabbits is characterized by glomerular deposits, the immunoglobulin (in eluates) of which reacts with non-basement membrane glomerular antigens. Moreover, rabbit antibodies to rat renal tubular antigens appear to bind directly to the glomerular capillary wall after intravenous infusion; again, a non-basement membrane glomerular antigen is apparently involved.

The autologous immune complex glomerulonephritis in rats originally described by Heymann is now felt to be caused, at least in part, by antibodies reacting directly with antigens in the glomerular capillary wall. Since this lesion has long been thought to be a model human membranous glomerulopathy, the experimental observations have caused a renewed evaluation of the immunopathogenesis of the human lesion.

In several experimental models, nephritogenic immune reactions involve nonglomerular antigens that are first trapped or planted within the glomeruli. As mentioned earlier, the autologous phase of experimental anti-GBM antibody-induced nephritis is a classic example of a planted or trapped foreign antigen (heterologous immunoglobulin) that later reacts with host antibody to cause glomerular injury. Antigenic material can also first be trapped or planted within the glomerular mesangium for subsequent interaction with antibody. We have recently shown that lectins, proteins with carbohydrate binding specificity, can bind to glycoproteins of the glomerular capillary wall and there serve as "planted" antigens for subsequent nephritogenic in situ immune complex formation. Potentially, the same events occur in humans who are subjected to many infective agents that contain lectin-like materials perhaps capable of binding to the glomerular capillary wall.

Classically, in situ nephritogenic immune reactions have been considered only in relation to the interaction of anti–basement membrane antibodies with their corresponding basement membrane antigens. This consideration should now be expanded to include immune reactions with non-basement membrane glomerular antigens and planted glomerular antigens as well.

Anti–Basement Membrane Antibody-induced Nephritis in Man

Anti-GBM antibody-induced glomerulonephritis. Linear IgG deposits similar to those seen in animal models of anti–basement membrane disease were identified in man beginning in the early 1960s. In 1967, Lerner et al.

clearly demonstrated the immunopathogenic role of anti-GBM antibodies in a series of such patients. These investigators demonstrated the presence of circulating anti-GBM antibodies and were able to transfer nephritis to subhuman primates with anti-GBM antibodies recovered from the patients' circulating blood and/or eluted from their kidneys. Even more convincing was the immediate recurrence of nephritis in a patient who was inadvertently given a renal transplant while his levels of circulating anti-GBM antibodies remained high.

Clinical, pathologic, and diagnostic features. Anti-GBM antibodies cause glomerulonephritis usually classed as rapidly progressive. About two-thirds of these patients also hemorrhage in the lung—the clinical presentation known as Goodpasture's syndrome (see the chapter on *Goodpasture's Syndrome*). Anti-TBM antibodies accompany the anti-GBM antibodies in about 70 percent of the patients. About two-thirds of them are males and about 60 percent are in the second and third decades of life, although patients below 10 and over 70 years of age, of both sexes, have been identified. The two most common presentations, rapidly progressive glomerulonephritis and Goodpasture's syndrome, often follow a prodromal flu-like illness, with a few patients having migratory arthritis or arthralgia as a prominent early complaint. When the presentation if that of Goodpasture's syndrome, pulmonary hemorrhage and renal symptoms often begin almost simultaneously, but either one may precede by several months. Pulmonary hemorrhage is usually episodic and may be mild to severe, occasionally leading to death from hypoxia. About three-fourths of the patients develop irreversible renal failure, and the mortality of those in the acute phase of the disease is perhaps 20 percent.

Morphologically, the glomeruli have varying degrees of proliferation, usually with severe and generalized crescent formation. Varying degrees of tublointerstitial change accompany the glomerular lesion and may correlate with the concomitant presence of anti-TBM antibodies. Diagnosis of anti-GBM glomerulonephritis is based on classical linear deposits of IgG detected along the GBM by immunofluorescence (Fig. 5). Less frequently, IgA or IgM may also be observed in a linear pattern. C3 accompanies the immunoglobulin deposit in about three-fourths of patients but may be more irregular and less striking than the linear immunoglobulin deposit. Elution study or assays for circulating anti-GBM antibodies should be done to confirm the diagnosis derived from immunofluorescence analysis. Nonspecific linear deposits are somtimes observed in normal kidneys, kidneys obtained at autopsy or following perfusion prior to transplantation, or from patients with diabetes mellitus.

Detection of circulating anti-GBM antibodies. Circulating anti-GBM antibodies are classically detected by indirect immunofluorescence studies using normal human kidney sections as a target. More recently, radioimmunoassays have been developed for detecting circulating anti-GBM antibodies. We have developed an assay using as an antigen the noncollagenous portion of the GBM remaining after collagenase digestion and extensive dialysis. All but 2 of 78 patients with immunopathologic evidence of anti-GBM antibody-induced Goodpasture's syndrome and 43 of 52 patients with anti-GBM antibody-induced nephritis alone had circulating antibodies according to this method. Only 2 of 392 patients with immune complex nephritis were positive and developed the antibody during the course of a membranous glomerulonephritis.

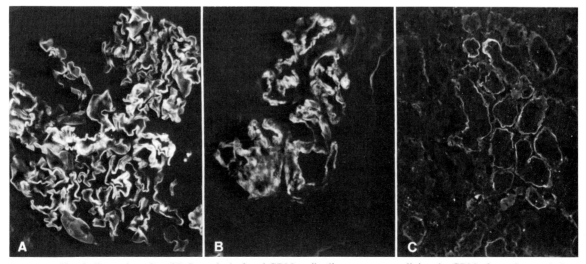

Fig. 5. (A) Classic linear deposits of IgG, typical of anti-GBM antibodies, are seen outlining the GBM of a patient early in the course of anti-GBM antibody-induced glomerulonephritis. (B) Somewhat irregular deposits of IgG are seen bound to the remnants of a corrugated and crumpled basement membrane of a patient with a more advanced stage of anti-GBM antibody-induced glomerulonephritis. (C) Anti-TBM antibodies are identified as continuous, circumferential, linear deposits outlining the TBMs of a portion of the renal tubules present in the section. Anti-TBM antibodies often are found in patients with anti-GBM antibody-induced nephritis and infrequently may occur primarily.

Of 56 patients with systemic lupus erythematosus, 4 also had circulating anti-GBM antibodies. Only one patient with negative renal immunofluorescence studies had anti-GBM antibodies, and this patient subsequently developed anti-GBM antibody-induced nephritis in a transplant, suggesting that the original tissue study was inadequate for diagnosis.

Antibody activity estimated by this assay does not differ significantly between patients with anti-basement membrane antibody-induced Goodpasture's syndrome and those with anti-GBM nephritis alone. The anti-GBM antibody response is usually transient, lasting only a few weeks to a few months, with only rare examples of recrudescence noted to date. No common antecedent events have been recognized, with only loose clinical associations to relate the onset of anti-GBM antibodies to such things as influenza A2 infection, damage from hydrocarbon solvent inhalation, renal injury or ischemia, drug nephrotoxicity, or neoplasia. The fact that individuals have antigenic differences in their renal basement membranes is now becoming evident. Some patients with hereditary nephritis of Alport's type appear to lack the usual nephritogenic antigens in their GBMs and may be susceptible to anti-GBM antibody formation when transplanted with a kidney containing normal GBM antigens. Although the exact nature of the nephritogenic GBM antigen is unknown, in both experimental studies and clinical observations it appears to be present in the noncollagenous glycoprotein portion of the basement membrane. Heterologous anticollagen antibodies are not particularly nephritogenic, and absorption of nephritogenic anti-GBM antibodies with collagen does not substantially reduce their nephrotoxicity. The finding of nephritogenic basement membrane antigens in normal urine and serum suggests that these materials are probably responsible for the normal state of immunologic tolerance to the basement membrane but conceivably could contribute to an anti-basement membrane immune response if reintroduced to the host in a nephritogenic manner.

Pulmonary involvement in anti-GBM antibody-induced glomerulonephritis. Anti–basement membrane antibodies are present along the alveolar basement membranes in patients with the Goodpasture's form of the disease. Antibodies eluted from the lungs of these patients react with both the alveolar basement membranes and GBM, indicating the cross-reactivity between these two basement membrane structures; however, neither the occurrence nor severity of pulmonary hemorrhage in patients with anti-GBM antibody-induced Goodpasture's syndrome correlates directly with the level of anti-GBM antibody detected by our radioimmunoassay. In some instances, the pulmonary hemorrhage seems to be precipitated by events such as fluid overload or pulmonary or systemic infection. Nephrectomy has been suggested as beneficial in patients with severe pulmonary hemorrhage of Goodpasture's type; however, the results have not been uniformly favorable. Nephrectomy has no immediate effect on the levels of anti-GBM antibody activity, although it may hasten somewhat its eventual disappearance. Since large doses of steroids are now considered therapeutic for acute pulmonary hemorrhage, nephrectomy is being considered only as a last resort.

Therapeutic considerations. The transient nature of the anti-basement membrane antibody response has led to therapies designed to blunt further antibody production and to hasten removal of residual circulating antibody. Combined intense immunosuppression and large volume plasmapheresis have been used for this purpose, with apparent benefit in some patients. Renal function has improved and pulmonary involvement regressed as antibody vanished, but since spontaneous remission also occasionally occurs, one must reserve judgment regarding the true benefit of such therapy until the results of controlled trials are available.

Transplantation while high levels of anti-basement membrane antibody persist can result in severe, recurrent glomerulonephritis. For this reason, most patients are observed for a period of time preceding transplantation until their circulating antibodies have disappeared or decreased to low levels. Then these individuals generally can be transplanted without great danger of recurrent nephritis, although exceptions do occur. A patient we recently evaluated who had well documented anti-basement membrane antibody nephritis received a transplant from an identical twin 2 years after the disappearance of circulating anti-GBM antibody. Within 3 months after transplantation (without immunosuppression), anti-GBM antibodies reappeared and bound to the GBM of the transplant. Graft function was maintained by the prompt institution of immunosuppression and plasmapheresis therapy.

Anti-TBM antibody-induced tubulointerstitial nephritis. In the last few years, anti-TBM antibodies have been identified associated with tubulointerstitial renal injury in some patients. The most frequent occurrence of anti-TBM antibodies is in association with anti-GBM antibodies, as described in a previous section. Anti-TBM antibodies have also been found in occasional patients with immune complex induced glomerulonephritis, in some patients with drug-induced tubulointerstitial nephritis, and in some recipients of renal transplants. At least two patients with possible primary anti-TBM antibody-induced tubulointerstitial nephritis have also been noted.

Anti-TBM antibodies complicating immune complex nephritis have been reported in a patient after severe poststreptococcal glomerulonephritis, and circulating anti-TBM antibodies were also observed. Anti-TBM antibodies have also complicated the immune complex nephritis of several children. In one child studied in our laboratory with intractable diarrhea early in life, immunofluorescence revealed granular glomerular immunoglobulin deposits consistent with immune complex induced glomerular injury; anti-TBM antibodies were also present. Subsequent elution studies recovered antibodies reactive with the TBM and the jejunal basement membrane as well as antibodies reactive with antigens in the brush border of the proximal renal tubule and on the surface of the jejunum.

Anti-TBM antibodies have also developed in some patients with methicillin-associated interstitial nephritis. In one instance, dimethoxyphenylpenicilloyl, a breakdown product of methicillin, was found bound to the TBM of the kidney, suggesting that a dimethoxyphenylpenicilloyl–TBM protein haptene conjugate had formed and induced antibodies reactive with the carrier (TBM) portion of the conjugate. Since anti-TBM antibodies are not found in most patients with methicillin-associated nephritis, probably they are not involved in the usual pathogenesis of this lesion. Anti-TBM antibodies have also been identified in patients with diphenylhydantoin-related interstitial nephritis.

Anti-TBM antibodies have most frequently been identified in patients after renal transplantation and appear to function in at least two ways. In one, the anti-TBM antibodies react with TBM antigens present in both the transplant and the native kidney, whereas in the other the anti-TBM antibodies react only with the TBM of the tranplant. The induction of antibody in the latter case is similar to that described earlier for cross-strain transplantation between Brown Norway and Lewis rats, in which "TBM antigen negative" Lewis rats developed anti-TBM antibodies when exposed to "TBM antigen positive" Brown Norway rat renal transplants.

CONCLUSIONS

Immune complex and anti-basement membrane antibody mechanisms account for most instances of glomerulonephritis in man. How frequently immune mechanisms will be found responsible for induction of tubulointerstitial nephritis remains to be determined. Immunofluorescent and serologic assays are available for detecting these immune mechanisms in renal tissue and should be applied to the study of all patients with glomerulonephritis as well as other patients suspected of having an immunologic component of their renal disease.

REFERENCES

Andres GA, McCluskey RT: Tubular and interstitial renal disease due to immunologic mechanisms. Kidney Int 7:271, 1975

Burkholder PM: Atlas of Human Glomerular Pathology. Hagerstown, Harper & Row, 1974

Cochrane CG, Koffler D: Immune complex disease in experimental animals and man. Adv Immunol 16:185, 1973

Germuth FG, Rodriguez E: Immunopathology of the renal glomerulus, in: Immune Complex Deposit and Antibasement Membrane Disease. Boston, Little, Brown, 1976

Glassock RJ, Bennett CM: The glomerulopathies, in Brenner BM, Rector FC Jr (eds): The Kidney. Philadelphia, W.B. Saunders, 1976

Koffler D: Immunopathogenesis of systemic lupus erythematosus. Annu Rev Med 25:149, 1974

Lockwood CM, Rees AJ, Pearson TA, et al: Immunosuppression and plasma-exchange in the treatment of Goodpasture's syndrome. Lancet 1:711, 1976

Unanue ER, Dixon FJ: Experimental glomerulonephritis: Immunologic events and pathogenetic mechanisms. Adv Immunol 6:1, 1967

Wilson CB, Dixon FJ: Anti-glomerular basement membrane antibody-induced glomerulonephritis. Kidney Int 3:74, 1973

Wilson CB, Dixon FJ: The renal response to immunological injury, in Brenner BM, Rector FC Jr (eds): The Kidney. Philadelphia, W.B. Saunders, 1976

Wilson CB, Dixon FJ: Renal injury from immune reactions involving antigens in or of the kidney, in Wilson CB, Brenner BM, Stein JH (eds): Contemporary Issues in Nephrology, vol 3. New York, Churchill Livingstone, 1979

Woodroffe AJ, Border WA, Theofilopoulos AN, et al: Detection of circulating immune complexes in patients with glomerulonephritis. Kidney Int 12:268, 1977

CAUSES OF PROLIFERATIVE GLOMERULONEPHRITIS

Marvin R. Garovoy and Terry B. Strom

Morphologic, clinical, and etiologic criteria have been utilized to classify the various categories of proliferative glomerulonephritis. We have chosen to utilize the last method for this discussion. Although this classification would also be appropriate to categorize the causes of the acute nephritic syndrome (see the chapter on *Acute Nephritis*), it should be emphasized that many of these entities could also present with rapidly progressive glomerulonephritis, the nephrotic syndrome, or other clinical syndromes.

Poststreptococcal glomerulonephritis is the classic example of acute glomerulonephritis and the acute nephritic syndrome. This entity is described in detail in the chapter on *Poststreptococcal Glomerulonephritis*. A burgeoning variety of infectious disease processes have also been causally linked to the acute nephritic syndrome (Table 1). Nonstreptococcal postinfective glomerulopathies tend to present with mild expressions of the acute nephritic syndrome and rapidly resolve without residua.

Nonstreptococcal bacterial infection (Table 1) can give rise to a proliferative glomerulonephritis. Infective endocarditis, most often associated with *Streptococcus viridans* or *Staphylococcus aureus,* has been long recognized as a cause of acute glomerulonephritis. Coagulase-negative *Staphylococcus albus* infections of ventriculoatrial shunts inserted for relief of hydrocephalus have been clearly implicated as a cause of glomerulonephritis. *Falciparum malaria,* leprosy, and secondary syphilis have been associated with an immune complex glomerulonephritis. A variety of other microbial diseases may give rise to acute glomerulonephritis. On rare occasions, the nephritic syndrome may occur in association with visceral abscesses. Hypocomplementemia is commonly found in association with these

Table 1
Causes of Proliferative Glomerulonephritis

Infectious diseases
   Poststreptococcal glomerulonephritis
   Nonpoststreptococcal glomerulonephritis
      Bacterial—infective endocarditis, "shunt nephritis," bacteremia, pneumococcal
        pneumonia, typhoid fever, secondary syphillis, leptospirosis.
      Viral—hepatitis B, infectious mononucleosis, cytomegalovirus, mumps, measles,
        varicella, vaccina, Echo and Coxsackie virus
      Parasitic—falciparum malaria, toxoplasmosis
      Rickettsial—typhus
Multisystem diseases—systemic lupus erythematosus, vasculitis, Henoch- Schonlein purpura,
   Goodpasture's syndrome, mixed essential cryoglobulinemia
Miscellaneous—Guillian-Barré syndrome, irradiation of Wilms' tumor, self-administered
   diphtheria-pertussis-tetanus immunization, serum sickness, narcotic addiction

entities. A rather heterogeneous assortment of glomerular alterations occur accompanying these conditions. In some of these states, presumptive identification of microbial antigen as a component of the intraglomerular immune complexes has been made. Antimicrobial therapy usually coincides with resolution of the clinical stimata of glomerulonephritis.

Viral diseases frequently are accompanied by an abnormal urinary sediment suggesting acute glomerulonephritis. Clinical and morphologic evidence have associated a large number of viral syndromes with acute glomerulonephritis and the acute nephritic syndrome. The role of the virus itself is not always clear. For example, individuals with several morphologic forms of glomerulonephritis, including IgA nephropathy (Berger's disease), focal proliferative glomerulonephritis, or membranoproliferative glomerulonephritis, may develop an abnormal urinary sediment coincident with viral infection. While infectious mononucleosis is often associated with mild hematuria or proteinuria, suggesting nephritis, it is difficult to absolutely exclude an associated infection with betahemolytic streptococci as causal. Hepatitis B virus has been clearly implicated as a cause of glomerulonephritis. A remarkably broad morphologic expression of this illness has been noted which includes a variety of patterns such as acute proliferative glomerulonephritis, vasculitis (polyarteritis nodosa), membranous glomerulonephritis, mesangiocapillary glomerulonephritis, and glomerular sclerosis.

In addition to postinfectious causes and a number of systemic diseases which may cause a proliferative glomerulonephritis, (Table 1) there are a number of miscellaneous causes, including irradiation of Wilms' tumor, Guillian-Barré syndrome, self-administration of diptheria-pertussis-tetanus vaccine, or narcotic addiction.

REFERENCES

Cameron JS: Bright's disease today: Pathogenesis and treatment of glomerulonephritis—I, II, III. Br Med J 4:87, 160, 217, 1972
Earle DP, Seegal D: Natural history of glomerulonephritis. J Chron Dis 5:3, 1957
Glassock RJ, Bennett CM: The glomerulopathies, in Brenner BM, Rector FC Jr (eds): The Kidney. Philadelphia, W.B. Saunders 1976
Maddox DA, Bennett CM, Deen WM, et al: Determinants of glomerular filtration in experimental glomerulonephritis. J Clin Invest 55:305, 1975
Merrill JP: Medical progress—glomerulonephritis (3 parts). N Engl J Med 290:257, 313, 373, 1974

POSTSTREPTOCOCCAL GLOMERULONEPHRITIS

Marvin R. Garovoy and Terry B. Strom

Acute poststreptococcal glomerulonephritis (APSGN) is often considered a classic form of immune complex mediated glomerulonephritis in which antigens derived from group A beta hemolytic strains of streptococci elicit an immunologic response culminating in pathologic and physiologic sequelae.

PATHOLOGY

By light microscopy the predominant findings are those of an endocapillary proliferative glomerulonephritis characterized by an increase in the endothelial and mesangial cell constituents of the glomerular tuft with a normal thickness to the basement membrane (see Fig. 1 in the chapter on *Light Microscopy*). This increase in cellular elements typically involves an entire glomerulus (diffuse process), with most glomeruli affected (generalized process), hence the designation of a generalized diffuse proliferative glomerulonephritis. Occasionally in severe cases, there will be proliferation of the epithelial cells of Bowman's capsule, resulting in crescents or an extracapillary proliferative glomerulonephritis (rapidly progressive poststreptococcal glomerulonephritis). In some cases the appearance of polymorphonuclear leukocytes indicates an exudative lesion. Focal glomerular hyalinization, lobular necrosis, frequent crescents, and prominent interstitial infiltration and fibrosis indicate a poor prognosis for complete healing.

With immunoflourescent staining techniques utilizing rabbit or goat anti–human immunoglobulin antiserum a granular or "lumpy-bumpy" deposition of antibodies along the capillary basement membrane is discerned. Most often C3 and IgG are found in these deposits, with occasional amounts of IgM and IgA on the basement membrane and in the mesangium. Properdin, factor B, and C1q have also been noted in small amounts. There are a few reports of a discontinuous linear staining pattern of IgG in patients biopsied long after the acute episode. There is no direct evidence that this represents anti–glomerular basement membrane antibody. Sequential renal biopsy specimens have revealed disappearance of both the immunoglobulins and ultrastructural deposits as clinical recovery ensues. There are, however, a few cases in which granular mesangial deposits of Ig and C3 have been noted to persist for months or years despite clinical healing.

Electron microscopy reveals discrete electron-dense deposits on the subepithelial aspect of the basement membrane (see Fig. 1 of the chapter on *Electron Microscopy*). These humps are especially frequent early in the clinical course but are usually not found more than 6 weeks after clinical onset.

EPIDEMIOLOGY

Although infection with strains of beta hemolytic group A streptococci are quite frequent, the nonsuppurative sequelae of glomerulonephritis and rheumatic fever are far less common. Rheumatic fever has a constant attack rate of nearly 3 percent and exclusively follows pharyngeal infections. Acute nephritis, on the other hand, has a varying attack rate of 1–10 percent and may follow either pharyngeal or skin infections. This difference in disease incidence has been related to both characteristics of the infecting organisms and the host immunologic response. While all strains of group A streptococci are capable of causing rheumatic fever, only a select few appear to be nephritogenic. Strains 12, 14, 49, 18, and 25 have been identified as causing acute nephritis following upper respiratory infections. Strains 2, 49, 55, 57, and 60 are noted primarily for their tendency to cause impetigo or pyoderma and nephritis. Only rarely do rheumatic fever and glomerulonephritis coexist.

Acute poststreptococcal glomerulonephritis (APSGN) is primarily a disease of children and young adults. It can occur either sporadically or in the form of regional epidemics (Great Lakes 1953, 1966). Most of the epidemics have been associated with impetigo-related strains with a predominance of affected males over females at a ratio approaching 2:1.

IMMUNOLOGY

The M proteins, located on the streptococcal cell wall, constitute the site of antigenic diversity enabling the differentiation of specific strains. Antibodies to this class of protein often persist for many years. In contrast, high titers or changing titers of antibody to the extracellular products of the beta hemolytic streptococcus, e.g., streptolysin O and S, hyaluronidase, and streptokinase, are useful indicators of recent streptococcal infection despite their offering little protection against subsequent infection. Antibodies to streptolysin O (ASO) ordinarily begin to rise 1–3 weeks after a streptococcal infection and reach a maximum in 3–5 weeks. Seventy to eighty percent of patients with proved streptococcal infection show significant increases in ASO titers. Many of the strains causing impetigo, however, produce very little ASO, and under these circumstances measurement of antibodies to DNAase and hyaluronidase are of special value in diagnosis. Elevated titers of anti-DNAase and antihyaluronidase antibodies are found in well over 90 percent of cases.

Serum complement (CH_{50} or C3 is almost invariably depressed during the acute phase due to a combination of decreased synthesis and increased consumption. With clinical quiescence the C3 levels slowly return to normal. Activation of the alternate as well as classical complement pathway is implied by finding the degree and duration of depression of the early complement components (C1q and C4) to be less than that of C3. Further, properdin and C3 are especially depressed in a subset of patients who possess a heat-labile, EDTA inhibitable factor capable of cleaving native C3.

Circulating cryoglobulins consisting of IgG alone or in combination with IgM and/or C3 have been reported in the serum and in the glomerular lesion of some patients. The common occurrence of cryoglobulins suggest that immune complexes are present in the circulation. Experimentally, autologous immunoglobulins altered by incubation with streptococci are capable of inducing cryoglobulins if reinjected into the circulation; however, since it has not yet been possible to demonstrate streptococcal antigen in these immune complexes, it has been proposed that a product of the streptococcus may have been "planted" in the glomerulus to initiate the immune response.

Using ferritin labeled antistreptococcal antibodies from patients with APSGN, antigenic material occurring in the mesangium and on the subendothelial aspects of the basement membrane have been detected but with little evidence of antigen in subepithelial electron-dense deposits. Streptococcal antigens have been detected in the mesangium 1 week after the disease begins but not at later periods, presumably because the antigenic sites are covered with excess antibody from the circulation.

The evidence strongly indicates an immune complex etiology for APSGN; however, the precise identification of the antigen–antibody system or the location of complex formation operating in this disease has not been fully elucidated.

HOST FACTORS

Studies in mice have provided data linking immune responsiveness and resistance or susceptibility to chemical and biological antigens to the murine major transplantation (H-2) antigen complex. Subsequently, a host of diseases in man have also been shown to be associated with the human HLA complex. These studies were undertaken in part because of the tacit assumption that putative HLA linked immure response genes analogous to the murine system would permit the development of certain disease processes. In 1975 Greenberg and colleagues linked in vitro responsiveness to the antigens SK/SD and the major histocompatibility complex. In comparison to 52 normal individuals whose lymphocytes proliferated in vitro in response to the antigen SK/SD, there were 47 individuals who showed a complete lack of response. HLA B5 was present in 30 percent of the responders versus 8 percent of nonresponders ($p < 0.05$). Data such as these suggest that the host factors responsible for control of the immune response to infectious agents such as streptococcus may subsequently be identified.

CLINICAL FEATURES

After a latent period of 1–2 weeks following a streptococcal infection, a typical patient may present with the acute onset of hematuria (smoky, rusty, cloudy urine), oliguria, and facial edema. Very short latent periods of only a few days generally are indicative of an exacerbation of preexisting disease. The facial edema is noticeably worse upon first arising and diminishes with prolonged upright posture. Systemic symptoms of fatigue, malaise, and anorexia are often described.

On physical examination there is nearly always mild to moderate hypertension but without the funduscopic vascular changes seen in chronic hypertensive states. The heart may be enlarged due to the circulatory congestion which develops secondary to the renal retention of sodium and water. Despite the expanded extracellular volume there is rarely frank cardiac failure. The kidneys are often tender due to stretching of the renal capsules, and trace pitting edema of the lower extremities may be evident.

Beta hemolytic streptococci frequently can be grown from the nose, throat, or skin of patients with untreated APSGN. Laboratory examination of a freshly voided specimen of urine will likely reveal a modestly concentrated urine with 1–3+ qualitative proteinuria and few red blood cell and hyaline casts. A full blown nephrotic syndrome has been found in nearly 20 percent of hospitalized patients. In addition, a mild normocytic normochromic anemia and an elevated sedmentation rate are characteristic findings. In the acute phase fibrin degradation products are found in the urine. Elevated levels of plasmin activity, factor VIII, and fibrinogen, if found, also tend to correlate with clinical severity.

There may be a mild to moderate decrease in glomerular filtration rate while renal blood flow is well maintained, producing a characteristically low filtration fraction. A dilutional hyponatremia may develop if during the period of oliguria fluid intake is maintained. With progressive renal impairment, hyperkalemia, acidosis, hyperphosphatemia, and hypocalcemia may ensue.

In addition, many subclinical cases may be discovered only upon examination of the urine sediment of family members of individuals with clearcut disease. In one epidemic (Red Lake 1966) over 50 percent of the patients with nephritis were entirely asymptomatic and were discovered only by routine surveillance for microscopic hematuria. Several cases have also been reported in which the clinical features of acute glomerulonephritis were present and confirmed by renal biopsy but in which urinalyses have been essentially normal.

COURSE AND THERAPY

APSGN has been shown to occur following a streptococcal infection even though appropriate antibiotic therapy had been instituted promptly. Once the renal lesion has developed there is no evidence that antibacterial therapy has any influence on the course or ultimate prognosis of the disease, but it does prevent suppurative complications and markedly reduces the likelihood of transmission of the nephritogenic organism to the contacts of the patient. Culture should be taken from members of the patient's family and other close contacts; if it is positive, a course of antibiotic therapy should be given to these individuals. Of the different routes and schedules of penicillin administration a single intramuscular injection of 600,000 units of benzathine penicillin is most convenient and very effective.

The key therapeutic problem is preventing or treating the life-threatening complications of the acute phase, namely, pulmonary edema, hypertensive encephalopathy, hyperkalemia, and uremia. Once these difficulties are avoided, characteristically the urine volume spontaneously increases, edema disappears, blood pressure falls to normal, cardiomegaly abates, and gross hematuria begins to subside.

The cause of hypertension in APSGN is not totally clear, but the frequently noted correlation with salt and water balance suggests that expansion of extracellular or intravascular volume plays an important part. Hypertension is often found in edematous patients and typically subsides as a spontaneous diuresis ensues. Antihypertensive therapy is not necessary in most patients, but persistent elevation of diastolic pressure to levels above 110 mm Hg or signs of impending or overt encephalopathy are indications for drug therapy. In most patients there will be no need for further antihypertensive therapy after a few days.

The manifestations of circulatory congestion, including peripheral edema, cardiomegaly, pulmonary congestion, and pulmonary edema, can be effectively treated by salt restriction and elevation of the head of the bed. Since the cardiac output remains essentially normal, digitalis is of little value except in the older patient suspected of having preexisting intrinsic myocardial disease.

The degree of impairment of renal function correlates well with the extent of glomerular hypercellularity; in the extreme cases, oliguria or anuria result from severe proliferation, thrombosis, and necrosis of glomerular tufts. Administration of corticosteroids or immunosuppressive agents has yielded little beneficial effect. It appears that the risk of treatment with these drugs outweighs any potential benefits. In the severely oliguric patient, water restriction is necessary and measures to prevent and treat hyperkalemia are vital. Curtailment of protein intake and repeated dialysis may also be necessary during the oliguric phase.

PROGNOSIS

Irreversible renal failure occurs in 0.5–2 percent of patients and manifests itself clinically by a prolonged period of severe oliguria or anuria. Over 90 percent of children and approximately 50 percent of adults with acute nephritis go on to complete healing of their renal lesions. In such patients proteinuria and sediment abnormalities usually disappear in 3–6 months. It has been stated that persistence of proteinuria beyond 1 year indicates that complete healing will not take place. The validity of this view, however, is open to question. The extent of the healing process can be assessed by repeated urinalyses and measurements of protein excretion. The renal lesion can be considered fully healed when 24 hour protein excretion is normal and when the urine sediment reverts to normal. Patients excreting abnormal amounts of protein should be studied for postural proteinuria by obtaining urine collected in the upright and recumbent positions. Excretion of excess protein in both positions implies continued disease activity, whereas excess excretion in only the upright position can be taken as a sign of healing.

The prognosis for complete healing appears to be different in children and adults. In a 10 year followup of 61 children affected during the Great Lakes epidemic of 1953, no instances of chronic or progressive renal disease were found. Following the epidemic of poststreptococcal acute glomerulonephritis (APSGN) involving 720 patients in South Trinidad in 1965 a progress report was issued; only 1.8 percent had persistent urine abnormalities and another 8 percent had abnormalities that were transient or occurred only after the patient assumed the lordotic position. In 1.4 percent hypertension was present, whereas only one patient had azotemia. The immediate outcome for sporadic poststreptococcal glomerulonephritis, in comparison to the epidemic variety, seems only slightly less favorable. Failure to heal after 3 years or longer was observed in 11 percent of 47 children reported with sporadic poststreptococcal glomerulonephritis. Differences in the rate of healing were predicted on the basis of age and renal morphology at the onset of the illness. The proportion of children observed to have proteinuria decreased progressively from 67 percent at 1 year to 14 percent at 3 years. Studies from New York University, however, have noted persistent and possibly progressive lesions in as many as one-third of hospitalized children with sporadic APSGN who were followed for 2 years or more. Overall, the prognosis is excellent for children albeit somewhat more guarded if the disease is severe enough to require hospitalization.

Under these circumstances, examination of a renal biopsy specimen may be a useful adjunct in prognosticating eventual recovery. In one study 12 of 36 adults with sproadic APSGN went on to develop chronic glomerulonephritis. Patients destined to develop chronic glomerulonephritis tended to show a more serious degree of cell proliferation and glomerular injury on biopsy than patients who eventually healed completely. Many other studies have also demonstrated the development of histological and clinical "chronicity." The studies of Baldwin and co-workers, in particular, showed the relatively less satisfactory rate of complete resolution in 168 hospitalized patients after a 10 year period of followup. The frequency of hypertension (89 percent), nephrotic syndrome (18 percent), and renal insufficienty (BUN > 30 mg/dl in 64 percent) at the onset of the disease reflected the clinical severity of presentation. Within 6 months 65 percent still had proteinuria. By 1 year less than 20 percent were still hypertensive. The incidence of elevated blood pressure, however, rose to 50 percent in those under observation 5 years or more. Clinical assessment suggested that renal function was restored roughly to normal in all patients by the end of the first year as assessed by the serum creatinine level. Thereafter clinical uremia developed in six patients over periods ranging from 2 to 12 years. In the remainder, one-third had mildly elevated creatinines ranging between 1.1 and 2 mg/dl. Of 36 biopsy specimens obtained 3–18 years after the onset of disease, 56 percent contained significant numbers of sclerotic glomeruli. Taking the entire patient population who had been followed for 2 years or more, proteinuria was present in 46 percent, hypertension in 42 percent, reduced glomerular filtration rate in 38 percent, and glomerular sclerosis in 50 percent. These data indicate an overall progression to chronic glomerular disease in 60 percent of adults with sporadic APSGN. These findings also suggest the possibility that some patients presenting with idiopathic chronic sclerosing glomerulonephritis previously had a subclinical episode of post streptococcal glomerulonephritis.

In conclusion, APSGN remains the prototype for immune complex mediated nephritis. Despite the uncertainty regarding the exact nature of the antigen or the primary site of immune complex formation, the entire spectrum of host response and glomerular alteration may be witnessed in this disease.

REFERENCES

Baldwin DS: Poststreptococcal glomerulonephritis. Am J Med 62:1, 1977

Dodge WF, Spargo BH, Bass JA, et al: The relationship between the clinical and pathologic features of poststreptococcal glomerulonephritis. Medicine (Baltimore) 47:227, 1968

Glassock RJ, Bennett CM: The glomerulopathies, in Brenner BM, Rector FC Jr (eds): The Kidney. Philadelphia,W. .B. Saunders, 1976, p 941

Kaplan EL, Anthony BF, Chapman SS, et al: Epidemic acute glomerulonephritis associated with type 49 streptococcal pyoderma. Am J Med 48:9, 1970

Kassirer JP, Schwartz WB: Acute glomerulonephritis. N Engl J Med 265:686, 736, 1961

Lawrence JR, Pollak VE, Pirani CL, et al: Histological and clinical evidence of post streptococcal glomerulonephritis in patients with the nephrotic syndrome. Medicine (Baltimore) 42:1, 1963

Potter EV, Bidh A, Sharrett S, et al: Clinical healing two to six years after poststreptococcal glomerulonephritis in Trinidad. N Engl J Med 48:9, 1978

MEMBRANOPROLIFERATIVE GLOMERULONEPHRITIS

Mark S. Schiffer and Alfred J. Fish

Membranoproliferative glomerulonephritis (MPGN) or mesangiocapillary glomerulonephritis is the major recognizable form of chronic glomerulonephritis which can lead to endstage renal disease. In 1965, West and Gottoff independently characterized this disease by the unique finding of chronic hypocomplementemia, although hypocomplementemia is not universally present. The morphological forms of MPGN by light microscopy include lobular glomerulonephritis and membranoproliferative glomerulonephritis with and without crescents. Electron microscopic distribution and nature of the immune deposits has led to the following classification of MPGN: type I has subendothelial and mesangial deposits; type II has dense intramembranous deposits; and type III combines both subendothelial and subepithelial deposits and basement membrane changes. The three types of MPGN have similar clinical features and will be considered together.

MPGN is prevalent in older children and adults, constituting 10 percent of glomerulonephritis in most biopsy series. It is infrequent in children under 8 years of age and adults over age 30. Habib's series of 105 cases and other large series of MPGN in children provide the most data regarding clinical features and prognosis; however, series which include adults and children show the disease process to be the same in both age groups.

PRESENTING RENAL MANIFESTATIONS AND CLINICAL COURSE

Clinical presentation is extremely varied, ranging from an acute and rapidly progressive onset to an insidious course which is asymptomatic until advanced renal insufficiency is evident. About one-third of the cases present in a manner resembling acute glomerulonephritis, with gross or microscopic hematuria and edema with hypertension. Many patients have decreased glomerular filtration as the initial nephritic episode subsides. The diagnosis of acute poststreptococcal glomerulonephritis is often mistakenly made, especially if an elevated ASO titer is detected. Almost 90 percent of patients present initially with some degree of hematuria. One-third have increased BUN. One-quarter of all children and a greater proportion of adults with MPGN are hypertensive. Two-thirds of patients with MPGN have the nephrotic syndrome on first presentation, overlapping with the nephritic group. The sustained absence of nephrotic syndrome is a favorable prognostic sign. Patients should be monitored for proteinuria. A few patients with MPGN have an asymptomatic presentation with only high blood pressure or an abnormal urinalysis.

MPGN is a nonsystemic disorder with immune complex mediated injury to the kidney only. Systemic complications relate to the presence of hypertension, nephrotic syndrome, and uremia. Patients with MPGN do not have fever, arthritis, skin lesions, or cardiopulmonary involvement, which are associated with other immune complex diseases. There is, however, one rare systemic condition in which MPGN occurs; patients with partial lipodystrophy, who may be recognized by the absence of subcutaneous fat, especially in the face, develop type II MPGN in association with decreased serum complement and a circulating complement activating factor. These patients can be studied prospectively for the development of hypocomplementemia and renal disease.

About 80 percent of patients with MPGN have marked depression of C3 and total hemolytic complement either at onset or during their course, although hypocomplementemia is most uniformly present in type II MPGN. There are marked fluctuations of C3 levels in type I patients. While early complement components are normal, frequently C3, properdin, and the terminal complement components are low, implicating the alternate pathway of complement activation in this disease. Most of the hypocomplementemic patients have a factor in their serum called C3 nephritic factor (C3 nef). Upon mixing with normal serum or injection into an animal, C3 nef will cause activation and breakdown of C3 via the alternate pathway. In addition, some patients with type I MPGN have depression of early complement components C1q and C4, indicating activation of the classical complement pathway.

Most urinary abnormalities are present from onset. Macroscopic hematuria may be present during the first year, followed by persistent microscopic hematuria. Two-thirds of patients with MPGN are nephrotic initially, and an additional 10 percent become nephrotic later in their course. The nephrotic syndrome often remits with persistence of lesser amounts of proteinuria. Of patients who are free of edema during the first year, one-half will remain so through their subsequent course. Some patients exhibit a silent phase of nephritis with normal urinalysis and normal renal function. Persistent hypocomplementemia, C3 nef activity, and renal biopsy findings have verified ongoing glomerulonephritic changes. The clinical course of patients with MPGN is progressive, leading to endstage renal failure in 5 percent of patients with each year of followup. Over half of patients have reached dialysis or transplant or die 10 years after onset. During the course of increasing azotemia, recurrent acute nephritic episodes may occur, and renal function may be regained after these episodes, only to be gradually lost over subsequent years.

Many clinical and pathological aspects of the disease have been analyzed as indicators of a favorable or unfavorable prognosis. Most clinical signs are not reliable in this regard; however, the absence of the nephrotic syndrome during the initial presentation and in subsequent followup has been found to carry a highly favorable prognosis. None of these patients were found to be progressing toward renal failure and represented 15 percent of Habib's cases. Among the majority of patients who are nephrotic, a small proportion experienced remission of proteinuria; these patients also fared better on followup than the remaining patients with persistent proteinuria. The degree of azotemia has been examined as a possible predictor of long-term renal function. Collectively the group of patients with initial azotemia have a poorer prognosis, only because a small proportion of these patients did not recover renal function during the first year of the disease.

Patients who had never been noted to be hypocomplementemic have been separated from the larger hypocomplementemic group in many studies on the hypothesis that complement activity could be correlated with activity of the disease; however, survival and preservation of renal function is not different in the hypocomplementemic and the normocomplementemic groups. Attempts to correlate long-term clinical outcome with renal histology have also been made. Among light microscopic findings, the extent of crescent formation has been found to be associated with rapidly progressive course. As in other glomerulonephritides, crescents result from inflammation and fibrin and possibly platelet deposition, which can lead to the destruction of the glomerulus. The poor prognosis of extensive crescent formation does not depend upon the position of deposits by electron microscopy; however, crescent formation is somewhat more common among patients with type II MPGN.

The clinical course of type II MPGN can be only partly contrasted with that of the remaining MPGN patients, since in the former presentation with hematuria and recurrences of macroscopic hematuria are twice as common. Conversely, patients with type I MPGN are more likely to be asymptomatic and discovered on routine urinalysis or in advanced chronic renal failure. Nearly equal percentages of type I and type II MPGN patients are in the nonnephrotic group with a better prognosis. Type II MPGN patients are more likely to have persistent nephrotic syndrome. Azotemia at onset of illness is more common in type II MPGN than type I. At the center where it was first described, type III MPGN (subendothelial deposits with basement membrane changes) constitutes 25 percent of MPGN patients. Their course as a group is not different from that of type I patients. In most series, type III patients have not been separated from types I and II MPGN.

Numerous patients with endstage renal failure and MPGN have received kidney transplants. MPGN can recur in the transplanted kidney despite the immunosuppressive therapy which transplant patients receive.

Complement depression and presence of C3 nef are not resolved by pretransplant nephrectomy and may persist following transplantation. Type II MPGN is more prone to recur in the transplanted kidney. Emerging information about clinical course, prognosis, and efficacy of treatment of MPGN is related to renal biopsy findings, including ultrastructural analysis. Every patient suspected of having MPGN should have a renal biopsy with preparation of the tissue for light, fluorescent, and electron microscopy.

PATHOGENESIS AND PATHOLOGY

Since granular deposits of C3 and immunoglobulin are found by immunofluorescence in type I MPGN, an immune complex pathogenesis has been proposed. Furthermore, circulating immune complexes have been detected in MPGN using the Raji cell and C1q binding assays; however, the antigenic components of these complexes have not been identified. Similar glomerular pathologic changes are seen in septic patients with chronic bacterial infection such as staphylococcal infection of ventriculoatrial shunts, or in subacute bacterial endocarditis. When the infections are treated to remove the course of chronic antigenemia, glomerular lesions heal (see the chapter on *Sarcoidosis*). MPGN, however, is not related to any known infectious insult. Preceding group A beta hemolytic streptococcal infection has not been documented serologically. In Poland, where a very high incidence of Australia antigenemia is present, an association with type I MPGN has been reported in a large series of patients; Australia antigen was observed by immunofluorescence in the glomerular lesions. It is possible that MPGN patients have an altered response to infection. The effects of multiple subclinical infections may result in glomerular immune complex injury.

The well documented occurrence of C3 depression prior to MPGN in partial lipodystrophy patients raises the possibility that the renal lesion is caused in some way by complement depression. Though these patients have recurrent infections, no link has been made between infections and type II MPGN. Possibly, MPGN patients are unable to clear immune complexes normally, while infectious agents are normally resisted. Miller and Nussenzweig have demonstrated the role of C3 in the dissolution of immune complexes. C3 nef has been considered a possible initiating factor in complement depression. The alteration in complement components in type I MPGN, along with the presence of C3 nef, has suggested that both the classical and alternative pathways of complement activation occurs. It has recently been discovered that C3 nef is an autoantibody reactive with activated C3. The relationship of these findings to the pathogenesis of type I MPGN remains unknown at present.

Despite the demonstration of circulating immune complexes in type II MPGN, the immunopathologic findings do not support an immune complex pathogenesis. Only C3 staining around dense deposits is demonstrated; however, other complement components and immunoglobulins are absent. Intramembranous dense deposits are also found in tubular basement membranes and Bowman's capsule. Because of the similar staining characteristics to glomerular basement membrane lamina densa material and an altered but similar amino acid and sugar composition, it has been postulated that the dense deposits may represent altered basement membrane material, synthesized in response to an immune injury.

MPGN is not a hereditary disorder and does not occur in other family members. The disease has not been associated with any of the major (*A* or *B* locus) HLA antigens; however, Friend has demonstrated an association with B cell alloantigens. Because of the linkage among genes controlling these antigens, the immune response, and several complement factors, this observation may be of pathogenetic significance. Additional factors not considered in detail here, including clotting factors and vasoactive amines, may be involved in the pathogenesis of MPGN and promote glomerular damage, with progression from immune complex deposition to cellular proliferation with inflammation on to glomerular destruction with scarring.

By light microscopy the appearance of kidneys with the three types of MPGN is similar. The two constant features are mesangial cellular proliferation and capillary wall widening. The latter includes the endothelial and epithelial cell, the true glomerular basement membrane, and any interposing structures or deposits. Most prominently, mesangial cell proliferation and an associated increase in intercellular mesangial matrix are evident. Expansion of the mesangial zones results in distortion of the glomerular basement membrane, displacing it peripherally. When mesangial expansion is extreme, marked alteration of glomerular

architecture with prominent lobulation occurs. The latter is found in all three types of MPGN. Glomerular capillary lumens are narrowed by intrinsic endothelial cell proliferation and by mesangial expansion (Fig. 1). Polymorphonuclear leukocytes may be seen within glomerular capillary lumens, and crescent formation may be present. The light microscopic classification into lobular MPGN, crescentic MPGN, and simple MPGN is found in all three types of MPGN; final pathologic analysis requires immunofluorescent and electron microscopy. The capillary wall in MPGN may have a double linear or "tram track" appearance with PAS or silver methenamine stain (Fig. 2). The inner (capillary) aspect of the double linear array represents mesangial matrix material laid down by mesangial cells which have become interposed between the endothelial cell and the glomerular basement membrane. Mesangial cells may expand to completely surround the capillary wall. The outer of the two lines is the true glomerular basement membrane and is of normal caliber and appearance in type I MPGN. (The double linear appearance is seen in most cases of MPGN type I and III and some cases of type II.) The intramembranous lesions of type II MPGN are not always seen by light microscopy but may appear as refractile widened portions of the glomerular and tubular basement membranes and Bowman's capsule. The dense intramembranous deposits are reactive with silver stain.

Fluorescent microscopy is important in distinguishing the various types of MPGN. In types I and III MPGN, granular subendothelial deposits in a peripheral lobular distribution are seen to contain C3, C4, IgG, IgM, and properdin (Fig. 3). Occasional subepithelial deposits are also found. The expanded mesangial zones are largely free of immune deposits, in contrast to other

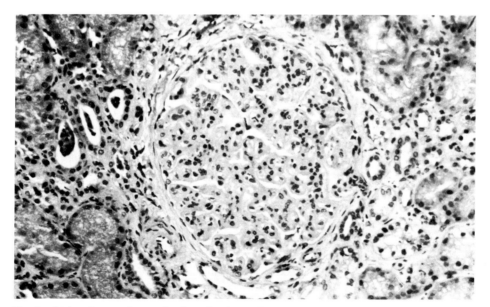

Fig. 1. Light microscopic examination of a glomerulus from a patient with type I MPGN showing marked endothelial and mesangial cell proliferation with glomerular capillary loop narrowing and lobulation. H & E. × 220.

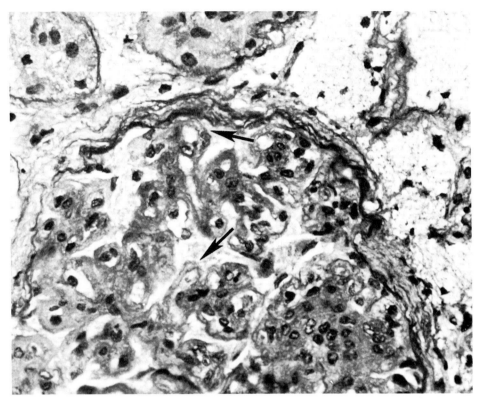

Fig. 2. Light microscopic examination of a portion of a glomerulus in type I MPGN showing splitting (arrows) and duplication of the glomerular basement membrane. PAS. × 540.

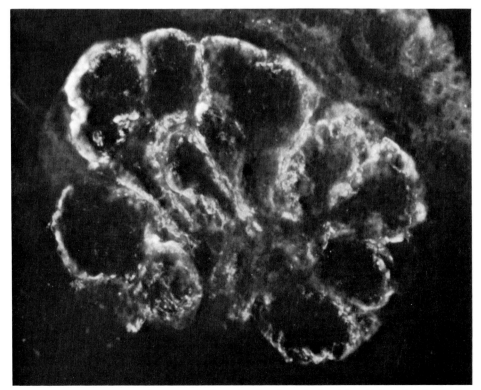

Fig. 3. Immunofluorescent microscopy findings showing the typical peripheral lobulation distribution of C3 in type I MPGN. × 350. [Reprinted with permission from Westberg NG, Naff GB, Boyer JT, Michael AF: Glomerular deposition of properdin in acute and chronic glomerulonephritis with hypocomplementemia. J Clin Invest 50:642, 1971.]

glomerulopathies with mesangial proliferation. In contrast, immunofluorescent staining in type II MPGN shows only a double linear staining pattern for C3 alone along the glomerular basement membrane. In addition, circular ring-like structures in the mesangium also stain for C3. The dense deposits themselves do not appear to contain immunoglobulins or complement components; however, the observed C3 staining appears only to surround but not include the dense deposits per se. Electron microscopy is required to definitively establish the type of MPGN. In type I MPGN mesangial proliferation and mesangial cell interposition along the glomerular capillary wall is prominent (Fig. 4). Electron-dense deposits are seen on the subendothelial side of the glomerular basement membrane; only occasional deposits in the mesangium and subepithelial loci are found. The true glomerular basement membrane is virtually normal in type I MPGN, except for focal splitting. In contrast, by electron microscopy typical immune deposits are not found in type II MPGN. Instead, electron-dense intramembranous deposits which appear to be fusiform widening of the lamina densa are evident. These intramembranous deposits have similar electron density to the lamina densa (Fig.

5). With peroxidase labeled antibodies, the absence of immunoglobulins and complement components within the dense intramembranous deposits and only scant C3 around the deposits is confirmed. Uniformly cases of type II MPGN have the dense deposits within the tubular basement membranes and Bowman's capsules as well. Type III MPGN has recently been described by the electron microscopic appearance of deposits on both sides of the glomerular basement membrane, which is widened but not uniformly dense and which has a frayed or striated appearance that can be highlighted by silver impregnation. Thus type III MPGN has immune deposits on either side of the glomerular basement membrane as in type I and alteration of the glomerular basement membrane itself, but the latter changes can be differentiated from the dense deposits characteristic of type II MPGN.

TREATMENT

No certain guidelines can be given for primary therapy of this inflammatory renal disease. Two forms of therapy for MPGN have been used by groups which have documented successful outcome in uncontrolled series. The two approaches are alternate day high-dose prednisone therapy or combination therapy with pred-

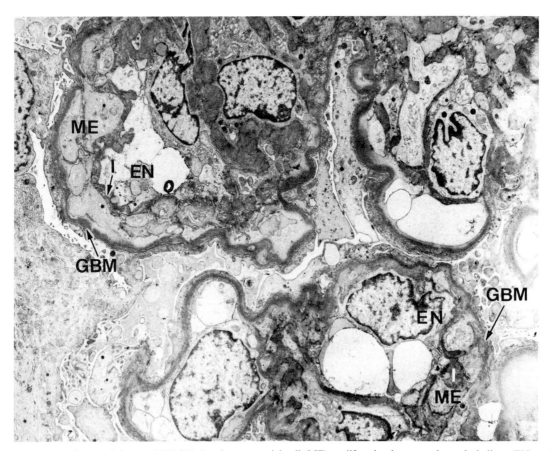

Fig. 4. Electron micrograph in type I MPGN showing mesangial cell (ME) proliferation between the endothelium (EN) and the glomerular basement membrane (GBM) with the interposition of mesangial matrix-like material (I). Original magnification × 5713. [Kindly provided by Dr. Robert Vernier.]

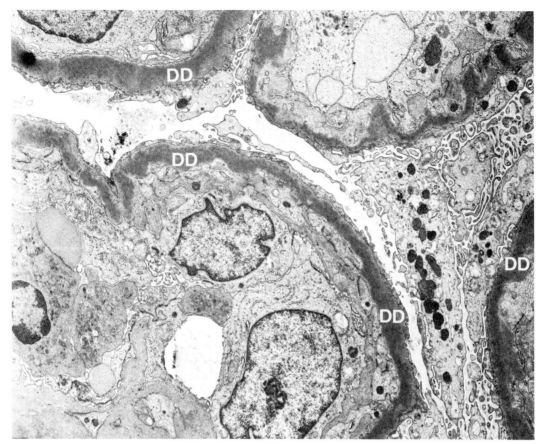

Fig. 5. Electron micrograph in type II MPGN showing a diffuse distribution of dense deposit (DD) material throughout the glomerular basement membrane. Original magnification × 6950. [Kindly provided by Dr. Robert L. Vernier.]

nisone, an alkylating agent, and anticoagulants. At present no controlled trial has been completed to support the efficacy of either form of treatment. Since controversy exists regarding the benefits of therapy in MPGN, the available data on this subject are detailed here.

West has treated a group of patients with prednisone using an alternate day dose of 1.5–2 mg/kg up to 80 mg for several years or longer. In eight patients followed with repeat biopsy for 3–9 years after institution of this regimen, documented histologic improvement occurred in all cases. Subendothelial deposits disappeared but intramembranous dense deposits persisted if previously present. Most glomeruli improved with diminution of hypercellularity. As noted by these investigators, this uncontrolled group of eight patients may represent a group with particularly nonaggressive MPGN, since during the interval prior to therapy renal function had not deteriorated, the average BUN remaining below 20 mg/dl. The International Study of Kidney Diseases in Children has undertaken a controlled trial of alternate day prednisone in children with MPGN using a slightly lower dose. The patients have been reevaluated with respect to renal function along with followup renal biopsies. Interim analysis of renal

function, with 27 patients followed for at least 2 years, failed to show significant advantage of prednisone therapy over a placebo. Both treated and untreated patients on repeat biopsy tended to show a diminution of mesangial hyperplasia.

Because of the role of coagulation mechanisms and platelets in the perpetuation of glomerular damage initiated by immune complex deposition, several groups have used combined immunosuppressive and anticoagulant therapy in MPGN. Kincaid-Smith has emphasized the role of anticoagulant therapy in the improvement of renal function and long-term prognosis. The addition of anticoagulants resulted in improved creatinine clearance in patients already being treated with immunosuppressive drugs. Currently, a controlled trial of the efficacy of the triad cyclophosphamide, warfarin, and dipyridamole in MPGN is being conducted in Australia. Early analysis shows no difference in proteinuria and other parameters related to therapy; however, there have been several more patients with deteriorating renal function in the "no treatment" group. This careful study may provide guidelines for therapy in the future. Other groups have also used combined immunosuppressive and anticoagulant therapy. Cameron has used corticosteroids, azathioprine, dipyridamole, and heparin (later changed to warfarin) in a group of patients with crescentic glomerulonephritis, including MPGN. In the most severe MPGN group, those with extensive crescents in more than 60 percent of glomeruli, 9 of 16 patients had improved renal function. The results were better than with the use of prednisone alone; however, the specific added benefit of anticoagulants cannot be determined from these series.

We currently do not treat MPGN patients with steroids or immunosuppressive therapy. We would, however, consider a short course of prednisone and azathioprine for patient with an aggressively inflammatory, crescentic lesion and a rapid progression toward renal failure. We await information of an adequately controlled study showing that any therapeutic regimen improves upon the natural history of this disorder. Additional general measures to control hypertension and alleviate the edema of fluid overload or nephrotic syndrome with diuretic therapy are of benefit. The usual approaches to managing chronic renal failure of MPGN include control of hyperphosphatemia, acidosis, and anemia. Despite the incidence of recurrent MPGN in the transplanted kidney, transplantation is of benefit to MPGN patients in chronic renal failure. The long-term survival of these grafts is uncertain at present.

REFERENCES

Antoine B, Faye C: The clinical course associated with dense deposits in the kidney basement membranes. Kidney Int 1:420, 1972

Gotoff SP, Fellers FX, Vawter GF, et al: The β1C globulin in childhood nephrotic syndrome. N Engl J Med 273:524, 1965

Habib R, Gubler M-C, Loirat C, et al: Dense deposit disease: A variant of membranoproliferative glomerulonephritis. Kidney Int 7:204, 1975

Habib R, Kleinknecht C, Gubler M-C, et al: Idiopathic membranoproliferative glomerulonephritis in children. Report of 105 cases. Clin Nephrol 1:194, 1973

Mandalenakis N, Mendoza N, Pirani CL, et al: Lobular glomerulonephritis and membranoproliferative glomerulonephritis. Medicine (Baltimore) 50:319, 1971

McAdams AJ, McEnery PT, West CD: Mesangiocapillary glomerulonephritis: Changes in glomerular morphology with long-term, alternate day prednisone therapy. J Pediatr 86:23, 1975

McLean RH, Geiger H, Burke B, et al: Recurrence of membranoproliferative glomerulonephritis following kidney transplantation serum complement component studies. Am J Med 60:60, 1976

Miller GW, Nussenzweig V: A new complement function: Solubilization of antigen-antibody aggregates. Proc Natl Acad Sci USA 72:418, 1975

Peters DK, Charlesworth JA, Sissons JGP, et al: Mesangiocapillary nephritis: Partial lipodystrophy and hypocomplementaemia. Lancet 2:535, 1973

West CD: Pathogenesis of membranoproliferative nephritis. Kidney Int 9:1, 1976

Westberg NG, Naff GB, Boyer JT, Michael AF: Glomerular deposition of properdin in acute and chronic glomerulonephritis with hypocomplementemia. J Clin Invest 50:642, 1971

EPIMEMBRANOUS NEPHROPATHY

Marvin Forland

Epimembranous nephropathy is a histopathologic entity characterized by lesions related to the presence of electron-dense deposits initially in the subepithelial area of the glomerular capillary wall which are believed to be of immune complex origin. The lesions may be idiopathic or associated with identifiable antigens of infectious, drug, neoplastic, or autoimmune origin (Table 1).

The addition of the prefix epi- to the earlier term, membranous nephropathy, makes more explicit the nature of the lesion. Epimembranous nephropathy is also preferable to the earlier designation, membranous glomerulonephritis, since the lesion does not have the proliferative or exudative features associated with a glomerular inflammatory process.

Bell introduced the term membranous glomerulonephritis in 1950 to describe renal disease of primarily glomerular localization with minimal proliferative changes. He included cases of lipoid nephrosis or "pure" nephrosis in this category, as well as those with clearcut glomerular capillary wall thickening. With the availability of electron microscopy, Farquhar was able to make the distinction between thickening of the capillary wall associated with epithelial foot process fusion or effacement in lipoid nephrosis and basement membrane thickening due to the addition of an irregular layer of dense, heterogeneous material on the epithelial side of the basement membrane in epimembranous nephropathy. Subsequently, distinct differences in pathology, natural history, and therapeutic response were described between epimembranous nephropathy and the nil or minimal change lesion associated with lipoid nephrosis. Immunofluorescence microscopy further confirmed the separation with the demonstration of the granular immunoglobulin deposits in epimembranous nephropathy and the lack of immunoglobulin deposition with a nil lesion.

INCIDENCE AND OCCURRENCE

Epimembranous nephropathy occurs primarily in adults, particularly in midlife, and has been found to be present in approximately one-quarter to one-third of adult patients with a diagnosis of idiopathic nephrotic syndrome undergoing renal biopsy. Its occurrence among children is far less common and accounts for approximately 5 percent of the idiopathic nephrotic group. A slight to major preponderance of males has been observed in most reported series of patients.

PATHOPHYSIOLOGY

The histopathology of epimembranous nephropathy closely resembles the experimental lesion resulting from the administration of a relatively small-sized antigen in just sufficient dosage to maintain a low-level antibody response with continuing antigen excess. The bovine serum albumin (BSA) rabbit model produces such a lesion when 1–5 mg BSA are given daily. It is postulated that the small, soluble immune complexes become trapped in the subepithelial area, where they are inadequate to initiate a significant inflammatory process due to their physical properties or localization. In the experimental model normal structure and function may return if the antigen administration is discontinued sufficiently early.

The analogy to the human lesion is supported by the increasing number of antigens which have been characterized by immunofluorescence microscopy or eluate studies of human renal biopsies. These include carcinoembryonic and other tumor antigens, hepatitis B, *Treponema pallidum,* and protozoal antigens. Recently developed techniques for detecting circulating immune complexes demonstrate such material in less than half the patients with membranous nephropathy.

PATHOLOGY

At the early stages of the disease, light microscopy reveals a rigid appearance of the glomeruli related to slight thickening of the capillary walls (see Fig. 4 of the chapter on *Light Microscopy*). Scattered, small, discrete electron-dense deposits are evident along the subepithelial surface of the glomerular basement membrane on electron microscopy. Proliferative, exudative, or necrotic changes are not present. Immunofluorescence studies show a diffuse granular pattern along the capillary surface with IgG and C′3 present (Fig. 1). IgA distribution may resemble IgG. IgM and fibrin may be present but irregularly distributed.

In more advanced lesions the capillary wall thickening is increased; methenamine silver stains demon-

Table 1

Clinical and Etiologic Associations With Epimembranous Nephropathy

Drugs and heavy metals
  Bismuth
  Gold
  Mercury
  Penicillamine
  Sulfadiazine silver
  Trimethadione
Infection
  Filariasis
  Hepatitis B
  Leprosy
  Malaria
  Schistosomiasis
  Syphilis —congenital, secondary
Neoplasia
  Carcinoma
  Lymphoma and Hodgkin's disease
  Sarcoma
Intrinsic or undefined antigens
  Renal tubular antigen
  Sarcoidosis
  Sickle-cell disease
  Sjögren's syndrome
  Systemic lupus erythematosus
Uncertain association
  Chronic allograft rejection
  Diabetes mellitus
  Renal vein thrombosis
  Rheumatoid arthritis

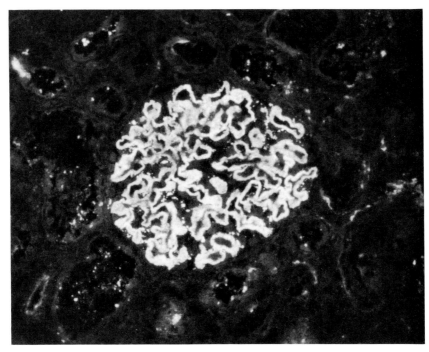

Fig. 1. Immunofluorescence microscopy demonstrating a heavy granular deposition of IgG along capillary walls in epimembranous nephropathy. × 250.

strate projections of basement membrane extending subepithelially and beginning to encompass large masses of periodic acid positive material believed to be immune complexes. This creates the characteristic "spike and dome" or "hairbrush" appearance of the outer surface of the capillary wall (Fig. 2). Tangential sections may show a bubbly appearance of the basement membrane related to irregularities of the lamina densa secondary to the deposits. On electron microscopy the basement membrane spikes are clearly delineated extending between the osmophilic deposits (see Fig. 3 of the chapter on *Electron Microscopy*). Fusion of the foot processes also usually is present. Heavy deposition of granular immunofluorescence material is now observed.

With further progression, portions of the glomerular tuft become sclerotic with occlusion of capillary lumina, adherence of loops, and eventual loss of glomeruli. The remaining discrete capillary walls may show a vacuolated appearance. Electron microscopy shows further capillary wall thickening with fusion of the spikes and complete enclosure of the deposits. The incorporated deposits may lose their electron density, become amorphous, and leave a markedly thickened, fenestrated, or scarred capillary basement membrane.

Ehrenreich and Churg have proposed a system of morphologic staging of epimembranous nephropathy. Stage 1 is characterized by scanty, small deposits; stage 2 is the fully manifest lesion with large, often contiguous deposits separated by narrow projections of basement membrane; stage 3 is an advanced lesion with deposits incorporated into a markedly thickened basement membrane with many spikes; stage 4 is characterized by an irregular, grossly thickened basement membrance with rarefied intramembranous deposits. A stage 5 has also been suggested for the endstage lesion with many obsolescent glomeruli. A recent study reports that the sequence of deposit deposition, incorporation, and ultimate clearing in some patients may occur at an electron microscopic level of resolution without appreciable spikes or glomerular basement membrane thickening on light microscopy. This evolution in ultrastructure alone was associated with a benign clinical course. Correlation between the stage of a lesion and the patient's clinical status generally has not been reliable, although stages 1 and 2 are considered by some as most likely to permit clinical remission. Glomerular filtration rate has been reported to correlate most closely with capillary wall thickening and proteinuria with the ultrastructural density of deposits and intensity of immunofluorescence staining.

CLINICAL AND LABORATORY FEATURES

Epimembranous nephropathy presents with nephrotic syndrome in most patients or asymptomatic proteinuria. Microscopic hematuria is seen in approximately half the patients, and macroscopic hematuria has been observed in children but appears to be rare among adults. Differential protein clearances generally show a nonselective pattern but may be highly selective with mild lesions. Serum complement levels are normal, except when the lesion is associated with systemic lupus erythematosus. Children typically have only a

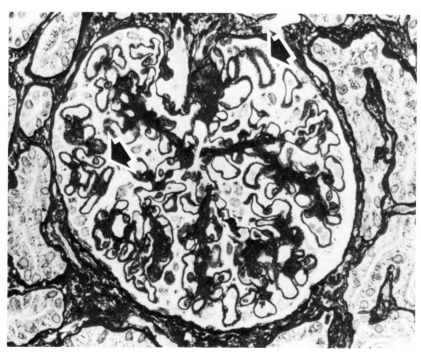

Fig. 2. "Spike and dome" or "hairbrush" appearance of the outer surface of the capillary wall (arrows) in epimembranous nephropathy. Methenamine silver–PAS. × 400.

moderate increase in cholesterol level, as well as marked hypoalbuminemia as compared to those with a minimal change lesion. Hypertension and azotemia are usual concomitants of progression of the lesion.

DIFFERENTIAL DIAGNOSIS

Epimembranous nephropathy must be a consideration in the differential diagnosis of any patient with proteinuria or nephrotic syndrome. It is associated with a wide range of etiologies, each apparently responsible for antigenic release and antibody formation. Systemic lupus erythematosus, carcinoma, hepatitis B antigen, and drug administration are among the most commonly recognized sources. Recent studies have demonstrated an association with carcinoma in approximately 10 percent of adult patients with nephrotic syndrome (see the chapter on *Renal Lesions in Malignancy*).

Approximately 70 percent of these patients with carcinoma and nephrotic syndrome have been found to have epimembranous nephropathy. A number of studies have demonstrated either tumor-associated antigens or antibodies to these antigens in the material eluted from renal biopsy tissue in tumor-associated epimembranous nephropathy. In addition to tumor-associated antigens, a possible role for fetal, viral, or autoimmune antibody complexes exists in such patients. Remission has been documented with successful resection of tumor, but the majority of patients have had a relatively rapid course associated with progressive carcinomatosis. Lung, colon, and stomach carcinomas have been the most frequently reported. The nephrotic syndrome associated with Hodgkin's disease has most often been associated with minimal change nephropathy, although epimembranous nephropathy has also been reported. Renal vein thrombosis has been considered to be a cause of epimembranous nephropathy, but more recent observations indicate it is more likely a consequence of nephrotic syndrome (see the chapter on *Renal Vein Thrombosis*).

A prospective study of patients with nephrotic syndrome has described renal vein thrombosis in over one-third of patients with epimembranous nephropathy or membranoproliferative glomerulonephritis, but others have failed to confirm this high frequency. In a review of the reported cases of renal vein thrombosis and nephrotic syndrome, epimembranous nephropathy contributed 51 of 87 cases (59 percent) and membranoproliferative glomerulonephritis 14 (16 percent). While evidence of a hypercoagulable state with an increased occurrence of thromboembolic phenomena has been well described in nephrotic syndrome regardless of etiology, the reasons for the predominant occurrence of renal vein thrombosis with epimembranous nephropathy remain unexplained.

Morphologically, the earlier stages of the lesions may be indistinguishable from the minimal change lesion by light microscopy. With progression, the light microscopic appearance may sometimes be confused with diabetic glomerulopathy or early amyloidosis, both causes of diffuse thickening of the glomerular basement membrane. Special staining techniques or electron microscopy particularly facilitate the establishment of the diagnosis by revealing the characteristic subepithelial deposits. The later stages may resemble membranoproliferative glomerulonephritis with light microscopy, but the normal mesangium and characteristic spike and dome pattern with PASM stain and lack of subendothelial deposits or basement membrane splitting and minimal proliferative changes are usually readily appreciated.

COURSE AND PROGNOSIS

Complete remission has been reported in about 20–25 percent of patients; in approximately half this has been independent of corticosteroid or immunosuppressive therapy. Complete clearing of immune complex deposits has been found on repeat renal biopsies in several patients with sustained remission, paralleling observations in the experimental model.

A variety of factors and findings have been suggested as influencing prognosis, both without treatment and in relationship to response to corticosteroid therapy. There is general agreement that pediatric patients are more likely to have spontaneous remissions and maintain stable renal function; only few cases of epimembranous nephropathy in childhood have been reported in which endstage renal disease has resulted. This advantage of youth has been true in groups compared with onset before and after age 30. Patients presenting with mild proteinuria appear to have a more favorable outlook than those with sufficient protein loss to result in nephrotic syndrome. Rowe and associates have found the degree of proteinuria at onset to be a better indicator of prognosis than the severity of histopathologic lesions on renal biopsy. Similar observations have been made in patients with mesangiocapillary glomerulonephritis and in the course of diabetic glomerulosclerosis. Less advanced staging of the histologic lesion also has been correlated with better prognosis by some but not all observers. Females have been found to have a better long-term prognosis in one study. The major factors at onset suggested as associated with high mortality have included massive proteinuria (greater than 10 g/day), severe hypoalbuminemia (less than 1.5 g/dl), diastolic hypertension, and sustained microscopic hematuria.

In patients presenting with nephrotic syndrome, approximately half will reach endstage renal disease within 10 years. Since the patients with proteinuria of lesser degree are apt to have a more benign course, Rowe et al. suggested that approximately one-third of adult patients with epimembranous nephropathy will have reached endstage renal disease within a 20 year period. Recurrence of the lesion following transplantation is described but rarely and has not emerged as a significant problem.

Superimposition of a rapidly progressive glomerulonephritis in a patient with nephrotic syndrome and epimembranous nephropathy has been observed. IgG eluates from the kidney were demonstrated to bind to human and monkey glomerular basement membrane, and the initial epimembranous nephropathy was postulated as a source for release of glomerular basement membrane antigens provoking an anti-GBM reaction.

THERAPY

The benefits of corticosteroids or immunosuppressive therapy have been difficult to evaluate in the treatment of epimembranous nephropathy because of its relatively slow rate of progression and the significant occurrence of spontaneous remission. In contrast to lipoid nephrosis, early uncontrolled studies failed to indicate therapeutic efficacy of glucocorticoids. A series of controlled studies have failed to demonstrate benefit from low-dose prednisone given for at least 6 months, prednisone and azathioprine for 2–6 months, and azathioprine or cyclophosphamide given alone for 1 year. A report by Lagrue et al. indicates greater than 50 percent remission in patients treated with chlorambucil alone.

Recent uncontrolled reports suggesting benefit from early and prolonged therapy with glucocorticoids have stimulated brisk correspondence from those with opposing views. The United States Collaborative Study of the Adult Nephrotic Syndrome has reported preliminary data demonstrating a reduction of proteinuria and less deterioration of GFR with a 2 month course of 2 mg/kg alternate day prednisone therapy as compared to a placebo treated group. While the corticosteroid treated group had a more marked diminution in proteinuria and higher number of remissions, relapses were the rule following cessation of therapy in most showing initial responses, and there was no difference between groups in the number remaining in remission at the time of the report; however, a doubling of serum creatinine occurred in only 1 of 34 treated patients and was seen in 11 of 38 patients without treatment. One in the latter group had died and five were on dialysis. These findings in two groups comparable in age, sex, severity of renal pathology, proteinuria, blood pressure, and duration of disease indicate the value of further followup and continued controlled clinical trials with perhaps a longer duration of therapy. The failure to induce complete remission but to maintain renal function with corticosteroids has been suggested in several earlier uncontrolled studies and is an important observation if confirmed.

Until firmer data are available, we reserve corticosteroid therapy for patients with the major features of nephrotic syndrome or fall in glomerular filtration rate.

REFERENCES

Ehrenreich T, Porush JG, Churg J, et al: Treatment of idiopathic membranous nephropathy. N Engl J Med 295:741, 1976

Germuth FG Jr, Rodriquez E: Immunopathology of the Renal Glomerulus. Boston, Little, Brown, 1973

Glassock RJ: The treatment of idiopathic membranous nephropathy in adults, in: Proceedings of the VIIth International Congress of Nephrology. Montreal, Presses de l'Universite de Montreal, 1978, p 425.

Habib R, Kleinknecht C, Gubler M-C: Extramembranous glomerulonephritis in children: Report of 50 cases. J Pediatr 82:754, 1973

Noel LH, Zanetti M, Droz D, et al: Long-term prognosis of idiopathic membranous glomerulonephritis. Am J Med 66:82, 1979

Row RG, Cameron JS, Turner DR et al: Membranous nephropathy. Long-term followup and association with neoplasia. Q J Med 44:207, 1975

RAPIDLY PROGRESSIVE GLOMERULONEPHRITIS

Allen I. Arieff

Rapidly progressive glomerulonephritis (RPGN) is a clinical pathologic syndrome that is characterized by an abrupt onset of azotemia which is often accompanied by oliguria, with a lack of tendency toward spontaneous recovery. RPGN is not a disease but rather a syndrome, which may be seen in association with several systemic disease states (Table 1). In addition, several systemic diseases may result in acute oliguric renal failure without glomerulonephritis. These include malignant hypertension, postpartum renal failure, scleroderma, interstitial hypersensitivity nephritis (usually drug related), atheroembolic renal disease, renal artery embolus, and acute renal failure.

The clinical characteristics of RPGN include a rapid onset of glomerulonephritis with azotemia, usually leading to loss of renal function within 6 months. There are no specific clinical signs or symptoms, although a history of upper respiratory infection is present in about 50 percent of cases. The physical findings are not different than those observed in patients with renal failure from other causes. Hypertension is not a consistent finding, nor is arthralgia. Urinalysis almost always reveals the presence of RBCs, WBCs, and RBC casts. There is a male sexual preponderance, and the age range extends from the late teens to the seventh decade, although most patients are males of age 30–50 years. Most patients have proteinuria of at least 2 g/day, with concomitant hypoaluminemia. Immunologic findings are variable. Total complement is generally normal, serum rheumatoid factor is positive in about 50 percent of cases, and the lupus erythematosus (LE) prep is usually negative.

Renal biopsy is necessary to establish the diagnosis of RPGN. There is a characteristic histologic pattern which includes extensive proliferation of the epithelial cells which line Bowman's space such that crescents are formed. These epithelial crescents (Fig. 1) probably should be present in at least 80 percent of glomeruli before the diagnosis of RPGN is made. In addition, most patients will have diffuse extracapillary proliferation. There may be endocapillary proliferation as well, particularly in patients with a history of streptococcal disease. Areas of necrosis and scarring may also be present. With a more extended illness, there may be organization of some crescents, and with time there is usually a tendency towards progressive sclerosis and fibrosis of glomeruli (Fig. 1).

Electron microscopy does not reveal a consistent pattern, and the changes may actually be related to the underlying disease processes. There may be subendothelial electron-dense deposits in some patients, but in others these are absent. The deposits may be located either endo- or extramembranously and often appear to consist of bundles of fine tubular structures seen in both longitudinal and transverse sections. There may be rupture of the basement membrane with wrinkling and cellular necrosis of capillary walls. Actual obstruction of capillary loops with platelet–fibrin thrombi may also be present.

The immunofluorescent findings are highly variable. There may be a linear deposition pattern suggestive of Goodpasture's syndrome, or there may be no evidence of deposits at all. At least four different patterns of immunoglobulin deposition have been described in patients with RPGN—31 percent were negative for IgG but positive for fibrin-related antigen (FRA) and/or C3, and 53 percent were distinctly positive for IgG and usually also positive for C3 and FRA. About 75 percent of the IgG positive group revealed a granular pattern,

Table 1
Systemic Disease Associated With Rapidly Progressive Glomerulonephritis

Goodpasture's syndrome
Polyarteritis nodosa
Systemic lupus erythematosus
Poststreptococcal glomerulonephritis
Henoch-Schönlein syndrome
Acute necrotizing vasculitis
Hypersensitivity angiitis
Wegener's granulomatosis
Infective endocarditis
Mixed cryoglobulinemia

whereas about 25 percent revealed linear deposits typical of an anti-GBM antibody pathogenesis. Approximately 16 percent of the biopsies were irregularly positive for IgG and/or C3. Glomerular deposition of FRA was found to some extent in about 80 percent of the cases.

It is apparent from the above that RPGN is a heterogeneous disorder, yet despite its obvious heterogeneous nature, attempts at therapy have been largely random, with no attempt to correlate treatment with other aspects of the disease. Many different therapeutic modalities have been employed. These have included steroids, immunosuppressive agents, antiplatelet

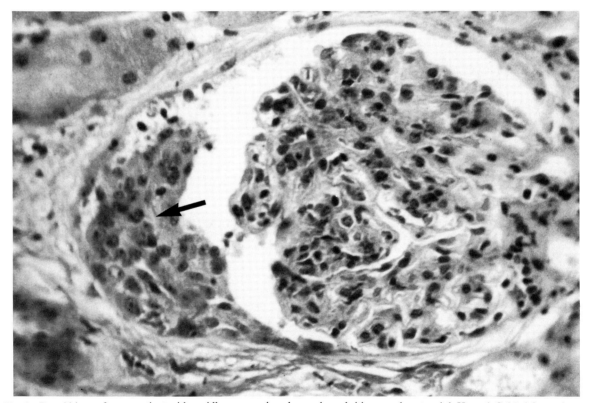

Fig. 1 Renal biopsy from a patient with rapidly progressive glomerulonephritis secondary to adult Henoch-Schönlein syndrome. There is early crescent formation (arrow) with focal infiltration (extracapillary) of the glomerulus. This patient's GFR fell as low as 16 ml/min, but rose to over 60 ml/min with anticoagulant therapy. Azan stain. × 450

agents, anticoagulants, plasmapheresis, extracorporeal immunoperfusion, and no therapy.

In general, in adults the natural history of the untreated disorder suggests a loss of renal function within 1 year in over 80 percent of patients. For example, in 11 large series comprising 154 patients, 88 percent lost all renal function within 1 year. Much of the literature on treatment of RPGN predates the rather extensive use of chronic dialysis and renal transplantation which is now common in the United States. Thus in many of the older studies the endpoint of RPGN was demise of the patient, whereas now (1980) most patients with endstage renal disease are treated with dialysis or renal transplantation.

Immunosuppressive therapy (steroids and immunosuppressive agents) have been used in various combinations to treat RPGN for over 15 years. The results are almost uniformly unsatisfactory. In four studies comprising 55 patients, over 85 percent died or became anephric within 1 year. Of the very few reported survivors, most either were under 16 years of age or had PRGN secondary to streptococcal disease. In the latter group of patients, RPGN is associated with a far more favorable prognosis. At present, the available evidence supports the concept that immunosuppressive therapy alone has no place in the treatment of RPGN. In patients whose RPGN is related to streptococcal disease, recovery is probably spontaneous and unrelated to therapy.

Anticoagulant and antithrombotic agents have been used in the treatment of RPGN for about 10 years. An understanding of the rationale for use of such agents involves a description of the role of the coagulation process in the pathophysiology of renal disease.

Involvement of the coagulation system in renal damage requires activation of intravascular coagulation in renal vessels. Agents which are known to trigger intravascular coagulation include tissue thromboplastin (activator), bacterial endotoxin, intravascular hemolysis, antigen–antibody complexes, particulate and colloidal matter, proteolytic enzymes, vasomotor activity, viruses, anoxemia, and endothelial damage in blood vessels.

The amount, type, and location of intravascular fibrin deposits are largely dependent on the condition of the vascular bed at the time the clotting mechanism is triggered. Known factors responsible for localization of fibrin deposits include amount and potency of procoagulants in the circulation, site of activation of the clotting mechanism, vasomotor-active agents (epinephrine, norepinephrine, histamine, serotonin), the fibrinolytic enzyme system, pregnancy, renal glomerular filtration, and endothelial damage in blood vessels.

The proximate activators of blood coagulation include three mechanisms: intrinsic system, extrinsic system, and complement.

The classical mechanism of complement activation involves the interaction of C1 with immunoglobulin aggregates, followed by the formation of the C3 convertase (C4,2) with subsequent initiation of the C3,9 sequence. Recently, an alternate pathway of complement activation has been defined that initiates the complement sequence at C3, bypassing the earlier components. According to McKay both endotoxin and immunoglobulins can activate this alternate mechanism.

The role of complement as a trigger to intravascular clotting may be very important in diseases in which fibrin deposits play a role in the pathogenesis of renal disease.

Each of the various mechanisms of fibrin deposition in the kidney apparently has a different effect on renal function. If the deposit obstructs the arteriolar or capillary lumen, ischemic necrosis follows. If a vein is obstructed, edema and hemorrhage are the major effects. If a vascular deposit is mural and nonocclusive, a diminished blood flow and/or glomerular filtration rate and albuminuria may result. If the deposit is extravascular, as in the capsular space, organization of the extravascular clot may result in a "crescent" with obliteration of the function of the nephron. This is felt to be the sequence in RPGN.

The intravascular or extravascular deposition of fibrin is always a secondary event and is indicative of a prior or primary etiologic factor. Knowledge of the mechanism by which fibrin is deposited may prove useful in selection of therapy. There are at least seven basic mechanisms, including thrombosis (intravascular coagulation); glomerular filtration—deposition of fibrin on the glomerular capillary basement membrane; hypertension with deposition of fibrin in walls of arteries and arterioles; leakage of blood (extravascular coagulation); glomerular endothelial damage (local intravascular coagulation); venous thrombosis; and uremia.

All of the above may be important in the pathogenesis of selected cases of RPGN. A pathogenetic association among activation of the coagulation system, fibrin deposition in arterioles, and the crescent formation and extracapillary proliferation typical of RPGN is suggested by the frequent finding of FRA in glomeruli and crescents by immunofluorescent studies and the presence of FRA in the urine. The focal gaps and discontinuities along glomerular basement membrane observed in association with crescents may be the route by which the large molecule of fibrinogen escapes into Bowman's space. Furthermore, the experimental production of similar lesions by intravascular coagulation supports such a relationship.

Several studies have demonstrated an inhibition of crescent formation in experimental nephritis by anticoagulants. The absence of antihemophilic globulin in the crescentic lesion suggests that the polymerization of the fibrinogen molecule may be occurring by thrombin independent mechanisms. Finally, several investigators have recently advanced the hypothesis that monocytes, machrophages, or inflammatory cells constitute the majority of the proliferating cells of the crescent rather than the conventional view of an epithelial cell origin for these cells. Polymerized fibrinogen itself or one of its derivatives acting on other plasma factors could be acting as a chemotactic factor under these circumstances.

With the above as background, several different investigators have with considerable success treated experimental RPGN in laboratory animals with anticoagulants. This led to the use of similar agents (heparin, dipyridimole, sulfinpyrazone, warfarin) to treat RPGN in man. Initial results suggested a therapeutic success exceeding 75 percent, but it is now apparent that less than half of such patients with RPGN will respond to anticoagulant therapy with an improvement in renal function to the point where dialysis will not be required. The usual regimen has been initial therapy with intravenous heparin infusion at about 1000 units/hour for about 2 weeks or until serum creatinine has stabilized. This has been followed by oral anticoagulants (warfarin) combined with agents which decrease platelet adhesiveness (dipyridamole, sulfinpyrazine, salicylate). The issue is somewhat clouded by the fact that most such patients were also simultaneously treated with immunosuppressive agents (steroids, azathioprine, cyclophosphamide).

Although anticoagulant therapy appears beneficial in many patients with RPGN, the potential complications are substantial. There have been reports of gastrointestinal hemorrhage, intramuscular bleeding, genitourinary bleeding, and pulmonary hemorrhage, with at least one death. Recent evidence suggests that the effects of heparin in treatment of RPGN may not be related to its anticoagulant effect but to some other pharmacologic action, such as inhibition of complement activation (see above discussion). Along these lines, several patients with RPGN have recently been treated with low-dosage heparin infusion (250 units/hour) such that clotting time is unaffected. In several case reports, low-dosage heparin infusion was as effective as high-dosage infusion in stabilzing or improving the renal function of patients with RPGN. If these early reports are confirmed, then regular use of low- rather than high-dosage heparin should diminish the incidence of hemorrhagic complications.

Plasmapheresis has been used in the treatment of a small number of cases of RPGN of diverse etiology. Compared to a loss of renal function in at least 80 percent of untreated patients, 73 percent of 22 patients treated with plasmapheresis showed an improvement in renal function

External immunoperfusion is conceptually similar to plasmapheresis, but rather than plasma exchange, blood is circulated extracorporeally through special columns designed to remove various pathogenetic substances. The columns may contain enzymes designed to degrade active complexes, such as DNA. This technique has not yet been used in human subjects; however it has been shown that extracorporeal perfusion of dog blood in vivo over a column containing deoxyribonuclease immobilized on activated nylon microspheres can degrade labeled DNA in vivo. Previous studies have demonstrated that various columns can absorb DNA and anti–bovine serum albumin. These studies suggest a future role of immunoperfusion in the treatment of RPGN.

It is apparent from the above discussion that rapidly progressive glomerulonephritis is not a homogeneous entity from a clinical, histological, or immunological viewpoint. It is rather a clinical syndrome characterized by rapid development of renal failure and widespread crescent formation. It can be found in association with a wide variety of known clinical conditions (Table 1). Histology and immunopathology, even in the "idiopathic" form, are extremely heterogeneous. It is no longer appropriate to describe therapeutic programs and recovery rates for rapidly progressive glomerulonephritis without defining the nature and extent of the renal lesions by immunofluorescence, electron microscopy, and routine histology.

REFERENCES

Arieff AI, Pinggera WF: Rapidly progressive glomerulonephritis treated with anticoagulants. Arch Intern Med 129:77, 1972

Brown CB, Turner D, Ogg CS, et al: Combined immunosuppression and anticoagulation in rapidly progressive glomerulonephritis. Lancet 2:1166, 1974

Cameron JS, Leathem A, Suc JM, et al: Are anticoagulants beneficial in the treatment of rapidly progressive glomerulonephritis? Proc Eur Dial Transplant Assoc 10:57, 1973

Glassock RJ: Clinico-pathologic spectrum and therapeutic strategies in "rapidly progressive" glomerulonephritis. Proc Clin Dial Transplant Forum 5:109, 1975

Kincaid-Smith P, Laver MC, Fairley KF, et al: Dipyridamole and anticoagulants in renal disease due to glomerular and vascular lesions: A new approach to therapy. Med J Aust 1:145, 1970

Kincaid-Smith P, Mathew TH, Becker EL: Glomerulonephritis with fibrin and crescent formation in Kincaid-Smith P, Mathew TH, Becker EL (eds): Glomerulonephritis: Morphology, Natural History, and Treatment, part II. New York, John Wiley & Sons, 1972, p 657

Kincaid-Smith P, d'Apice AJF: Plasmapheresis in rapidly progressive glomerulonephritis. Am J Med 65:564, 1978

McKay DG: Blood coagulation and renal disease, in Kincaid-Smith P, Mathew TH, Becker EL (eds): Glomerulonephritis: Morphology, Natural History, and Treatment, part II. New York, John Wiley & Sons, 1973, p 771

Terman DS, Tavel A, Tavel T, et al: Degradation of circulating DNA by extracorporeal circulation over nuclease immobilized on nylon microcapsules. J Clin Invest 57:1201, 1976

Vassalli P, McCluskey RT: Pathogenetic role of the coagulation process in glomerular diseases of immunologic origin, in Hamburger J, Crosnier J, Maxwell MH (eds): Advances in Nephrology, vol I. Chicago, Year Book Medical, 1971, p 47

GOODPASTURE'S SYNDROME*

Curtis B. Wilson

The term "Goodpasture's syndrome" is used to describe the coincident occurrence of glomerulonephritis and varying degrees of pulmonary hemorrhage, with or without pulmonary failure. Goodpasture's syndrome is most commonly caused by antibodies that react specifically with the basement membranes of the glomerulus and alveolus, although nonspecific deposition of circulating immune complexes in the glomerular and alveolar vasculature can cause a similar clinical disease.

The pulmonary capillary bed, then, may sustain damage by immunopathologic mechanisms like those that cause most glomerulonephritis. These mechanisms involve the production of antibodies reactive with structural glomerular antigens, for example, the glomerular basement membrane (GBM). In addition, the glomerulus can be injured by circulating antigen–antibody complexes which form as part of the body's normal immunologic surveillance or in association with autoimmune disease and then become trapped in the glomerular filter. Perhaps as much as 80 percent of all glomerulonephritis is caused by the immune complex mechanism, and 3–5 percent is caused by anti-GBM antibodies. Either of these mechanisms can induce tissue injury through a series of systems including complement, polymorphonuclear leukocytes, vasoactive amines, and the Hagemann factor systems of coagulation and kinin formation.

ANTI–BASEMENT MEMBRANE ANTIBODY-INDUCED GOODPASTURE'S SYNDROME

Anti-GBM antibodies generally induce rapidly progressive glomerulonephritis, and pulmonary hemorrhage (Goodpasture's syndrome) also develops in about two-thirds of these patients. The pulmonary hemorrhage is generally episodic but may be severe enough to result in hypoxia and death; however, milder and occasionally self-remitting forms of the disease are being identified, as well as clinical manifestations confined largely or solely to the lung. The frequency with which anti–basement membrane antibodies are responsible for so-called idiopathic pulmonary hemosiderosis is yet to be determined.

The evidence that anti-GBM antibodies cause glomerulonephritis is most convincing. These antibodies can be identified in these patient's kidneys by using immunofluorescence, and the antibodies recovered from their circulations or their kidneys can be used to transfer nephritis to subhuman primates. Even better proof is the immediate recurrence of anti-GBM anti-

body-induced nephritis in renal transplants of patients with residual high levels of circulating anti-GBM antibody. Antibodies similar to or cross-reactive with those of the GBM are almost certainly involved in the pulmonary injury of anti-GBM antibody-associated Goodpasture's syndrome as well; however, here the evidence is less direct. Anti–basement membrane antibodies can be demonstrated in the alveolar basement membrane by immunofluorescence, and antibodies reactive with both the alveolar basement membrane and the GBM can be recovered in eluates from lung tissue of affected individuals. Experimentally, antibodies against lung tissue cause both glomerulonephritis and pulmonary hemorrhage. All in all, however, it is more difficult to induce lung injury than glomerular injury by these experimental maneuvers, and the lung disease of anti–basement membrane antibody-induced Goodpasture's syndrome has not yet been transferred to monkeys satisfactorily. The reasons could be qualitative and quantitative differences in the anti–basement membrane antibodies, the associated mediator systems, or perhaps the inaccessibility of the alveolar basement membrane antigens to circulating antibody. Clinical observations suggest that additional factors, such as fluid overload and systemic or pulmonary infection, etc., may contribute in an as yet undefined way to the pneumotoxicity of anti–basement membrane antibodies.

The events responsible for the induction of the anti–basement membrane response are poorly understood. Some but not particularly compelling associations have been observed between the occurrence of anti–basement membrane antibody disease and such events as influenza A2 infection, hydrocarbon solvent inhalation, renal ischemia, drug toxicity, and neoplasia. The fact that the anti–basement membrane response is generally self-limited, lasting only weeks to months, suggests that the stimulus for formation of the antibody is also brief and therefore potentially identifiable. Whether infectious or toxic environmental stimuli alter basement membrane antigens, perhaps in the lung, thereby rendering them immunogenic, is unknown. Conversely, such events might lead to the uncovering of normally sequestered antigens for reaction of anti–basement membrane anti-bodies formed for some other reason. Basement membrane antigens have been identified in the urine (and in the serum) and used to induce anti–basement membrane antibodies in experimental animals. Conceivably such antigens could be a stimulus in man, under appropriate circumstances.

The diagnosis of anti–basement membrane antibody-induced Goodpasture's syndrome is based on a combination of immunofluorescence and elution studies of renal and pulmonary tissue and is supported by the demonstration of circulating anti–basement membrane antibodies. Anti–basement membrane antibodies are found as typical linear deposits of immunoglobulin (almost always IgG) along the GBM and alveolar basement membranes (Fig. 1). Since immunoglobulin (usually accompanied by albumin) can sometimes accumu-

*This is publication 1607 from the Department of Immunopathology, Research Institute of Scripps Clinic, 10666 N. Torrey Pines Rd., La Jolla, Calif. This work was supported in part by USPHS Grants AM-20043, AM-18626, and AI-07007 and BRS Grant RRO-5514.

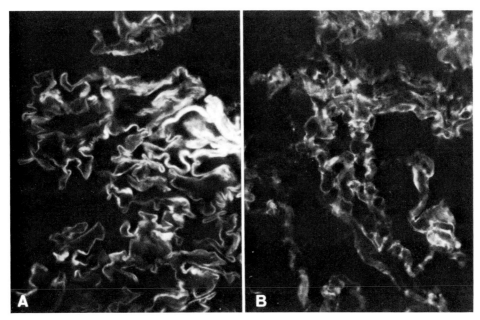

Fig. 1. (A) Linear deposits of IgG observed along the GBM of a patient with Goodpasture's syndrome. (B) Anti–alveolar basement membrane antibodies observed as linear deposits of IgG in the lung.

late nonspecifically in basement membranes, the immunofluorescence studies should always be confirmed by demonstrating the antibody's specificity in an elution study or by detecting anti–basement membrane antibodies in the circulation. The immunoglobulin deposits are generally accompanied by C3 and other complement components, suggesting complement's role in mediating the injury. Interestingly, however, about one-fourth of such patients lack detectable C3 deposits, suggesting that noncomplement mediator pathways may also be involved.

Circulating anti–basement membrane antibodies can be detected by indirect immunofluorescence using normal kidney or lung sections as a target. More recently, radioimmunoassays have been used to locate and quantitate the anti-GBM antibodies. A radioimmunoassay has been developed in our laboratory that utilizes the noncollagenous glycoproteins that remain after collagenase digestion of the GBM to interact with the antibodies we wish to find in the patient's serum. This assay seems to be very effective in detecting and monitoring anti–basement membrane antibody levels. To date, the test has been positive in 76 of 78 patients with well documented anti–basement membrane antibody-induced Goodpasture's syndrome. Since serum samples are generally not available at the onset of disease, it is unknown if the overall severity of clinical involvement relates directly to the amount of antibody produced or not; however, there seems to be little correlation between the episodic occurrence of pulmonary hemorrhage and the level of anti-GBM antibody present. That is, episodes of pulmonary hemorrhage can occur at any time during the usually finite period of

antibody production. Antibody usually tends to disappear after several weeks or months, but it sometimes persists for 2–3 years. As far as we know, bilateral nephrectomy has no immediate effect on anti-GBM antibody levels, although the levels may decrease more rapidly thereafter than in nonnephrectomized patients.

A small but interesting group of patients has been recognized by radioimmunoassay whose levels of circulating anti-GBM antibody are moderate and whose lung lesions are often severe but who develop only mild, usually nonprogressive renal problems. At least one such patient has had three distinct episodes of pulmonary hemorrhage and mild nephritis over a period of 10 years. Patients are also beginning to be identified in whom the clinical involvement is confined entirely to the lung, with a presentation of idiopathic pulmonary hemosiderosis. In at least two of these patients, however, anti–basement membrane antibodies have been identified in the kidney by using immunofluorescense. It is unknown why the antibody fails to induce sufficient renal injury to be detected clinically; however, the observations would suggest that the anti–basement membrane antibodies in this instance are directed predominantly toward lung basement membrane antigens.

Patients with anti–basement membrane antibody-induced Goodpasture's syndrome generally have severe and rapidly progressive nephritic courses, characterized histologically by severe, proliferative, and crescentic forms of glomerulonephritis. A prodromal period of flu-like illness may be noted, and occasionally the disease begins with migratory arthralgia or arthritis. Nephrotic syndrome is unusual. The onset of renal or pulmonary problems may be simultaneous or separated by periods of up to 1 year. The disease is somewhat more common in males than in females and is most frequent in individuals between 15 and 35 years of age. The age range in both sexes, however, varies from below 10 to over 70. Hemoptysis is generally episodic and when severe may lead to death through hypoxia. Anemia of a microcytic hypochromic type is general and may be severe, with evidence of pulmonary sequestration of red cells. Radiographic studies detect often rapidly fluctuating, diffuse, fluffy densities throughout the lung fields (Fig 2). Renal failure requiring dialysis develops in about three-quarters of the patients, and death occurs in the acute phases of the disease in about 20 percent.

Although still a very serious disease, anti–basement membrane antibody-associated Goodpasture's syndrome now resolves in a more favorable manner than before. The improved management of chronic renal failure through dialysis, as well as the use of high-dose steroids for the management of pulmonary hemorrhage and the recognition of greater numbers of patients with milder forms of the disease, probably contribute to this apparent lessening of morbidity and mortality. There has been enthusiasm recently for combining plasmapheresis with immunosuppression to rapidly lower the patient's content of circulating anti–basement membrane antibodies and thereby minimize their immunopathogenic effect (Fig. 3). Some patients have responded well to this form of therapy, in some instances even regaining sufficient renal function to maintain life after undergoing a period of dialysis. Since this treatment is as yet uncontrolled, its true value is difficult to assess; however, the theory is reasonable and deserves careful further evaluation. In addition to lowering levels of circulating anti–basement membrane antibodies, plasmapheresis may also alter the levels of circulating mediators of inflammation such as the complement and coagulation proteins and thus contribute to any therapeutic benefit.

As noted earlier, the incidence of pulmonary hemorrhage in patients with anti–basement membrane antibody-induced Goodpasture's syndrome is episodic and the severity varies. In some instances non-immunologic factors, such as fluid overload or infection, seem to be the cause. Management, then, should include a search for and correction of any such factors. Steriod administration is thought to be of benefit in controlling some episodes of pulmonary hemorrhage. For more persistent attacks, immunosuppression and plasma exchange have been tried and found helpful in some patients. Again, assessment of the true value of this combined therapy awaits controlled trials.

Bilateral nephrectomy, if beneficial for patients with life-threatening pulmonary hemorrhage, as reported, acts in a manner that is not clear. As noted earlier, nephrectomy has no immediate effect on levels of circulating anti–basement membrane antibodies, and no controlled observations are available. In reviewing results of a series of nephrectomized and unnephrectomized patients, one finds that severe pulmonary hemorrhage can occur after nephrectomy, suggesting that its effect is, at least, uncertain. In view of this unpredictable outcome and the occasional spontaneous recovery of renal function in these patients, nephrectomy as therapy for acute pulmonary hemorrhage should be considered only as a last resort.

When dealing with patients who have anti–basement membrane antibody-induced Goodpasture's syndrome, the clinician may ultimately face the problem of renal transplantation. It is clear that severe anti–basement membrane antibody-induced nephritis may recur when a transplant is placed in a recipient with high levels of circulating anti-GBM antibodies.

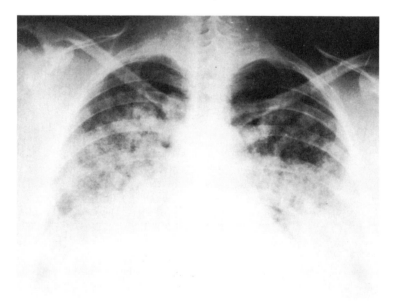

Fig. 2. Diffuse, bilateral, fluffy infiltrates are seen in a chest x-ray during an episode of acute pulmonary hemorrhage with hemoptysis in a patient with Goodpasture's syndrome.

Therefore most of these patients are observed for a period of time prior to transplantation until their circulating antibody levels are low or undetectable. At that time, these patients generally can be transplanted without great danger of recurrent nephritis. Exceptions do occur; one patient with documented Goodpasture's syndrome whom we evaluated recently received a transplant from an identical twin 2 years after the disappearance of circulating anti-GBM antibodies. Within 3 months after transplantation (without immunosuppression), anti-GBM antibodies reappeared in her circulation and were found affixed to the renal transplant. Institution of immunosuppressive and plasmapheresis therapy at that point decreased the antibody activity and maintained graft function sufficiently to avoid a return to dialysis.

IMMUNE COMPLEX INDUCED GOODPASTURE'S SYNDROME

Immune complexes deposited in glomeruli are now believed to cause most forms of glomerulonephritis in man. Immune complex glomerulonephritis may sometimes be accompanied by pulmonary involvement, leading to the clinical presentation of Goodpasture's syndrome. Such an example would be the combined glomerular and pulmonary injury seen in the widespread systemic immune complex deposition of patients with systemic lupus erythematosus. Goodpasture's syndrome has also been observed in patients with cryoglobulinemia and in patients with immune complex nephritis of unknown causes. On occasion, the lung may be the source of antigen for the formation of circulating immune complexes, with subsequent deposition in the kidneys and the initiation of a nephritic process. Antigens associated with pulmonary infections, neoplasia, or other involvements such as sarcoidosis have been identified or suggested.

In experimental chronic serum sickness nephritis induced by repeated immunization of rabbits with bovine serum albumin, circulating immune complexes form daily. Although the majority of these complexes are removed relatively harmlessly by the reticuloendothelial system, a small percentage deposit in the kidney and, to a lesser extent, the lung. Indeed, pulmonary lesions in addition to glomerulonephritis have been reported in rabbits with experimental chronic serum sickness. Factors influencing the particular site or tissue in which immune complexes localize are poorly understood but seem to include immune complex size, determined in part by the relative antigen:antibody ratio, changes in vascular permeability caused by immune release of vasoactive materials, and the hemodynamics of blood flow, etc. It should also be noted that once deposited, immune complexes remain in equilibrium with antigen or antibody from the circulation so that their composition may be continually modified.

A growing number of exogenous and endogenous antigens have been identified in immune complex deposits in man and include antigens from many infectious agents as well as antigens from such sources as nuclear materials in patients with systemic lupus erythemato-

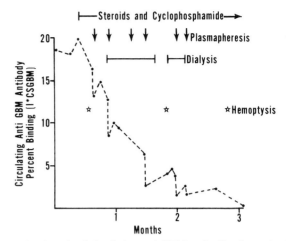

Fig. 3. Levels of circulating anti-GBM antibodies determined by radioimmunoassay correlated with the patient's course and clinical management, including plasmapheresis with exchange of 4 liters of plasma on six occasions.

sus, in bodily tissues in persons, autoimmune diseases, and neoplasm-associated antigens. Diagnosis of immune complex disease is based on using immunofluorescence to detect granular immunoglobulin deposits, generally associated with complement, in the vessels of affected tissue. These deposits can also be visualized through the electron microscope as dense deposits. The fact that they are immune complexes is confirmed by identifying the specific antigen–antibody system involved. Serologic studies of such a patient may reveal a depressed concentration of serum complement components and the presence of cryoglobulins. Methods are evolving to detect circulating immune complexes as a means of diagnosing these patients' disease and in monitoring their therapy.

The clinical disorders most commonly associated with immune complex forms of Goodpasture's syndrome are systemic lupus erythematosus and other systemic vasculitides. Wegener's granulomatosis is a form of vasculitis that frequently involves pulmonary and renal symptoms. Limited immunopathologic and electron microscopic studies have suggested the presence of renal immune complex deposits in these patients, although the deposits, if present, are scant. Hypersensitivity angiitis, particularly of the Henoch-Schönlein type, may cause severe renal involvement in addition to pulmonary manifestations. Mixed cryoglobulinemia can also lead to pulmonary and renal disease, occasionally manifesting itself as Goodpasture's syndrome. As more is understood about immune complex disorders, the frequency with which this mechanism leads to combined renal and pulmonary involvement will be further delineated. As yet, however, immune complex disorders account for only a small portion of patients with Goodpasture's syndrome.

The management of patients with immune complex induced Goodpasture's syndrome should be appropriate for their underlying systemic immune complex disorder, be it systemic lupus erythematosus, vasculitis, Wegener's granulomatosis, etc. Too few examples of primary immune complex induced glomerulonephritis complicated by pulmonary hemorrhage have yet been identified to advocate any specific therapeutic modality.

GOODPASTURE'S SYNDROME OF UNCERTAIN ETIOLOGY

In spite of the advances made in immunopathologic study of renal and pulmonary tissue, not all individuals who present clinically with Goodpasture's syndrome can be classified immunopathologically as to cause of disease. That is, immunofluorescence study of renal or lung biopsies does not always reveal the presence of either anti–basement membrane antibodies or immune complex deposits in some of the patients who, nevertheless, usually have rapidly progressive glomerulonephritis complicated by pulmonary hemorrhage. Similarly, the sera of these patients may be negative for circulating anti–basement membrane antibodies and immune complexes. These negative findings could represent merely inadequate sensitivity of the diagnostic method employed or the involvement of immune or nonimmune mechanisms other than those tested in a small percentage of patients with apparent Goodpasture's syndrome.

REFERENCES

Beirne GJ, Wagnild JP, Zimmerman SW, et al: Idiopathic crescentic glomerulonephritis. Medicine (Baltimore) 56:349, 1977

Benoit FL, Rulon DB, Theil GB, et al: Goodpasture's syndrome: A clinicopathologic entity. Am J Med 37:424, 1964

Johnson JP, Whitman W, Briggs WA, et al: Plasmapheresis and immunosuppressive agents in antibasement membrane antibody-induced Goodpasture's syndrome. Am J Med 65:354, 1978

Lockwood CM, Rees AJ, Pearson TA, et al: Immunosuppression and plasma-exchange in the treatment of Goodpasture's syndrome. Lancet 1:711, 1976

Martinez JS, Kohler PF: Variant "Goodpasture's syndrome"? The need for immunologic criteria in rapidly progressive glomerulonephritis and hemorrhagic pneumonitis. Ann Intern Med 75:67, 1971

Wilson CB: Immunologic diseases of the lung and kidney (Goodpasture's syndrome), in Fishman AP (ed): Pulmonary Diseases, New York, McGraw-Hill, 1979, p 699

Wilson CB, Dixon FJ: Anti-glomerular basement membrane antibody-induced glomerulonephritis. Kidney Int 3:74, 1973

Wilson CB, Dixon FJ: The renal response to immunological injury, in Brenner BM, Rector FC Jr (eds): The Kidney. Philadelphia, W.B. Saunders, 1976

FOCAL GLOMERULONEPHRITIS

Thomas F. Ferris

Focal glomerulonephritis describes a renal inflammation which, unlike the more usual diffuse glomerulonephritis, is restricted to either certain glomeruli (focal involvement) or to lobular segments of an individual glomerulus (local involvement). The inflammation can be necrotizing (Fig. 1), in which case glomeruli may become hyalinized with reduction in glomerular filtration rate or may consist only of a proliferative response in segments of glomeruli without capillary necrosis (Fig. 2). Focal glomerulonephritis was described initially in association with certain systemic diseases, i.e., bacterial endocarditis, systemic lupus erythematosus, hypersensitivity angiitis, Wegener's granulomatosis, Henoch-Schönlein purpura, and Goodpasture's syndrome. When associated with these diseases the renal lesions are of the necrotizing type. When the lesions were first described in bacterial endocarditis they were thought to represent emboli to the kidney from the cardiac vegetation; however, it is now clear that focal glomerulonephritis is caused by immunological injury to the glomerulus (see the chapter on *Anaphylactoid Purpura Nephritis*).

CLINICAL FINDINGS

In the absence of a systemic disease, focal glomerulonephritis usually presents in children and young adults with recurrent episodes of gross hematuria following either exercise or an upper respiratory infection; however, a similar clinical presentation may occur with diffuse glomerulonephritis or in the absence of glomerular pathology; thus the diagnosis of focal glomerulonephritis should be restricted to those patients in whom focal glomerular changes have been demonstrated by renal biopsy.

The disease is most common in children and young adults, with a predominance in males. The condition is alarming to the patient and may be associated with back pain and renal colic caused by clots in the ureter and bladder. In some patients there is a low-grade fever and an erythematous rash, but in most there are no symptoms of systemic illness. The hematuria may persist for several days or weeks; in other instances it may clear immediately, only to recur at a subsequent time. Between attacks some patients have complete clearing of the hematuria, whereas others have persistent microscopic hematuria. Blood pressure and renal function are normal, and usually the proteinuria is minimal, under 500 mg/24 hours. In children who have been followed for many years following episodes of hematuria, the condition is benign with no evidence of development of chronic renal failure. The condition has been called idiopathic hematuria, benign hematuria, or recurrent hematuria. In approximately one-third of adults having a similar clinical history in whom a focal glomerulonephritis is suspected, the renal biopsy will reveal a diffuse form of glomerulonephritis. In the author's experience, these patients usually have heavier proteinuria, i.e., greater than 1 g/24 hours, but others have found that some patients with focal glomerulonephritis will have greater than 500 mg proteinuria/24 hours. In patients with diffuse glomerulonephritis or the necrotizing form of focal glomerulonephritis, the prognosis must be guarded. Most series indicate that with diffuse glomerulonephritis the combination of gross

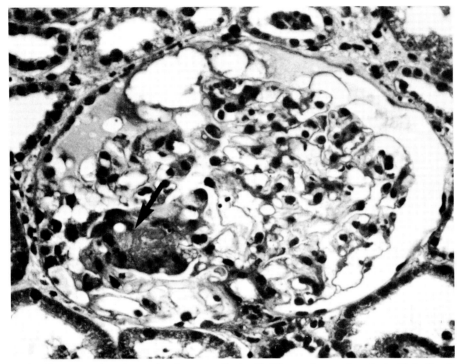

Fig. 1. Representative glomerulus from a patient with Wegener's granulomatosis. Note the focal necrosis of a segment of the glomerulus with normal architecture elsewhere.

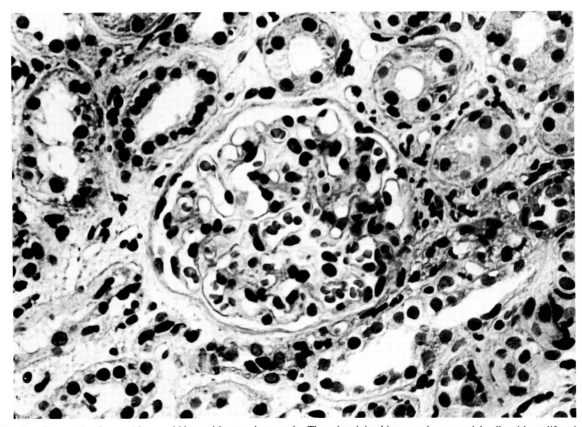

Fig. 2. Glomerulus from a 16 year old boy with gross hematuria. There is minimal increase in mesangial cells with proliferation of matrix.

hematuria, normal blood pressure, and normal renal function is usually associated with a good prognosis. In the few patients with focal glomerulonephritis where deterioration of renal function occurred, the process is slowly progressive. Approximately 20–30 percent of patients with gross hematuria and RBC casts will have no evidence of glomerular pathology on biopsy. Since a similar clinical picture can occur with a bleeding source in the renal pelvis, ureter, or bladder, the finding of red blood cell casts in the spun sediment is important in confirming the renal origin of the hematuria. A urological evaluation is indicated if red blood cell casts are not seen to exclude the genitourinary tract as the source of the bleeding and to confirm that the hematuria is present in the urine from both kidneys. Having excluded the GU tract as a source of the bleeding, repeated cystoscopies are not indicated with subsequent episodes of hematuria.

PATHOLOGY AND IMMUNOPATHOLOGY

The pathology affects glomeruli locally or can be confined to one or two lobules of a glomerulus. The changes are usually proliferative, frequently at the periphery of a lobule. In the necrotizing form of the disease there is capillary necrosis with epithelial crescent formation within Bowman's capsule and fibrosis and hyalinization at sites of necrosis. The renal inter-stitium is usually normal, although infiltration of lymphocytes and plasma cells may occur in the interstitium. Although focal proliferation of glomerular epithelial and endothelial cells may occur, the proliferation is usually of mesangial cells with increase in mesangial matrix (Fig. 3). Electron microscopy has revealed the presence of electron-dense deposits in the mesangium with great variability among glomeruli in the extent of mesangial matrix. Berger was the first to note mesangial deposits of IgA, IgG, and β1C globulin in patients with focal glomerulonephritis and gross hematuria; properdin, a component of the alternate pathway of complement activation, also was found in about 50 percent of these patients. The combination of gross hematuria, focal glomerulonephritis, and IgA and IgG deposits in the mesangium has come to be described as Berger's syndrome; however, IgA and IgG deposits are found in the mesangium in other forms of glomerulonephritis, so that the presence of IgA deposits within the mesangium is not pathognomonic of the syndrome. What role IgA plays in focal glomerulonephritis is not known, although there have been reports of elevated serum IgA concentration in some patients with the disease. When focal glomerulonephritis is present with SLE or Henoch-Schönlein purpura, IgA is frequently found in the mesangium. There is evidence that the mesangial cell is

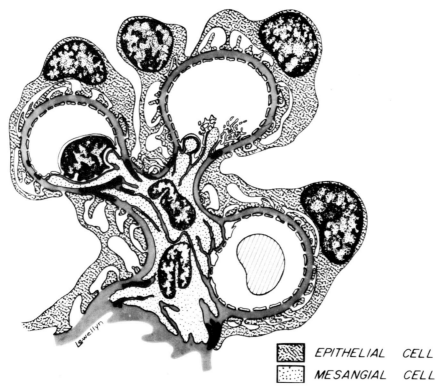

EPITHELIAL CELL

MESANGIAL CELL

Fig. 3. Schematic drawing of a glomerulus demonstrating mesangial and epithelial cells. The mesangial cells may proliferate and project into the capillary lumen in mesangioproliferative glomerulonephritis, as demonstrated in the upper two capillaries, or may not alter the capillary lumen, as illustrated in the bottom right capillary. [Reprinted from Kidney International with permission—Vernier RL, Resnick JS, Mauer SM: Recurrent hematuria and focal nephritis. Kidney Int 7:224, 1975.]

involved in the glomerular reaction, since substances such as carbon particles or antigen–antibody complexes with molecular weights greater than 1,000,000 daltons become localized in the mesangium when injected into experimental animals. Interestingly, when glomerulonephritis is induced by injections of bovine serum albumin into rabbits, the larger antigen–antibody complexes lodge in the mesangium, in which case the glomerular pathology is focal and proteinuria not striking. When the immune complex deposits have lower molecular weights they are more apt to deposit in the glomerular capillary loop accompanied by a diffuse inflammatory reaction and heavy proteinuria. Since gross hematuria with focal glomerulonephritis frequently follows an upper respiratory infection, viral antigens may be the cause of the condition in some instances. Why hematuria is so prominent and so frequently follows exercise is not known. Exercise induces microscopic hematuria in normal individuals; thus the hematuria seen with focal glomerulonephritis may be an exaggeration of this phenomenon.

TREATMENT

Since the condition is self-limited and benign, no treatment is usually needed; however, when focal necrotizing glomerulonephritis is found on a renal biopsy, a careful history should be elicited to exclude a systemic cause of the condition, since specific therapy directed at the systemic disease may be indicated. Patients and parents of children with focal nonnecrotizing glomerulonephritis must be reassured of the benign course, since hematuria is frightening. Some have reported that steroids cause cessation of the hematuria, but they rarely are needed, since the hematuria usually subsides in 3–4 days. Frequent urological evaluations should be avoided once the diagnosis has been established.

REFERENCES

Berger J: IgA glomerular deposits in renal disease. Transplant Proc 1:939, 1969

Ferris TF, Gordon P, Kashgarian M, et al: Recurrent hematuria and focal nephritis. N Engl J Med 276:770, 1967

Heptinstall RN: Pathology of the Kidney (ed 2). Boston, Little, Brown, 1974

Vernier RL, Resnick JS, Mauer SM: Recurrent hematuria and focal glomerulonephritis. Kidney Int 7:224, 1975

FOCAL GLOMERULAR SCLEROSIS

Mark S. Schiffer and Alfred J. Fish

Although focal glomerular sclerosis (FGS) is a descriptive pathologic term, the occurrence of this lesion associated with idiopathic nephrotic syndrome merits consideration as a separate clinical entity. In a less specific sense, focally sclerotic glomeruli can occur in pyelonephritis, diabetic nephropathy, hypertensive nephropathy, Alport's syndrome, and endstage kidney disease; additional pathological and clinical findings clearly separate these groups from the proteinuric patients with FGS.

About 80 percent of patients with FGS demonstrate segmental involvement of some glomeruli, termed focal segmental glomerular sclerosis. This entity can be differentiated from global glomerular sclerosis both clinically and pathologically.

About 40 percent of adults and 15 percent of children with idiopathic nephrotic syndrome have FGS. Less commonly, some patients with asymptomatic proteinuria also demonstrate this lesion by kidney biopsy.

PATHOLOGY

The characteristic lesion in FGS is a focal, segmental, nonproliferative capillary sclerosis (Fig. 1A). In addition, within the sclerotic lesion are often hypereosinophilic hyaline deposits, foam cells, and adhesions to Bowman's capsule. As Rich noted in 1957, only the juxtamedullary glomeruli may be affected early in the disease; thus a superficial cortical biopsy is inadequate to rule out FGS. Nonsclerotic glomerular segments and nonsclerotic glomeruli manifest the changes seen in minimal lesion nephrotic syndrome (MLNS) which may include a slight increase of mesangial cells and matrix. Some specimens display a mesangial proliferative lesion in nonsclerotic segments. Tubular and interstitial changes are mild except in relation to totally sclerosed glomeruli. Interstitial inflammatory changes may also develop during the course of the disease. In patients with progressive FGS, serial biopsies show an increasing proportion of totally sclerosed glomeruli and increasing sclerosis of the remaining ones. Interstitial fibrosis and vascular changes are late findings.

By electron microscopy, in both nonsclerotic and segmentally sclerotic glomeruli, epithelial cell swelling and degeneration with fusion and loss of the foot processes are evident. Near areas of sclerosis, thickening of the glomerular basement membrane and electron dense deposits in the paramesangial subendothelium may be seen. Immunofluorescent microscopy reveals that the proteins deposited in focal sclerotic lesions include immunoglobulins M and G, complement components, and fibrin (Fig. 1B).

In patients with global glomerular sclerosis, totally sclerosed glomeruli coexist with glomeruli that are nearly normal by light microscopy. Light microscopy reveals interstitial changes in relation to the sclerotic glomeruli. With proteinuria, electron microscopy reveals epithelial cell foot process fusion in functioning glomeruli. By fluorescent microscopy, the nonsclerotic glomeruli appear normal, while the sclerotic glomeruli stain for IgM, C3, and properdin, as do endstage glomeruli from any cause. When considering this lesion, one must be aware that about 10 percent of glomeruli may be sclerosed in the normal kidney, and higher percentages of glomeruli may be involuted in the young infant and the elderly.

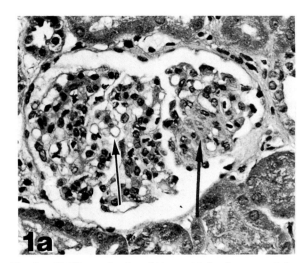
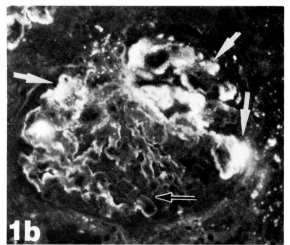

Fig. 1. (A) Glomerulus from kidney with focal segmental glomerular sclerosis. Thick arrow indicates a sclerotic segment. Thin arrow indicates a normal segment. Other segments display varying degrees of mesangial proliferation. H & E. × 300. (B) Glomerulus with segmental sclerosis stained for IgM. White arrows indicate IgM in sclerotic segments. Black arrow indicates minimal IgM deposits along capillary wall. Fluorescent microscopy. × 300.

PATHOGENESIS

Most patients with FGS have nephrotic syndrome and focal segmental sclerosis by biopsy early in the course of the disease, while most patients with minimal lesion nephrotic syndrome show no progressive pathologic alteration despite years of recurrent disease. Some investigators have suggested that glomerular segments with mesangial proliferation may be superceded by sclerosis and that the mesangial proliferative lesion is a precursor of FGS. On the other hand, some workers have shown a continuum of pathology from minimal lesion nephrotic syndrome to FGS, with intermediate stages showing sclerosis only by electron microscopy. By analogy, rats with experimental nephrotic syndrome produced with aminonucleoside of puromycin develop focal sclerosis with characteristic light microscopic and fluorescent changes after several months, during which time only minimal lesion changes were evident. Habib concludes that FGS can evolve from minimal lesion nephrotic syndrome, but in most cases it occurs in a separate patient population.

CLINICAL FEATURES

Clinical presentation of patients with FGS is similar to that of patients with minimal lesion nephrotic syndrome; nephrotic syndrome may remit or partially remit spontaneously. These patients are not nephritic, macroscopic hematuria is rarely seen, and GFR is normal early in the course, except when severe hypovolemia is present. Most adults and nearly all children present with normal blood pressure. Persistent microscopic hematuria does not reliably predict the presence of FGS at the onset. The disease can be more clearly separated clinically by its persistence, progression, and lack of response to steroid therapy.

Patients with FGS suffer complications common to all nephrotic patients. Gram-positive or gram-negative bacterial infections, including septicemia, pneumonia, cellulitis, peritonitis, and meningitis may develop; this susceptibility to infection is due in part to urinary loss of C3 proactivator (factor B), a component of the alternate complement pathway, a heat-labile opsonin active in phagocytosis. As in other nephrotic patients, in FGS a hypercoaguable state is present with the risk of thrombotic and embolic complications.

Most patients with FGS steadily progress toward renal failure. Proteinuria persists, though it may decrease as glomerular filtration decreases. Uremia, acidosis, hypertension, and endstage renal disease usually occur 5–7 years after the onset of the disease; however, those patients whose proteinuria remits with steroid therapy as outlined below are exempt from this grave prognosis. Renal transplantation has been successfully performed in these patients, although some develop nephrotic syndrome again.

THERAPY

Prior to therapy, all adolescent and adult patients should be completely evaluated, including kidney biopsy. We recommend one course of prednisone 60 mg/m² in divided doses for 4 weeks. A very few patients with FGS who are not steroid responsive will respond to an alkylating agent such as cyclophosphamide or chlorambucil. Patients with FGS who have responded to a course of steroids and then relapse will likely respond again. Patients who were initially responsive and became "late responders" upon exacerbation have a chance of response to subsequent courses of steroids or alkylating agents. Incomplete remissions with therapy are difficult to evaluate, as they occur spontaneously in the course of the disease.

Since nonresponsiveness to steroids is likely in FGS, the risk must be considered before treating patients such as the elderly who are particularly susceptible to steroid toxicity. Likewise, the small potential added benefit of cyclophosphamide for a steroid non-responsive patient should be considered before using that agent in a varicella susceptible individual.

In contrast to patients with FGS, most patients with global glomerular sclerosis respond completely to steroids; these patients often undergo relapses but remain steroid responsive on retreatment.

CONCLUSION

FGS is an entity associated with nephrotic syndrome clinically and with segmental glomerular scarring pathologically. The disorder is usually unresponsive to steroid therapy and leads to renal failure in most patients. The pathogenesis is unknown.

REFERENCES

Glasser RJ, Velosa JA, Michael AF: Experimental model of focal sclerosis. I. Relationship to protein excretion in aminonucleoside nephrosis. Lab Invest 36:519, 1977

Habib R: Focal glomerular sclerosis. Kidney Int 4:355, 1973

Hyman LR, Burkholder PM: Focal sclerosing glomerulopathy with segmental hyalinosis, a clinicopathologic analysis. Lab Invest 28:533, 1973

Lim VS, Sibley R, Spargo B: Adult lipoid nephrosis: Clinicopathological correlations. Ann Intern Med 81:314, 1974

Rich AR: A hitherto undescribed vulnerability of the juxtamedullary glomeruli in the lipoid nephrosis. Bull Johns Hopkins Hosp 100:173, 1957

Siegel NJ, Kashgarian M, Spargo BH, et al: Minimal change and focal sclerotic lesions in lipoid nephrosis. Nephron 13:125, 1974

SYSTEMIC LUPUS ERYTHEMATOSUS

James V. Donadio, Jr.

In 1922, Keith and Rowntree made the first observations of the importance of renal involvement in patients with systemic lupus erythematosus (SLE). Today, with the aid of percutaneous renal biopsy, the various forms of lupus renal disease can be classified for diagnostic and therapeutic purposes.

HISTOPATHOLOGY

The morphologic classification of lupus nephritis is based primarily on glomerular changes and may be arbitrarily divided into the following four categories: (1) mesangial lupus nephritis; (2) mild (focal) proliferative lupus nephritis; (3) severe (diffuse) proliferative lupus nephritis; and (4) membranous lupus nephropathy.

In mesangial lupus nephritis the glomeruli may show a slight, irregular increase in mesangial cells and matrix. Other features which are characteristic of proliferative lupus nephritis are not found, and the tubules, interstitium, and arteries are essentially normal. By immunofluorescence, deposits of IgG and C3 are found diffusely throughout the mesangial region and usually in all glomeruli (Fig. 1). Occasionally granular deposits of IgG may be found in segments of the glomerular capillary walls. On electron microscopy, electron-dense

deposits are present in mesangial areas and usually in all glomeruli. Less commonly, small deposits may also be seen within the glomerular basement membrane or in a subendothelial position, particularly in the paramesangial region.

Mild (focal) and severe (diffuse) proliferative lupus nephritis are characterized by similar histologic changes and differ mainly in the extent of involvement of individual glomeruli and by the percentage of glomeruli involved. Perhaps more important than classifying a biopsy as focal or diffuse proliferative nephritis is to point out the specific features of morphologically active lesions (Fig. 2). The pleomorphic nature of the glomerular changes (when compared with other forms of glomerulopathies) is striking. The most characteristic glomerular lesion is one that is segmental or local (one or two lobules) and exhibits the following features on light microscopy; cellular proliferation and swelling (mesangial and endothelial cells); thickening of the capillary wall (fibrinoid deposition or the so-called "wire loops"); karyorrhexis; increase in mesangial matrix (deposits); swelling of visceral and parietal epithelial cells (frequent cellular and cytoplasmic adhesions to Bowman's capsule); and evidence of immune deposits in subendothelial, subepithelial, and mesangial regions with special histochemical stains, immunofluorescence, and electron microscopy. Frequently seen within active glomerular lesions are polymorphonuclear leukocytes and hyaline thrombi. Hematoxyphil bodies and diffuse extracapillary proliferation, or crescent formation, are not frequently observed.

Renal biopsy specimens are classified as mild (focal) proliferative lupus nephritis when less than 50 percent of the total area of glomerular tufts are affected with the inflammatory changes of activity as described. In many instances, only 10–20 percent of glomeruli show segmental proliferative lesions while the other glomeruli may show only slight irregular increase in mesangial cells and matrix. On immunofluorescence, deposits of IgG and C3 are present in mesangial regions of most glomeruli, even in those appearing normal on histologic examination, and there may be segmental, granular capillary wall staining with IgG and C3. On electron microscopy, electron-dense deposits are found in the mesangial region of most glomeruli and usually scattered in a subendothelial location, especially if a glomerulus under examination contains a proliferative lesion in peripheral capillary loops.

In severe (diffuse) proliferative lupus nephritis, proliferative glomerular changes involving 90 percent or more of glomeruli are usually present with segmental or lobular accentuations of the tufts, variable glomerular scarring, interstitial fibrosis and tubular atrophy, and usually focal interstitial infiltration with plasma cells and lymphocytes. Crescent formation may be found especially when peripheral capillaries are involved with active lesions. On immunofluorescence, deposits of IgG and C3 are found in broad and irregular patterns diffusely throughout the glomerular capillary walls and

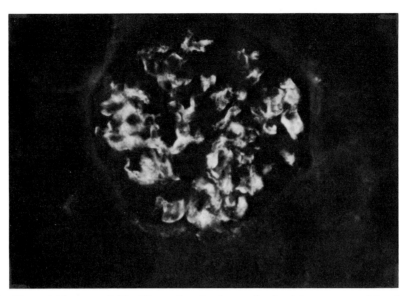

Fig. 1. Mesangial lupus nephritis. Glomerulus showing predominant lumpy mesangial pattern and segmental staining of capillary walls with anti-IgG (anti–human IgG). × 250.

within the mesangium. There is variable staining of these immunoreactants of tubular basement membranes, epithelial cell nuclei, and peritubular capillaries. On electron microscopy, there are various changes that involve diffuse mesangial cell hyperplasia and matrix increase, with segmental areas of mesangial interposition, variable endothelial cell swelling, both large and small electron-dense deposits in subendothelial and mesangial regions, and variably in intramembranous and subepithelial locations.

In membranous lupus nephropathy (Fig. 3), histopathologic changes include diffuse glomerular capillary wall thickening with only mild local increase in mesangial cells and matrix and no proliferation of other intracapillary or extracapillary cells on light microscopy. On immunofluorescence, deposits of IgG and C3 are observed in a characteristic granular pattern along glomerular capillary walls. On electron microscopy, electron-dense deposits are found in subepithelial and intraglomerular basement membrane locations; scattered mesangial deposits may also be present, but subepithelial and intramembranous deposits should predominate.

Several other immunofluorescent and electron microscopic findings have been observed in lupus nephritis which are probably not relevant to classification. These include (1) the frequent finding of C1q, C4, and properdin in glomeruli, suggesting activation of both the classical and alternate pathways of complement activation; (2) variable presence of IgA and IgM in glomeruli, and the rare findings of IgE; (3) electron-dense deposits which contain crystalline "fingerprint" patterns and microtubular arrays, usually abundant in the cytoplasm of endothelial cells.

Tubular and interstitial lesions usually coexist with glomerular lesions and are focal in nature. Occasionally,

a patient with SLE will have a primary tubulointerstitial nephritis with minimal glomerular changes. In either instance, the lesions are represented by interstitial infiltration of mononuclear and polymorphonuclear cells, thickening of the tubular basement membrane (TBM), and interstitial fibrosis and tubular atrophy. On immunofluorescence (Fig. 4), IgG and C3 deposits are located along the TBM and epithelial cell nuclei preferentially in proximal convoluted tubules, in the walls of peritubular capillaries, and in the interstitium. On electron microscopy, electron-dense deposits are found on the interstitial and epithelial sides of and within the TBM, the peritubular capillaries, and in the interstitium.

PATHOGENESIS

Today, there is a large body of evidence that the above-described pathologic processes of lupus nephropathy are mediated at least in part by immunological mechanisms. In fact, SLE has often been described as the prototype of immune complex disease. The deposition of circulating immune complexes and the subsequent immune injury involves incompletely understood mediators present in serum, body fluids, and circulating cells. The production and release of physiologic agents such as vasoactive amines, enzymatic constituents of neutrophilic leukocytes, platelets, basophils, and mast cells have been shown to be critical events in the initiation of tissue injury resulting from antigen–antibody interaction in experimental models of nephritis. In addition, the activation of the complement system plays a central role in immune renal disease from the standpoint of producing injury by coordinating the physiologic and cellular mediators. By way of elution studies of isolated glomeruli obtained from kidneys at autopsy, two types of immune complexes have been identified with certainty in human lupus nephritis: single stranded DNA (sDNA)–anti-sDNA and double stranded or native

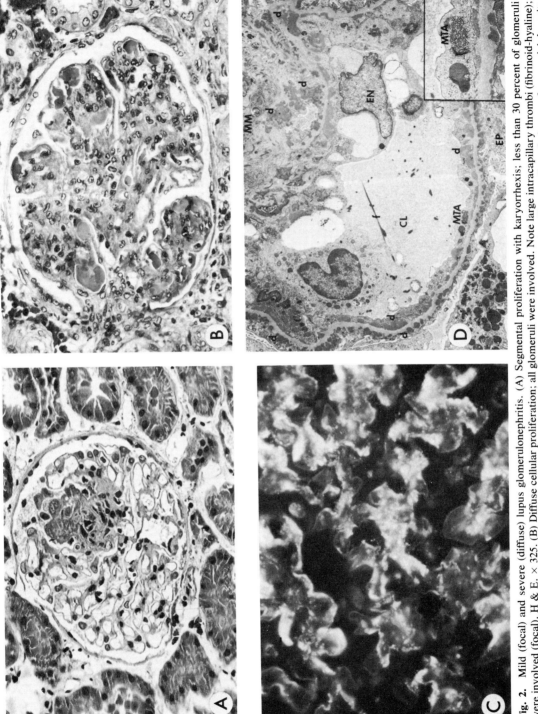

Fig. 2. Mild (focal) and severe (diffuse) lupus glomerulonephritis. (A) Segmental proliferation with karyorrhexis: less than 30 percent of glomeruli were involved (focal). H & E. × 325. (B) Diffuse cellular proliferation: all glomeruli were involved. Note large intracapillary thrombi (fibrinoid-hyaline); capillary walls are thickened. H & E. × 400. (C) Glomerulus showing broad and irregular staining of capillary walls and clumps of mesangial deposits with (anti–human IgG). × 625. (D) Electron micrograph showing electron-dense deposits (d) in mesangium (MM) and on either side of basement membrane. Note microtubular array (MTA) (inset) and fibrin strand (f) in capillary lumen (CL). EP, visceral epithelial cytoplasm; EN, endothelial cell. × 7500. [Reprinted by permission from Wagoner RD, Holley KE: Parenchymal renal disease: Clinical and pathologic features, in Knox FG (ed): Textbook of Renal Pathophysiology. Hagerstown, Harper & Row, 1978, p 226.]

317

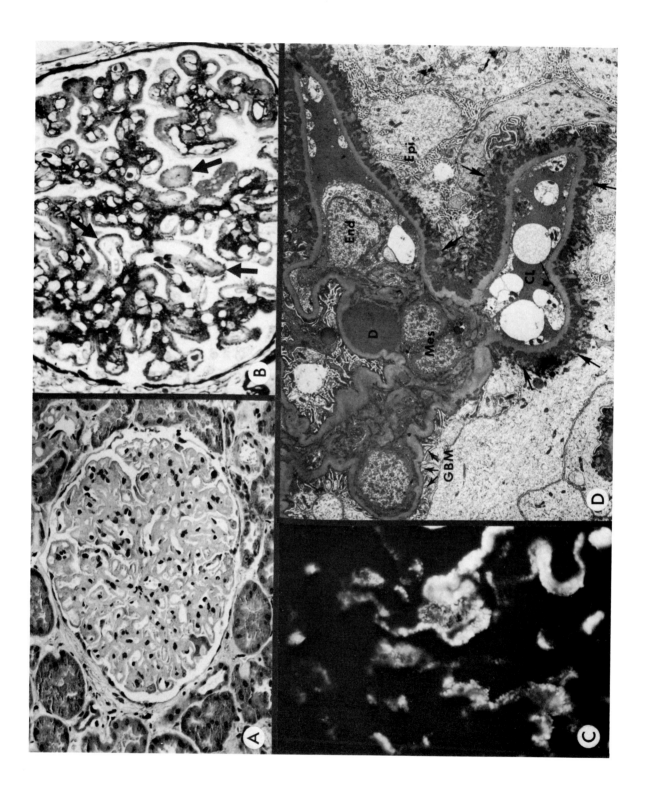

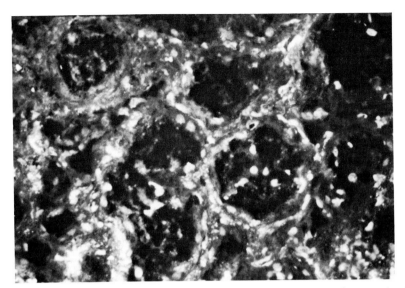

Fig. 4. Tubulointerstitial nephritis showing segmental tubular basement membrane and epithelial cell nuclear fluorescence with anti-IgG. × 250.

DNA (nDNA)–anti-nDNA complexes. Complexes involving components of cryoglobulins and idiotypic IgG antibodies have also been identified in human renal eluates.

Further work into the mechanisms of lupus nephropathy should include studies of the accurate measurement of immune complexes in the circulation and the correlation with disease activity, cellular immune mechanisms, antibody responses, possible sources of additional antigens, and the renal deposition and biologic activity of immune reactants. Along these lines, it has been shown recently that antibodies against DNA eluted from nephritic kidneys have a much higher avidity than do serum anti-DNA antibodies for DNA. This observation might provide insight as to why severe glomerulonephritis develops in some patients but not in others although both groups may have high levels of circulating anti-DNA antibodies.

The well known female sex predilection for SLE led to recent investigations of sex hormones in modulating the expression of murine lupus in the New Zealand black/white hybrid mouse (NZB/W). This animal invariably develops a progressive form of immune complex nephritis. Androgens suppressed and estrogens accelerated the disease in animals treated at 2 weeks of age, long before they ordinarily develop antinuclear

antibodies. If animals were treated after the disease developed, androgens still ameliorated the nephritis and survival was prolonged without affecting anti-DNA antibody synthesis. To date, no trials using androgens to modify severe human lupus renal disease have been reported.

CLINICOPATHOLOGIC CORRELATIONS

Each patient with a suspected or confirmed diagnosis of SLE should have careful assessment of his or her renal status by way of the following clinical renal tests: (1) urinalysis with examination of urine sediment and measurement of qualitative protein on first morning voided urine samples, (2) 24 hour measurement of total protein in the urine if qualitative proteinuria is found, and (3) renal function preferably measured by a clearance technique to estimate glomerular filtration rate.

Microscopic hematuria, pyuria, cylindruria, and lipiduria are frequent manifestations of renal involvement. Finding erythrocytes and erythrocyte or blood casts in the urine sediment is particularly indicative of glomerular injury; however, in a few patients with mesangial lupus nephritis and with the focal and diffuse proliferative forms of nephritis, no erythrocytes, leukocytes, or cellular casts have been found in the urine at the time when a renal biopsy was accomplished. Urinary sediment abnormalities may occur in the pres-

---

Fig. 3 (left). Membranous lupus nephropathy. (A) Glomerulus showing diffuse thickening of capillary walls and mesangial expansion. H & E. Original magnification, × 400. (B) Glomerulus showing diffusely thickened capillary walls due to subepithelial deposits and basement membrane "spikes" (arrows) Methenamine silver. Original magnification, × 640. (C) Glomerulus showing diffuse, granular capillary wall fluorescence with anti-IgG. Original Magnification, × 400.(D) Electron micrograph showing glomerular capillary wall markedly thickened by subepithelial electron-dense deposits several layers deep interspersed by basement membrane "spikes" (arrows), areas of irregularly thickened glomerular basement membranes without deposits (GBM with arrows), and a large mesangial deposit (D). CL, capillary lumen; Mes, mesangial cell; End, endothelial cell; Epi, visceral epithelial cell. Original magnification × 6250. [From Donadio JV, Burgess JH, Holley KE: Membranous lupus nephropathy: A clinicopathologic study. Medicine 56:527, 1977. Reprinted by permission, © 1977 The Williams & Wilkins Co, Baltimore.]

ence of mild or heavy proteinuria and with normal or impaired glomerular filtration rate. Thus such abnormalities do not predict the type or extent of glomerular injury; however, an abnormal urine sediment alone may be the earliest sign of renal involvement. Also, in general, heavy amounts of urinary protein and impaired glomerular filtration rate are associated with the more severe proliferative lesions.

If renal tests are abnormal, then renal biopsy should be performed, preferably by percutaneous technique, with subsequent categorization of the renal lesion.

TREATMENT AND PROGNOSIS

The treatment of lupus nephritis should be considered in the context of the total treatment of the disease. Adrenocorticoids (mainly oral prednisone) are the primary agents used today in treating lupus nephritis. Recommended dosages and durations of steroid treatment are various, consisting of single, multiple, or every other day dosage schedules. No one method of treatment is demonstrably superior to any other; however, when there are severe systemic manifestations of the disease, divided dose schedules are preferable, and when one is planning to use high doses of prednisone (for example, 60 mg/day) for several months, then changeover to a single daily dose schedule is preferred once the systemic manifestations are under control. Careful attention should also be given to adjunctive treatment such as sodium-restricted diets, antihypertensive and diuretic agents in the presence of hypertension, and sodium restriction when high doses of prednisone are being administered. Also, salicylates, extra rest, skin care, and antimalarial drugs should be used when appropriate for the control of systemic manifestations of the disease.

Only rarely do patients with mesangial lupus nephritis develop severe renal disease later in their course, and high doses of prednisone therapy are not advisable. Nevertheless, patients with this form of nephropathy should be tested regularly in order to detect evidence of aggravation of their renal disease as soon as possible. The 5 year survival rate of patients with mesangial lupus nephritis is approximately 80 percent and death from renal failure is uncommon. The dosage of prednisone used to treat these patients is that which is required to control extrarenal manifestations of their disease.

In patients with mild (focal) proliferative lupus nephritis, prognosis is worse because the disease may progress to a more severe, diffuse form (approximately 25 percent of patients). The 5 year survival rate of patients with mild (focal) proliferative lupus nephritis is about 65 percent, and most deaths are from nonrenal causes, though endstage renal disease does occur in this group. A short course (1 month) of high-dosage prednisone therapy, 60 mg/day, with rapid tapering to a level required to control extrarenal manifestations, is probably the treatment of choice. As in the group of

patients with mesangial lupus nephritis, careful followup examinations are necessary to detect change in the disease course.

In severe (diffuse) proliferative lupus nephritis, high dosages of prednisone have been shown to favorably alter the course of the disease; however, there is not a single control study available to substantiate this statement, and the treatment of such patients remains an unsettled issue in clinical medicine. Until 1970, the reported 5 year survival rate of adult patients with this severe form of lupus nephropathy was 25 percent. In more recent reports, treatment with prednisone alone and with combinations of prednisone and azathioprine, cyclophosphamide, or nitrogen mustard provided better 2 year survival rates than did the steroid treatment of the older studies; however, these shorter term survival data, showing greater improvement more recently, must be tempered by the knowledge that there was great variability in patient selection, criteria used to define disease activity (including biopsy classification and interpretation), and treatment. Today, clinicians have a better appreciation of the potency of high-dosage prednisone treatment. Bacterial sepsis and other opportunistic infections (for example, cytomegalovirus, *Pneumocystis carinii*, herpes simplex, and fungal) in patients receiving high dosages of prednisone, with or without cytotoxic agents, are responsible for many deaths of patients with diffuse proliferative lupus nephritis, most of whom are in renal failure. Because of the demonstrated failure of high-dosage prednisone, with or without cytotoxic drugs, to benefit patients with advanced lupus renal disease, perhaps it would be better not to use these agents in this situation so as not to further jeopardize chances for successful dialysis or renal transplantation by placing such patients at additional risk from serious infection. In terms of the improved survival reported in recent years in patients with diffuse proliferative lupus nephritis, there is no study that adequately demonstrates that the improvement was due to the addition of cytotoxic drugs to prednisone treatment, such as the addition of azathioprine, cyclophosphamide, or nitrogen mustard, the drugs most often used; however, in a recent prospective study of patients with diffuse proliferative lupus nephritis the effectiveness of cyclophosphamide was evaluated—26 patients received prednisone(average dose 40 mg/day) and 24 received combined prednisone (average dose 29 mg/day) and cyclophosphamide (average dose 107 mg/day) for 6 months. Most of the patients improved (84 percent) after 6 months of treatment with either program. Early disease progression, ending mainly in endstage renal disease, occurred with equal frequency in both treatment groups in patients with already advanced renal disease. In a 4 year followup, there was a higher incidence and average rate of clinical recurrence of nephritis in the original prednsione treated group than in the combined drug treated group; however, the proportion of patients alive after 4 years with stable or improved renal function was similar in the two treatment groups (60 percent). Nevertheless, if the difference in renal flares between treatment groups continues with further observations, then combined, short-term treatment with prednisone and cyclophosphamide may reduce the rate of progression to endstage renal disease, which is still the major consequence of diffuse proliferative lupus nephritis.

In membranous lupus nephropathy, prednisone treatment does not appear to influence either proteinuria or renal function. The 5 year survival rate of these patients is approximately 80 percent with most dying patients succumbing to cardiovascular illnesses. Most patients with membranous lupus nephropathy have a relatively benign and stable renal course but otherwise have typical SLE. This suggests that the renal pathogenesis may be different from that of the proliferative forms of lupus nephritis.

In patients with primary tubulointerstitial nephritis, the effect of the interstitial inflammation and tubular deposits on renal function and the evolution of the disease remains to be evaluated. Impaired glomerular filtration rate, glucosuria (with normal blood sugar levels), and aminoaciduria have been reported in several patients. The influence of steroid therapy on this lesion is indeterminate.

REFERENCES

Brentjens JR, Sepulveda M, Baliah T, et al: Interstitial immune complex disease in patients with systemic lupus erythematosus. Kidney Int 7:342, 1975

Donadio JV Jr, Burgess JH, Holley KE: Membranous lupus nephropathy: A clinicopathologic study. Medicine (Baltimore) 56:527, 1977

Donadio JV Jr, Holley KE, Ferguson RH, et al: Treatment of diffuse proliferative lupus nephritis with prednisone and combined prednisone and cyclophosphamide. N Eng J Med 299:1151, 1978

Dubois EL: Lupus Erythematosus: A Review of the Current Status of Discoid and Systemic Lupus Erythematosus and Their Variants (ed 2). Los Angeles, University of Southern California Press, 1974

Keith NM, Rowntree LG: A study of the renal complications of disseminated lupus erythematosus: Report of four cases. Trans Assoc Am Physicians 37:487,1922

McCluskey RT: Lupus nephritis, in Sommers SC (ed): Pathology Annual. New York, Appleton-Century-Crofts, 1973, pp 125–144

Pirani CL, Manaligod JR: The kidneys in collagen disease, in Mostofi FK, Smith DE (eds): The Kidney. Baltimore, Williams & Wilkins, 1966, p 147

Wagoner RD, Holley KE: Parenchymal renal disease: Clinical and pathologic features, in Knox FG (ed): Textbook of Renal Pathophysiology. Hagerstown, Harper & Row, 1978, p 226

Winfield JB, Faiferman I, Koffler D: Avidity of anti-DNA antibodies in serum and IgG glomerular eluates from patients with systemic lupus erythematosus: Association of high avidity antinative DNA antibody with glomerulonephritis. J Clin Invest 59:90, 1977

DIABETES MELLITUS

Allen I. Arieff

It has been estimated that the total population likely to develop endstage renal disease in the United States each year is about 53,000. Of these, about 3200 (6 percent) will have renal disease related to diabetes mellitus. Additionally, among diabetic patients who are below the age of 40, the incidence is about 20 percent. Furthermore, other renal diseases which are commonly associated with diabetes, such as pyelonephritis, renal arteriosclerosis, and papillary necrosis, probably account for an additional 10 percent of diabetes-related deaths. Other causes of renal insufficiency, such as contrast agent induced acute renal failure and obstructive neprhopathy due to vesical dysfunction, also contribute to the loss of renal function in diabetic patients.

Most reviews of renal involvement in diabetes mellitus have stressed the pathophysiology, pathological changes, and clinical manifestations of diabetic nephropathy. There is a paucity of information available on the treatment of such disorders. Although there is yet no definitive therapy for diabetic nephropathy, there are several therapeutic approaches which, by correcting other complications associated with diabetes, may arrest the course of progressive renal failure. The role of "control" of blood glucose levels in preventing the occurrence of diabetic nephropathy, despite a vast array of clinical and laboratory studies, remains unclear. Two of the more promising recent experimental therapeutic advances in the treatment of diabetes mellitus, the "artificial pancreas" and pancreatic islet cell transplantation, may finally shed some light on this problem. Until a new major therapeutic advance is made, patients with endstage diabetic nephropathy must be treated with dialysis and/or renal transplantation. Both of these techniques are associated with major difficulties which have yet to be resolved.

PATHOLOGY OF DIABETIC NEPHROPATHY

The most common glomerular lesion is diffuse intercapillary glomerulosclerosis, which is characterized by an increasing accumulation of PAS positive staining matrix within the mesangium. Simultaneously, the glomerular capillary wall may become thickened and may be identified with PAS stains. This latter feature may make the lesion difficult to distinguish from that of membranous glomerulopathy. As the mesangium becomes increasingly expanded by the accumulation of eosinophilic matrix material, the adjacent capillary lumina may become obliterated, eventually leading to glomerular hyalinization. The severity of this diffuse form of intercapillary glomerulosclerosis has been found to correlate reasonably well with the clinical manifestations of diabetic nephropathy.

A second variety of glomerular change, nodular glomerulosclerosis, is characterized by the diabetic nodule originally described by Kimmelstiel and Wilson. Such nodules are seen in the glomeruli of about half of all patients with the diffuse lesion. Of variable size generally, the fully developed lesion may be an almost spherical mass which is PAS positive (Fig. 1). With increasing size, these nodules will often encroach on the patency of adjacent capillaries, but owing to their focal nature they may not have major functional consequences. The presence of nodules correlates only poorly with the clinical severity of diabetic nephropathy.

Exudative glomerular lesions are probably least specific for diabetes. Similar lesions may be observed in arteriosclerosis and are rarely observed in various forms of glomerulonephritis. Typically, the lesion is seen at the periphery of a lobule, where because of its crescentic shape it is known by the descriptive name of hyaline cap.

The major renal arteries and their intrarenal branches are arteriosclerotic in a high proportion of patients with diabetes. These arteriosclerotic lesions do not appear to be substantially different from those observed in nondiabetic individuals.

Various tubular lesions have been described in diabetic nephropathy. The only specific change, the Armanni-Ebstein lesion, is characterized by pale-staining glycogen-laden cells in the pars recta segment of the proximal tubule. A common autopsy finding in the preinsulin era, it is rarely seen today.

By the time glomerulosclerosis is visible by light microscopy, glomerular basement membrane (GBM) thickness is significantly increased. While the GBM retains its fibrillar structure and clearly defined borders, "moth-eaten" areas appear in the most advanced stages of the disease. Increasing amounts of mesangial matrix may occupy the center of a lobular stalk. These are the lesions that characterize the nodular variety of diabetic glomerulosclerosis. As the mesangial matrix continues to increase, mesangial cellularity decreases and the fully developed nodule tends to be acellular. Surrounding capillary loops are usually compressed but occasionally may be greatly dilated. By contrast with the uniformly consistent abnormalities in the GBM and mesangium in diabetic glomerulosclerosis, the epithelial cells may appear healthy and their foot processes discreet. Once proteinuria appears, a variable patchy obliteration of foot processes usually appears.

Diffuse linear localization of immunoglobulin G (IgG) along the GBM is the most frequently described immunofluorescence microscopic finding and has been reported in most patients with diabetic nephropathy. The immunofluorescence findings resemble the ribbon-like deposition if IgG described in anti-GBM glomerulonephritis insofar as the distribution of IgG is concerned. Additionally, IgM, fibrinogen, albumin, and the third component of complement (C3) have been demonstrated in a similar distribution in some cases. The significance of these findings is uncertain.

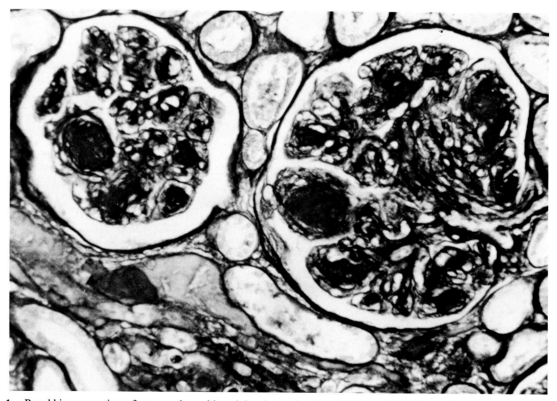

Fig. 1. Renal biopsy specimen from a patient with nodular glomerulosclerosis (Kimmelstiel-Wilson disease). There are nodules in most of the glomerular tufts, with obliteration of capillary loops.

CLINICAL CHARACTERISTICS OF DIABETIC NEPHROPATHY

In general, diabetes mellitus must be present for at least 10 years before proteinuria first appears. This late appearance of overt nephropathy is usually preceded by substantial morphological changes in glomeruli.

Proteinuria, which is regarded as the clinical hallmark of diabetic nephropathy, is invariably associated with morphological evidence of diabetic nephropathy. The corollary of this statement is, however, not true. Advanced diabetic glomerulosclerosis has been found on biopsy studies of patients in the absence of proteinuria. Thus the use of proteinuria as a marker tends to underestimate the prevalence of diabetic glomerulosclerosis in diabetic populations. Prospective studies of large juvenile diabetic populations have demonstrated that about 50 percent of these subjects will have proteinuria after 30 years of the disease. A particularly unfavorable course is likely to ensue when proteinuria exceeds 3 g/day, and the nephrotic syndrome becomes manifest. Such patients also tend to have massive edema, which is often refractive to diuretic therapy. Finally, heavy proteinuria tends persist even when the GFR declines to levels below 10 ml/min.

The diagnosis of underlying diabetic glomerulosclerosis as the cause of nephrotic syndrome in the diabetic patient is somewhat simplified by the frequent coexistence of diabetic retinopathy in such patients. This is usually such a consistent finding that performance of a diagnostic renal biopsy should almost have always be entertained in a diabetic subject who has nephrotic syndrome without retinopathy, particularly when diabetes has been present for less than 10 years. The occurrence of other primary glomerulopathies, such as minimal change disease, membraneous glomerulopathy, and proliferative glomerulonephritis, has been reported under such circumstances.

Once renal function has declined to a point where azotemia develops, deterioration is irrevocable, leading to endstage renal failure. The morphological changes of diabetic glomerulosclerosis usually correlate well with clinical severity of the disease of this stage. Both peripheral neuropathy and retinopathy are generally present in most diabetic patients by this time. Cardiovascular disorders are common, and these, along with stroke, account for the majority of fatalities in such patients. The need for dialysis or transplantation therapy in endstage renal failure patients thus occurs at a time when formidable extrarenal complications of the diabetic state are prevalent.

TREATMENT OF DIABETIC NEPHROPATHY

Insulin has been used to treat or prevent the complications of diabetes for about 50 years. To date, therapy with many different insulin regimens has failed to prevent the development of diabetic nephropathy. It may be that perhaps optimal regulation of carbohydrate metabolism requires around-the-clock maintenance of near-normal levels of plasma glucose, although the actual data are not very convincing.

The principles of management of diabetic patients with edema, hypertension, and renal insufficiency do not differ substantially from those in nondiabetic subjects. There are, however, a number of adverse effects of commonly used drugs which are unique to the diabetic patients and deserve special emphasis. The thiazide diuretics and furosemide have been shown to produce modest worsening of glucose tolerance in diabetic hypertensives. Nonetheless, there appears to be a consensus favoring continued usage of these agents provided vigilance for hyperglycemic episodes is maintained. The nonselective beta blocker propranolol may block the epinephrine-induced tachycardia which occurs in response to insulin-induced hypoglycemia. The net effect is to possibly mask one of the symptoms by which the patient may recognize hypoglycemia.

OTHER CONDITIONS AFFECTING THE KIDNEY

Nephrotoxic acute renal failure is now a well recognized complication of the intravascular administration of radiographic contrast agents to subjects with diabetic nephropathy. More than 77 diabetic subjects with contrast agent induced acute renal failure have been reported in the literature during the last decade, as well as a substantial number of cases in patients with other systemic diseases. Close inspection of the clinical features of such reported patients usually reveals underlying diabetic nephropathy, often with preexisting proteinuria, hypertension, or azotemia.

Renal papillary necrosis is an ischemic infarction of the inner medulla and renal papilla of the kidney which is most often associated with obstructive nephropathy, analgesic abuse, alcoholism, sickle-cell disease, or diabetes mellitus (see the chapter on *Urinary Tract Infections*). The disease most often begins as a febrile illness associated with dysuria, chills, flank pain, and renal colic. The urine usually contains many red and white blood cells and bacteria. There usually is necrosis of the renal papilla, which sloughing of the papillary tip, so that the urine may contain fragments of such tissue. In many cases of renal papillary necrosis, there is a rapid (less than 1 week) loss of renal function, with oligoanuria. Intravenous pyelography may reveal separation of the papillae, with a characteristic "ring" sign caused by destruction of the papillary tip. Another possible clinical course of papillary necrosis is the subacute form with evidence of severe recurrent urinary tract infections, often accompanied by renal calculus formation. The subacute form may remit following fluid and antibiotic therapy, but the usual pattern is that of recurrent attacks with progressive loss of renal function.

Neurogenic vesical obstruction is a complication of diabetic neuropathy of undertermined frequency which may lead to renal failure. The outstanding clinical feature is the insidious nature of the bladder paralysis. The earliest manifestations are an abnormal cystometrogram and an enlarged bladder, often without residual urine. In men, the clinical picture may easily be confused with prostatic obstruction. Although the duration of diabetes may vary considerably, most patients with vesical dysfunctions are known to have been diabetic for at least 10 years, virtually all have diabetic autonomic neuropathy, and many also have underlying diabetic nephropathy with azotemia. The dangers of such a condition include infection, pyelonephritis, and obstructive nephropathy. Because of the ever-present danger of infection, there is a natural reluctance to catheterize the diabetic patient; however, if obstruction is not relieved, renal failure will likely ensue.

DIALYSIS OF DIABETIC PATIENTS

There is now a cumulative experience of about 20 years of dialytic therapy in the treatment of diabetic patient. Taking into account the obvious limitations of combining series of patients from different institutions, it is still probably useful to compare the results of dialysis in diabetic versus nondiabetic uremic subjects. In Fig. 2 are shown the results of several patient series, all published after 1975, of diabetic patients who have been followed for at least 3 years. These are compared with data on over 25,000 nondiabetic subjects who were also followed for 3 years. In diabetic patients, survival rates for the first, second, and third years are about 61 percent, 40 percent, and 38 percent, respectively. It has been suggested that chronic peritoneal dialysis may be a more suitable mode of therapy than is hemodialysis for diabetic patients. Data to support such a concept are not available, although in diabetic patients who have acute renal failure, treatment with

peritoneal dialysis is at least as effective as is hemodialysis. Despite hazards of combining data from several series of patients, it is apparent that—whatever figures are used—gross mortality statistics show that among dialysis patients there is a substantially higher death rate for diabetic subjects than for nondiabetic subjects (Fig. 2). Among the causes of death in such patients, cardiac disease, particularly myocardial infarction, uremia, infection, and stroke account for the high mortality.

The efficacy of dialysis in such patients will become at least partly dependent on the "quality of life" desired by the patients and/or their physicians. A partial evaluation of this elusive commodity can be ascertained by determining the complications suffered by diabetic uremic patients treated with dialysis. Diabetic patients on dialysis average about 3.5 days/month of hospitalization (versus 1.8 days/month in nondiabetic patients). About 35 percent of diabetic patients are blind prior to starting dialysis, and about 98 percent have evidence of retinopathy. Evidence available thus far suggests that after patients are begun on dialysis retinopathy will continue to progress, with about 60 percent of diabetic patients becoming blind within 3 years of dialysis. Similarly, symptoms of diabetic neuropathy continue to progress during dialysis.

TRANSPLANTATION IN DIABETIC PATIENTS

The generally poor results obtained with dialytic therapy in uremic diabetic patients have led to the increased use of renal transplantation as a therapeutic

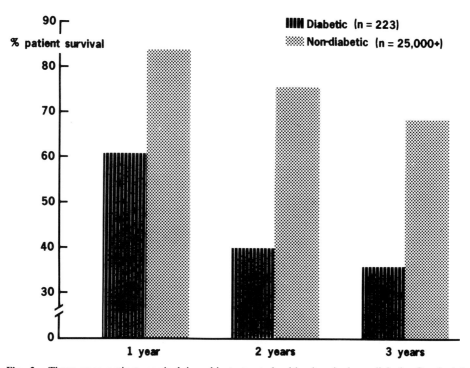

Fig. 2. Three year patient survival in subjects treated with chronic hemodialysis. Survival is compared in diabetic versus nondiabetic individuals, using data published in the period 1975–1978. It is clear that after 3 years survival is almost double in normal individuals when compared to those whose renal failure is due to diabetes mellitus. [Reprinted with permission from Arieff AI, in Brenner BM, Rector FC (eds): The Kidney, Philadelphia, W.B. Saunders, 1980, Chap 36.]

modality. Figure 3 compares the patient survival in diabetic subjects treated with chronic hemodialysis versus those receiving a cadaveric renal transplant. It can be seen that patient survival for the initial 3 years after transplant is not different than results obtained with chronic hemodialysis, After 3 years, patient survival is 39 percent in patients receiving cadaveric renal grafts versus 38 percent in those treated with hemodialysis (Fig. 3). It must be pointed out that in these comparisons no attempt has been made to match patients with respect to age, associated illness, or severity of diabetes. It is apparent that neither cadaveric renal transplantation nor dialysis is as effective a therapeutic modality in diabetic patients as is chronic hemodialysis in nondiabetic subjects (Fig. 2).

The success of transplantation of related nondiabetic donor kidneys into diabetic subjects has been greater than that obtained with cadaveric donors, as has been the case in nondiabetic recipients. The 3 year patient survival is about 40 percent in diabetic patients receiving cadaver kidney transplants versus about 80 percent for related donors. In addition, the 1–4 year survival rates are essentially the same for diabetic related donor transplants as for nondiabetic subjects similarly treated.

Within the initial 6 month posttransplant period, the major causes of death have been infection and acute myocardial infarction. After 6 months, most deaths were also due to infection and myocardial infarction, but in addition several patients died of stroke, urological complications (neurogenic bladder, ruptured cystotomy, ureteral necrosis, ileal bladder leak), ruptured aortic aneurysm, and suicide.

Urological complications are somewhat more prevalent in diabetic than in nondiabetic transplant recipients. Such complications include ureteral stenosis, ureteral necrosis, bladder leakage, and neurogenic bladder and represent a significant cause of morbidity and mortality.

It has been the general experience that at least 30 percent of diabetic patients are blind at the time treatment (dialysis or renal transplantation) for endstage renal disease is required, and chronic hemodialysis does not seem to affect the progression of diabetic retinopathy. Current information suggests that about 60 percent of diabetic subjects will be blind within 3 years of initiation of dialytic therapy. By contrast, the effects of renal transplant on visual status in diabetic subjects are not well defined. Studies show that 1–2 years after renal transplantation, there has been stabilization of vision at

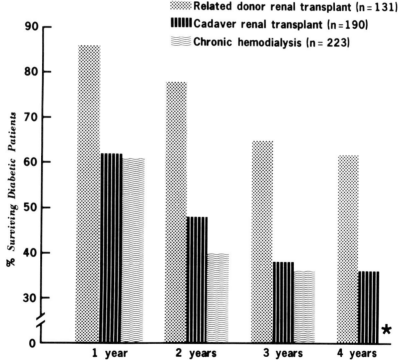

Fig. 3. Four year patient survival compared in diabetic patients with endstage renal failure who were treated with either chronic hemodialysis or renal transplantation; data compiled from articles published 1975–1978. It is apparent that survival is not different after 3 years in patients treated with chronic hemodialysis versus those receiving cadaveric renal transplantation. Survival in patients treated with related donor renal transplantation is almost double that of the other therapeutic modalities but must be viewed with caution because the data represent only two medical centers. *Data not available. [Reprinted with permission from Arieff AI, in Brenner BM, Rector FC (eds): The Kidney. Philadelphia, W.B. Saunders, 1980, Chap 36.]

the pretransplant level, without evidence of further deterioration. Recent data suggest that there will be stabilization of vision for at least 2 years after renal transplant with a well functioning renal allograft. In general, it would then appear that renal transplantation, either cadaveric or related donor, will often arrest the progression of diabetic retinopathy. The arrest of visual deterioration may be superior to the results obtained with chronic hemodialysis. If similar results are reported from other medical centers, it would represent a compelling advantage of renal transplantation over chronic hemodialysis, since gross survival figures for the two therapeutic modalities are not different.

A matter of concern is the effect of diabetes on the transplanted kidney. Only limited data are available and for only a 2 year followup period. Most evidence suggests that in diabetic patients nephropathy does not develop until diabetes has been present for 15–20 years. Thus it is perhaps unreasonable to expect that transplanted kidneys which have been in a diabetic environment for less than 10 years would show any evidence of diabetic nephropathy.

Examination by light microscopy has been carried out in kidneys transplanted into 12 diabetic subjects with endstage renal disease. Findings were compared to those present in age-matched nondiabetic patients who had received renal transplants for a similar time period. All allografts had been functional for at least 2 years. In 10 of the 12 diabetic subjects, renal biopsy of the transplanted kidneys revealed obvious deposition of PAS-positive hyaline refractile material in arteriorial walls.

The lesions were most often seen in glomerular arterioles, and in six of ten specimens there was hyaline change in both afferent and efferent arterioles. The deposition of hyaline material appeared to begin as a circumferential layering of the arteriolar subendothelial space, and it often extended between strands of a disrupted internal elastic lamina. In more advanced lesions, hyaline material appeared to replace the entire vessel wall. Interlobular arteries were usually, but not always, spared from hyaline change.

In the nondiabetic transplant recipients, there were occasional glomerular arterioles which showed hyaline deposits indistinguishable from those seen in the diabetic group. Two of these patients had received a related and one a cadaver donor graft. One of these patients had endstage chronic rejection, and the other two had no other major renal pathologic alterations, had normal renal function, and were normotensive. All three of these patients, however, had had their transplanted kidney for at least 5 years. None of the nondiabetic subjects had both afferent and efferent arteriolar hyalinzation. The arteriolar lesion was not found in any of the 23 nondiabetic patients with transplants in place for less than 5 years. The ten diabetic patients who had hyaline lesions all had their transplants for less than 5 years.

The interpretation of the above pathological findings is still conjectural. There are changes in normal kidneys transplanted into diabetic recipients which resemble diabetic nephropathy. Only 1 of 12 such patients developed a lesion which resembled nodular diabetic glomerulosclerosis. At this time there has not been a single reported instance where a renal allograft has undergone functional deterioration because of "diabetic" nephropathy. Thus at our present level of knowledge the possibility of recurrent diabetic nephropathy should not be construed as a contraindication to renal transplantation in a diabetic subject with endstage renal disease. Since the 4 year survival of cadaveric kidneys transplanted into diabetic recipients is less than 20 percent (Fig. 3), it is not certain that recurrent diabetic nephropathy will ever be a clincally important consideration.

There is a substantial body of experimental data on the effects of transplantation of a normal kidney into a diabetic animal. In rats with streptozotocin-induced diabetes for at least 6 months, glomerular lesions develop. In the early stages these lesions are characterized by thickening of the PAS-positive mesangial matrix, which extends to the hilus of the glomerulus and surrounds the intraglomerular portion of the afferent and efferent arterioles. In addition, glomerular hyaline deposits of PAS-positive material frequently develop. After 10–16 months of diabetes, progressive thickening of the mesangium culminates in sclerosis of glomerular tufts.

When kidneys from diabetic rats (streptozotocin induced) are transplanted into normal recipients, within 2 months there is noted the disappearance of IgG, Igm, and C3 deposits from the mesangium. There is also an arrest or reversal of glomerular mesangial thickening, which is the major finding on light microscopy in the kidneys of diabetic rats. Conversely, kidneys which are transplanted from normal to diabetic rats develop, over a period of 2 months, mesangial thickening with deposition of immunoglobulins and complement in the mesangium. The above changes are not observed when normal kidneys are transplanted into normal rats.

Additional studies are available which deal with the effects of correction of experimental diabetes on the lesions of experimental diabetic nephropathy. Normalization of blood glucose can be accomplished by transplantation of pancreatic islet cells into the diabetic (streptozotocin induced) Lewis rat. In these rats, there is a regression of both the light microscopic and immunopathologic glomerular lesions of experimental diabetic nephropathy. These and subsequent studies strongly suggested that there was renal mesangial dysfunction induced by some metabolic alteration associated with diabetes; however, although the glomerulopathy associated with longstanding diabetes in the rat bears some resemblance to that seen in man, there are several important differences as well. These morphologic differences raise serious questions as to the relevance of these animal models to the glomerulopathy observed in humans.

OTHER THERAPY FOR DIABETIC NEPHROPATHY

During the 50 years since insulin use became widespread, there has been essentially no promising pharmacological therapy for the treatment of diabetic nephropathy. Regimens which have been attempted include the following.

Immunosuppressive agents. These drugs have been used to treat wide variety of renal diseases, despite the lack of evidence of their efficacy. One would not think that such agents (steroids, antimetabolites) would be efficacious in the treatment of diabetic nephropathy. There has apparently been very little clinical experience employing these preparations in diabetic patients with renal disease, but despite this fact there are frequent allusions to their ineffectiveness. The few clinical and experimental reports that are available attest to the fact that such therapy appears to be unwarranted in diabetic patients.

Anticoagulant and antithrombotic agents. In recent years, such agents have been used to treat a variety of primary and secondary renal lesions. The common denominator of all such lesions appears to be a secondary activation of the clotting system, resulting in platelet–fibrin thrombi in small vessels and trapping of fibrin in glomerular capillaries. In several patients with diabetes mellitus, fibrin has been recognized within glomerular capillaries. These patients had stable renal function but had proteinuria at the time of biopsy. The presence of fibrin was demonstrated by immunofluorescence and electron microscopy, but the significance of this finding is now known. The patients also had decreased platelet survival and elevated levels of urinary fibrin degradation products. Therapeutic trials of heparin have been very limited in patients with diabetic nephropathy, but these preliminary data suggest some degree of improvement in the glomerular histological picture although not in GFR.

Pituitary ablation. This technique, employing surgery, cryogenic methods, or radiation, has been employed frequently to treat the retinal complications of diabetes mellitus. Little information is available on the effects of such therapy on the renal lesions of diabetes. Some studies suggest that pituitary ablation may be followed by significant improvement of the renal histological picture, although effects on GFR are variable and arteriosclerotic lesions are unaffected. These initial findings have yet to be confirmed.

Conservative management. Supportive principles of management of diabetic patients with renal insufficiency do not differ substantially from those of other patients with renal failure (see the chapter on *Conservative Therapy*).

KIDNEY, WATER, AND ELECTROLYTE METABOLISM IN DIABETIC COMA

Diabetic Ketoacidosis

Diabetic ketoacidosis is an acute metabolic disorder which is most common in "Juvenile" or growth onset diabetic patients. These patients are generally insulin dependent, and most lack effective beta cell function. The exact mechanism which triggers an episode of diabetic ketoacidosis is uncertain, although such a response is often aggravated by infection or other acute stress. Recurrent episodes of diabetic ketoacidosis appear to be related to a stressful circumstance, such as acute infection, myocardial infarction, emotional upset, or, more commonly, omission of an insulin dose. All of these conditions may lead to lack of insulin effect, which can result in abnormalities of fat, protein, and carbohydrate metabolism, The primary abnormalities in substrate metabolism may lead to secondary derangements in water, electrolyte, and acid–base metabolism. It is these secondary irregularities which may ultimately pose a threat to survival of the patient.

Concomitant with the presence of hyperketonemia, glucose accumulates in extracellular fluid. The increased load of ketone bodies, particularly the strong acids beta hydroxybutric acid and acetoacetic acid, may result in a severe metabolic acidosis, while hyperglycemia will lead to an osmotic diuresis with loss of water and electrolytes in the urine. The consequences of such water and electrolyte depletion, coupled with metabolic acidosis, include a fall in extracellular volume, decreased cardiac output, a decrease in renal concentrating ability, an increase in viscosity of the blood, and a fall in arterial blood pressure. Azotemia is the usual rule in patients with diabetic ketoacidosis and there is a marked fall in both GFR and renal blood flow (RBF). In general, both GFR and RBF have returned almost to normal values within 3 weeks after correction of metabolic acidosis, but in a substantial number of patients persistence of renal failure has been observed. The acute renal failure generally has a less severe course than that observed in acute renal failure from most other causes, but some patients have required hemodialysis, and several deaths have been reported.

The impaired renal function which may accompany diabetic ketoacidosis has both pathophysiologic and therapeutic implications. Normal subjects can excrete glucose at a rate of about 32 g/hour (175 mmole/hour) when renal function is not impaired. In patients with diabetic ketoacidosis, maximal excretion of glucose is only about 19 g/hour. The marked decrease in glucose excretion resulting from ketoacidosis can lead to increasing hyperglycemia and hyperosmolality. Ability to excrete ketoacids will also be impaired by the fall in GFR, leading to increasing acidosis. Inability of the kidney to elaborate a maximally concentrated urine, perhaps as a consequence of osmotic (glucose) diuresis and/or potassium depletion, can result in a greater degree of dehydration than would otherwise be expected. Generally, each gram of glucose lost in the urine obligates about 21 ml of water. Thus although the fundamental derangements leading to diabetic ketoacidosis are related to impaired insulin effect, the resulting impairments in renal perfusion and renal handling of salt and water are largely responsible for the progression of dehydration, acidosis, and electrolyte depletion.

Following the initiation of hyperglycemia and hyperketonemia in patients with diabetic ketoacidosis, the maximal rate of glucose reabsorption by the kidney will be exceeded. Glucose will then appear in the urine in increasing amounts, and there will be an osmotic diuresis, with the now largely nonreabsorbable solute glucose preventing the reabsorption of both water and sodium salts. The loss of solute during glucose osmotic diuresis differs in at least two important respects from the electrolyte loss which occurs during other settings associated with increased urine flow. During other types of osmotic diuresis, most anion lost in the urine is chloride, and urinary losses of potassium are minimal; however, during glucose osmotic diuresis associated with diabetic ketoacidosis, most anion lost in urine is not chloride but consists of potassium and sodium salts of ketoacid anions, i.e., acetoacetate and beta hydroxybutyrate. Thus urinary losses of sodium will substantially exceed those of chloride.

Generally speaking, during osmotic diuresis with a nonreabsorbable solute, urinary losses of potassium, although increased, are quite modest compared to losses of sodium and chloride; however, such is not the case in patients with diabetic ketoacidosis. Balance studies in the latter reveal urinary potassium losses to be about 70 percent of sodium losses. The reasons for this kaliuresis include the following:

1. The presence of metabolic acidosis leads to an increased excretion of acid anions in urine. These anions must be titrated with a cation, and in the presence of maximal stimulation for sodium reabsorption additional amounts of potassium will be excreted into the urine.
2. There is increased lean tissue breakdown due to insulin deficiency and the hyperadrenalcorticoid state.
3. Usually, severe secondary hyperaldosteronism will be present, which would tend to enhance renal losses of potassium.
4. Many patients have protracted vomiting, which can result in substantial loss of potassium.

Hyperosmolar Coma with Hyperglycemia (Nonketotic Coma)

Nonketotic coma is a syndrome characterized by severe hyperglycemia and dehydration in the absence of ketoacidosis. Diagnostic criteria include a plasma osmolality of at least 350 mOsm/kg H_2O, with plasma glucose over 600 mg/dl, in the absence of ketoacidosis (plasma Acetest reaction less than 2+ at a 1:1 dilution) and depression of sensorium to at least the level of stupor.

Nonketotic coma has been reported to occur in association with many precipitating events, including hemodialysis, peritoneal dialysis, burns parenteral hyperalimentation, administration of many drugs (including diphenylhydantoin, thiazide and furosemide diuretics, azathiaprine, steroids, and diazoxide), pancreatitis, infection, hyperthyroidism, and excessive carbohydrate intake. In some patients, no precipitating event can be identified.

The presence of hyperglycemia (plasma glucose greater than 600 mg/dl) without ketoacidosis (plasma Acetest less than 2+ at a 1:1 dilution) is the hallmark of nonketotic coma. Reasons for the absence of ketoacidosis in such patients have been the subject of much recent investigation. At present, there is ample evidence that several different mechanisms may be operative in different patients. The reasons for failure of ketoacidosis to occur will probably differ considerably from one patient to another.

Sustained hyperglycemia without ketoacidosis has at least two prominent sequelae: (1) osmotic diuresis with loss of water and electrolytes in the urine, and (2) absence of symptoms associated with metabolic acidosis, allowing more prolonged dehydration to occur. The osmotic diuresis differs somewhat from that observed in patients with diabetic ketoacidosis. There is a disproportionately larger loss of water than of solute, losses of potassium are less marked, and anions lost in urine are largely chloride rather than acid anions.

Although patients with nonketotic coma often have metabolic acidosis, the severity does not approach that usually observed in patients with diabetic ketoacidosis, and thus loss of acid anions in the urine should not be as great. The lesser urinary loss of anions is associated, as expected, with less urinary loss of potassium. Emesis is not as prominent a feature of nonketotic coma as it is in diabetic ketoacidosis, where repeated episodes of vomiting may contribute substantially to potassium loss.

The protracted osmotic diuresis associated with nonketotic coma may continue for periods of many weeks, but as long as the patient is able to obtain adequate quantities of water he can maintain extracellular volume relatively intact. The only consistent symptom as dehydration progresses is that of increasing unresponsiveness. Thus largely because of the duration of prodromal manifestations the mean water deficit in patients with diabetic ketoacidosis is about 4.4 liters, whereas in nonketotic coma it is greater than 9 liters. The loss of electrolytes in patients with nonketotic coma is substantially less than in patients with diabetic ketoacidosis. The loss of each liter of water is accompanied by a loss of about 60 mEq of monovalent cation (Na^+ or K^+). In general, patients with nonketotic coma have fluid losses which approximate 24 percent of total body water, with this loss being about equally divided between intracellular and extracellular compartments.

Most patients with nonketotic coma present with azotemia (BUN > 60 mg/dl; serum creatinine > 4 mg/dl) which is both renal and prerenal in origin. After the patients have been stabilized for several days, the mean creatinine clearance is below 50 ml/min, far less than normal. Autopsy studies of kidneys of patients who have died after an episode of nonketotic coma usually have revealed preexisting renal functional impairment. Most often, these patients had pyelonephritis, nephrosclerosis, glomerulosclerosis, or renal vein thrombosis, and most also had small, shrunken kidneys.

Despite the extensive dehydration in patients with nonketotic coma, most have an adequate urine output when first evaluated, and this is probably related to the glucose osmotic diuresis. When patients are treated with insulin, causing an abrupt decline in plasma glucose concentration, oliguria may ensue. Furthermore, acute renal failure often follows the oliguria. When the oliguria has been promptly treated with adequate volume expansion combined with intravenous loop diuretics (ethacrynic acid or fuorsemide), however, acute renal failure usually has not occurred.

It is a common conception that patients with nonketotic coma have normal blood pH; however, more than one-half such patients have metabolic acidosis, with a mean plasma bicarbonate of less than 14 mEq/liter and unmeasured anion concentration above 35 mEq/liter.

It may be that there are other endogenous organic acids which can produce metabolic acidosis. Recently, experiments have been carried out in patients with metabolic acidosis and increased anion gap. It was found that about half of the acid anions present in blood of such patients were not accounted for by commonly measured substances such as lactate, acetoacetate, and beta hydroxybutyrate. In all probability, the metabolic acidosis present in many patients with nonketotic coma represents the cumulative effect of modest elevations in serum lactate levels, acute renal insufficiency, cellular breakdown with release of organic acids into the circulation, and accumulation of as yet unidentified organic acid anions, such as short chain fatty acids.

REFERENCES

Arieff AI, in Brenner BM, Rector FC Jr (eds): The Kidney. Philadelphia, W.B. Saunders, 1980, Chap 36

Arieff AI, Carroll HJ: Nonketotic hyperosmolar coma with hyperglycemia: Clinical features, pathophysiology, renal function, acid-base balance, plasma-cerebrospinal fluid equilibria and the effects of therapy in 37 cases. Medicine (Baltimore) 51:73, 1972

Balodimos MC: Diabetic nephropathy, in Marble A, White P, Bradley RF, et al (eds): Diabetic Nephropathy (ed 11). Philadelphia, Lea & Febiger, 1971, p 526

Gellman DD, Pirani CL, Soothill JF, et al: Diabetic nephropathy: A clinical and pathologic study based on renal biopsies. Medicine (Baltimore) 38:321, 1959

Goldstein DA, Massry SG: Diabetic nephropathy: Clinical course and effect of hemodialysis. Nephron 20:286, 1978

Kahan M, Goldberg PD, Mandell EE: Neurogenic vesical dysfunction and diabetes mellitus. NY State J Med 70:2448, 1970

Kussman MJ, Goldstein HH, Gleason RE: The clinical course of diabetic nephropathy. JAMA 236:1861, 1976

Mauer SM, Steffes MW, Michael AF, et al: Studies of diabetic nephropathy in animals and man. Diabetes 25 [Suppl 2]: 850, 1976

Najarian JS, Sutherland DER, Simmons RL, et al: Kidney transplantation for the uremic diabetic patients. Surgery 144:682, 1977

SCLERODERMA

Robert T. Kunau, Jr.

Scleroderma (progressive systemic sclerosis) is a disorder characterized by alterations in the connective tissue and blood vessels. Although the etiology would appear to be immunologic in nature, the precise cause is unclear. In addition to the characteristic skin findings, visceral involvement is common, particularly of the gastrointestinal tract, lungs, heart, and kidney. As expected, the prognosis of the patient is usually dependent upon the nature and severity of the visceral lesions.

The incidence of renal involvement in scleroderma is difficult to determine, since uniform dianostic criteria have not been employed. In a large series followed for 10 years, some degree of renal involvement manifest by either proteinuria, azotemia, or hypertension was present in 45 percent of patients. Of further interest is that renal scleroderma accounted for over 40 percent of the deaths in autopsied cases. Renal involvement usually appears several years after other clinical presentation(s) of the disease, with proteinuria being the earliest and most common laboratory manifestation. Although the proteinuria is usually present in small amounts, on occasion the nephrotic syndrome may develop. The urinary sediment is commonly benign, frequently demonstrating only modest hematuria.

The clinical presentation of renal scleroderma may take on several forms. In some patients, the course may be indolent with slow deterioration of renal function; however, in approximately 15–20 percent of patients, renal involvement is characterized by a unique clinical presentation. The latter is characterized by the sudden onset of malignant hypertension, frequently associated with congestive heart failure, and a rapid loss of renal function within a brief time interval. Other patients may present in an identical fashion with rapid deterioration of renal function but without hypertension. The difference in the normotensive and hypertensive groups may, at least in part, be related to the elevated levels of plasma renin observed in the latter group. Although the reason for the sudden dramatic impairment in renal function is unclear, extensive visceral involvement, infection, dehydration, or a pericardial effusion may be preceding events. In addition, this clinical course occurs more commonly in patients who previously had hypertension, proteinuria, or azotemia.

Two types of sclerodermatous involvement of the renal vasculature have been described. The chronic form occurs primarily in patients who have had scleroderma for some time. The vascular lesions in this type are usually limited to the arcuate and larger interlobular arteries where sclerotic intimal thickening may be noted. There may also be diffuse ischemic tubular and glomerular atrophy and interstitial fibrosis. In the acute form of the disease, characteristic findings are again most evident in the smaller arcuate and interlobular arteries (Fig. 1). In these vessels intimal proliferation is observed with the deposition of a mucinous material

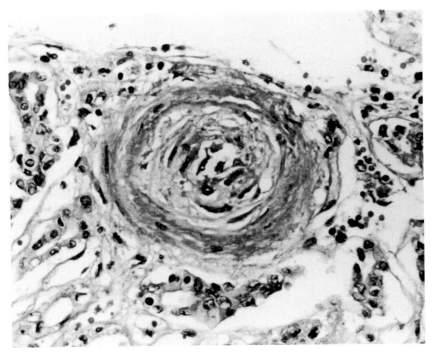

Fig. 1. Characteristic acute changes observed in interlobular artery in scleroderma.

possessing finely collagenous appearance which has staining characteristics suggestive of glycoproteins and acid and neutral mucopolysaccharides. This intimal proliferation may be so extensive as to compromise or occlude the lumen. The findings seen in the interlobular and arcuate vessels are not observed in smaller arterioles, although fibroblastic intimal proliferation may be present in these latter vessels. A variety of glomerular changes may on occasion be seen, but they are of doubtful specificity. Among the changes observed are mesangial proliferation, localized thickening of capillary walls, epithelial crescents, and fibrinoid necrosis. Most glomeruli, however, demonstrate only ischemic contraction. As anticipated from the elevated renin levels, hyperplasia of the juxtaglomerular apparatus may be seen in some patients.

Although similarities between the intrarenal histologic lesions of scleroderma and malignant hypertension have been noted, several notable differences have been reported. First, adventitial fibrosis around the intralobular arteries can be seen in scleroderma but is not observed in hypertension. Tubular atrophy is more common, and small infarcts less so, in malignant hypertension than in scleroderma. In the sclerodermatous kidney, the interlobular arteries usually show the most extensive changes, whereas malignant hypertension primarily involves smaller arteries and arterioles.

There is not uniform arrgrement regarding the nature of the immunofluorescent findings seen in the kidney in this disorder. The immunoglobulin IgM and complement have been observed in the vascular wall,

while the immunoglobulins IgG and IgA and fibrinogen are seen less frequently. IgM and complement may be seen in both the intima and the media and are not restricted to areas of necrosis. In the glomeruli the serum components may be localized in a segmental pattern along the peripheral capillary walls or in the mesangium. Antinuclear antibodies have been eluted from kidneys possessing the histologic changes of scleroderma and present a speckled and nucleolar pattern when studied by indirect immunofluorescence.

The treatment of the renal lesion of scleroderma is, at best, extremely difficult. Agents—e.g., reserpine—which have been used to relieve the vasospastic component of scleroderma in other arteries have not proven to be of merit when administered into the renal artery. Corticosteroids are of no benefit, although it seems unlikely that they are detrimental, as some investigators have previously concluded. D-Penicillamine may inhibit the synthesis of collagen cross-links and effect softening of the skin lesions, but there is no evidence that it diminishes the severity of the visceral lesions. The clinical efficacy of other agents which inhibit collagen cross-linkage remains to be fully defined.

At the present time, effective therapy of any hypertensive tendency which may be present—in particular, control of the blood pressure of patients with malignant hypertension—is felt to be important. Although the malignant hypertension can result from an increase in renin production, the use of propranolol to reduce the renin level should be used with caution if cardiac failure is also present. The characteristic resistant nature of the hypertension in these patients at times will require the use of potent antihypertensive medication, such as minoxidil. Bilateral nephrectomy has been suggested as a means to control the hypertension and to lessen the mortality of hemodialyzed patients. Recent evidence would indicate, however, that some degree of renal function may return in the patient with severe hypertension and renal insufficiency if the blood pressure is adequately controlled and the patients are supported for a time with hemodialysis. Bilateral nephrectomy therefore should not be performed without a careful determination of the degree of restoration of renal function and control of blood pressure after an appropriate interval on hemodialysis.

Hemodialysis in the patient with scleroderma at times is technically difficult because of the arterial lesions and frequent clotting of shunts. Transplantation has been performed in several instances and, though it has been successful in some patients, sclerodermatous lesions have appeared in the grafted kidney in others.

REFERENCES

Cannon PJ, Hassar M, Case D, et al: The relationship of hypertension and renal failure in scleroderma (progressive systemic sclerosis) to structural and functional abnormalities of the renal cortical circulation. Medicine (Baltimore) 53:1, 1974

LeRoy EC, Fleischmann RM: The management of renal scleroderma. Experience with dialysis, nephrectomy and transplantation. AM J Med 64:974, 1978

McCoy RC, Tisher CC, Pepe PF, et al: The kidney in progressive systemic sclerosis. Lab Invest 35:124, 1976

Merino GE, Sutherland DER, Kjellstrand CM, et al: Renal transplantation for progressive systemic sclerosis with renal failure. AM J Surg 133:745, 1977

Richardson JA: Hemodialysis and kidney transplantation for renal failure from scleroderma. Arthritis Rheum 16:265, 1973

Sellers AL, Rosen VJ: The kidney in progressive systemic sclerosis. Contr Nephrol 7:166, 1977

Stone RA, Tisher CC, Hawkins HK, et al: Juxtaglomerular hyperplasia and hyperreninemia in progressive systemic sclerosis complicated by acute renal failure. AM J Med 56:119, 1974

Wasner C, Cooke CR, Fries JF: Successful medical treatment of scleroderma renal crisis. N Engl J Med 299:873, 1978

VASCULITIC SYNDROMES OF CLASSIC POLYARTERITIS NODOSA AND HYPERSENSITIVITY VASCULITIS

Robert T. Kunau, Jr.

Numerous attempts have been made to classify the necrotizing vasculitides into separate and clearly definable categories based upon either clinical or pathogenic criteria. Such a separation has proved difficult, since there is considerable overlap in the manner in which these disorders present clinically and since it is now apparent that identical etiologic factors may produce several different clinical syndromes.

In the present discussion, the salient features of the renal lesions of two variants of the systemic necrotizing vasculitides are presented. The two variants discussed are classic polyarteritis nodosa, an entity which involves small- and medium-sized muscular arteries, and the entity variously classified as hypersensitivity vasculitis (angiitis) or the microscopic form of polyarteritis. The latter entity typically involves smaller arteries, arterioles, venules, and capillaries. It should be stressed that both classic polyarteritis nodosa and hypersensitivity vasculitis are part of larger subgroups of the necrotizing vasculiticles and may share certain features with other members of their respective subgroup.

The current theory is that the etiology of most of the vasculitic syndromes has an immunologic basis, i.e., the lesions are the consequence of the deposition of immune complexes in blood vessel walls or a cell-mediated immune reaction. In the former circumstance, for example, soluble antigen–antibody complexes are assumed to be deposited in the vessel wall. Complement components are then activated, some of which serving as chemotactic factors for polymorphonuclear leukocytes. As these cells infiltrate the vessel wall, intracytoplasmic lysosomal enzymes are released, resulting in damage to and necrosis of the vessel wall. As a consequence, thrombosis, hemorrhage, and ischemic changes in the tissue distal to the lesion can occur. The character of the pathologic lesion induced depends not only upon the nature of the immunologic mechanism involved but also upon hemodynamic factors which tend to predispose to the preferential localization of the immunologic damage in certain areas of the vasculature.

Recently, it has become apparent that patients with hepatitis B antigen associated vasculitis may present clinically with classic polyarteritis, with hypersensitivity vasculitis, or with a vasculitic syndrome which is typical of neither. Snydromes suggestive of either hypersensitivity vasculitis or classic polyarteritis nodosa have also been reported in drug abusers, particularly those who have used methamphetamine. Hypersensitivity vasculitis can be noted in patients who have a history of a preceeding drug ingestion—e.g., sulfonamides, penicillin—whereas an allergic history is unusual in patients with classic polyarteritis nodosa.

CLASSIC POLYARTERITIS NODOSA

In this entity, males are affected approximately twice as frequently as females, with the highest incidence occurring in the sixth decade. Malaise, fever, and weight loss are frequent constitutional findings. Arthralgias, abdominal pain, and mononeuritis multiplex are common clinical features. Cardiac abnormalities related to coronary arteritis may also be noted, whereas lung, spleen, and skin involvements are unusual. Hypertension, perhaps renin mediated, occurs in over 60 percent of patients and can dominate the clinical picture. A microangiopathic hemolytic anemia, leukocytosis, eosinophilia, and elevated sedimentation rate may also be observed. The renal manifestations, observed in 70 percent or more of patients, are related to infarction of renal mass distal to an arterial lesion or to ischemia. Loin pain and hematuria are common consequences of renal infarction, and hypertension can result from vessel occlusion. Proteinuria may be seen but is rarely present in quantities sufficient to result in a nephrotic picture.

The kidneys from patients with classic polyarteritis nodosa may be so extensively infarcted that only small areas of normal tissue are present, surrounded by regions of infarcted or ischemic tissue. As stated above, small- and medium-sized muscular arteries are involved in classic polyarteritis nodosa; hence in the kidney the arcuate and interlobar arteries are primarily afflicted (Fig. 1). The lesions are usually most prominent at points of vessel bifurcation. In the involved arteries, inflammatory lesions of various stages, from acute to healed, may be seen at one time, with areas of vasculitis interspersed between segments of normal vessel. The acute lesion is characterized by necrosis of variable portions of the vessel wall with replacement by fibrin-like material—hence the term fibrinoid necrosis. In this process, the internal elastic membrane is destroyed. The necrosis of the vessel wall is accompanied by an inflammatory response with polymorphs, eosinophils, and mononuclear cells being particularly prominent. The vessel walls may be weakened in the area of the lesion, with the result that aneurysms are formed. In addition, thrombosis may also occur in the diseased vessel. Healing occurs with the replacement of the necrotic areas by fibrous tissue but without significant regeneration of the muscle. In areas in which infarcts are not present, the tissue may histologically appear quite normal or demonstrate changes of gradual ischemia. The latter changes include tubular atrophy, shrinkage of the glomerular tuft, and hypertrophy of the juxtaglomerular apparatus. Examination of case reports which appear to be consistent with classic polyarteritis nodosa without hypertension indicate the occasional presence of patchy fibrinoid necrosis of the glomerular tufts, epithelial crescent formation, and endothelial cell proliferation, but the rarity of these observations suggests that they are not part of the typical histologic picture. Renal immunofluorescent and electron microscopic studies to date have not demonstrated a characteristic pattern. Finally, it should be recognized that the histologic findings may also reflect the effect of severe hypertension if the latter is present.

The diagnosis of polyarteritis nodosa within the kidney may be suspected by the character of the clinical presentation but must be confirmed by the demonstration of the arterial lesion. Renal involvement may be suggested by two findings commonly seen with renal angiography, (1) the presence of multiple small intrarenal aneurysms seen in 85 percent of cases (Fig. 2), usually associated with vascular irregularity, and (2) a mottled nephrogram, a manifestation of ischemic infarcts. Although suggestive, the presence of intrarenal microaneurysms should not be considered diagnostic of classic polyarteritis nodosa, since they can be seen in other disease entities as well.

Recently, significant advances have been made in the therapy of patients with classic polyarteritis nodosa. Remissions have been induced with the use of corticosteroids and azathioprine or cyclophosphamide. In patients with corticosteroid resistant disease, the addition of cyclophosphamide has resulted in disappearance of all aneurysms as judged by angiography and amelioration or improvement of all clinical symptoms.

HYPERSENSITIVY VASCULITIS

The clinical presentation of patients with hypersensitivity vasculitis may be similar to that noted in patients with classic polyarteritis nodosa. Hypertension and intestinal involvement are less frequently observed, but

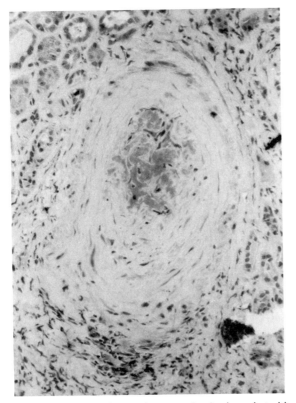

Fig. 1. Arcuate-sized muscular artery in classic periarteritis nodosa showing fibrosis of the destroyed muscular wall and an organizing luminal thrombus. Original magnification × 250.

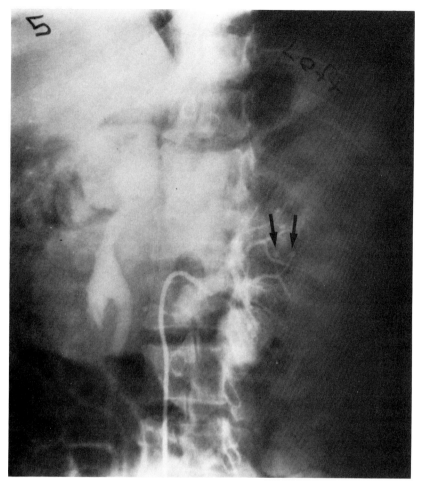

Fig. 2. Intrarenal aneurysms seen in left kidney after selective angiography.

pulmonary, cardiac, and skin disease are more commonly seen in hypersensitivity vasculitis than in classic polyarteritis nodosa.

In hypersensitivity vasculitis, renal involvement may present as an acute glomerulonephritis with hematuria, cellular casts, and proteinuria. Depending upon the extent of glomerular involvement and the severity of the lesions, the patients may present clinically with acute renal failure or follow a course similar to rapidly progressive glomerulonephritis. In other patients, the clinical course is more indolent, with slower progression being noted.

Gross inspection of the kidney reveals a normal-sized or somewhat enlarged organ with small petechial hemorrhages on the surface. Microscopically, fibrinoid necrosis is seen in the smaller interlobular arteries, arterioles, venules, and capillaries. The most pronounced alterations, however, are seen in the glomeruli. The extent of glomerular involvement is quite variable. In some instances only a few glomeruli are involved,

whereas in other cases the majority of glomeruli are afflicted. The most characteristic finding is the presence of fibrinoid necrosis, which may involve all or only part of a glomerular tuft (Fig. 3). In conjunction with the necrosis, proliferation of the cells within the tuft is frequently noted. Red cells and fibrin are frequently seen in Bowman's capsule, and epithelial crescents are common. On occasion, periglomerular granulomatous lesions surrounding fibrosing glomeruli, interstitial round cell infiltration, and hemorrhage may be present. Again as with the classic form, no consistent immunofluorescent or electron microscopic feature has been reported.

Since hypersensitivity vasculitis may be self-limited, evaluation of the effectiveness of any therapeutic modality is difficult. Thus any decision to treat these patients should be based upon the severity and extent of the vasculitis. Corticosteroids and appropriate immunosuppressive agents deserve consideration if the disease is progressive and the patient is deteriorating.

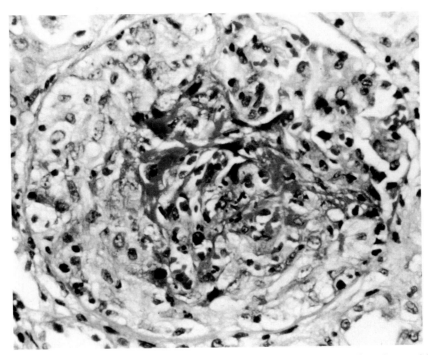

Fig. 3. Glomerulus in hypersensitivity vasculitis showing necrosis of the tuft and an epithelial crescent within Bowman's space. × 250.

REFERENCES

Davson J, Ball J, Platt R: The kidney in periarteritis nodosa. Q J Med 17:175, 1948

Duffy J, Lidsky MD, Sharp JT, et al: Polyarthritis, polyarteritis and hepatitis. Medicine (Baltimore) 55:19, 1976

Fauci AS, Doppman JL, Wolff SM: Cyclophophamide-induced remissions in advanced polyarteritis nodosa. AM J Med 64:890, 1978

Fauci AS, Haynes BF, Katz P: The spectrum of vasculitis. Clinical, pathologic, immunologic and therapeutic considerations. Ann Intern Med 89:660, 1978

Heptinstall RH: Polyarteritis (periarteritis) nodosa and rheumatoid arthritis, in: Pathology of the Kidney. Boston, Little, Brown, 1966, p 507

Sergent JS, Lockshin MD, Christian CL, et al: Vasculitis with hepatitis B antigenemia: Long-term observations in nine patients. Medicine (Baltimore) 55:1, 1976

Zeek PM: Periarteritis nodosa and other forms of necrotizing angiitis. N Engl J Med 248:764, 1951

CRYOGLOBULINEMIA

John J. Bardgette

Cryoglobulins are immunoglobulins or immunoglobulin complexes which reversibly precipitate at temperatures below 37°C. Cryoglobulinemia frequently accompanies the renal disease seen with systemic lupus erythematosus or following a streptococcal infection, but the present chapter will be limited to a consideration of the renal disease which attends cryoglobulinemia in the absence of other disease entities, i.e., essential cryoglobulinemia. The varieties of cryoglobulins are divided into three categories. Type I cryoglobulins are single monoclonal immunoglobulins. Type II cryoglobulins are complexes of a monoclonal immunoglobulin and polyclonal immunoglobulins. Owing to the presence of both monoclonal and polyclonal immunoglobulins, type II cryoglobulins are called mixed cryoglobulins. Type III cryoglobulins are composed of one or more polyclonal immunoglobulins. Although renal disease may occur with all three types of cryoglobulins, the renal disease which occurs with essential cryoglobulinemia is usually asscociated with type II or III cryoglobulinemia.

EPIDEMIOLOGY

The mean age of patients with essential cryoglobulinemia and renal disease is 35 years, with a range of 19 to 66 years. There is a preponderance of women among individuals with essential cryoglobulinemia with or without renal disease. The sex incidence of those with renal disease is not available.

PATHOGENESIS

The role of cryoglobulins in the pathogenesis of renal disease is incompletely understood, but several pieces of evidence suggest that cryoglobulins behave as immune complexes and that their deposition is responsible for renal injury. Electron microscopic and immunofluorescent studies of kidneys from cryoglobulinemic patients show electron-dense deposits and granular deposits, respectively, reminiscent of the deposits seen in experimental immune complex nephritis. Further, injection of cryoglobulin complexes from affected patients into experimental animals produces renal lesions which resemble the glomerulonephritis of cryoglobulinemia.

CLINICAL MANIFESTATIONS

Cutaneous symptoms and signs—Raynaud's phenomenon, dependent purpura, distal necrosis, livedo, urticaria, and leg ulcers—are the most common presenting symptoms as well as the most common manifestations of cryoglobulinemia. Infrequently renal failure or laboratory abnormalities may prompt diagnostic inquiry. Arthralgias, hepatosplenomegaly, and lymph node enlargement commonly occur. Abdominal pain, gastrointestinal hemorrhage, and intestinal infarction may be encountered.

Cryoglobulins are said to be present in 15 percent of patients with idiopathic renal disease. Patients manifest renal injury in several distinct patterns. An acute nephritic syndrome with gross hematuria and anuric renal failure may develop. Detection of proteinuria and microscpic hematuria may prompt investigation. The syndrome of rapidly progressive glomerulonephritis may occur. In some patients a history of weight gain and edema formation lead to the detection of the nephrotic syndrome, renal insufficiency, and cryoglobulinemia.

Serum complement levels are often reduced when renal disease is active. Mild leukopenia, an increased erythrocyte sedimentation rate, rheumatoid factor activity in the cryoprecipitates and less commonly in the serum, polyclonal hyperglobulinemia, and antinuclear antibodies may be found. The presence of hepatic disease, often associated with evidence of hepatitis B virus, should be sought.

PATHOLOGY

Light microscopy shows diffuse glomerulonephritis characterized by an increase in mesangial matrix material and an increase in mesangial and endothelial cellularity. The glomerular capillaries may be infiltrated with polymorphonuclear leukocytes, and the capillary lumina may contain hyaline thrombi. Epithelial crescents are seen with the clinical syndrome of rapidly progressive glomerulonephritis. Interstitial inflammation and necrotizing arteritis may be present.

Electron microscopy reveals subendothelial dense deposits and less frequently subepithelial deposits. Some workers have noted that these deposits have a distinctive fibrillar appearance. Immunofluorescent studies show positive glomerular staining for immunoglobulins and C'3 in a granular pattern. The types of immunoglobulins found in the kidney are usually similar to those present in circulating cryoglobulins.

THERAPY AND PROGNOSIS

A consistently effective therapy for the renal manifestations of cryoglobulinemia has not been found. Corticosteroids, immunosuppressive agents, and splenectomy have been used with limited success. The utility of plasmapheresis for the renal disease of essential cryoblobulinemia is not known, but this mode of therapy seems worthy of consideration. Avoidance of long periods of standing is useful for dependent pupura, and exposure to cold should be avoided.

The serum levels of cryoglobulins correlate roughly with clinical renal abnormalities and the severity of glomerular proliferation, but in many patients improvement in all measures of disease activity may occur without a reduction in the cryoglobulin level.

The ultimate course of renal disease is unpredictable. In some patients a rapidly downhill course occurs, while in others modest renal functional impairment may persist for years without further deterioration.

REFERENCES

Adam C, Morel-Maroger L, Richet G: Cryoglobulins in glomerulonephritis not related to systemic disease. Kidney Int 3:334, 1973

Brouet J, Clauvel J-PD, Danon F, et al: Biologic and clinical significance of cryoglobulins. Am J Med 57:775, 1974

Feiner H, Gallo G: Ultrastructure in glomerulonephritis associated with cryoglobulinemia. Am J Pathol 88:145, 1977

Grey H, Kohler P: Cryoimmunoglobulins. Semin Hematol 10:87, 1973

Meltzer M, Franklin EC, Elias K, et al: Cryoglobulinemia—A clinical and laboratory study. Am J Med 40:837, 1966

RENAL LESIONS IN MALIGNANCY

H. John Reineck

A wide variety of renal lesions has been reported in association with extrarenal malignancies. This list includes acute urate nephropathy, ureteral obstruction, renal vein thrombosis, amyloidosis, cryoglobulinemia, lymphomatosis infiltration, and lesions associated with dysproteinemias, primarily multiple myeloma and Waldenström's macroglobulinemia. These entities are discussed elsewhere, and this chapter is devoted to glomerulopathies occurring in patients with malignancy.

These lesions usually manifest as the nephrotic syndrome, and the clinical significance of this association is reflected in a recent review which reports that 11 percent of adult patients with the nephrotic syndrome harbor a malignancy. Pathologically, these glomerulopathies are of two general types—immune complex mediated disease and lipoid nephrosis or "minimal change" nephrotic syndrome. Although some overlap exists, carcinomas are generally associated with the former group of diseases, and lymphomas, primarily Hodgkin's disease, are seen with the latter lesions. This interesting separation is substantiated by the finding that 20 of 21 patients with carcinomas and the nephrotic syndrome had evidence of immune complex disease by immunofluorescence and electron microscopy, while only 5 of 18 patients with malignant lymphomas (15 with Hodgkin's disease) had these findings.

The immune complex glomerulopathy seen with carcinoma is primarily of the membranous variety. Focal and diffuse proliferative, as well as extracapillary glomerulonephritis, have also been reported. These lesions may occur with carcinomas of virtually any histologic type and origin, though tumors of the lung and gastrointestinal tract predominate.

The precise pathogenesis of carcinoma related glomerulonephritis is not entirely clear. The immune complex nature of this disease is supported by the high incidence of soluble circulating immune complexes in patients with neoplastic disease. The nature of these complexes is uncertain, however, The most widely accepted view holds that they are comprised of tumor antigen–antibody aggregates. In support of this concept are observations describing both tumor-specific antibody and tumor antigens identified from involved glomeruli. Other theories include tumor related virus antigen–antibody complexes and the development of antibodies against normal tissue. This latter view gains credibility from the high incidence of autoantibodies in patients with carcinoma.

Nephrotic syndrome with lipoid nephrosis or "minimal change" disease has been described with several lymphoproliferative diseases but is especially prevalent in patients with Hodgkin's disease, particularly those with the mixed cellular type. Suggesting that this association is of more than chance occurrence are the impressive coincident onset of both diseases and the simulatenous remissions of both disorders. The pathogenesis of lipoid nephrosis is obscure. Because of its association with Hodgkin's disease, its frequent remission during measles infection, and its response to steroids and cytotoxic drugs, a role for T lymphocytes has been invoked. The most attractive hypothesis involves the elaboration of a glomerular toxic lymphokine by these cells. Accordingly in Hodgkin's disease, a T cell proliferative disorder, such a substance could explain altered glomerular capillary permeability to protein. Unfortunately, the existence of this postulated toxin remains, to date, unconfirmed.

REFERENCES

Eagen JW, Lewis EJ: Glomerulpathies of neoplasia. Kidney Int 11:297, 1977

Lee JC, Yamauchi H, Hopper J: The association of cancer and the nephrotic syndrome. Ann Intern Med 64:41, 1966

Moorthy AV, Zummerman SW, Burkholder PM: Nephrotic syndrome in Hodgkin's disease: Evidence for pathogenesis alternative to immune complex deposition. Am J Physiol 61:471, 1976

Ozawa T, Pluss R, Lacher J, et al: Endogenous immune complex nephropathy associated with malignancy: I. Studies on the nature and immunopathogenic significance of glomerular bound antigen and antibody, isolation and characterization of tumor specific antigen and antibody and circulating immune complexes. Q J Med 44:523, 1975

Shalhoub RJ: Pathogenesis of lipoid nephrosis: A disorder of T cell function. Lancet 2:556, 1974

MULTIPLE MYELOMA

John J. Bardgette and Steven Z. Fadem

Multiple myeloma is an hematopoietic neoplasm characterized by proliferation of plasma cells which overproduce a single form of immunoglobulin. Excepting genitourinary neoplasms, multiple myeloma is the malignancy most likely to result in renal dysfunction. Although multiple myeloma may have diverse systemic extrarenal consequences, its effects are often intimately linked to the kidney. This relationship has important diagnostic and prognostic import. The first recognition of multiple myeloma around 1846 underscores this linkage, for it was then that a London physician, William MacIntyre, saw a patient suffering severe bone pain who excreted urine with unusual characteristics. In association with MacIntyre, Henry Bence Jones described the now well known thermal properties of the urinary protein (Bence Jones protein) which this patient excreted.

CLINICAL

Myeloma affects men and women equally but appears to have a greater predilection for blacks than whites. The onset of symptoms most commonly occurs in the sixth decade of life, and it is unusual for the disease to afflict individuals before the age of 40 years. These epidemiologic characteristics apply equally to those individuals with multiple myeloma who have renal dysfunction.

The most prominent early symptoms are skeletal pain, which may be evanescent or persistent, weakness, and easy fatigability. Epistaxis or gastrointestinal hemorrhage occurs in a sizable minority of individuals. Weight loss may occur. A variety of neurologic symptoms may be present, but these are uncommon early manifestations. Pallor, bone tenderness, and less commonly hepatosplenomegaly are found on examination.

LABORATORY

Abnormalities of serum and urine proteins are the laboratory hallmarks of multiple myeloma. Monoclonal immunoglobulins or Bence Jones protein in urine and/or serum have been found in 99 percent of patients. When sought, Bence Jones proteinuria is present in 50 percent of cases, and in 25 percent of cases Bence Jones proteinuria may be the only protein abnormality. Detection and characterization of protein abnormalities requires electrophoresis and immunoelectrophoresis. Concentration of the urine prior to immunoelectrophoresis may be necessary in order to detect Bence Jones protein. The classical heat test is neither as specific nor as sensitive as the electrophoretic method.

Proteinuria may be discovered by conventional Albustix testing, but this test is insensitive to Bence Jones protein. Thus screening for Bence Jones protein should be performed with the sulfosalicylic precipitation method. Examination of the urinary sediment may show a few white blood cells as well as hyaline and granular casts. When myeloma cells are diligently sought in urine, they are found with surprising frequency.

The other common laboratory findings include anemia and an elevated erythrocyte sedimentation rate. Hypercalcemia frequently accompanies multiple myeloma, being present in 30 percent of patients at the time of diagnosis and in an additional 30 percent during the course of the disease. Leukopenia and thrombocytopenia occasionally occur, and hyperuricemia may also be seen.

The anion gap (serum sodium minus the sum of chloride plus bicarbonate) is frequently low in patients with multiple myeloma. Although the overlap is considerable, fewer than 2 percent of controls will have anion gaps of less than six, whereas over 25 percent of patients with multiple myeloma may have such low values. The phenomenon of a low anion gap in multiple myeloma is presumably due to the presence of cationic paraproteins in the serum of these patients. It is of interest to note that the development of metabolic acidosis in such patients would result in a "normal" anion gap.

RENAL MANIFESTATIONS

Renal functional impairment is frequently present at the time of initial presentation. In one large series in which serum creatinine was available, more than half of patients had an elevated serum creatinine at the time of initial evaluation. In another series, 35 of 421 patients had serum creatinine values greater than 2 mg/dl at the time of diagnosis.

The presence of renal disease has a profound influence on the prognosis of patients with multiple myeloma. In one large series of patients, those with a blood urea nitrogen value below 20 mg/dl had a median survival of 37 months, whereas those with a blood urea nitrogen greater than 40 mg/dl had a median survival of only 2 months.

Acute Renal Failure

The frequency of acute renal failure is increased in multiple myeloma. DeFronzo et al. reported a 7 percent incidence of abrupt deterioration of renal function in a group of 187 myeloma patients. The age and sex distribution of this group was typical of myeloma.

Although acute renal failure commonly makes its appearance after the diagnosis of multiple myeloma, renal failure may be the most prominent initial manifestation of the disease. In 5 of the 14 patients reported by DeFronzo et al. the diagnoses of multiple myeloma and acute renal failure were made simultaneously. In the remaining patients a variable period of up to 6 years intervened between the diagnosis of myeloma and the development of renal failure. In elderly patients acute renal failure of inapparent cause should stimulate consideration of the presence of multiple myeloma.

There is evidence that the pattern of and predisposing factors to acute renal failure in multiple myeloma are changing. Earlier work noted the development of acute renal failure on a background of chronic renal

functional impairment in almost 50 percent of cases of myeloma with acute renal failure. In contrast, a recent study noted the development of acute renal failure exclusively in patients free of previous renal insufficiency. Similarly, etiologic associations appear to be changing. Past authors frequently attributed the onset of acute renal insufficiency to the effects of intravenous pyelography and dehydration. More recently, however, the presence of hypercalcemia and the administration of nephrotoxic antibiotics have assumed major roles as causative factors.

The precise relationship between Bence Jones proteinuria and renal failure is unknown, but it should be noted that 10 of the 11 patients with acute renal failure reported by DeFronzo et al. had Bence Jones proteinuria. A similar high incidence of Bence Jones proteinuria has been observed in preceding case reports of acute renal failure. The reason for this apparent relationship between Bence Jones proteinuria and acute renal failure is not clear. In vitro studies demonstrate a propensity of these proteins to precipitate at high concentrations as well as decreased solubility at acid pH. In view of the physiologic functions of the distal nephron—i.e., concentration and acidification—these observations lead naturally to speculation that precipitation of Bence Jones protein is the major contributing cause of acute renal failure. Other studies suggest that these proteins may have a direct toxic effect on renal tubular cells. It is of interest to note that injection of light chains into experimental animals can produce a form of acute renal dysfunction which has many resemblances to the disease seen in man.

The role of intravenous pyelography in precipitating acute renal failure is ambiguous. Although there are multiple instances in which functional impairment ensued after pyelography, review of large series of patients with multiple myeloma undergoing intravenous pyelography has not shown an increased incidence of acute renal failure. Prudence, however, would dictate that studies employing contrast agents be restricted to those occasions when information of essential therapeutic import can be obtained. Since dehydration may aggravate the nephrotoxic effect of pyelography, the conventional practice of restricting fluids prior to renal or other radiographic studies should be avoided.

Histologic examination shows features of acute tubular necrosis, diffuse tubular atrophy with intratubular casts, or tubular atrophy and/or calcification. The presence of intratubular casts is not invariable, however, a fact which is hard to reconcile with pathogenic theories that ascribe primacy to the role of intratubular precipitation of Bence Jones protein in the development of acute renal failure.

Myeloma Kidney

Myeloma kidney refers to a constellation of characteristic renal pathologic findings which include tubular atrophy and dilatation, eosinophilic lamellated intratubular casts with giant cell reactions surrounding the tubule, and interstitial fibrosis (Fig. 1). Glomeruli are generally normal. These histologic findings are usually associated with impairment of glomerular filtration. The severity of impairment of glomerular filtration parallels roughly the severity of the injury as determined by histology. Similarly the presence of Bence Jones protein in the urine is strongly correlated with the severity of renal insufficiency. There are exceptions to these correlations, however, and occasional patients may have marked depression of creatinine clearance in the absence of striking histologic findings and without the presence of Bence Jones proteinuria.

Renal Tubular Dysfunction

Multiple myeloma has been associated with several forms of renal tubular defects, including the Fanconi syndrome and distal renal tubular acidosis.

The full array of abnormalities present in the Fanconi syndrome may occur: hyperchloremic acidosis, hypophosphatemia, osteomalacia, glycosuria, hypouricemia, hypokalemia, and aminoaciduria.

Although the Fanconi syndrome has been described in fewer than 20 patients with multiple myeloma, the relationship has diagnostic importance. In most patients appearance of the Fanconi syndrome has preceded the diagnosis of multiple myeloma; in a few patients the two diagnoses have been made concurrently; but in no instance has the Fanconi syndrome developed subsequent to the discovery of multiple myeloma. In many of these patients Bence Jones proteinuria may antedate a conclusive diagnosis of multiple myeloma by several years. Thus patients with otherwise unexplained Fanconi syndrome should be followed carefully to evaluate for the development of a plasma cell dyscrasia. When

the light chains excreted by patients with Fanconi syndrome are typed, they are of the kappa type; the precise significance of this observation is not known.

Several considerations suggest that light chains may play a pathogenetic role in the tubular dysfunction which accompanies myeloma. Physiologic studies indicate that light chains, molecular weight approximately 22,000, are freely filtered by the glomerulus and subsequently are reabsorbed and catabolized by proximal tubular cells. Urinary excretion of light chains, in the absence of manifest multiple myeloma, is associated with renal tubular defects. Pathologic examination of the kidney shows degenerative changes of the proximal tubular cells, and in almost one-half of reported patients intracytoplasmic crystalline deposits have been found in tubular cells.

Urinary acidification defects have rarely been sought in a large group of patients with myeloma, but when ammonium chloride loading has been performed nearly 50 percent of patients have had some form of abnormal acidification. Almost all of these patients with acidifying defects have Bence Jones proteinuria. The majority of patients from this subset also have electrolytes and blood gases indicative of renal tubular acidosis. These observations suggest an intimate relationship between the presence of Bence Jones proteinuria and tubular dysfuntion. On the other hand, it should be noted that many patients with Bence Jones proteinuria are able to maximally acidify the urine.

Amyloidosis and Nephrotic Syndrome

Clinical series have noted an increased frequency of amyloidosis in multiple myeloma. As many as 5 percent of patients with multiple myeloma have evi-

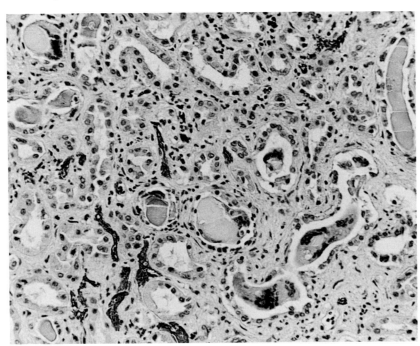

Fig. 1. Myeloma kidney. There is tubular atrophy, lamellated intratubular casts with giant cell formation, and interstitial fibrosis.

dence of amyloidosis. Those with light chain myeloma may also have an increased frequency of amyloidosis. Orthostatic hypotension, purpura, macroglossia, hepatomegaly, and carpal tunnel syndrome are clinical features suggestive of amyloidosis. Ten percent of individuals with multiple myeloma and systemic amyloidosis have nephrotic syndrome.

Because a large component of urinary protein in multiple myeloma may be low molecular weight protein, proteinuria per se does not imply abnormal glomerular permeability to protein. If the nephrotic syndrome occurs in patients with multiple myeloma in the absence of renal amyloidosis, it is presumably due to unrelated glomerular disease.

In a group of 35 patients studied by DeFronzo et al. all but 2 had increased protein excretion, but only 4 excreted albumin in amounts greater than 600 mg/24 hours. Biopsy in these 4 patients showed 2 with amyloidosis, 1 with glomerulonephritis, and 1 with minimal abnormalities; 11 patients excreted more than 1 gram of Bence Jones protein per day.

Hypercalcemia

As mentioned above, hypercalcemia is a common manifestation of multiple myeloma. The pathogenesis of hypercalcemia in multiple myeloma remains uncertain, but (1) direct invasion of bone by plasma cells with resultant bone dissolution and (2) production of a humoral substance by plasma cells which resorb bone are two possible mechanisms. This latter mechanism is thought to be mediated by osteoclastic activating factor (OAF), which has been detected in plasma cells from myeloma patients.

Hypercalcemia may alter renal function in these patients in several ways. It may cause a syndrome of nephrogenic diabetes insipidus with resultant polyuria and polydipsia. Because dehydration may contribute to the development of acute renal failure in multiple myeloma, the consequences of hypercalcemia are particularly perilous. Hypercalcemia may cause renal vasoconstriction. Hypercalcemia, whether via its dehydrating potential or through its vasoconstrictor properties, is at present a frequent cause of acute renal deterioration in myeloma patients. Prompt treatment of hypercalcemia can reverse the functional impairment.

Urinary Infections

Patients with multiple myeloma are more susceptible to a variety of infections. This propensity is reflected in an increased number of urinary tract infections. Urinary infections account for more than half of the infections encountered in myeloma patients, and as expected gram-negative organisms predominate. There are several factors which predispose these individuals to the development of urinary infection. The disease itself probably alters normal antimicrobial defenses. Infection frequently coincides with the insertion of bladder catheters. Thus fastidious attention to aseptic technique should be given when bladder catheterization is necessary. Myeloma patients are prone to develop neurogenic bladder dysfunction. Finally, in males, age confers an increased likelihood of prostatic hypertrophy.

Hyperuricemia

Mild hyperuricemia is not uncommon in multiple myeloma, but it is a rare cause of renal dysfunction in this population. Prophylactic therapy with the xanthine oxidase inhibitor allopurinol prevents the acute renal failure which may follow cytotoxic therapy.

THERAPY

Treatment of the systemic extrarenal manifestations of multiple myeloma should be conducted by an individual experienced in the management of this disease. There is no specific treatment for the renal disease associated with multiple myeloma. Due attention, however, should be given to appropriate hydration, avoidance of needless contrast studies, careful use of potentially nephrotoxic antibiotics, and prompt detection and treatment of hypercalcemia. The experience with dialysis for patients with multiple myeloma and renal failure is not extensive, but early reports are encouraging.

REFERENCES

DeFronzo RA, Cooke CR, Wright JR, et al: Renal function in patients with multiple myeloma. Medicine (Baltimore) 57:151, 1978

DeFronzo RA, Humphrey RL, Wright JR: Acute renal failure in multiple myeloma. Medicine (Baltimore) 54:209, 1975

Emmett M, Narin RG: Clinical use of the anion gap. Medicine (Baltimore) 56:38, 1977

Koss MN, Pirani CL, Osserman EF: Experimental Bence Jones cast nephropathy. Lab Invest 34:579, 1976

Maldonado JE, Velosa JA, Kyle RA, et al: Fanconi syndrome in adults: A manifestation of a latent form of myeloma. Am J Med 58:354, 1975

Pringle JP, Graham RC, Bernier GM: Detection of myeloma cells in urine sediment. Blood 43:137, 1974

AMYLOIDOSIS

Marvin Forland

Systemic amyloidosis is a disease process related to the deposition of a fibrillar extracellular glycoprotein in varying organ systems throughout the body. Its manifestations reflect the functional impairment induced by its accumulation in the particular tissue.

CLASSIFICATION AND PATHOGENESIS

Early classification of amyloidosis was based on its idiopathic (primary) presence with usual localization to the heart, tongue, nerves, skin, and joints, its secondary appearance in association with chronic suppurative processes with preferential localization to the liver, spleen, kidney, and adrenal glands, or its association with multiple myeloma; however, anatomical patterns have not been reliable, and refinements in molecular biology have permitted a more fundamental understanding of the pathogenesis and a classification based on the biochemical nature of the amyloid fibril. The "primary" and myeloma-associated forms are related to deposition of light chain immunoglobulins (AL protein) or their proteolytically derived fragments; the usual "secondary" variant and some familial forms have a unique protein known as amyloid A (AA) protein as a major component. The forms of amyloidosis occurring with advanced age or as a localized tumor are not associated with renal involvement.

Primary amyloidosis and myeloma-associated amyloidosis are usually associated with the deposition of fibrils derived from light chain immunoglobulins, most frequently the variable fragment. The amyloid fibrils, as in other forms, are mixed with a plasma derived (P) component, an α_1 glycoprotein present in normal sera. The presence of a similar monoclonal, usually Bence Jones protein of apparent origin from a common clone of immunoglobulin synthesizing cells has been reported in the urine and/or blood of 50–90 percent of patients in this group. Multiple myeloma or occult plasma cell dyscrasia are usually the associated conditions if any are identifiable. Approximately 10–15 percent of patients with typical multiple myeloma develop amyloidosis. Encroachment by the infiltrate most often is manifested in the heart, tongue, nerves, smooth and skeletal muscle, skin, and joint ligaments.

Secondary amyloidosis has been associated with chronic infections, rheumatoid arthritis, Hodgkin's disease, and familial Mediterranean fever. A low molecular weight protein (7000–9000 daltons) termed amyloid A (AA) has been found to be the major component of these fibrils. A substance has been detected in human serum (SAA) which is immunologically related to AA and which appears to be an acute phase reactant. Acute transient rises in SAA are observed with infection, fever, and pregnancy. The origin and factors leading to conversion and deposition of precursors in the tissue remain unknown. Elevations in monoclonal serum immunoglobulin concentrations are seen in more than half of these patients but are usually IgG, IgA, IgD, or IgM rather than light chains. Organs most frequently involved are the liver, spleen, kidney, and adrenal glands.

As many as 30 percent of patients present with a mixed pattern. This heterogeneity may be manifested clinically by the distribution of the amyloid as well as biochemically with the desposition and coexistence of both light chain fragments and AA protein.

The common denominator in the varying forms of amyloidosis appears to be the production of a protein capable of undergoing transformation into a β pleated sheet fibril and hence assuming the physiocochemical properties, including staining reactions, of amyloid. The plasma cell is clearly the origin of the AL protein. The cell source of the AA protein remains speculative, but its production appears related to an immune stimulus.

RENAL MANIFESTATIONS

Evidence of renal infiltration is one of the most common and potentially threatening manifestations of systemic amyloidosis. Proteinuria is the most frequent finding and was present in 86 percent of patients in a recent review; manifestations of renal amyloid were the presenting findings in more than half. Proteinuria and associated hypoalbuminemia are often sufficiently marked to result in nephrotic syndrome. In reported renal biopsy reviews in this country, amyloidosis was found in 3–13 percent of adults presenting with nephrotic syndrome. Geographic variations in prevalence are marked, and a similar review from Turkey reported 62 percent of adults with nephrotic syndrome had amyloidosis due to the high incidence of familial Mediterranean fever. Reports from developing nations indicate similarly high incidence rates of amyloidosis related to tuberculosis and other chronic infections. Renal amyloidosis in the United States tends to be more prevalent in males above age 50.

CLINICAL AND LABORATORY FINDINGS

Preservation of selective proteinuria has been reported with renal amyloidosis, but Bence Jones proteinuria is often present as a diagnostic clue. Increase in renal size is usually described, but normal or contracted kidneys are not rare. Contrary to early descriptions, hypertension may develop as renal insufficiency progresses. Maintenance of glomerular filtration rate and serum creatinine level is often surprisingly good despite massive glomerular amyloid replacement; however, functional deterioration may be relatively rapid once renal insufficiency becomes manifest.

Hypoalbuminemia may be particularly severe because of impaired albumin synthesis related to small bowel involvement compromising amino acid absorption and hepatic amyloidosis impairing protein synthetic ability. Abnormalities in renal tubular function result from the peritubular deposition of amyloid or associated light chain proteinuria. Renal tubular acidosis and nephrogenic diabetes insipidus have been reported in association with renal amyloidosis.

Amyloidosis is one of the renal lesions associated with a higher incidence of renal vein thrombosis. This may present with a rapid worsening of nephrotic syndrome, particularly edema of the lower extremities, embolization, or the sudden development of oliguric renal failure.

DIAGNOSIS

Diagnosis is best established by tissue biopsy with selection of the site based on the patient's physical and laboratory findings. Renal biopsy has provided an 85–95 percent diagnostic yield and is particularly useful in the patient with proteinuria. The risks of renal biopsy do not appear increased in these patients, as has been described with liver biopsy. Amyloid may be found in the arterioles of the rectal submucosa in as many as 75 percent of patients, and this appears to be the most useful site for blind biopsy. Liver biopsy has been helpful in approximately 50 percent and gingival biopsy in only 20 percent. The intravenous Congo red test is no longer used as a screening procedure due to an unacceptably high incidence of false negative results.

The identification of amyloid fibrils in the urinary

sediment by electron microscopy has been suggested as a diagnostic means which might supercede renal biopsy; however, the recent reports of fibrils ultrastructurally indistinguishable from amyloid fibrils in both amyloidotic and control urine sediments and the failure to produce specific confirmation of urinary amyloid by a variety of techniques necessitates a reexamination of this approach.

PATHOLOGY

With large amounts of amyloid deposition the kidney is enlarged, waxy, and pink or gray in appearance, with a firm, rubbery consistency. With far advanced renal involvement, the kidney may be pale and contracted.

On light microscopy amyloidosis is characterized by a diffuse increase in glomerular extracellular material with moderate variability between glomeruli and within segments of the individual glomerulus (Fig. 1). There is usually no significant cellular proliferation. The material is eosinophilic, smooth, and homogeneous and stains weakly violaceous with PAS and is negative with silver methenamine. Dichromic birefringence with Congo red produces a brilliant apple green with polarized light and is characteristic and of major diagnostic value. Metachromasia with methyl or crystal violet and intense fluoresence with Thioflavin-T are also characteristic.

The early deposition is in the mesangium and later between the endothelial cells and glomerular basement membrane. With progression there is an irregular narrowing of the capillary lumen with retention of the central ring of endothelial cells. Eventually the deposition results in capillary occlusion and obsolescence of the glomerulus.

Methenamine stains may show hairbrush-like argyrophilic projections from the epithelial surface of the irregularly thickened capillary wall in areas of amyloid deposition. It has been suggested these represent parallel arrangements of the amyloid spicules and contrast to the usually nonargyrophilic properties of the amyloid.

Amyloid deposition is frequently present in vessels of all sizes, particularly the arterioles and interlobular arteries, and is most abundant in the media and subendothelial areas. It also may be noted in the peritubular basement membranes; however, vacuolar changes and lipid deposition characteristic of massive proteinuria are more prominent. Interstitial deposition of amyloid may be massive.

Nodular diabetic glomerulosclerosis and the lobular form of membranoproliferative glomerulonephritis may be differential considerations and are readily distinguished from amyloid by their silver methenamine positivity and negative birefringence with Congo red.

On electron microscopy the infiltrate is found to be composed of randomly arranged nonbranching 70–90 Å wide fibrils (Fig. 2). In the early stages these are seen in the mesangium and in close proximity to the basement membrane, particularly in the subendothelial area. They are also evident in the peritubular basement membrane, vessel walls, and between interstitial cells.

Immunofluorescence results have varied widely in reported series, without a distinctive pattern emerging. Glomerular and interstitial fluorescence has been re-

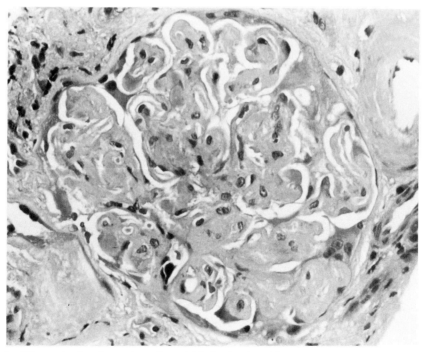

Fig. 1. Glomerulus in advanced renal amyloidosis showing diffuse thickening of the capillary walls with near-obliteration of many capillary lumina. H & E. × 400. [Courtesy of Dr. G. A. Bannayan.]

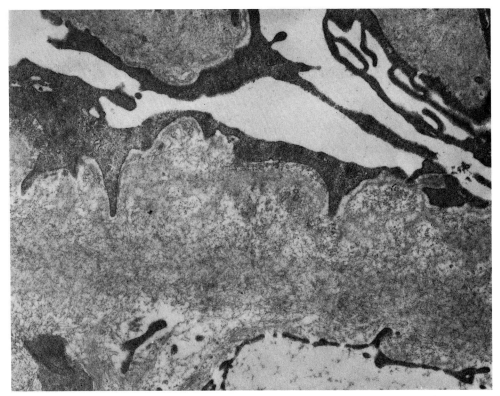

Fig. 2. High power electron microscopy of thickened glomerular capillary wall in renal amyloidosis demonstrating typical fibrillar arrangement of amyloid. × 22,500. [Courtesy of Dr. G. A. Bannayan.]

ported with the use of specific antisera to light chain immunoglobulins.

PROGNOSIS AND TREATMENT

Renal insufficiency is a major cause of mortality and approaches 50 percent in most series. Endstage renal disease is reached in 1–4 years in patients with nephrotic syndrome secondary to amyloidosis, although occasional prolonged courses have been reported in patients with mild proteinuria and even in some with nephrotic syndrome.

Successful treatment of the primary disease and removal of the antigenic stimulus in patients with secondary amyloidosis has been followed by clearing of hepatic amyloid infiltrates and resolution of proteinuria despite persistence of mesangial amyloid deposition.

In patients with amyloidosis and Bence Jones paraproteinuria, or plasma cell dyscrasia without skeletal lesions or a diagnosis of multiple myeloma, clinical and laboratory improvement has been reported with melphalan alone or in combination with prednisone and fluoxymesterone. Such trials are still in an investigation stage in the management of primary amyloidosis. The use of colchicine is also undergoing clinical trials because of its reported success in controlling the clinical manifestations of familial Mediterranean fever.

Renal transplantation has been accomplished successfully in some patients with amyloidosis with sus-

tained function and without evidence of recurrence on biopsy for up to 10 years; however, there are reports of biopsy evidence of recurrence at 6 months and 3½ years after transplantation.

REFERENCES

Cohen AS: Amyloidosis, in Buchanan WW, Dick WC (eds): Recent Advances in Rheumatology. Edinburgh, Churchill Livingstone, 1976, p 19

Glenner GG, Page DL: Amyloid, amyloidosis and amyloidogenesis. Int Rev Exp Pathol 15:1, 1976

Isobe T, Osserman EF: Patterns of amyloidosis and their associations with plasma-cell dyscrasia, monoclonal immunoglobins and Bence Jones proteins. N Engl J Med 290:473, 1974

Jones NF: Renal amyloidosis: Pathogenesis and therapy. Clin Nephrol 6:459, 1976

Kyle RA, Bayrd ED: Amyloidosis. Medicine (Baltimore) 54:271, 1975

Pruzanski W: Amyloidogenesis—Theories and facts. J Rheumatol 4:219, 1977

Shirahama T, Skinner M, Cohen AS, et al: Uncertain value of urinary sediments in the diagnosis of amyloidosis. N Engl J Med 297:821, 1977

Triger DR, Joekes AM: Renal amyloidosis—A fourteen year follow-up. Q J Med 42:15, 1973

MACROGLOBULINEMIA

Stephen Z. Fadem and Meyer D. Lifschitz

Macroglobulinemia usually presents clinically as anemia, a bleeding disorder, lymphadenopathy and hepatosplenomegaly, associated with an elevated erythrocyte sedimentation rate, and an increase in IgM protein on immunoelectrophoresis. The increased IgM is produced by lymphocytoid-like cells, and many of the clinical symtoms are due to the consequences of this circulating immunoglobulin. The clinical symptoms differ from multiple myeloma in that bone involvement is rare, the hypervisocosity syndrome and cryoglobulinemia are common, and lymphoid hyperplasia is present. Although the kidney is at times involved in macroglobulinemia, the frequency is presently felt to be less than 30 percent; even when renal involvement is present it is usually less pressing clinically than other symptoms.

With respect to the kidney, macroglobulinemia involves chiefly the glomerulus, and intratubular casts, characteristic of the "myeloma kidney," are rare. In part, the difference may be related to the size of the respective proteins: the protein of macroglobulinemia has a molecular weight of approximately 1,000,000 daltons, while the Bence Jones proteins characteristically have a molecular weight of approximately 24,000 daltons. Thus the M proteins are not filterable and may lodge in the glomerular capillary, where they interfere with kidney function. Bence Jones proteinuria occurs in 10–15 percent of patients with macroglobulinemia but usually is not clinically significant.

The hypervisocity syndrome is one of the chief clinical manifestations of macroglobulinemia and is characterized by visual impairment, a characteristic "sausage shaped" appearance of retinal veins, central nervous system changes which may lead to focal abnormalities or even coma, and circulatory overload. Renal involvement, aside from the secondary effect of congestive heart failure, also includes an acidifying and concentrating defect, although it is not clear whether the increase in paraproteins or the hyperviscosity per se is responsible for these abnormalities. About one-third of IgM proteins form unstable precipitates in the cold, called cryoglobulins. Thus macroglobulinemia may be associated with a secondary cryoglobulinemia which may present as Raynaud's phenomenon, dependent purpura, cold insensitivity, or vasculopathy. Glomerular disorders may accompany secondary cryoglobulinemia as well as primary cryoglobulenemia, as described in the chapter on *Cryoglobulinemia*.

Amyloidosis is less common in macroglobulinemia than in myeloma, but it does occur and may be responsible for renal pathology. Rarely, plasma cell invasion of the kidney parenchyma can occur to the extent of increasing kidney size, and in at least one instance, a patient with macroglobulinemia presented with an abdominal mass which was found to be a kidney infiltrated with plasma cells (Fig. 1). While most cases of renal failure in macroglobulinemia are insidious in onset, patients have been known to have a rapidly progressive course.

In a study of 19 patients with IgM monoclonal gammopathy, 17 had Waldenström's macroglobulinemia; 4 of these patients had associated cryoglobulinemia, of which 2 had monoclonal IgM, and the other 2 had a mixed cryoglobulin, IgM–IgG. Proteinuria of some degree was present in all of the patients. In 12 it was minimal, and in two-thirds of these patients there was a small but detectable amount of Bence Jones protein. Of the 17 macroglobulinemia patients, 7 had more than 2 grams of protein in the urine, and 2 patients had the nephrotic syndrome. There were 7 patients who presented with BUN levels greater than 50 mg/dl, and in 7 the BUN was between 20 and 50 mg/dl; 5 patients had BUN levels less than 20 mg/dl. There were 8 patients who had no renal lesion except for a mild interstitial infiltrate; among the other 11, 3 had amyloidosis. None of the patients with amyloidosis presented with BUN levels greater than 50 mg/dl or with the nephrotic syndrome. The majority of the remaining patients had intraglomerular deposits. These deposits were proximal to the inner surface of the glomerular basement membrane and in some instances completely occluded the capillary lumen. The basement membrane was intact. Differential immunofluorescent staining demonstrated IgM proteins, with intracapillary deposits staining negative for IgG and IgA. In contrast to IgG–IgM essential cryoglobulinemia, immunofluorescent staining for complement was negative. In some cases the glomerular pathology was attributable to the presence of thrombi occluding the glomerular capillaries, and consisting entirely of IgM proteins. Tubular casts rarely occurred, distinguishing macroglobulinemia from myeloma.

Proliferative glomerular lesions have rarely been described in macroglobulinemia, and it has been suggested that the passive deposition of circulating IgM complexes, rather than any immunologically mediated response, accounts for the glomerulopathy in most patients with renal involvement.

The mainstay of therapy involves the use of cytotoxic agents, and specifics regarding the treatment of this neoplasm have been described elsewhere in this series. Plasmapheresis has been well established as a valuable adjunct to therapy and is useful in alleviating the symptoms caused by the associated hyperviscosity syndrome. Since hyperviscosity may lead to congestive heart failure, fluid restriction is frequently necessary. Renal failure induced by radiographic contrast agents has not to date been reported in macroglobulinemia, and hypercalcemia and hyperuricemia usually do not occur. The cold-induced vasculopathy must be managed symptomatically, as in essential cryoglobulinemia or chronic cold-agglutinin disease. Hemodialysis may be employed if endstage renal failure develops.

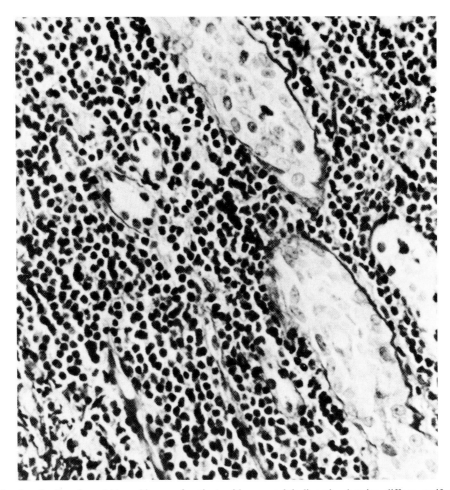

Fig. 1. Section from kidney biopsy of patient with macroglobulinemia showing diffuse, uniform interstitial infiltrate of lymphoid plasma cells. This involvement is more severe than that usually found in such patients. [Reprinted with permission from Grossman ME, Bia MJ, Goldwein MI, Hill G, et al: Giant kidneys in Waldenström's macroglobulinemia. Arch Int Med 137:1613, 1977. Copyright 1977, American Medical Association.]

In summary, macroglobulinemia is a neoplastic disorder characterized by the abnormal production of monoclonal IgM proteins. These proteins account for the hyperviscosity symptoms and the frequent cryoprecipitates. The renal disorders are mainly related to the passive deposition of circulating IgM complexes in the glomerular capillaries and may lead to hematuria and proteinuria, to the nephrotic syndrome, or to chronic renal failure.

REFERENCES

Forget BG, Squires JW, Sheldon H: Waldenström's macroglobulinemia with generalized amyloidosis. Arch Int Med 118:363–375, 1966

Grossman ME, Bia MJ, Goldwein MI, Hill G, et al: Giant kidneys in Waldenström's macroglobulinemia. Arch Int Med 137:1613, 1977

Mackenzie MR, Fudenberg HH: Macroglobulinemia: Analysis of forty patients. Blood 39:874–889, 1972

Morel-Maroger L, Basch A, Davon F, et al: Pathology of the kidney in Waldenström's macroglobulinemia. N Engl J Med 282:123–129, 1970

Morel-Maroger L, Verroust P: Glomerular lesions in dysproteinemias. Kidney Int 5:249–251, 1974

Verroust P, Mery J-P, Morel-Maroger L, et al: Glomerular lesions in monoclonal gammopathies and mixed essential cryoglobulinemias IgG-IgM. Adv Nephrol 1:161–194, 1971

ANAPHYLACTOID PURPURA NEPHRITIS

Mark S. Schiffer and Alfred J. Fish

Anaphylactoid purpura (AP) or Henoch-Schönlein purpura is a syndrome characterized by purpuric skin lesions, hemorrhagic gastroenteropathy, and arthritis. In addition, one-third to one-half of patients with anaphylactoid purpura have renal involvement. Long-term (chronic) morbidity and mortality of AP is due solely to the nephritis. The syndrome is more common in children, but it does occur in adults with similar clinical features.

NONRENAL MANIFESTATIONS

Small erythematous lesions appear from the elbows to the hands and from the waist to the feet. Early lesions can be urticarial or macular. The lesions may become hemorrhagic and darken as they gradually fade over several weeks. As with other aspects of the disease, the lesions can recur. Skin biopsy of lesions shows perivascular inflammation. Immunofluorescence reveals IgA in the small dermal vessels and the dermal epidermal junctions of both lesions and clinically uninvolved skin.

Arthralgia and arthritis are mild, self-limiting, and nondeforming. The small bowel can be involved by vasculitis, causing edema and petechial hemorrhage and giving rise to cramping, melena, and intestinal protein loss. The bowel does not ulcerate, and necrosis does not occur in the absence of intussuception. The edematous bowel can become intussucepted at the ileal–cecal area, usually requiring surgical management.

Nonrenal manifestations rarely require antiinflammatory therapy; however, the abdominal lesions and symptoms do respond to corticosteroids. If abdominal cramping is intractable and disabling, it can be treated with a short course of steroids.

PRESENTING RENAL MANIFESTATIONS

The initial signs of nephropathy usually appear during the first 3 months of the syndrome. Rarely, the renal manifestations can precede the purpuric lesions, making the diagnosis obscure. Eighty percent of patients with nephropathy have gross hematuria at some time, in addition to prolonged microscopic hematuria. One-half of the patients with renal involvement have the nephrotic syndrome, and the remainder have lesser degrees of proteinuria. A small percentage of children and a greater percentage of adults with the syndrome are hypertensive. Early in the course of kidney involvement, function can range from normal to progressive renal insufficiency.

Serum complement determinations are generally normal. Individual complement components can be transiently decreased, and C3 proactivator (factor B) can be transiently elevated. Serum immunoglobulin and fibrin levels are normal. Thrombocytopenia is not found. Coagulation profile is normal except for the hypercoagulability that accompanies the nephrotic state.

RENAL PATHOLOGY

AP nephritis is a proliferative glomerulonephritis (Fig. 1A). Crescent formation is a prominent feature and may appear even in cases where the glomerular involvement is focal and mild. There is proliferation of glomerular epithelial, endothelial, and mesangial cells. Extraglomerular arterioles are not commonly involved by vasculitis. Immunofluorescence (Fig. 1B) reveals IgG, IgA, and fibrin in the mesangium and focally along the capillary loops; C3 and properdin are similarly observed. Fibrin may be found in early lesions in the absence of immunoglobulins. Electron microscopy shows basement membrane splitting and dense deposits

in the basement membrane, particularly adjacent to the mesangium. Further deposits are seen in the mesangium along with increase of mesangial matrix, mesangial cell proliferation, and infiltration of polymorphonuclear leukocytes.

PATHOGENESIS

No etiologic agent has been identified in AP. The syndrome can be temporally linked to upper respiratory infection in many cases. Evidence for infection by viruses or group A beta hemolytic streptococcal infection is inconsistent. Although some patients have been exposed to a wide variety of drugs prior to the onset of the syndrome, hypersensitivity to specific agents is not a proven cause of AP. The positive immunofluorescent findings of granular mesangial deposits suggest an antibody–antigen immune complex pathogenesis. Evidence of cryoglobulinemia has been inconsistent. The early presence of fibrin in glomerular lesions suggests the etiologic role of the clotting system. It is likely that AP can result from a variety of etiologic factors.

After the initial presentation, it has been noted that immunofluorescence remains positive for prolonged periods. Perhaps the trapping of fibrin and other serum proteins predisposes some of these patients to progressive glomerular destruction.

CLINICAL COURSE

There is some correlation between the degree of clinical renal involvement and severity of changes on renal biopsy.

The correlation of outcome with the initial renal findings is complicated by the recurrence of acute features of this disease. Recurrent macroscopic hematuria is frequently observed with or without the reappearance of purpura. Aside from renal failure, the most severe acute clinical signs of nephropathy usually occur in the first several months of the disease.

Ten to twenty percent of children—and probably a higher percentage of adults—with AP nephritis progress to renal failure several years after onset. Among those that do, the initial kidney biopsy usually demonstrates crescents in 50 percent or more of the glomeruli. The initial presentation with nephrotic syndrome, prolonged nephritis with macroscopic hematuria, and hypertension is a poor prognostic sign.

Acute recurrences of active AP nephritis may occur within the first 2 years after initial presentation; however, patients with AP nephritis are subject to further renal deterioration for many years after the initial presentation. Therefore all patients with AP nephritis should have periodic monitoring of renal function and urine protein excretion.

TREATMENT

Treatment has been attempted with corticosteroids, azathioprine, and several other agents, but no controlled studies have been carried out to demonstrate the efficacy of these therapeutic trials. Although the gastrointestinal symptoms quickly subside, the introduction of steroids with or without azathioprine is not associated with prompt cessation of hematuria or pro-

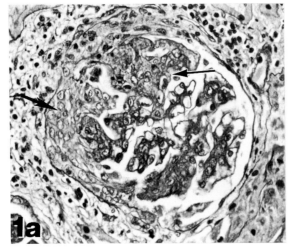 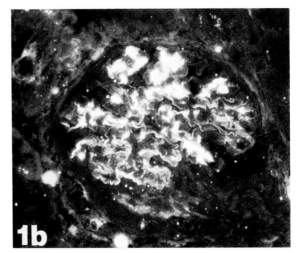

Fig. 1. (A) Glomerulus from kidney with AP nephritis. Thick arrow indicates cellular crescent. Thin arrow indicates glomerular cell proliferation. PAS stain. × 250. (B) Glomerulus in AP stained for IgA, predominantly in mesangial pattern with focal capillary wall staining. Fluorescent microscopy. × 250.

teinuria or immediate improvement of renal function. In published series, only the patients with more severely involved kidneys have been treated with immunosuppressive therapy. Because of the poor prognosis of patients with severe renal involvement, we currently recommend the use of prednisone and azathioprine therapy in patients with ongoing nephrotic syndrome or persistent decline of creatinine clearance and severe histologic involvement. After an initial month of divided dose steroid and daily azathioprine therapy, steroids are changed to an alternate day schedule with continuation of azathioprine. The patients are monitored closely, and if they are improved or stable a repeat kidney biopsy is performed with the aim to discontinue immunosuppressive therapy in 12–18 months.

Patients with endstage renal failure due to AP nephritis have received renal transplants successfully.

REFERENCES

Ballard HS, Eisinger RP, Gallo E: Renal manifestations of the Henoch-Schoenlein syndrome in adults. Am J Med 49:328, 1970

Counahan R, Winterborg MH, White RHR, et al: Prognosis of Henoch-Schönlein nephritis in children. Br Med J 2:11, 1977

Garcia-Fuentes M, Chantler C, Williams DG: Cryoglobulinaemia in Henoch-Schönlein purpura. Br Med J 2:165, 1977

Kobayashi O, Wada H, Okawa K, et al: Schönlein-Henoch's syndrome in children. Contrib Nephrol 4:48, 1977

Levy M, Broyer M, Arsan A, et al: Anaphylactoid purpura nephritis in childhood: Natural history and immunopathology. Adv Nephrol 6:185, 1976

Urizar RE, Michael AF, Sisson S, et al: Anaphylactoid purpura: II. Immunofluorescent and electron microscopic studies of the glomerular lesions. Lab Invest 19:437, 1968

WEGENER'S GRANULOMATOSIS

John J. Bardgette

Wegener's granulomatosis is an uncommon systemic disease of unknown etiology involving the upper and lower respiratory tracts and kidneys. The distinguishing features of the disorder include necrotizing granulomata, diffuse segmental vasculitis of both arteries and veins, and glomerulitis.

EPIDEMIOLOGY

A predilection for men exists which in some series has been twice that of women. The patient is usually in the fourth or fifth decade of life, but the age range extends from 6 months to 75 five years. There is no known geographic, racial, or ethnic predisposition.

ETIOLOGY

The etiology of Wegener's granulomatosis remains obscure. Although immunologic derangements have been postulated as the cause of this entity, there is no firm evidence to support this explanation.

CLINICAL MANIFESTATIONS

The manifestations of Wegener's granulomatosis are myriad, but the presenting complaints usually focus on pulmonary and otolaryngologic symptoms. A typical history is one of the insidious onset of fever, anorexia, and symptoms referable to the upper respiratory tract—sinusitis, rhinorrhea, epistaxis, earache, and hearing loss—and lower respiratory tract symptoms—cough, hemoptysis, dyspnea, and pleuritic chest pain. Examination reveals nasal mucosal crusting, nasopharyngeal ulceration, saddle nose deformities, and otitis media. Eventually multiple organs may be involved, including skin, eyes, heart, lungs, and kidneys.

Eighty percent of patients with Wegener's granulomatosis have renal involvement. In the early stages of the disease, symptoms and signs indicative of renal disease are conspicuous by their absence, however. Renal disease announces itself with the appearance of proteinuria, hematuria, and urinary sediment abnormalities including red blood cell casts. Clinically, the renal disease may be manifested as oliguric renal failure, rapidly progressive glomerulonephritis, or the nephrotic syndrome. Functional impairment may initially be absent, but once it appears progressive deterioration, often fulminant, is the rule. The renal disease does not spontaneously remit. Hypertension is characteristically absent.

LABORATORY MANIFESTATIONS

Most patients exhibit normocytic normochromic anemia, leukocytosis, hyperglobulinemia, and an increased erythrocyte sedimentation rate. In many individuals the serum concentration of IgA is elevated. Circulating immune complexes have been found in three of five patients so studied. Eosinophilia is rare in Wegener's granulomatosis. The serum complement level is typically in the normal range, even in the presence of active renal disease.

RENAL PATHOLOGY

Light microscopy reveals focal, segmental glomerulonephritis, at times conjoined to necrotizing vasculitis and a granulomatous reaction around blood vessels or glomeruli (Fig. 1). The number of glomeruli involved may vary from few to nearly all. Epithelial cell proliferation, fibrinoid necrosis, and the presence of inflammatory cells in Bowman's space are notable. Crescent formation may also be a feature. Evidence of past renal injury, as manifested by segmental glomerular sclerosis,

may coexist with active lesions. There is rough correlation between the presence and severity of clinical renal disease and the activity and severity of the light microscopic findings, but occasionally histologic abnormalities are present in the absence of clinically apparent disease.

Electron microscopy may show the presence of finely granular, homogeneous electron-dense deposits beneath the glomerular epithelium. Rarely such deposits have a subendothelial location. In many patients, however, no electron-dense deposits are demonstrable. Immunofluorescent staining usually indicates the presence of complement and IgG in a granular pattern along the glomerular capillaries. The presence and pattern of electron-dense deposits and of immunoglobulin and complement deposition in the kidney suggest that immune complex deposition may be responsible for the renal lesion of Wegener's granulomatosis. Therapy with immunosuppressive agents, as described below, suppresses glomerular proliferation and eliminates basement membrane deposits. The renal pathologic findings in Wegener's granulomatosis are not pathognomonic and cannot be differentiated from many other focal glomerulitides.

PROGNOSIS AND THERAPY

The patient with untreated Wegener's granulomatosis has a dismal prognosis. Ninety percent of untreated patients die within 2 years, renal failure being the major cause of death. Therapeutic advances in the preceding two decades have dispelled the pessimism which formerly attended the diagnosis of Wegener's

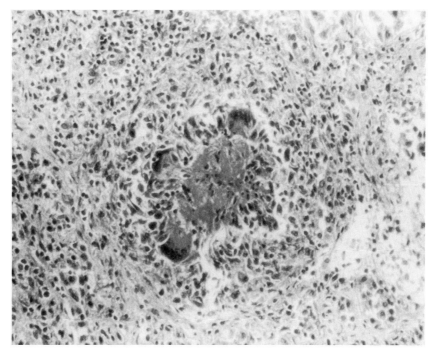

Fig. 1. Demonstration of a noncaseating granuloma within a glomerulus from a patient with Wegener's granulomatosis.

granulomatosis. Initial attempts to modify the disease with corticosteroid administration were associated with occasional favorable responses, but these responses were at best temporary, and corticosteroids do not seem to have altered the inexorably fatal course of the disease. The advent of immunosuppressive therapy for these patients, however, has brought striking and lasting therapeutic responses. In the largest reported series, therapy with cyclophosphamide produced a remission in 17 of 21 patients. With this agent, remissions lasting up to 5 years have been achieved. The necessary duration of therapy has not been established, but in several patients cyclophosphamide therapy has been discontinued and disease-free intervals of greater than 2 years have been seen. When relapses occur, reinstitution of immunosuppressive therapy again produces both clinical and laboratory improvement. Hemodialysis is indicated for those patients with severe renal functional impairment. A response to immunosuppressive therapy cannot be expected in all patients who have severely impaired renal function. If the other manifestations of the disease are controlled, renal transplantation can be considered. Successful transplantation with no evidence of recurrent glomerulonephritis 2 years following transplantation has been reported. Short-term treatment with corticosteroids may be useful for some disease manifestations, particularly pericarditis, skin lesions, and ocular abnormalities. Local measures and antibiotics are indicated when appropriate for otolaryngologic complications.

REFERENCES

Drachman DA: Neurological complications of Wegener's granulomatosis. Neurology 8:45, 1963

Fauci AS, Balow JE, Brown R, et al: Successful renal transplantation in Wegener's granulomatosis. Am J Med 60:437, 1976

Godman GC, Churg J: Wegener's granulomatosis. Pathology and review of the literature. Arch Pathol 58:533, 1954

Haynes BF, Fishman ML, Fauci AS, et al: The ocular manifestations of Wegener's granulomatosis. Am J Med 63:131, 1977

Horn RG, Fauci AS, Rosenthal AS, et al: Renal biopsy pathology in Wegener's granulomatosis. Am J Pathol 74:423, 1974

Walton EW: Giant cell granuloma of the respiratory tract. Br Med J 2:265, 1958

Wolff SM, Fauci AS, Horn RG, et al: Wegener's granulomatosis. Ann Intern Med 81:513, 1974

IMMUNE COMPLEX NEPHRITIS ASSOCIATED WITH SYSTEMIC INFECTIONS

Robert A. Gutman

Many—perhaps most—infections can precipitate glomerular injury and related disease. Experimental and clinical evidence suggest that a common initiating event is the development of soluble circulating immune complexes (IC) composed of antigen from the infectious agent and antibody from the host. Chronic infections, especially those in which the blood is constantly seeded by foreign antigen, seem most likely to be associated with IC glomerulonephritis (GN). Infections by almost all classes of pathogens have been implicated, including extracellular and intracellular bacteria, fungi, viruses, protozoa, and helminths. The biological events surrounding the development of GN in these patients are similar to those observed in experimental animals which are given repeated injections of foreign protein or, alternatively, are carriers of a chronic (usually viral) infection. A state of sustained but limited antibody response with persistence of excess antigen and resulting "equivalency" state appears to be necessary in order to develop immune complex solubility and resulting capillary damage. The clinical and renal response to the formation of the complexes depends on the number, size, and solubility of the complexes, the persistence of the antigen exposure, and the host's ability to mount an inflammatory response. The clinical presentation may be dominated by extrarenal phenomena including arthritis, arthralgias, vasculitis, purpura, rash, fever, and weight loss. The renal injury may be manifested largely as nephritis with hematuria, red blood cell casts, reduction of glomerular filtration, and hypertension; as nephrosis with proteinuria and generalized edema and with little change of GFR or blood pressure; or as a combination of nephritic and nephrotic phenomena. Accompanying serological abnormalities may mimic those of systemic lupus erythematosus and include a general increase in serum globulin, reduction of complement levels, a small increase of antinuclear antibody, and high titers of rheumatoid factor and cryoglobulin.

Detailed examination of renal tissue has been done in only a few cases. Light microscopy usually reveals changes of proliferative GN, but the severity, precise glomerular localization, and degree of accompanying membranous thickening, sclerosis, obliteration, or crescent formation varies widely. In some cases, there is only glomerular membranous thickening with virtually no evident proliferation. Those cases which have been generally accepted as examples of IC GN have immunofluorescent evidence of granular or lumpy deposition of serum immune globulins, usually IgM or IgG, and serum complement. Coincident with immunofluorescent evidence, electron microscopy, where performed, reveals electron-dense deposits beneath (subendothelial), within (intramembranous), or above (subepithelial) the glomerular basement membrane.

Taken together these clinical, serological, and microscopic phenomena are generally regarded as evidence that an infection has precipitated immune complex disease. Firmer evidence requires demonstration that the complexes contain the foreign protein and antibody to that protein. Although such demonstration has been rare, a number of such cases have been reported. Other chronic diseases in which foreign antigen is present, notably cancer, may also cause IC GN (see the chapter on *Renal Lesions in Malignancy*).

There are other mechanisms of renal injury associated with systemic infections. These include shock, hemolysis, embolic phenomena, and hematogenous dissemination of bacteria or fungi. Viral infections may lead to cytopathic changes of renal parenchyma. Immunological sequelae may not be limited to IC formation. Infection with *Streptococcus pneumoniae* has been reported to activate the alternate pathway toward complement activity, and infections with agents bearing antigens common to the kidney could conceivably initiate formation of autoantibodies.

These other mechanisms notwithstanding, IC GN seems the most common expression of renal injury during infection. Table 1 lists many of the organisms or infectious diseases in which IC GN has been proven or suspected. Where complexes found in the circulation or on glomerular basement membranes contain antigen of the invading organism or antibody directed toward that antigen, the evidence may be considered strong; in the other cases there is limited clinical, serological, or histological evidence of the same phenomena. Four infections associated with IC GN are discussed in some detail because of the frequency or the special interest of the association.

BACTERIAL ENDOCARDITIS

In the past, renal disease associated with bacterial endocarditis, exclusive of large renal infarctions, was considered the result of microemboli. Historically and for this reason, the term "focal embolic glomerulonephritis" was used in this circumstance. It remains possible that fibrin originating in cardiac vegetations is responsible for some of the lesions, but most attempts to demonstrate bacteria lodged within the glomerulus have failed. Available evidence supports the thesis that clinically significant GN in patients with either acute or subacute bacterial endocarditis is the consequence of circulating soluble immune complexes. Immunofluorescence microscopy reveals granular or lumpy deposition of IgM and complement in most cases. IgG and IgA have also been noted. In a few well studied patients, elution of the glomerular membranes yielded antibody against the infecting organism or there was evidence by immunofluorescence of bacterial antigen within the deposits.

The clinical presentation and course of the IC GN of bacterial endocarditis is variable. In most cases, nephritis rather than nephrosis dominates the clinical presentation. Severe renal failure has been reported, but more commonly reduction of glomerular filtration rate is mild and recovery occurs when there is successful eradication of the infection. Virtually every organism known to cause endocarditis has been found in patients with this syndrome. Indeed, recent data suggest that most patients with endocarditis have detectable levels of circulating immune complexes whether or not GN is discovered. Older literature and several well documented recent cases have emphasized the apparent increased incidence of GN during the "immunological phase" of endocarditis when blood cultures may be negative. This seems to occur more readily in patients with subacute, right-sided endocarditis.

There are other nonsuppurative clinical manifestations of bacterial endocarditis which also may be the consequence of immune complex formation. Osler nodes, petechial hemorrhages, Roth spots, and Janeway lesions may represent peripheral inflammatory reactions to their deposition. Stronger evidence has been provided recently that thrombocytopenic purpura and generalized vasculitis have the same pathogenesis as the GN of endocarditis.

The laboratory findings in those endocarditis patients who have GN reflect a state of chronic immunologic stimulation. Serum complement activity and individual components of the complement system are

Table 1
Infections Causing Immune Complex Glomerulonephritis

Strong Evidence	Some Evidence
Syphilis	*Streptococcus pneumoniae*
Endocarditis	*Salmonella typhosa*
Staphylococcus aureus	*Yersinia enterocolitica*
Streptococcus viridans	*Klebsiella pneumoniae*
Culture negative	Leprosy
Other	Tuberculosis
Infected ventriculoatrial shunts	*Candida parapsilosis*
Staphylococcus albus	Schistosomiasis
Corynebacterium bovis	Infectious mononucleosis
Osteomyelitis (usually *S. aureus*)	(Epstein-Barr virus)
Quartan malaria	Mumps
Falciparum malaria	Varicella
Toxoplasmosis	ECHO-9 virus
Rubeola with subacute sclerosing	Coxsackie B virus
panencephalitis	
Hepatitis B	Dengue fever

usually found to be reduced in contrast to the normal values in patients with uncomplicated endocarditis. Cryoglobulins may be noted in large amounts. Antinuclear antibody has been found, but titers are usually much lower than in patients with SLE. As with other infections causing GN, fibrinogen and serum immune globulins may be elevated. Rheumatoid factor (anti-IgG), especially as determined by latex flocculation, is markedly elevated in about 30–50 percent of patients with endocarditis, but the frequency is not greater in those who have acquired GN as a consequence of their infection.

The histological severity of the GN of endocarditis varies from focal and mesangial to diffuse, generalized proliferation with severe exudation and necrosis. Immune deposits may be located anywhere within or on the glomerular basement membrane. Those patients who have GN with acute (usually *S. aureus*) endocarditis are more likely to have large subepithelial deposits which by electron microscopy are remarkably similar to the deposits seen in poststreptococcal GN. In contrast, the glomerular membranes of patients with GN associated with less invasive and therefore more chronic infections, including those which are culture negative, appear to be more likely to have subendothelial deposits resembling those seen in patients with SLE.

Several authors have emphasized the similarity of the course, serology, and renal manifestations between some patients with endocarditis, especially if blood cultures are negative, and some with SLE. This similarity has led to inappropriate therapy of some patients with bacterial endocarditis.

SYPHILIS

Active infections with *Treponema pallidum* has been known for almost 150 years to cause renal disease. Nephrotic syndrome is the usual presentation. The pathogenesis of the renal injury has been variously ascribed to the presence of the organisms in the renal parenchyma, the arsenicals used to treat the infection, or to a "renal Jarisch-Herxheimer reaction." More recently, convincing evidence has been provided that this is another example of immunologic injury caused by circulating antigen–antibody complexes.

Syphilitic nephrosis is an uncommon complication of the infection. Its occurrence is generally limited to those patients with either the congenital or acquired secondary forms of the illness, the two conditions in which there is a large host burden of the organism. In secondary syphilis, the nephrosis is self-limited, probably because of the tendency for the infection to become latent, thus changing the ratio of antibody to antigen. Syphilitic nephrosis disappears quickly after institution of appropriate therapy. In contrast to the renal reaction to endocarditis, there is little or no evidence of nephritis; the sediment usually contains no red cell casts and few if any red cells. The glomerular filtration rate is not affected, and hypertension is not described.

Laboratory findings are those of nephrotic syndrome. There is significant proteinuria, generally over 3.5 g/day in adults, hypoalbuminemia, hypercholesterolemia, and elevated α_2 globulin. The urine sediment contains fat, tubular epithelial cells and hyaline and granular casts. The erythrocyte sedimentation rate is usually high. There is a positive venereal disease research laboratory (VDRL) test and reactive fluorescent treponemal antibody absorption (RTA-ABS). In contrast to those patients with immune complex renal injury in association with endocarditis, there is little serological evidence of sustained immunological stimulation. The serum complement is normal, the latex fixation is negative, and antinuclear antibody has not been found.

The light microscopic findings of syphilitic nephrosis are those of mild proliferative GN. The increased cellularity is largely mesangial. There is little or no exudation or necrosis. Proximal tubular cells appear swollen and may contain hyaline droplets. By fluorescence microscopy, there are lumpy deposits of IgG and occasionally of complement. Electron microscopy supports the thesis that IC deposits are present in the areas of positive immunofluorescent staining. Most deposits are subepithelial in location. In addition, epithelial foot processes are swollen. Elution of immunoglobulin from affected renal tissue reacts specifically with treponemal antigen, evidence that the deposits are indeed antigen–antibody complexes induced by syphilis.

HEPATITIS B

Since discovery of the specific viral surface antigen associated with type B of hepatitis (HB$_s$ Ag), there has been a dramatic increase of our awareness of the scope of diseases which it may cause. Infected patients may experience a short, temporarily debilitating icteric illness followed by complete resolution; there may be a fatal and rapid liver destruction; or chronic, persistent, and aggressive hepatitis may be the dominant feature. More recently evidence has accumulated that some patients may be afflicted by a persistent nonhepatic immunologic illness including arthralgias, vasculitis, and GN. Polyarteritis (periarteritis) nodosa in particular is very commonly associated with persistent antigenemia and/or detectable levels of anti-HB$_s$ Ag.

Glomerulonephritis without accompanying evidence of systemic vasculitis and often without evidence of hepatic disease has been described in association with circulating immune complexes containing HB$_s$ Ag. Usually the patients present with nephrotic syndrome, but nephritis, hypertension, and renal failure have occurred as well. In a survey of 52 sequential renal biopsies from children with both nephrosis and nephritis other than acute GN, 32 were found to have immunofluorescent evidence of IC GN with HB$_s$ Ag within the deposits.

Other than laboratory findings of chronic hepatitis B infection, nephrosis, or nephritis, there appear to be no distinctive serological findings; however, only a few authors have presented information regarding complement levels, antinuclear antibody, or latex fixation.

The histologic pattern by light microscopy in these patients generally varies between changes indistinguishable from those of membranous GN to focal, mesangial, or mild proliferative GN. Rarely glomerular obliteration and renal failure have been noted. Severe or rapidly progressive GN with crescent formation has been described only in association with the polyarteritis syndrome. Immunofluorescence microscopy has revealed IgG complement and HB$_s$ Ag in granular distribution along capillary loops and mesangial areas. In most instances, electron microscopy has shown the deposits to be intramembranous. In several cases, electron microscopy has also shown virus-like forms in the renal tissue.

QUARTAN MALARIA

Infection of African children by *Plasmodium malariae*, the protozoan responsible for quartan malaria, has been known to cause nephrotic syndrome since the beginning of this century. Recently several investigators have provided renal immunofluorescent evidence of immune complex disease involving plasmodial antigen. Quartan malaria often causes a chronic, almost undetectable parasitemia in children of endemic areas. In this respect it is more indolent than other malarial infections, and there may be more prolonged liberation of antigen, perhaps increasing the chance of development of soluble antigen–antibody complexes; however, renal disease and soluble antigens have also been described in patients infected with *P. falciparum*.

Most of the children present with clinical findings indistinguishable from other forms of nephrotic syndrome; however, many are hypertensive, and a few progress to renal failure, though it has not been possible to rule out associated poststreptococcal GN in these patients. It is not clear that treatment of the infection improves the renal disease.

Laboratory findings reflect the severity of the nephrotic syndrome or renal failure. There are few reports of serum immunoglobulins, complement, or other phase reactants. The children of the endemic area who have malarial nephrosis are most easily distinguished from their peers who have ordinary lipoid nephrosis by the greatly reduced selectivity of their proteinuria.

As with other infection-related IC GN, there is variation in the histological reaction. Most of the renal biopsies have proliferative changes, but segmental sclerosis and membranous thickening have been emphasized by some authors. Immunofluorescence microscopy has shown IgG and IgM in equal proportions and in a granular or finely granular pattern along basement membranes. Complement and malarial antigens are also present. The electron microscopic changes are also variable, but there appears to be a predilection for subepithelial distribution of deposits.

CONCLUSION

Perhaps the most intriguing aspect of infectious causes of glomerulonephritis is that taken together, the phenomena encompass the entire clinical and histological expression of human renal disease. Discovery of a relation between an infection and its renal consequences has required modern skills and diligent search. It therefore is conceivable that the cause of many other human renal diseases may yield to further discovery of persistent, unrecognized, and otherwise mild infections.

REFERENCES

Braunstein GD, Lewis EJ, Galvanck EG, et al: The nephrotic syndrome associated with secondary syphilis: An immune deposit disease. Am J Med 48:643, 1970

Brzosko WJ, Nararewicz T, Krawczynski K, et al: Glomerulonephritis associated with hepatitis-B surface antigen immune complexes in children. Lancet 2:477, 1974

Gutman RA, Striker GE, Gilliland BC, et al: The immune complex glomerulonephritis of bacterial endocarditis. Medicine (Baltimore) 51:1, 1972

Hendrickse RG, Adeniyi A, Edington GM, et al: Quartan malarial nephrotic syndrome. Lancet 1:1143, 1972

SARCOIDOSIS

Domenic A. Sica

Sarcoidosis is a multisystem disease of unknown etiology in which organ involvement usually occurs secondary to granuloma formation which results in replacement and destruction of normal parenchymal architecture. The organ systems most commonly involved include lung, lymphatics, liver, muscle, and skin, although virtually any organ system, including the kidney, may be involved.

The diagnosis of sarcoidosis is often difficult. Common findings include hilar adenopathy, hypercalcemia, abnormalities of liver function tests, especially elevations in alkaline phosphatase activity, hypergammaglobulinemia, and elevation of the erythrocyte sedimentation rate. Immunologic abnormalities are common and include impaired delayed hypersensitivity with cutaneous anergy and Kviem-Siltzbach skin test reactivity. Recent studies have reported increased levels of serum lysozyme and enhanced angiotensin converting enzyme activity. All of these findings are highly nonspecific, and various combinations of these abnormalities may be seen in a variety of diseases. Thus the diagnosis of sarcoidosis usually depends on the demonstration of noncaseating epitheloid granulomas in one or more organs in the absence of evidence for other granulomatous diseases.

As mentioned above, organ system involvement in sarcoidosis is generally due to tissue replacement and destruction by granuloma formation. The pathophysiology of renal involvement may be much more complex, however. Table 1 lists the various renal lesions which may occur in association with sarcoidosis.

Table 1
Renal Involvement in Sarcoidosis

Renal Lesion	Pathophysiology	Manifestations
Reversible azotemia	Hypercalcemia	Renal insufficiency
Nephrolithiasis—	Hypercalciuria	Renal colic
Nephrocalcinosis		Infection
		Obstruction
		Renal insufficiency
Granulomatous involvement	Parenchymal replacement	Renal insufficiency
Glomerulopathies	Immune complex disease	Proteinuria
		Hematuria
		Renal insufficiency
Obliterative arteritis	Granulomatous vasculitis	Hypertension
		Renal insufficiency
Tubular abnormalities	Hypercalcemia	Polyuria, polydipsia
Nephrogenic diabetes insipidus	Nephrocalcinosis	
	Granulomatous nephritis	
Renal tubular acidosis	Hypergammaglobulinemia	Hyperchloremic acidosis
	Nephrocalcinosis	

Hypercalcemia is a relatively common finding in sarcoidosis, occurring in 15–25 percent of patients with this condition. Increased sensitivity to vitamin D is thought to result in increased gastrointestinal calcium absorption, a theory supported by recent reports of low serum parathyroid hormone levels. Levels of 1,25-dihydroxycholecalciferol have been reported as normal and elevated. In view of this mechanism it is not surprising that hypercalcemia is most prominent during the summer months, when sunlight exposure increases vitamin D synthesis. Hypercalcemia may lead to reversible diminution in GFR, probably by mediating renal vasoconstriction and decreased renal blood flow.

Nephrolithiasis and *nephrocalcinosis* are also common complications of sarcoidosis and correlate with the occurrence of hypercalciuria, a finding more common than hypercalcemia. This increased urinary calcium excretion is also secondary to gastrointestinal hypersensitivity to vitamin D and accordingly is magnified during summer months. In addition, the depression of parathyroid hormone secretion diminishes tubular calcium reabsorption and thereby increases urinary calcium excretion. When nephrolithiasis complicates sarcoidosis, its manifestations do not differ from those seen with other causes of renal calculi—obstruction, infection, renal colic, and possibly renal insufficiency. Nephrocalcinosis may also occur in sarcoidosis and may present as a benign radiologic curiosity or may be associated with significant impairment of renal function. In addition, as will be discussed below, renal tubular abnormalities may result from nephrocalcinosis, even in the absences of compromised GFR.

Granulomatous infiltration of the renal parenchyma has been reported to occur in 17–25 percent of patients with sarcoidosis. This tissue replacement is seldom extensive, however, and only a few cases of renal failure from such a mechanism have been reported.

Numerous *glomerulopathies* have been documented in the course of sarcoidosis. These include membranous nephropathy, focal glomerulonephritis, and membranoproliferative glomerulonephritis. Whether these entities occur as a manifestation of sarcoidosis or represent chance coexistence is not clear. A recent report of circulating immune complexes in patients with sarcoidosis, however, suggests that these glomerular lesions may be a consequence of sarcoidosis.

Obliterative arteritis has been documented in a few patients with sarcoidosis. Pathologically, the lesion is characterized by granulomatous involvement of the renal arterioles and clinically may be manifest by renal insufficiency and severe hypertension.

Finally, renal involvement in sarcoidosis may present with *tubular abnormalities*. Nephrogenic diabetes insipidus occurs in patients with sarcoidosis and may be caused by a number of pathogenic mechanisms. Hypercalcemia per se may lead to this condition. Nephrocalcinosis and its attendant interstitial involvement may cause ADH resistance, and, rarely, granulomatous interstitial nephritis underlies the defect in distal water reabsorption. In considering the diagnosis of polyuria in patients with sarcoidosis, it should also be kept in mind that sarcoid may involve the central nervous system and therefore cause central diabetes insipidus. Renal tubular acidosis has also been reported in sarcoidosis. The most likely explanation for this occurrence is either hypergammaglobulinemia or nephrocalcinosis.

REFERENCES

Bolton WK, Atun NO: Reversible renal failure from isolated granulomatous renal sarcoidosis. Clin Nephol 5:88, 1976

Coburn JW, Hobbs C: Granulomatous sarcoid nephritis. Am J Med 42:273, 1967

Cushard WG, Simon AB: Parathyroid function in sarcoidosis. N Engl J Med 286:395, 1972

Falls WF, Randall R: Nonhypercalcemic sarcoid nephropathy. Arch Intern Med 130:285, 1972

McCoy RC, Tisher C: Glomerulonephritis associated with sarcoidosis. Am J Pathol 68:339, 1972

GOUT

Allan E. Nickel

Uric acid is a relatively insoluble endproduct of purine metabolism in primates and a few other species which have lost the degradative enzyme uricase. In these species (including man) the kidney has assumed the major excretory role of uric acid elimination, although under normal conditions small amounts are also excreted by the gastrointestinal tract. Thus there are essentially two factors which control the circulating pool of uric acid—purine degradation to uric acid and uric acid excretion by the kidney. Numerous factors affect purine degradation, and this topic is beyond the scope of this chapter. The renal handling of uric acid is discussed in the chapter on *Organic Anion Secretion and Urate Handling by the Kidney*, and only uric acid induced renal abnormalities will be discussed here.

As noted earlier, uric acid is relatively insoluble, and its propensity to precipitate in synovial joints is well known. Precipitation within the kidney, although less common, can be an equally or even more serious complication of hyperuricemia. At physiologic pH (7.4), 98 percent of uric acid exists in the form of the monovalent monosodium urate, whereas at a urinary pH of 5.5 more than 50 percent exists in its neutral form. Therefore throughout most of the nephrons monosodium urate is deposited when crystallization occurs, while in the collecting system, where an acid pH is normally maintained by hydrogen ion secretion, neutral uric acid is the crystallization product. Crystallization of monosodium urate is therefore primarily dependent upon the serum urate concentration and renal concentrating ability, whereas crystallization of uric acid is mainly dependent on urinary uric acid concentration and urinary pH.

With these concepts in mind it should be noted that there are three basic types of renal abnormalities caused by uric acid and its salts: (1) acute uric acid nephropathy, (2) gouty nephropathy, and (3) renal stone disease.

Acute uric acid nephropathy is a form of acute renal failure caused by precipitation of a large load of uric acid within the distal collecting system. The culprit in this entity is uric acid, with little or no contribution from monosodium urate. The intratubular crystallization of uric acid causes tubular obstruction and a rapid decline in renal function. This pnenomenon usually occurs in a setting in which there is a high purine degradation rate, volume depletion, and/or an acidic urine. Clinically, this entity is seen in a relatively pure form during effective chemotherapy or radiation thera-

py of myeloproliferative or lymphoproliferative malignancies. Similar acute episodes have been reported in patients with hereditary defects in purine metabolism which lead to chronic overproduction of uric acid. Additionally, uric acid precipitation may play a role in the acute renal failure associated with rhabdomyolysis, although other factors are obviously also important. Regardless of its cause, acute uric acid nephropathy is nearly always preventable by inhibition of uric acid production with allopurinol and maintenance of adequate hydration. Once the nephropathy is established, treatment consists of alkaline diuresis with bicarbonate and administration of a carbonic anhydrase inhibitor such as Diamox. The response to this regimen is usually rapid, and permanent renal insufficiency is uncommon if it is treated promptly and appropriately.

The second form of uric acid induced renal disease in *chronic uric acid nephropathy, gouty nephropathy,* or, more appropriately, *urate nephropathy.* For over a century it has been appreciated that there is a high incidence of renal abnormalities in patients with hyperuricemia and gout. Pathologically the kidneys show a relatively nonspecific medullary scarring. If they are properly processed to preserve crystals, however, monosodium urate deposits can be seen within these lesions (Fig. 1). This is the unique finding in urate nephropathy. In addition to these deposits, tubular atrophy is common. In large autopsy series of gouty patients, however, the most common lesion found in nephrosclerosis. These observations have therefore raised the question of which abnormality is primary, i.e., whether renal disease of some other cause may lead to or be associated with hyperuricemia and gout or whether the hyperuricemia is primary, leading to structural renal damage and hence hypertension and/or renal insufficiency.

Data gathered from the era prior to modern effective treatment of gout clearly established that progressive renal impairment was rarely the cause of death in patients with many years of gout and major renal urate deposits. The predominant lesion in autopsied patients, as noted earlier, is nephrosclerosis, and most of these individuals had hypertension. Although hypertension is the most plausible explanation for this high incidence of nephrosclerosis, some have proposed that hypertension may be induced in some manner by the renal urate deposits. Many patients with similar deposits are normotensive, however, casting doubt on this theory. Therefore at present there is scant evidence to support urate nephropathy as a significant source of renal insufficiency in the vast majority of gouty patients. Despite this conclusion, there are reports suggesting that prolonged severe hyperuricemia (> 12 mg/dl) may be associated with progressive renal insufficiency in a minority of patients. Therefore at present most authorities recommend that patients with marked chronic hyperuricemia be treated with allopurinol unless circumstances dictate otherwise.

Another controversial issue surrounding gouty nephropathy centers on the role of hyperuricemia in the

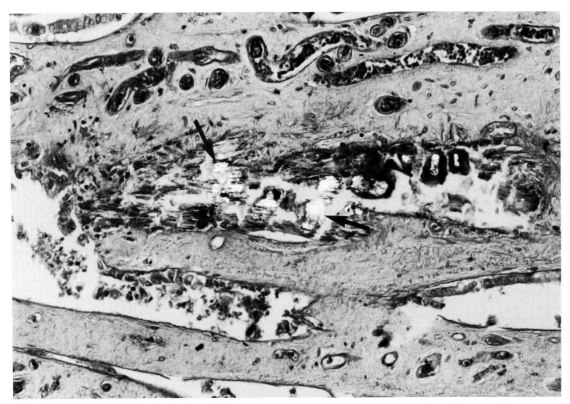

Fig. 1. Inner medulla with scarring, tubular damage, and urate crystals (arrow). [Tissue section kindly provided by Dr. Kim Solez.]

progression of renal diseases of any cause. In general, uric acid clearance is maintained at a normal level by increased tubular urate secretion until the GFR falls below about 40 ml/min. Thereafter, rising serum uric acid levels occur due to decreased clearance of the urate. Although this hyperuricemia is nearly always mild (< 10 mg/dl), some investigators have suggested this may contribute to the progression of renal insufficiency by interstitial urate crystallization; however, at about the same degree of renal insufficiency that hyperuricemia becomes manifest, diminished concentrating ability is also noted. Therefore although serum levels of urate may be elevated, the medullary concentration may be decreased or unchanged, and there may be no more tendency to crystallize urate under these conditions than existed prior to the deterioration in renal function. Studies to evaluate this general problem are few, but to date no effect of normalization of serum urate on the progression of renal insufficiency has been documented. Although more data are needed, unless symptomatic from gout or stone disease (both of which are rare in this population) these patients probably need not be treated with allopurinol.

The third form of uric acid induced renal abnormality is *renal stone disease* (see the chapter on *Renal Stones*). Pure uric acid stones are relatively uncommon and account for less than 10 percent of all renal stones in the United States. These radiolucent stones are usually formed in the setting of chronic hyperuricosuria and mild dehydration with acidic urine. In general, the stones are small in size and frequently appear in the urine as "gravel." This disease is readily treated with allopurinol to diminish uric acid production and excretion and increased hydration to diminish the tubular uric acid concentration.

Of possibly greater importance, however, is the recent finding of hyperuricosuria in many patients with calcium oxalate nephrolithiasis. Coe has shown the incidence of stone episodes in these individuals is greatly diminished by treatment with allopurinol alone. Various mechanisms have been proposed to explain the manner in which hyperuricosuria might enhance calcium oxalate stone formation. At present no mechanism is clearly established.

REFERENCES

Berger L, Yu T: Renal function in gout. IV. An analysis of 524 gouty subjects including long term follow-up studies. Am J Med 59:605, 1975

Coe FL: Hyperuricosuric calcium oxalate nephrolithiasis. Kidney Int 13:418, 1978

Emmerson BT, Row PG: An evaluation of the pathogenesis of the gouty kidney. Kidney Int 8:65, 1975

Rieselbach RE, Bentzel CJ, Cotlove E, et al: Uric acid excretion and renal function in the acute hyperuricemia of leukemia: Pathogenesis and therapy of uric acid nephropathy. Am J Med 37:872, 1964

INTERSTITIAL DISEASE

Richard Parker and William M. Bennett

Disease of the renal interstitium has been attributed primarily to upper urinary tract infection. In recent years it has become widely recognized that infection is only one of many etiologies of acute and chronic interstitial changes in the renal parenchyma. The recognized causes of these pathologic findings are listed in Tables 1 and 2. Recent studies have emphasized a relatively minor role for infection in the pathogenesis of interstitial nephritis.

DEFINITION OF INTERSTITIAL DISEASE

The interstitium of the normal kidney appears sparse due to the close apposition of the renal tubules. When the kidney is examined histologically with the use of reticulum stains, fine fibrils composing the support structure of the interstitium are seen. These fibrils become more evident in situations where nephrons are damaged or lost with disease. Depending on the etiology, the interstitium may demonstrate edema, cellular infiltrate, fibrosis, or tumor cells. These pathologic findings can occur singly or in combination.

Interstitial disease is usually categorized as either acute or chronic. This distinction is usually made on the basis of the evolution of the clinical picture. The rapidity of the clinical onset and associated signs and symptoms need to be used in classification rather than the pathologic description, since the cellular infiltrate is frequently similar in both acute and chronic interstitial nephritis. The most consistent morphologic distinction between acute and chronic disease is the degree of interstitial fibrosis.

ACUTE INTERSTITIAL NEPHRITIS

The term acute interstitial nephritis has been primarily used to describe the renal pathologic findings associated with acute systemic bacterial infection, most commonly those secondary to streptococcus or diphtheria. More recently, however, the term has been used to describe the clinicopathologic syndrome associated with renal dysfunction developing in patients exposed to a growing list of drugs (Table 1). The development of acute renal failure following exposure to these drugs most likely represents a hypersensitivity phenomenon. There is no demonstrable relationship between toxicity and drug dosage.

Methicillin Nephritis

Acute renal insufficiency following exposure to methicillin provides a model for the clinicopathologic entity of acute interstitial nephritis. The presentation of patients with methicillin nephritis is diverse and varies from transient abnormalities of the urinary sediment to frank renal failure requiring support by dialysis. Hematuria (both gross and microscopic), fever, and eosinophilia are seen in more than 80 percent of patients. A generalized and pruritic morbilliform rash has been described in approximately 20 percent of patients. Although 50 percent of patients develop azotemia, only 20 percent are oliguric. The interval between the insti-

Table 1
Drugs Associated With Acute Interstitial Nephritis

Penicillin and its analogues
Rifampin
Sulfonamides
Cephalosporins
Phenindione
Azathioprine
Diphenylhydantoin
Furosemide
Thiazide diuretics
Sulfinpyrazone
Allopurinol

tution of methicillin therapy and the onset of signs and symptoms of nephritis ranges from 2 to 44 days, with a mean of 17 days; however, azotemia and oliguria have been reported during the first week of therapy. In some patients, eosinophils can be demonstrated in the urinary sediment. Abnormalities of renal function may persist for relatively protracted periods. Persistent renal dysfunction for a mean of 45 days following discontinuation of methicillin has been reported.

In spite of the potential severity of the acute renal failure, recovery is the rule. Only 7 percent of the reported patients have had azotemia 1 year after methicillin exposure. None of these patients has required chronic dialysis or transplantation. Management of the acute phase consists of withdrawal of the offending

Table 2
Causes of Interstitial Nephritis

Toxic	Analgesic associated nephropathy, lead,* cadmium*
Anatomic abnormalities	Urinary tract obstruction, vesicoureteral reflux
Metabolic	Urate nephropathy, hypercalcemic nephropathy, hypokalemic nephropathy
Vascular disorders	Sequelae of acute vasomotor nephropathy, nephrosclerosis, sickle-cell disease
Neoplastic disorders	Multiple myeloma, lymphoma, leukemia
Environmental factors	Balkan nephropathy
Immunologic	Sjögren's syndrome, transplant rejection†
Hereditary diseases	Medullary sponge kidney,‡ medullary cystic disease,§ hereditary nephritis‖

*See the chapter on *Toxic Nephopathy.*
†See the chapter on *Renal Transplantation.*
‡See the chapter on *Medullary Sponge Kidney.*
§See the chapter on *Medullary Cystic Disease.*
‖See the chapter on *Alport's Syndrome (Hereditary Nephritis).*

Modified with permission from Suki W, Eknoyan G: Tubulo-interstitial disease, in Brenner BM, Rector FC (eds): The Kidney. Philadelphia, W.B. Saunders, 1976.

agent along with the conventional supportive management of acute renal failure. The use of high-dose steroids such as prednisone 30–60 mg/day has been recommended; however, since these patients frequently have severe infections, the use of steroid therapy may be hazardous. The use of steroids should be reserved for cases in which renal function is significantly impaired.

Acute interstitial nephritis has been documented in those patients who have been biopsied. The interstitium is involved with a cellular infiltrate of lymphocytes, plasma cells, and eosinophils (Fig. 1). In addition to the cellular infiltrate, interstitial edema is also prominent. The glomeruli are normal in the acute phase of the interstitial process.

Immunofluorescent examination of the biopsy may reveal variable deposition of IgG, complement, and fibrinogen. IgG and complement have been demonstrated in a continuous linear pattern along the tubular basement membrane. In addition, dimethoxyphenlpenicilloyl (DPO)—an antigenic determinant of methicillin—has been found on the tubular basement membrane in a similar linear pattern. Border et al. have found circulating anti–tubular basement membrane antibodies in a patient with methicillin nephritis, suggesting that the acute interstitial disease has an immunologic pathogenesis. It must be noted that methicillin nephritis is the only acute interstitial nephritis in which the above observations of a circulating anti–tubular basement membrane antibody have been made. It is not clear whether all cases of methicillin nephritis have a similar pathogenesis.

The other drugs listed in Table 1 may produce a disease process identical to that seen in methicillin nephritis. With the exception of the potential presence of DPO along the tubular basement membrane, the clinical or pathologic picture does not allow for differentiation.

CHRONIC INTERSTITIAL NEPHRITIS

Significant chronic interstitial changes may be the end result of a great number of pathologic processes. These changes frequently occur in the absence of glomerular pathology. The resulting pathologic picture was for a long time termed chronic pyelonephritis; however, as shown in Table 2, many causes other than infection are now recognized as etiologic in chronic interstitial nephritis. There is now considerable evidence to suggest that bacterial infection of the kidney only rarely causes renal insufficiency in the adult population in the absence of other primary causes of interstitial disease.

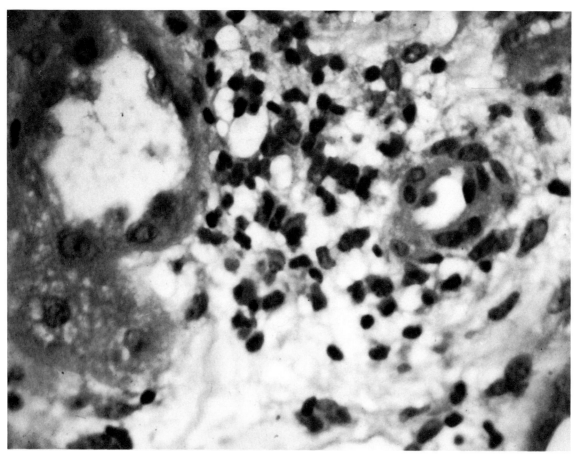

Fig. 1. Methicillin interstitial nephritis. Cellular infiltrate of lymphocytes and eosinophils.

Thus many processes can produce a common histologic picture due to the restricted number of interstitial responses to injury. The failure to appreciate the nonspecific nature of the renal parenchymal changes called chronic pyelonephritis has led to widespread acceptance of the central role of infection in the pathogenesis of chronic interstitial nephritis. Careful evaluation of the presentation and course of patients with interstitial nephritis will, in the great majority of cases, allow for the determination of the specific etiology of the renal failure. Murray and Goldberg were seemingly able to define the etiology in 89 percent of their 101 patients with interstitial nephritis. In none of these patients was infection felt to play a primary role.

Clinical Features

Just as the final pathologic picture is similar in the majority of cases of interstitial disease, the clinical features are often not distinctive. Chronic interstitial nephritis may have a paucity of signs and symptoms prior to advanced stages of renal insufficiency. As opposed to glomerular disorders, gross hematuria, edema, and the nephrotic syndrome are infrequent. The clinical picture is usually dominated by the systemic illness that is etiologic in the renal disease. The initial diagnosis of renal insufficiency is often made at a time when the BUN and serum creatinine are markedly abnormal. Other common findings at the time of diagnosis are anemia and hypertension.

A number of physiologic abnormalities may accompany chronic interstitial nephritis. The earliest detectable abnormality is an inability to maximally concentrate the urine. Other features include disorders of urine acidification and an impaired ability to conserve sodium. Proteinuria, as determined by dipstick, may be present; however, 24-hour urine excretion rarely exceeds 2.5 g. The proteinuria consists primarily of small molecular weight peptides which escape reabsorption due to tubular disease.

Abnormalities of the urinary sediment are varied. Moderate to marked pyuria is the rule. Cellular casts are rare except during periods of acute infection, when white blood cell casts may be seen. Microscopic hematuria of a minimal to moderate degree is common. Gross hematuria is not a common feature of the interstitial nephrititis. The urinary sediment is often surprisingly bland considering the severity of the physiologic derangement.

The intravenous urograms in patients with chronic interstitial nephritis fall into one of four categories. In mild disease they may be normal. Evidence of papillary necrosis is seen in 5 percent of patients. If only patients with analgesic associated nephropathy are considered, this figure increases to approximately 20 percent. Specific abnormalities are seen in those cases associated with stones or other anatomic abnormalities. The majority of patients have nonspecific findings which include irregularly spaced indentations on the outline of the kidney associated with papillary scarring and an overall reduction in kidney size.

Pathology

The most striking feature of the histology in chronic interstitial nephritis is the cellular infiltrate (Fig. 2). The cells are primarily lymphocytes and plasma cells. The polymorphonuclear leukocytes and eosinophils that are commonly seen in acute disease are not found in chronic cases. The interstitium is involved with varying degrees of fibrosis and scarring. Depending upon the underlying etiology, there may be specific interstitial infiltrates such as amyloid, neoplastic cells, or urate deposits. The pathologic appearance of the glomeruli is important in distinguishing primary interstitial disease from glomerular disease. The glomeruli that are outside of areas of fibrosis and scarring are generally normal. Other more involved glomeruli may show thickening of Bowman's capsule, periglomerular fibrosis, or generalized sclerosis and hyalinization. Arteries and arterioles located in areas of scarring may show medial changes and intimal proliferation. These vascular changes may be worsened by concomitant nephrosclerosis. Depending on the underlying cause, papillary necrosis may dominate the pathologic picture.

ANALGESIC-ASSOCIATED NEPHROPATHY

In 1975 Murray and Goldberg reported that ingestion of large quantities of analgesic mixtures was responsible for chronic interstitial nephritis in 20 percent of a large series of patients. Since then, many other workers have confirmed these findings and have emphasized the primary etiolgic role of excessive analgesic ingestion. It is now apparent that what was previously thought to be a significant cause of chronic renal failure only in Europe and Australia is of major importance in the United States as well.

Phenacetin has been considered the compound in analgesic mixtures most likely responsible for the renal lesions of analgesic nephropathy. While the role of this agent cannot be denied, evidence has accumulated from animal investigations as well as clinical studies that other analgesic compounds are also potentially nephrotoxic. Aspirin and acetaminophen have attracted much investigational interest. Evidence for their role in producing renal dysfunction will be presented below.

Clinical Features of Analgesic-associated Nephropathy

Most of the clinical data available have been generated from reports evaluating patients with a well defined exposure history. A total ingestion of 3 kg or more of the index compound or a yearly intake of 1 gram or more for 3 years has been thought necessary to produce clinical nephropathy. It is important to note that these minimum exposure requirements do not address the risk incurred with the ingestion of smaller total doses.

The typical patient with analgesic-associated nephropathy is a middle-aged female with a long history of headaches and abdominal or back pain. A family history of analgesic abuse can frequently be obtained. Gastrointestinal symptoms are common, as is anemia out of proportion to the degree of renal failure. Hyper-

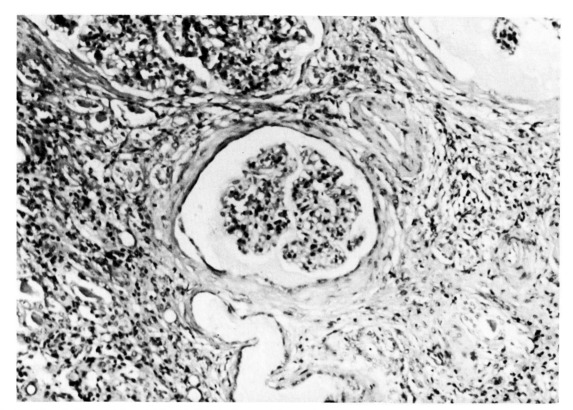

Fig. 2. Chronic interstitial nephritis. Marked infiltrate with round cells. Extensive interstitial fibrosis can be seen. The glomerular tuft is minimally involved, although significant periglomerular fibrosis is present.

tension is seen in approximately 50 percent of patients at the time of diagnosis.

Papillary necrosis is considered the sine qua non in the pathologic diagnosis of analgesic nephropathy; however, less than 50 percent of patients have demonstrated the classic radiographic findings of papillary necrosis. Similarly, clinically symptomatic papillary necrosis is relatively uncommon compared with pathological find-

ings. Thus the risk of underdiagnosis of analgesic nephropathy is substantial if clinical or radiographic evidence of papillary necrosis is demanded.

The history of drug ingestion obtained from patients is variable and often difficult to extract. The most common pattern is the habitual ingestion of drugs containing both phenacetin and aspirin. Table 3 lists the most common proprietary analgesic drugs containing

Table 3
Amounts of Various Analgesic Drugs That Constitute Abuse, Expressed in
Amounts of Phenacetin or Acetaminophen

Proprietary Name	Index Drug in Combination*		No. of Tablets to Provide 0.1 g/day	No. of Years to Provide 3.0 kg at Ten Tablets/Day
	Phenacetin	Acetaminophen		
Darvon	+		6	5
Compound	+		7	6
Empirin	+		8	7
Fiorinal	+		6	5
Norgesic	+		6	5
Sk-65	+		6	5
Percodan	+		6	5
Excedrin		+	11	9
Vanquish		+	6	5

*Phenacetin and acetaminophen are used only as indices of amount of consumption, not necessarily to imply that they are the primary nephrotoxin.

Reprinted from Kidney International with permission—Murray TG, Goldberg M: Analgesic associated nephropathy in the USA: Epidemologic, clinical and pathogenic features. Kid Int 13:64, 1978.

phenacetin or aspirin available in the United States. It is apparent that cumulative doses of either aspirin or phenacetin sufficient to place a patient at risk can easily be achieved with chronic analgesic intake.

The urinary sediment and renal function data are similar to those seen in other forms of chronic interstitial nephritis. Acute papillary necrosis is likely to be associated with gross hematuria, renal colic, or upper urinary tract infection.

The clinical course is dependent on whether analgesic abuse is continued. It appears that if the drugs are discontinued at a time prior to endstage renal disease, renal function may stabilize or improve. Continued ingestion is associated with the development of renal failure and the need for dialysis or transplantation.

Pathology

As noted above, the frequency of papillary necrosis helps to separate analgesic-associated nephropathy from other forms of chronic interstitial disease (Fig. 3). The renal cortical findings of interstitial fibrosis, scarring, and cellular infiltrate are thought to be secondary to the papillary necrosis. Interstitial changes are most prominent at the corticomedullary junction.

Pathogenesis

The initial event in the pathogenesis of interstitial nephritis is thought to be papillary necrosis. It is not clear whether the necrosis is secondary to vascular damage or due to a direct toxic effect of the drugs. In high doses phenacetin and aspirin given alone can produce papillary necrosis in the rat. When the drugs are administered together, papillary necrosis results with lower doses of both drugs. The toxic role of acetaminophen is not completely understood; however, phenacetin is nearly completely metabolized to acetaminophen within 1 hour of ingestion. This suggests that the toxic effect of phenacetin may be mediated by acetaminophen or, more likely, a metabolite of acetaminophen. Dehydration has been shown to potentiate the papillary necrosis produced by analgesics.

Following filtration of the drug a medullary concentration gradient for acetaminophen from tubular lumen to interstitium is established. Aspirin is also concentrated within the tubular lumen of the nephron, but the evidence for a functionally significant medullary gradient is conflicting. The exact cellular mechanism for the toxic effect of analgesic drugs is not known. Acetaminophen is a powerful oxidizing agent. It is possible that oxidative damage results following the depletion of intracellular reducing agents. Aspirin could enhance this oxidative damage by its ability to inhibit the hexose monophosphate shunt, the primary means by which cells maintain their intracellular concentration of reducing agents. Oxidative damage may result from the binding of activated drug metabolites to intracellular

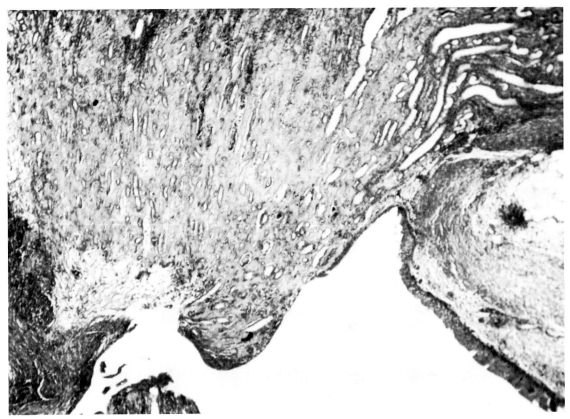

Fig. 3. Papillary necrosis in a kidney from a patient with analgesic associated nephropathy. The delineation between necrotic and viable tissue is evident.

macromolecules with resulting cellular damage and necrosis.

OTHER CAUSES OF INTERSTITIAL NEPHRITIS
Anatomic Abnormalities

Obstruction within the urinary tract or vesicoureteral reflux accounts for a relatively high percentage of patients developing chronic interstitial nephritis. Complete obstruction is not necessary, since the pathologic changes may result from vesicoureteral reflux alone. Although urinary tract infection is common in the patient with obstructive uropathy, infection is not required in order for pathologic lesions to develop. The pathogenesis of the interstitial changes observed in obstructive uropathy may relate to impaired venous drainage from the kidney.

Urate Nephropathy

Renal parenchymal involvement in gout is frequent; however, there is a poor correlation between histologic change and functional impairment. Because of this poor correlation, there is continuing controversy regarding the necessity of reducing serum uric acid in patients with asymptomatic hyperuricemia for the purpose of preserving renal function.

Urate nephropathy may be acute or chronic. Acute disease is seen almost exclusively in patients with lymphoproliferative or myeloproliferative disorders, frequently in association with cytotoxic therapy. In this instance, the clinical presentation is that of acute renal failure due to obstruction of renal tubules by precipitated uric acid.

Chronic urate nephropathy is variably associated with clinical gout. The only specific histologic finding in chronic urate nephropathy is the presence of urate deposits in the renal interstitium. The deposits are requently associated with a foreign body giant cell reaction. Other changes of tubular atrophy, cellular infiltrate, and arteriolosclerosis are nonspecific and similar to those seen in other forms of interstitial nephritis. Glomerular lesions are minimal. The role of obstruction and infection subsequent to uric acid stones in the development of interstitial changes is not known but is probably minor in most cases.

Most recent studies suggest that renal function in patients with asymptomatic hyperuricemia is well preserved. The earliest functional change is in urinary concentrating and acidifying ability. The urinary sediment is nondiagnostic with the possible exception of urate crystals, which are sometimes present when the urine is acidic. The severity of renal involvement and its tendency toward progression are dependent upon the duration and degree of hyperuricemia.

Vascular Disorders

Lesions of the renal vasculature, either extrarenal or within the renal parenchyma, result in varying degrees of interstitial fibrosis, scarring, and tubular degeneration. Acute renal failure in the form of vasomotor nephropathy is associated with interstitial edema and a monomuclear cell infiltrate. Followup biopsies of patients recovering from acute renal failure have shown interstitial fibrosis in some reported cases.

Although arteriolar nephrosclerosis usually occurs with hypertension, elevated blood pressure is sometimes absent. The vascular changes are accompanied by interstitial fibrosis along with variable degrees of tubular atrophy.

Sickle-cell disease is associated with a glomerulopathy as well as interstitial fibrosis and tubular atrophy. The abnormalities of urinary concentration and dilution that occur in this disease are thought to be due to these interstitial and tubular changes.

Neoplastic Disorders

The renal parenchyma may be infiltrated by a variety of tumors, usually of hematopoietic or lymphoproliferative origin. With the exception of multiple myeloma, renal insufficiency is not a common result of renal parenchymal tumor involvement. Renal pathologic findings primarily consist of interstitial infiltration with leukemic or lymphomatous cells. If renal insufficiency does result from this infiltration, improvement in function may be seen following chemotherapy or irradiation.

Hypercalcemic Nephropathy

The renal functional and morphologic changes associated with hypercalcemia are dependent both on the degree and duration of the elevation in serum calcium. Histologic changes are evident throughout the nephron. As a result of tubular cell damage, necrotic debris accumulates within tubular lumina and provides a nidus for calcification and subsequent tubular obstruction. This obstructive process eventually results in dilatation and atrophy of the tubule. Because it occurs most often in the distal nephron, atrophy and scarring of the entire cortical segment draining into an involved collecting duct may occur. This most likely accounts for the histologic picture of alternating areas of normal and wedge-shaped scars seen in advanced hypercalcemic nephropathy. While the parenchymal scarring is most likely secondary to the above sequence of events, it is also possible that stones with secondary obstruction and infection contribute to the pathology. Within the areas of interstitial nephritis a lymphocytic cellular infiltrate is present along with variable degrees of glomerular hyalinization. Glomeruli outside the areas of scarring may show minimal involvement.

As with most other interstitial nephritides, the earliest functional change is an impairment in urine concentrating ability. In part, this may be due to inhibition of adenylcyclase activity by calcium. Because the actions of ADH in the kidney are mediated by the adenylcyclase–cyclic AMP system, the antidiuretic effect of ADH is diminished by excess calcium. In addition, the suppression of ADH activity serves to inhibit the accumulation of urea in the renal medulla, thus further impairing concentrating ability. Sodium wasting with a tendency to dehydration is frequently seen in hypercalcemic states. This may result from inhibition of a Na^+ K^+ activated ATPase. This enzyme plays an important role in the transcellular movement of sodium ions within the nephron. Renal blood flow and the glomerular filtration rate are also decreased by elevations in the serum calcium.

It is of interest that calcium induced alterations in

renal function occur following the acute intravenous injection of the ion. This observation suggests a poor correlation between renal functional and morphologic changes.

Hypokalemic Nephropathy

The relationship between interstitial nephritis and hypokalemia is well established in animal models (see also the chapter on *Clinical Disorders of Potassium Metabolism*). In man the evidence that irreversible structural lesions result from hypokalemia is less certain. It is established that in response to hypokalemia, vacuolation of the renal tubular cells does occur. This is considered a characteristic but not invariable accompanyment of potassium depletion. The vacuolar lesions are primarily of the proximal tubule but may also be seen in the distal nephron. In contrast to the rat, no characteristic medullary lesions have been described in man. These vacuolar lesions are reversible with potassium repletion.

Chronic changes of interstitial scarring and fibrosis are described as the pathologic correlates of irreversible hypokalemic nephropathy. It is not certain, however, what role parenchymal renal infection plays in the development of these chronic changes. At present, the data supporting a cause and effect relationship between hypokalemic nephropathy and renal infection are not convincing. Infection does not provide an adequate explanation for the chronic irreversible changes of kaliopenic nephropathy. The duration and severity of hypokalemia required to produce permanent structural changes are unknown.

From a functional standpoint, the most consistent abnormality is a decrease in the concentrating ability of the kidney. The mechanism for this defect is unknown. Conflicting data exist supporting both an abnormality in the countercurrent concentrating system and a decrease in the permeability of the collecting ducts to water. In the early stages, the concentrating defect is reversible by the replenishment of potassium.

Balkan Nephropathy

An endemic form of chronic interstitial nephritis occurs in a localized area that encompasses portions of Yugoslavia, Bulgaria, and Romania. The histopathologic picture is that of interstitial nephritis with tubular atrophy, extensive fibrosis, and a modest degree of cellular infiltration.

This disease occurs in approximately 20 percent of the population living within the endemic area. It has been demonstrated to occur within families. Most investigators, however, feel that the disease is acquired rather than inherited.

As with other forms of chronic interstitial nephritis, it is insidious in its onset. Progression to endstage renal disease is the rule. A decrease in the concentrating ability is the first functional abnormality noted. Mild proteinuria and a nonspecific urinary sediment are characteristic.

The etiology of this unqiue form of renal disease remains unknown. The bulk of evidence supports some unidentified environmental toxin as the most likely cause.

Sjögren's Syndrome

Sjögren's syndrome is a disorder of unknown etiology. Most consider it an abnormality of altered immunity. It is characterized by dryness of the eyes and mouth, salivary gland enlargement, and, in 30 percent of patients, inflammatory joint disease that resembles rheumatoid arthritis. In addition, there occurs within the kidney an interstitial nephritis of varying severity and clinical significance.

The renal histologic picture is that of a mononuclear cell infiltrate of the interstitium associated with tubular atrophy and interstitial fibrosis. The cellular infiltrate is primarily lymphocytic and similar to that seen in the salivary and lacrimal glands.

Clinically significant renal dysfunction is uncommon. Concentrating ability is altered in the early stages of renal involvement. Renal acidification disorders may occur and are manifested by renal tubular acidosis. Proteinuria of less than 1 gram has been noted in 5 percent of patients.

REFERENCES

Border WA, Lehman DH, Egan JD, et al: Antitubular basement membrane antibodies in methicillin-associated interstitial nephritis. N Engl J Med 291:381, 1974

Ditlove J, Weidman P, Bernstein M, et al: Methicillin nephritis. Medicine (Baltimore) 56:483, 1977

Freedman LR: Natural history of urinary infection in adults. Kidney Int 8:S96, 1975

Klinenberg JR, Gonick HC, Dornfeld L: Renal function abnormalities in patients with asymptomatic hyperuricemia. Arthritis Rheum 18 [Nov–Dec Suppl], 1975

Murray TG, Goldberg M: Chronic interstitial nephritis: Etiologic factors. Ann Intern Med 82:453, 1975

Murray TG, Goldberg M: Analgesic associated nephropathy in the U.S.A.: Epidemiologic, clinical and pathogenetic features. Kidney Int 13:64, 1978

Ooi BS, Wellington J, First MR, et al: Acute interstitial nephritis. A clinical and pathologic study based on renal biopsies. Am J Med 59:614, 1975

Suki W, Eknoyan G: Tubulo-interstitial disease, in Brenner BM, Rector FC (eds): The Kidney. Philadelphia, W.B. Saunders, 1976

TOXIC NEPHROPATHY

N. Lameire

Among a number of reasons why the kidney is especially vulnerable to injury by toxins, three must be emphasized. First, the kidney has a rich blood supply which amounts to 20 percent of cardiac output; consequently, a major intrarenal vascular endothelial surface is exposed to large amounts of circulating toxins or drugs. Second, the renal countercurrent mechanism produces hypertonicity in the medullary and papillary interstitium, so that high local concentrations of potentially noxious agents may be achieved. Third, impaired renal function interferes with the elimination of certain toxins, since the kidney functions as an obligatory route for the elimination of many toxins or drugs.

Nephrotoxicity can result from a combination of several mechanisms. These mechanisms represent a wide spectrum of clinical nephrologic syndromes, which of course can be induced by a variety of nontoxic causes, so that a nephrotoxic etiology is not always easily recognized. The diagnosis of toxic nephropathy depends primarily on the completeness of the patient's history, where particular attention should be given to the careful search for any of the known nephrotoxins in the environment. Information on surreptitious drug abuse must be obtained from family members or other relatives. It is perhaps most appropriate to approach the problem of toxic nephropathy based on a classification of the different clinical symptom complexes which may be produced by various nephrotoxins.

The patient presenting a toxic nephropathy may present with acute renal failure, chronic renal failure, nephrotic syndrome, or specific tubular disorders. The classification and causes of these syndromes are listed in Table 1.

NEPHROTOXIC ACUTE RENAL FAILURE

This syndrome is characterized by an abrupt decline in renal function with a rise in blood urea nitrogen and serum creatinine. The patient may present with either oliguric or nonoliguric acute renal failure. Several subgroups in this syndrome may be recognized.

Acute Tubular Necrosis

Nephrotoxins incriminated as causes of this syndrome are listed in Table 1. While this list is not exhaustive, it does indicate the variety of toxins responsible for acute tubular necrosis.

Numerous chemical agents can cause acute tubular necrosis.

Heavy metals. Among the intoxications with heavy metals, mercury poisoning is the most classic example in this group. Intoxication by inorganic Hg salts (most frequently bichloride of Hg) occurs accidently, in industrial poisoning or laboratory contamination with mercury, in cases of suicide, or following its use as an abortifacient. It appears that Hg initiates cellular destruction by combining with the sulfhydryl groups of protein in the mitochondrial membrane. The earliest changes appear in the middle and terminal portions of the proximal tubule, at least in the experimental animal challenged with moderate doses of mercury.

In severe Hg intoxication the whole proximal convoluted tubule may show extensive cellular necrosis, the lumens being filled with granular eosinophilic cytoplasm. In the recovery phase, the epithelium of the proximal convoluted tubules regains its normal appearance.

Organic Hg compounds producing nephrotoxicity include mercurichrome, mercury-containing dermatological preparations, and a variety of mercurial diuretics. The histological lesions with these compounds are very similar to those observed with inorganic Hg salts. The clinical picture of acute mercury poisoning consists of severe gastrointestinal symptoms in association with oliguric acute renal failure, occurring after a few hours of ingestion and persisting for an average of 15 days.

The mortality rate is very high after massive ingestion. The therapy of the mercury ingestion is similar to treatment of most other heavy metal poisonings and includes induction of emesis, administration of charcoal, and injections of BAL (2,3-dimercaprol). In anuria BAL is retained by the kidney, but it can be removed by hemodialysis.

Acute oliguric renal failure occurs frequently after bismuth intoxication. Renal histology is characterized by proximal tubular necrosis with distinctive inclusion bodies in the nucleus and cytoplasm of the epithelial cells. Beneficial effects of BAL therapy have not yet been demonstrated.

Arsenic poisoning with acute renal failure occurs in persons exposed to certain fertilizers containing the metal, in agricultural sprays, or in workers in the petroleum industry exposed to arsin gas (AsH_3). Exchange transfusion and BAL administration have been recommended.

Gold salts are used in the treatment of rheumatoid arthritis and systemic lupus erythematosus. Most frequently, a subacute renal failure and nephrotoc syndrome are observed in this setting. Fatal anuric renal failure, however, has also been reported. BAL can be an effective therapeutic agent.

Acute nephrotoxic renal failure in man has been reported after exposure to silver, ingestion of large doses of ferrous sulfate or antimony salts, and acute copper intoxication.

Uranium salts are quite often used to study experimental renal failure, but no convincing report exists on acute nephrotoxic renal failure after accidental or industrial exposure to uranium salts in man.

Halogenated hydrocarbons. Carbon tetrachloride (CCl_4), widely used as a household cleaning agent, appears to be hepato- and nephrotoxic. Tubular necrosis is localized in the proximal tubule, both limbs of Henle's loop, and rarely in the distal tubule.

The clinical picture is characterized by the combination of subconjunctival or periorbital hemorrhages, gastrointestinal symptoms, toxic hepatitis with jaundice, and oligoanuric acute renal failure. The onset of renal abnormalities is often insidious, and a delay of up to 1 week after exposure is quite typical. Owing to the associated hepatic failure, resulting in a lower BUN, serum creatinine is a more reliable guide to the course of the renal failure. Carbon tetrachloride intoxication is one of the few causes of acute toxic renal failure where moderate hypertension is present. Standard management of acute hepatic and renal failure should be initiated. It is very questionable whether CCl_4 can be removed by early hemodialysis.

Approximately the same acute hepato- and nephrotoxic lesions occur after exposure to both tri- and tetrachloroethylene, used during dry cleaning of clothes.

Ethylene glycol is used in automobile antifreeze, lacquers, cosmetics, flavoring extracts, and textiles. Renal functional impairment is seemingly related to intrarenal crystallization of the metabolic endproduct, oxalic acid. Direct tubular toxicity of ethylene glycol, however, is also a possible explanation for the renal failure. The clinical picture is characterized by central nervous system manifestations, gastrointestinal symptoms, and signs of cardiopulmonary distress with pulmonary edema. Abrupt total anuria is frequent, and this renal failure is characterized by very severe metabolic acidosis. Prompt dialysis to remove the circulating ethylene glycol and administration of alkali has been advocated by some clinicians. Both diethylene glycol

Table 1
Classification of Toxic Nephropathies

Acute renal failure
  Acute tubular necrosis
    Heavy metals—mercury, bismuth, arsenic, gold, silver, ferrous sulfate, antimony
    salts, copper, uranium salts
    Halogenated hydrocarbons—carbon tetrachloride, glycols
    Contrast media
    Antimicrobial agents—cephalosporins, aminoglycosides (gentamicin, tobramycin and
    amikacin, polymyxin B–E), sulfonamides, penicillin-G, semisynthetic penicillins,
    viomycin and capreomycin, cotrimoxazole, tetracyclines
  Acute interstitial nephritis
    Penicillins
    Methicillin
    Sulfonamides, cephalosporins, phenindione, azathioprine, diphenylhydantoin,
    allopurinol, furosemide, thiazides, sulfinpyrazone
  Acute glomerulonephritis and acute intrarenal angiitis
    Penicillin G
    Organic solvents
    Amphetamines
  Acute prerenal failure and disturbances of body fluids
    Tetracyclines
    Steroids, diuretics, hyperalimentation
    Diuretics, Na$^+$ salts (polystyrene sulfonate, penicillins)
  Acute postrenal failure
    Crystal precipitation—sulfonamides, uric acid, oxalate, ethylene glycol,
    methoxyflurane
    Nephrocalcinosis—Worcestershire sauce, Milk–alkali syndrome, phosphate salts

Chronic renal failure
  Chronic interstitial nephritis
    Analgesic nephropathy
    Lead
    Cadmium
    Beryllium
    Radiation nephritis
  Chronic glomerulonephritis
    Heroin addiction
    Drug-induced SLE

Nephrotic syndrome
  Penicillamine
  Gold salts
  Anticonvulsants, tolbutamide, perchlorate, probenecid, EDTA, polyvinyl alcohol, Hg,
  Br salts, snake venom, allergens

Disorders of tubular function
  Fanconi's syndrome
    Outdated tetracyclines
    Streptozotocin
  Renal tubular acidosis and metabolic alkalosis
    Amphotericin B, 6-mercaptopurine, sulfonamides, outdated tetracyclines,
    streptozotocin, heavy metals
    Licorice
    Penicillins
  Disturbances in water transport
    Increased water excretion—lithium, demeclocycline, methoxyflurane, sulfonylurea,
    osmotic diuretics
    Impaired water excretion—vasopressin, oxytocin, chlorpropamide, diuretics,
    cyclophosphamide, vincristine, Tegretol, clofibrate, carbamazepine

and propylene glycol also produce a similar clinical picture.

Contrast media. Nephrotoxicity is occasionally caused by contrast media and is clearly related to the dosage of organic iodine. Postulated mechanisms of nephrotoxicity include direct cellular toxicity, a fall in renal blood flow, osmotic diuresis, obstructive crystalluria (mostly urate precipitation), and a hypersensitivity reaction. Acute renal failure following routine intravenous pyelography is fortunately rare. The frequent use of the drip infusion technique, however, has been associated with an increased incidence of acute renal failure or accentuation of an underlying renal insufficienty. Complications most often occur in dehydrated patients, particularly those suffering from multiple myeloma, renal amyloidosis, and diabetes.

It is known that the overall renal response to an acute osmotic load of contrast material is vasoconstriction. The uricosuric effect of the organic iodides may also contribute to nephrotoxicity. The incidence of nephrotoxicity after angiography varies from 0.3 to to over 4 percent.

Cholecystographic agents are lipid soluble, iodinated carboxylic acids that may cause tubular necrosis, particularly when biliary elimination is impaired. This acute tubular necrosis has been frequently seen following bunamyodyl cholecystography and is much less frequent following the use of iopanoic acid. Testing for hypersensitivity, adequate maintenance of diuresis, and careful monitoring of iodide dosage constitute the best prevention of iodide nephrotoxicity.

Antimicrobial agents. Acute tubular necrosis occurs rarely following the use of sulfonamides, penicillin-G and semisynthetic penicillins, the antituberculous compounds (viomycin and cappreomycin), cotrimoxazole (sulfamethoxazole and trimethoprim), and tetracycline. In contrast, this complication is more frequent with some cephalosporins, aminoglycosides, polymyxin B, and colistin.

Dosage-related nephrotoxicity due to cephaloridine has been clearly demonstrated in animals and man. In animals, it has been shown to cause proximal tubular damage. Characteristically, patients who develop nephrotoxicity secondary to cephaloridine therapy have received excessive dosages (over 6 g/day) and have decreased renal function associated with either advanced age or preexisting renal disease without appropriate dosage reduction. Cefazolin and cephalothin have caused dose related tubular damage in rats and rabbits, but the lesions are much less severe and much higher doses must be used than with cephaloridine. Relatively mild and reversible tubular necrosis has been described in man due to the cephalosporins other than cephaloridine, but it is rare and its mechanism is unknown.

Since it has been suggested that cephalosporins may enhance the nephrotoxicity of aminoglycoside antibiotics, it is advisable to monitor renal function carefully in patients receiving this combination of drugs.

The aminoglycosides include streptomycin, neomycin, kanamycin, gentamicin, and newer agents such as tobramycin, amikacin, sisomicin, and spectinomycin. The aminoglycosides are extremely useful in the management of severe bacterial infections, but their potential nephrotoxicity has created great concern among clinicians. Overt proximal tubular necrosis occurs rarely in patients treated with streptomycin, and the nephrotoxocity that complicated early experience with this agent has been virtually abolished by purification of the parent compound. Neomycin is highly nephrotoxic, but it is almost always used orally because it is relatively nonabsorbable. Acute tubular necrosis, however, may occur with administration of large oral doses in the presence of gastrointestinal disease or preexisting impaired renal function. Continued therapy with kanamycin, as in the treatment of tuberculosis, causes oliguric renal failure in 10 percent of cases.

The administration of gentamicin results in nephrotoxic injury in man and in a variety of experimental animals. It has been claimed that nephrotoxicity occurs when renal excretory function is already compromised or massive doses are given. Gentamicin therapy, however, is associated with a high incidence of renal impairment even in patients with previously normal renal function. Ultrastructural abnormalities of the proximal tubule have been demonstrated following administration to animals of doses of gentamicin equivalent to the dose employed clinically. Gentamicin is excreted predominantly by glomerular filtration. The drug is bound to renal tissue, and both experimental animals and man concentrate the drug up to 20 times the serum levels in the renal cortex; however, a close relation between total cortical drug concentration and nephrotoxicity has not been demonstrated. Characteristic ultrastructural lesions in both men and animals have been described in the epithelial cells of the proximal tubule, where the lysosomes contain a lamellated appearance of myeloid bodies. It is suggested that these myeloid bodies are the morphologic expression of an interaction of the polycationic compound with acid lipoproteins in the lysosomal matrix. Further, a recent study in Munich Wistar rats demonstrated a reduction of 50 percent in glomerular capillary ultrafiltration coefficient without obvious histologic abnormalities of the glomerulary capillary wall after gentamicin.

Combination of the anesthetic methoxyflurane and gentamicin, on one hand, and sodium deficiency and diuretic therapy, on the other, potentiates the gentamicin-induced renal failure. The clinical incidence of gentamicin nephrotoxicity ranges from 2–10 percent and it is often expressed as a nonoliguric acute tubular necrosis. In animals, decreased urinary osmolality and vasopressin-resistant polyuria precede the rise in BUN and creatinine.

In general, changes are reversible after discontinuation of the drug, but substantial damage requiring dialysis and a prolonged recovery phase may be observed.

A higher frequency of gentamicin-induced renal failure in association with other antibiotics, notably cephalosporin, has been noted. A 20 percent prevalence of renal damage in patients on cephalosporin–gentamicin therapy, as compared to 3.4 percent with carbenicillin–gentamicin, has been reported. The role of the cephalosporins in enhancing this nephrotoxicity is unclear, and animal studies have still not resolved this problem. In any case, gentamicin with its low rate of toxicity and definite therapeutic value is a vital part of the clinician's therapeutic armamentarium, but recognition of high-risk patients, monitoring of serum creatinine levels, and measurement of serum levels of gentamicin is advisable. In the presence of renal dysfunction, either the normal dosage must be reduced or the intervals between drug administration must be increased. In patients with renal failure who are on dialysis, the unpredictability of serum drug levels has been well documented and rather special dosage programs should be used.

Two new semisynthetic derivatives of aminoglycosides, tobramycin and amikacin, have been produced in an attempt to find agents which are resistant to bacterial enzymatic inactivation. The renal toxicity of tobramycin is low, the worldwide experience being only 1.5 percent. The histologic lesions after drug administration to animals are similar to those produced by gentamicin. Amikacin is resistant to many of the bacterial R factor mediated enzymes that inactivate kanamycin and gentamicin. Recent prospective comparative clinical studies of the nephrotoxicity of amikacin and gentamicin revealed a slightly lower incidence among amikacin treated patients. Both tobramycin and amikacin should be used with caution in patients with depressed renal function, and all the aforementioned warnings concerning the use of gentamicin should be applied to tobramycin and amikacin.

All polymyxins may produce renal damage, and the nephrotoxicity may be mediated through the drug's action as a surfactant on renal tubular cells. At a dose of 3 mg/kg/day polymyxin B may cause decreased glomerular filtration rate in patients with previously normal renal function. Tubular necrosis occurs with higher doses in both aminals and man. The nephrotoxicity of colistimethate is relatively frequent (20 percent) and is dose related; therefore this drug should be used only when other, less toxic antibiotics are not therapeutically indicated.

Acute Interstitial Nephritis
See the preceding chapter (Interstitial Disease).
Acute Glomerulonephritis and Acute Necrotizing Angiitis
A clinical picture of acute glomerulonephritis on a nephrotoxic basis may occasionally be observed. Isolated proliferative glomerulonephritis in association with Henoch-Schönlein purpura has been described with penicillin-G therapy. Recently, an increased incidence of exposure to a variety of organic solvents in patients suffering from Goodpasture's syndrome has also been reported.

Necrotizing renal angiitis due to intravenous drug abuse, particularly amphetamines, must be suspected when a combination of severe oliguric acute renal failure and severe hypertension occurs. Visceral angiography may be diagnosed by the presence of aneurysmal changes in the arteries of the abdominal viscera, including the kidneys.

Acute Toxic Prerenal Failure and Disturbances of Body Fluids
A rise in BUN level independent of renal function can be produced by steoid therapy, tetracycline, diuretics, and hyperalimentation solutions. Azotemia caused by tetracyclines is due to their antianabolic effect on protein metabolism. It has been postulated that with decreased utilization of amino acids in protein synthesis, an additional load of protein metabolites becomes available for renal excretion and accounts for the rise in BUN.

A major increase in sodium intake may occur by ingestion of sodium containing pharmacological agents, such as the semisynthetic penicillins and sodium polystyrene sulfonate (Kayexalate).

Acute Postrenal Failure—Toxic Obstructive Nephropathy
Toxic obstructive nephropathy may be caused by either intrarenal crystal deposition or precipitation of crystals within the collecting system. A first example is the intrarenal precipitation caused by the older sulfonamides—sulfapyridine, sulfathiazole, and sulfadiazine. Their solubility in the urine depends on tubular fluid concentration, the urinary pH and temperature, and their intrinsic solubility properties. Crystalluria has also occurred following dextran administration. Intrarenal obstruction may also be produced by precipitation of uric acid within the tubular lumen. This is frequently observed secondary to chemotherapy in patients with hematologic neoplasms. Prevention of this disorder consists of the pretreatment of the patient with allopurinol, together with an increased fluid intake and alkalinization of the urine with sodium bicarbonate.

Intrarenal oxalate deposition occurs from the metabolism of such compounds as ethylene glycol, methoxyflurane, and rarely ascorbic acid. Several cases of obstructive renal failure have been observed following methoxyflurane anesthesia. This acute renal failure is characterized by two phases. A first polyuric period is caused by a state of nephrogenic diabetes insipidus due to the accumulation of inorganic fluoride. A second period of prolonged anuria may subsequently occur, and renal biopsy shows extensive deposition of caldium oxalate crystal in the renal tissue. Other causes of toxic intrarenal nephrocalcinosis include excessive intake of Worcestershire sauce, the milk–alkali syndrome, and the intravenous use of phosphate salts in the emergency treatment of hypercalcemia. Extrarenal ureteral obstruction caused by retroperitoneal fibrosis may follow prolonged ingestion of methysergide, a serotonin antagonist used in the treatment of migraine.

TOXIC CHRONIC RENAL DAMAGE
Two pathological entities can be included in the syndrome of toxic chronic renal failure; the lesions are predominantly localized either in the interstitium, producing interstitial nephritis, or in the glomerulus, re-

sulting in chronic glomerulonephritis. Drug-induced nephrotic syndrome may also be placed in this second category. Chronic interstitial nephritis occurs with analgesic abuse, lead, cadmium, and beryllium intoxication, and after certain forms of radiation therapy.

Chronic Interstitial Nephritis

This general topic and the clinical syndrome of analgesic associated nephropathy are discussed in the preceding chapter.

The chronic interstitial nephritis occurring in lead poisoning is often obscured by the more striking systemic manifestations. Major sources of lead include ingestion of contaminated foods, drinking water, or medications. Pica is the leading cause of lead poisoning in young children and in adults. Chronic lead nephropathy has been endemic in some parts of the United States, associated with the use of illegally distilled alcohol. Lead accumulates in proximal tubular cells, and its rate of excretion is quite delayed. After chronic exposure to lead in man, interstitial fibrosis, ischemic changes in the glomeruli, and fibrosis of arteriolar walls are noted. Intranuclear of cytoplasmic inclusions in proximal tubular cells have been found in biopsies of patients with this disorder and may persist for long periods of time. Patients with chronic lead nephropathy manifest a lower uric acid clearance at any given level of creatinine clearance, and clinical gout with arthritis may occur in as many as 50 percent of the patients. Treatment of lead nephropathy includes immediate removal of the source of the metal and an attempt of increase the urinary lead excretion by disodium calcium EDTA.

Chronic exposure of workers in the cadmium industry to cadmium fumes results in chronic interstitial nephritis. A proteinuria of the tubular type, characterized by low molecular weight components, results from proximal tubule damage occurs and can be associated with Fanconi's syndrome and an impaired urinary concentrating ability. Most patients have a decreased plasma uric acid level due to an increased uric acid clearance. The presence of painful osteomalacia may be a clue to the diagnosis.

The nephrotoxic dose resulting in an interstitial nephritis following irradiation is in excess of 2500 R over a few weeks. Both acute and chronic radiation nephritis are often complicated by the development of malignant hypertension. Although the interstitial changes are the most striking features, the earliest lesions in chronic radiation nephritis are glomerular and vascular. It must be emphasized that patients with chronic radiation nephritis can present without evidence of an acute radiation syndrome. The chronic renal disease may lead to terminal renal failure after a period of approximately 10 years.

Chronic Glomerulonephritis

Focal glomerulosclerosis and mesangiocapillary glomerulonephritis with progressive renal failure has been found with increasing incidence in heroin addicts. The prognosis is poor, with 75 percent of these patients developing endstage renal failure within 4 years of the onset of proteinuria. All forms of treatment appear to be ineffective. A relationship with hepatitis virus cannot be excluded, although it is also probable that the disease reflects an immune response to contaminants in street heroin or to other infectious agents. A number of drugs may cause a clinical syndrome indistinguishable from systemic lupus erythematosus (SLE). Although there is a low incidence of renal manifestations in the drug-induced syndrome, both procainamide and hydralazine may produce renal complications.

TOXIC NEPHROTIC SYNDROME

The aminonucleoside of puromycin, a chemotherapeutic agent, is used as a standard model to produce experimental nephrotic syndrome. In man, a toxic type of nephrotic syndrome has been described following use of a number of unrelated drugs or toxins, including the anticonvulsants (trimethadione, ethadione, or paramethadione), tolbutamide, perchlorate, probenecid, EDTA, polyvinyl alcohol, organic compounds of mercury, bismuth, and gold, and snake venom. A number of cases of multiple recurrences of nephrotic syndrome associated with pollen allergy have been reported. Two common drugs used in the treatment of rheumatoid arthritis cause the nephrotic syndrome: organic gold salts and penicillamine. The mechanism of penicillamine-induced glomerular damage is presumed to be immunologic and probably involves circulating immune complexes. Stopping the penicillamine results in improvement in the nephrotic syndrome and normalization of the renal biopsy. The nephrotic syndrome produced by gold therapy is characterized pathologically by membranous nephropathy. Electron-dense deposits are seen within the glomerular basement membrane, and immunoglobulins may be found on immunofluorescent examination. The nephrotic syndrome usually recedes when gold treatment is stopped.

DISORDERS OF TUBULAR FUNCTION

A number of specific syndromes of tubular dysfunction have been reported with various nephrotoxins. They are usually reversible once the exposure is stopped. A full review of these disorders can be found in other chapters.

Fanconi's syndrome. A characteristic syndrome has occurred in man in association with degraded tetracyclines. Recovery ensued within 4 weeks after discontinuing the antibiotic. The syndrome has been reproduced in animals as well. Streptozotocin, a cancer chemotherapeutic agent, has caused a Fanconi syndrome with renal tubular acidosis and, in some patients, anuria.

Renal tubular acidosis and metabolic alkalosis. An impairment in hydrogen ion transport has been reported in association with amphotericin B, mercaptopurine, sulfonamides, degraded tetracyclines, streptozotocin, heavy metals such as lead, mercury, and bismuth, and toluene sniffing. The defect has involved both the proximal and distal tubule and was reversible in most instances. Lactic acidosis is a serious complication of the use of phenformin, an oral hypoglycemic agent. Metabolic alkalosis can be the result of heavy use of licorice due to its mineralocorticoid-like properties. A recently recognized cause of "toxic hypokalemic metabolic alkalosis" is the administration of large doses of penicillins, particularly carbenicillin. The penicillin moiety, acting as a nonreabsorbable anion within the nephron, may increase the negativity of the distal tubular lumen leading to the passive excretion of potassium and hydrogen ions.

Disturbances in renal water transport. The syndrome of vasopressin resistant polyuria occurs during or after exposure to lithium salts, demeclocycline, methoxyflurane, certain sulfonylurea compounds, and osmotic diuretics, like mannitol. On the other hand, many drugs may interfere with renal water excretion, and these effects may be independent of the primary pharmacologic action of the drug. Besides vasopressin itself, a growing number of pharmaceutical agents share the ability to decrease maximum free water clearance. This group includes oxytocin, chlorpropamide, diuretics, cyclophosphamide, vincristine, tegretol, clofibrate, and carbamazepine.

REFERENCES

Appel GB, Neu HC: Nephrotoxicity of antimicrobial agents. N Engl J Med 296:663, 722, 784, 1977

Bennett WM, Plamp C, Porter GA: Drug-related syndromes in clinical nephrology. Ann Intern Med 87:582, 1977

Lant AF: Renal excretion and nephrotoxicity of drugs, in Black D (ed): Renal Disease. Oxford, Blackwell Scientific, 1972, p 591

Maher JF: Toxic nephropathy, in Brenner BM, Rector FC Jr (eds): The Kidney, Philadelphia, W.B. Saunders, 1977, p 1355

Nanra RS, Kincaid-Smith P: Chronic effects of analgesics on the kidney, in Edwards KDG (ed): Drugs Affecting Kidney Function and Metabolism. Basel, S. Karger, 1972, p 285

Schreiner GE: Toxic nephropathy due to drugs solvents and metals, in Edwards KDG (ed): Drugs Affecting Kidney Function and Metabolism. Basel, S. Karger, 1972, p 248

POLYCYSTIC RENAL DISEASE

Michael J. Hanley

Polycystic renal disease (PRD) is a hereditary disorder with two distinct subtypes. The adult form of the disorder is a relatively common condition transmitted in an autosomal dominant pattern generally resulting in renal insufficiency in middle age. The infantile form of the disorder is a rare disease transmitted in an autosomal recessive pattern generally resulting in renal insufficiency in childhood. In each subtype there is clinical and morphologic heterogeneity.

Not all renal cysts constitute PRD. The classification of cysts leans strongly on morphologic and radio-

logic observations. Some cystic abnormalities are developmental and others acquired; some are heritable and others sporadic. Cysts can and do arise at any time during life, they can arise in any part of a nephron, and they can be characterized as harmless or destructive.

A cyst is defined as a cavity lined with epithelium and filled with fluid or semisolid material. The other cystic disorders are usually easily separable from PRD. Renal dysplasia is a developmental defect associated with ureteral and lower urinary tract obstruction. Renal cortical cysts are not heritable. Medullary, extraparenchymal, and miscellaneous cystic disorders are usually easily separated from PRD. PRD is a hereditary disorder with diffuse involvement of both kidneys.

Genitically, PRD is an autosomal dominant disorder with a high degree of penetrance which approaches 100 percent in the eighth and ninth decades of life. The lack of a family history in a large number of cases suggests that there exists a relatively high rate of spontaneous mutations. The disease is relatively uncommon in blacks, and there is a strong association with other heritable conditions, such as myotonic dystrophy, Peutz-Jeghers syndrome, and spherocytosis.

Except for its genetic transmission, the etiology of PRD and the cause of the cyst formation is unknown. There is no evidence that the disorder represents a developmental or continuing metabolic abnormality. Obstruction does not appear to play a role early in the evolution of the disease, but secondary tubular obstruction may contribute to the formation of cysts in the later stages. In the U.S., PRD is the third most common cause of renal failure in adults, accounting for 6 percent of endstage renal disease.

Infantile PRD refers to a group of rare hereditary disorders that occur primarily in childhood but that can affect older children and adults. All forms are transmitted by an autosomal inheritance, and all forms are accompanied by hepatic abnormalities. The essential renal lesion appears to be enlargement of the cortical collecting tubules with cellular hyperplasia. The evidence points to an abnormality acquired later in gestation, perhaps on previously normal nephrons and ducts. It has been suggested that tubular injury occurs initially and that the cyst formation is predominantly a response of the immature kidney. Even if this hypothesis is true, the cause of the initial tubular injury and the nature of its perpetuation remains unclear. In the infantile disease the presence of associated hepatic dysfunction and recessive inheritance suggests a generalized enzyme defect.

The adult form of PRD is characterized by (1) recognition after the second decade, (2) bilateral distribution, (3) positive family history, (4) cysts of varying sizes scattered through both kidneys, (5) progressive renal failure, and (6) cystic liver in one-third of patients. The earliest and most common symptom of PRD is lumbar pain or heaviness, which preceeds the development of flank masses and renal impairment. The pain may be severe if caused by sudden cyst rupture, intracystic hemorrhage, or infection. Colicky pain usually represents obstruction secondary to stone formation. Hematuria can also be a presenting symptom. Gross hematuria is usually caused by cyst rupture into the renal pelvis, but microscopic hematuria is the more common initial finding. Hypertension is a frequent feature of PRD, although this usually occurs later in the course of the disease. Proteinuria is usually encountered in patients with PRD, but cases of nephrotic syndrome are rare. Urinary examination in asymptomatic patients characteristically shows an inability to maximally concentrate the urine with mild proteinuria and hematuria.

The most common clinical expression of infantile PRD is large kidneys and oliguria in the newborn. Despite neonatal oliguria, death from renal failure is unusual. Some infants have enlarged livers, and hepatic involvement with infantile PRD is the rule. Renal insufficiency begins early in childhood, but its progression is variable. Urinalysis proteinuria, RBCs, and WBCs without apparent infection. Laboratory findings are those of chronic renal failure, with hypertension and congestive heart failure being characteristic in the course of the disease. Progressive hepatic disease in older children with mild or inapparent renal involvement is sometimes regarded as a separate disease, but the point is unclear. The one characteristic radiologic finding in older infants, children, and adults with this disorder is medullary ducta ectasia. This radiologic pattern is indistinguishable from medullary sponge kidney but separable on the basis of age, incidence, and clinical implications. Infantile PRD is usually fatal in childhood, but there are some instances of prolonged survival.

Pathologic examination of polycystic kidneys shows them to be grossly enlarged but not overly deformed (Fig. 1). The kidneys usually contain numerous irregularly clustered small cysts in childhood, but adults show hundreds of larger, scattered cysts of varying sizes. The cysts usually contain a yellow fluid, but some may be filled with blood or pus. Scaring and adhesions from repeated bouts of infection are also characteristic. On cut sections the cysts are found throughout the renal parenchyma and vary in size from 1 mm to more than 5 cm. Microdissections in adult kidneys have shown that cysts may arise in any part of the nephron. Tubular cysts usually communicate with the nephron, although occasional cysts may lack luminal connection. Glomerular cysts are often noncommunicating. On microscopic examination the cysts are found to be lined with a single layer of epithelium, and interstitial fibroses are usually encountered in the renal parenchyma (Fig. 2). In PRD cysts are frequently found in other organs. Hepatic involvement occurs in one-third of the cases, but portal hypertension is rare. Aneurysms of the cerebral arteries are found in 10–20 percent of autopsied patients with polycystic kidneys. Cysts have also been reported in the pancreas, spleen, thyroid, and ovary.

Whether the cysts are acquired through the action of some toxin or are developmental in origin remains an open question. The cysts appear to be massively

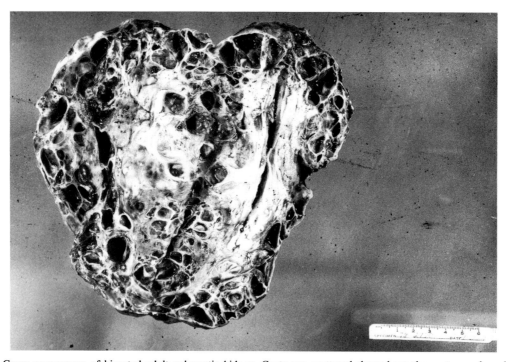

Fig. 1. Gross appearance of bisected adult polycystic kidney. Cysts are scattered throughout the cortex and medulla with marked distortion of the renal architecture.

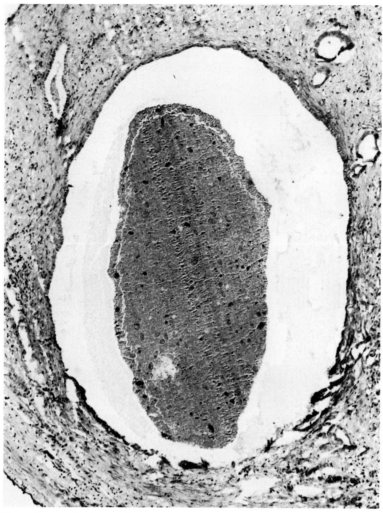

Fig. 2. Photomicrograph of a cyst from an adult with polycystic renal disease. Note the lining of the cyst cavity by a single layer of cuboidal epithelium. The cyst cavity is filled with semisolid proteinaceous material.

distended nephron segments and can arise from any portion of the nephron. How the cysts grow is unknown, but the fluid accumulation could arise from glomerular filtration and/or fluid secretion into the cysts. Obstruction of the nephrons does not seem to play a role, since the hydrostatic pressure in the cyst does not appear to be greater than in adjacent nephrons. Whether or not abnormally distendible basement membranes are the cause of dilitation is not known. Diphenylamine and diphenylthiazole, when administered to adult rats, cause cysts to develop. In micropuncture studies it was shown that the hydrostatic pressure in the cystic tubules was the same as normal nephrons, that salt and water reabsorption was normal, and that there was no distal obstruction to urine flow. These findings suggest that cysts develop as a consequence of aberrant structural derangements of the basement membrane, but no abnormalities were found on electron microscopic study of this structive. The acquired nature of the tubular defect is inferred by the fact that the renal cysts

disappeared when the drugs were removed from the diet. The diagnosis of polycystic renal disease rests on the physical examination, the family history, and especially on the radiographic findings (Fig. 3). Intravenous pyelography with nephrotomograms will usually demonstrate the characteristic findings of PRD. Expansion of the renal cortex, displacement of the calyces, and individual cysts can usually be easily identified in the affected patients. Contrast studies should be cautiously performed in polycystic patients with hyperuricemia, since renal failure has been reported secondary to uric acid crystalization. Isotopic studies and ultrasound have been utilized in the diagnosis of PRD, but to date the direct contrast studies remain the "gold standard." Retrograde pyelography, in general, should not be used in the diagnosis of PRD, the only exception being a high index of suspicion that obstruction by stone, clot, or tumor is present.

In the early stages of the disease renal function is usually normal despite the appearance of multiple cysts

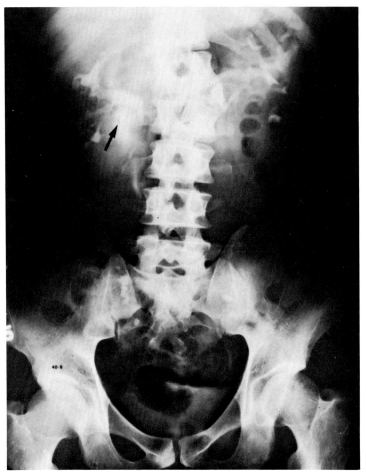

Fig. 3. X-ray contrast study from an adult with polycystic renal disease. Note the distorted architecture and the extrapelvic collection of contrast material (arrow).

on contrast study. Mild proteinuria and microscopic hematuria are frequently observed, but glycosuria is not a feature of PRD. It has been reported that asymptomatic patients with PRD have an inability to normally concentrate the urine despite a normal creatinine clearance. The test may prove to be a useful screening procedure for family members of affected individuals but is certainly not diagnostic. Hyperuricemia and erythrocytosis can be observed in patients with PRD. The cause and incidence of the hyperuricemia is unknown, but the erythrocytosis is due presumably to increased erythropoietin production.

There is no specific treatment for patients with PRD. Management in general should be conservative and individualized. Mild hypertension should be managed with Aldomet or propranolol, if possible. Severe hypertension should be treated aggressively with combination drug therapy, including diuretics. Infection is a problem in patients with PRD. This is due primarily to the difficulty encountered in treating infected cysts, since antibiotics have difficulty in penetrating the cyst cavity. Attempts must be made to avoid urinary tract

infections, and they should be treated aggressively for prolonged periods if they occur. Renal hemorrhage and gross hematuria usually responds to bedrest and sedation. Persistent or massive hemorrhage should suggest renal stone or tumor. Rapid enlargement or rupture of cysts can occasionally resemble peritonitis. When renal failure eventually occurs, dialysis and transplantation become the modes of therapy. To the patient on dialysis the remnant polycystic kidney usually represents a mixed blessing. On one hand, cysts have the potential to become infected, but on the other, the remnant frequently excretes relatively large volumes of urine, reducing the need for ultrafiltration, and produces erythropoietin, which lessens the severity of anemia. These considerations become especially important if the patient is a candidate for transplantation. If the patient is to receive a living related donor allograft, bilateral nephrectomy is usually performed prior to transplantation.

Recipients of cadaver kidneys will undergo nephrectomy if these patients have large kidneys, bacteriuria, or multiple episodes of urinary tract infection. Patients with small kidneys and no difficulty with infection are usually not nephrectomized prior to cadaveric transplantation. At the present time there is no evidence that polycystic disease recurs in the cadaveric transplant.

REFERENCES

Berstein J: The classification of renal cysts. Nephron 11:91, 1973

Berstein J: A classification of renal cysts, in Bardner KD Jr (ed): Cystic Diseases of the Kidney. New York, John Wiley & Sons, 1976

Bernstein J: Polycystic disease, in Edelman CM Jr (ed): Pediatric Kidney Disease, vol 2. Boston, Little, Brown, 1978

Carone FA, Rowland RG, Perlman SG, et al: The pathogenesis of drug-induced renal cystic disease. Kidney Int 5:411, 1974

Comfort MW, Gray HK, Dahlin DC, et al: Polycystic disease of the liver: A study of 24 cases. Gastroenterology 20:60, 1952

Grantham JJ: Polycystic renal disease, in Earley LE, Gottschalk CW (eds): Strauss and Welt's Diseases of the Kidney, vol 2. Boston, Little, Brown, 1979

MEDULLARY CYSTIC DISEASE

Michael J. Hanley

Medullary cystic disease (MCD) is a disorder characterized by multiple cysts in the renal medulla and the insidious onset of anemia and uremia, usually becoming clinically manifest in the third decade of life. Familial juvenile nephronophthisis (FJN) is a childhood renal disease characterized by polyuria, growth failure, and progressive renal failure. Medullary cysts are found in the great majority of the patients. Although morphologically and clinically similar, the diseases may be separable on the basis of age of onset and genetic transmission. MCD usually expresses itself in young adulthood and appears in many cases to be an autosomal dominant disorder. The genetics of MCD is complicated by the relatively high incidence of supposed new dominant mutations producing the renal defect. FJN is an autosomal recessive disorder characterized by onset in childhood and the occasional association of nonrenal abnormalities. For many years the similarities between the two disorders were not recognized, and care should therefore be exercised in reviewing older literature on MCD and FJN. MCD was the entity commonly referred to in the American literature, while FJN was emphasized in the European literature. It has become increasingly clear in recent years that macroscopic cysts are not present in all cases but that microscopic cysts and cystic dilitations are usually present in both conditions.

MCD affects young adults, with no sexual predilection. The most common presenting manifestations are those of chronic uremia. The anemia is normochromic and normocytic and in most instances is proportional to the degree of renal insufficiency present. There are some isolated reports of anemia not explainable by the renal insufficiency, but these have not been well characterized. The earliest manifestations observed by otherwise asymptomatic patients are polyuria and nocturia reflecting an inability to concentrate the urine. The childhood form (FJN) accounts for two-thirds of the reported cases, and a history of consanguinity is usually present. In general, evidence for an abnormality in heterozygous carriers is inconclusive, although a concentrating defect has been documented in some unaffected parents and siblings of documented cases. The ratio of unaffected to affected siblings seems unexpectedly high in many family studies, but this may merely reflect a literature bias of reporting cases with an especially good family history. The pathogenesis of the disorder is entirely unknown. The primary renal defect appears to be in the distal nephron. Evidence for this supposition rests on observations in patients who have not progressed to renal insufficiency. Some of these patients exhibit urinary concentrating defects and distal acidification defects. Disordered proximal tubular function (glycosuria or aminoaciduria) is not characteristic in this syndrome. It is assumed that the genetic abnormality brings about progressive tubular damage which results in secondary glomerular and interstitial damage. The disease has not been reported to recur in transplanted kidneys, which is evidence against a circulating nephrotoxic agent.

The clinical features of MCD–FJN are similar. Children generally present with growth retardation in addition to the polyuria, polydypsia, anemia, and azotemia seen in adult patients. The renal concentrating defect occurs independently of renal failure, but definitive data about the specific nature of the tubular defect are generally lacking because the majority of the patients are first seen because of renal insufficiency. Two-thirds of the patients exhibit salt wasting but persistent hypokalemia and defective acidification have also been reported in a smaller percentage of cases. The urinalysis is only minimally abnormal, with the most common finding being low-grade proteinuria. Blood pressure is normal except in patients with substantial renal insufficiency. Bone changes and growth retardation are usually manifested only when young children are severely affected. Laboratory data generally reflect only chronic renal insufficiency (i.e., increased BUN, serum creatinine, and serum phosphorus and decreased serum calcium and bicarbonate). Anemia is invariably present, and the alkaline phosphatase is generally elevated in children. Physical examination is unremarkable unless signs of uremia are present. Radiologic studies have added little to our understanding of the disorder. This is due in part to the advanced state of renal insufficiency at the time of initial evaluation. Intravenous pyelography and renal arteriograms generally only show small shrunken kidneys with a thin cortex and diminished blood flow. Cysts appear as lucencies in the neph. graphic phase of the study.

At autopsy the kidneys are small with a thin cortex. The unique pathologic feature of this disorder is the presence of multiple cysts usually located in the outer cortex just below the corticomedullory junction. Renal biopsies early in the disease may show little or no specific change. The characteristic morphologic abnormality in advanced cases is tubular atrophy out of proportion to glomerular damage. The striking medullary cysts are located within the distal convoluted tubules and collecting ducts. These cysts do freely communicate with other portions of the nephron. The cysts are lined with a flattened epithelium and sometimes contain scanty amorphous eosinophilic material. In cases of MCD identified because of sibling involvement, cysts are not invariably present. The absence of cysts in some cases demonstrates that medullary cysts are not necessary for the full expression of the disorder. Pathologic examination of the renal blood vessels shows no specific changes, but the interstitium does show leukocytic infiltration and gives the appearance of a chronic pyelonephritis.

The differential diagnosis of MCD includes all forms of chronic renal failure. The evaluation of a patient with azotemia, anemia, and a concentrating defect is by no means specific for MCD unless a family history or pathologic material is also available. Autosomal recessive polycystic disease (see the preceding chapter) is a disorder which affects older children and adults with varying degrees of renal impairment and is definitely another consideration in many instances. MCD can usually be differentaited from medullary sponge kidney (see the following chapter) because the latter disorder generally produces no renal functional impairment but does frequently produce nephrocalcinosis and nephrolithiasis, which are uncharacteristic of MCD.

There is no known method of preventing progression of renal failure in MCD. Salt wasting and acidosis require appropriate amounts of NaCl and $NaHCO_3$. Renal failure is managed by dialysis, and the patients are candidates for transplantation. It goes without saying that care must be exercised in the selection of living related donors.

The prognosis is uniformly poor. The average time span between clinical recognition and renal failure is 4 years, with no difference between the recessive and dominant disease.

REFERENCES

Bernstein J, Gardner KD Jr: Familial juvenile nephronophthisis—Medullary cystic disease, in Edelmann CM (ed): Pediatric Kidney Disease. Boston, Little, Brown, 1978
Gardner KD Jr: The medullary cystic diseases: The nephronophthisis–cystic renal medulla complex and medullary sponge kidney, in Early LE, Gottschalk CW (eds): Strauss and Welt's Diseases of the Kidney (ed 3). Boston, Little, Brown, 1979

MEDULLARY SPONGE KIDNEY

Michael J. Hanley

Medullary sponge kidney (MSK) is a renal cystic disorder characterized by dilatation of the collecting ducts and cyst formation in the medullary inner papillary pyramids. Histologic changes do not extend beyond the corticomedullary junction. As far as can be ascertained, MSK is entirely asymptomatic unless accompanied by complications of passage of or obstruction by stones or by the development of pyelonephritis. Whether or not hematuria occurs in the absense of stones remains unknown. The true incidence of the disorder is unknown because the diagnosis is dependent on intravenous pyelography, which is unlikely to be performed in asymptomatic cases. The data available seem to indicate no sexual, racial, or familial preponderance. Most reported cases of MSK occur sporadically, but the characteristic radiologic appearance has also been reported in other hereditable disorders, including polycystic liver disease.

MSK is most certainly a developmental defect, although the exact nature of such a defect is unclear. Sometime during development, ductal arborizations become dilated and undergo a cystic transformation. This view is supported by the few cases followed serially over many years, but it cannot be proved because of the absence of information in the newborn.

The diagnosis of MSK is largely dependent on radiologic examination, often performed for evaluation of nephrolithiasis or pyelonephritis. On plain films the characteristic features are enlargement of one or both kidneys (33 percent of cases) and the presence of a variable number of radiopaque calculi. On intravenous pyelography the density of contrast material is normal (in the absense of pyelonephritis or hydronephrosis), with the early appearance and delayed emptying of contrast medium filled cavities (Fig. 1). The cavities are confined to the papillary pyramids, producing enlargement of the involved pyramids and corresponding calyces. Retrograde pyelography seldom reveals as many cavities as intravenous pyelography. Reports of long-term followup indicate that the pattern of changes in individual cases tends to remain constant. In instances in which changes do occur, they appear to be the result of complications, infection, or obstruction due to stone formation. Although the collecting system appearance remains constant, there is an increase in size and number of calculi with time in 50 percent of patients with this disorder.

The gross and microscopic appearance of the uncomplicated case is characteristic. The kidneys are normal to moderately enlarged. The lesions are limited to the pyramids, which are enlarged and which bulge into the calyces. The papillary region shows varying number of cavities filled with semiliquid material and calculi. Microscopically there is dilatation of collecting ducts, cysts connected to tubules, and isolated cysts. Stones are most often apatite, and the cysts are lined

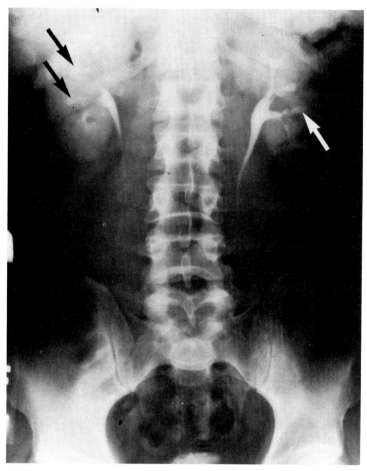

Fig. 1. Medullary sponge kidney during pyelography. Dye filled cavities are seen in all papillae.

with transitional epithelium. The histologic changes of pyelonephritis are found in cases with this complication.

The diagnosis of MSK is made by demonstration of the characteristic radiologic appearance together with the exclusion of other developmental or familial renal cystic disease and acquired renal disease associated with medullary cavitation. Other renal cystic diseases can usually be easily eliminated by their clinical course, i.e., renal function impairment. Calyceal diverticula, pyelonephritic cysts, and papillary necrosis can usually be differentiated by other radiologic criteria. Renal TB can mimic MSK, but the cavitary lesions need not be confined to the medulla in renal tuberculosis. Urine culture, chest x-ray, and skin testing are mandatory in all cases to rule out this potentially treatable renal lesion in someone suspected of having MSK. Nephrocalcinosis can also have various etiologies (renal tubular acidosis, hyperparathyroidism, etc.), and these should also be excluded.

Since uncomplicated cases are asymptomatic, no therapy is required. In those cases complicated by hematuria, nephrolithiasis, or pyelonephritis, conservative management is in order, since the disease is bilateral and all attempts must be made to preserve renal function. In uncomplicated cases renal function is

generally normal, but some reduction in concentrating ability and impaired net acid excretion have been reported and probably reflect medullary damage secondary to complications of the disease.

REFERENCES

Ekstrom T, Engfeldt B, Lagergren C, et al: Medullary sponge kidney, in: Proceedings of the third International Congress of Nephrology, Washington, D.C., vol. 2. Basel, S. Karger, 1966, p 54

Hayslett JP: Medullary sponge kidney, in Edelman CM (ed): Pediatric Kidney Disease. Boston, Little, Brown, 1978

Strauss MB: Microcystic disease of the renal medulla, in Strauss MB, Welt LG (eds): Diseases of the Kidney (ed 2). Boston, Little, Brown, 1971

ALPORT'S SYNDROME (HEREDITARY NEPHRITIS)

Thomas A. Golper and William M. Bennett

Alport first noted the association of hereditary nephritis with deafness in 1927. In 1954 lens defects were added to the syndrome, making a triad of associated abnormalities. Hereditary nephritis probably encompasses several distinct clinical entities related only in the sense that they are familial. Evaluations of small pedigrees and nonuniform identifying criteria explain the inexactness of the arbitrary term, hereditary nephritis. Since the basic membrane defects and genetics are not yet understood, there is no certainty that hereditary nephritis is pathogenetically and/or genetically homogeneous.

INCIDENCE AND GENETICS

About 2 percent of all glomerulopathies are ultimately diagnosed as hereditary nephritis. The true sex ratio of involvement is important for understanding the genetic transmission. Unfortunately, male predominance, equal incidence, and 2:1 female predominance have all been observed. The 2:1 female predominant ratio reported by O'Neill and colleagues is from the largest kindred studied. There is general agreement that males have more severe phenotypic expression. Affected males appear to have a low incidence of affected sons. Affected females often have an excess of both affected sons and affected daughters. Therefore dominant transmission seems certain.

Three genetic theories have active proponents: (1) partial sex (X)-linked dominant, (2) autosomal dominant with reduced genetic penetrance in males and an unfavorable intrauterine environment in affected mothers which increases the gene penetrance in their sons as compared to their daughters, and (3) autosomal dominant with the mutant gene-bearing chromosome preferentially segregating with the X chromosome.

Again, more than one explanation may be valid, since so many variants have been described. Furthermore, Shaw and Kallen postulate that 18 percent of all newborns heterozygous with the Alport syndrome genotype may be new mutants. As the therapy for endstage renal disease enhances survivorship and reproductive performance, population dynamics will be influenced and more exact genetic understanding may be achieved.

PATHOGENESIS

Spear explains the disorder through a structural gene abnormality that governs the composition of basement membrane collagen. The nephropathy may be the result of phenotypes reflecting genetic heterogeneity, explaining why some kindreds are clinically different. The glomerular basement membrane (GBM) as well as the basement membranes of the lens capsule, tectorial membrane of the organ of Corti, and Descemet's membrane have very similar biochemical composition, characterized by the presence of large amounts of hydroxylysine, hydroxyproline, and glycine as well as disulfide bonds.

Alternatively, an immune pathogenesis can be postulated. Despite the frequently negative serological studies and glomerular immunofluorescence, several lines of evidence prevent the exclusion of an immunological pathogenesis. Miyoshi and colleagues have noted an unusually high incidence of antithyroid antibodies in patients with Alport's syndrome and in their unaffected relatives. The ultrastructural lesion of the GBM has features consistent with resorption of immune deposits. Specifically, electron-dense granulations of 500 Å are seen within the GBM. Halo-like clear areas around the particles have an appearance similar to resolving immune deposits being incorporated in GBM, as is seen in membranous glomerulopathy or resolving poststreptococcal glomerulonephritis. Also, C3 degradation factor has been observed frequently in hereditary nephritis.

CLINICAL AND LABORATORY FINDINGS

The clinical presentation varies with the kindred. The disease usually begins in childhood or adolescence and appears earlier in males. Microscopic hematuria, occurring in 80–100 percent of individuals, may be intermittent or constant. Gross hematuria may be seen following exercise, nonspecific upper respiratory infections, ingestion of certain foods or spontaneously. There is no special relationship to streptococcal infections. Red blood cell casts are seen in 18 percent of cases. Mild intermittent proteinuria occurs in 40–100 percent and, with time, becomes persistent. Proteinuria has been reported only in the presence of hematuria. Nephrotic syndrome may occur and, in some kindreds, occurs in over half the affected cases. Sterile pyuria is quite variable but important in that infectious pyelonephritis may supervene and aggravate the condition. Progressive renal failure develops until endstage renal disease is reached, usually between the ages of 25 and 40 years. The later the initial presentation of symptoms, the better the prognosis and clinical course. Hypertension is not a prominent feature, but a mild form is a usual late finding.

Bilateral symmetrical sensory nerve deafness can often be the first symptom. Between 0 and 100 percent of patients have deafness, the overall incidence being about 35 percent. Some kindreds demonstrate a parallel severity of renal disease and deafness, while in others there is no clear relationship. The incidence, rapidity of progression, and severity of deafness is generally greater in males. Frequently, only an audiometric examination reveals a hearing deficit in affected females. Audiograms are flat (12 percent), trough shaped (47 percent), or sloping to a more severe loss in the higher frequencies (41 percent). Deafness can occur as an isolated finding or in association with renal disease.

Fifteen percent of the affected patients suffer from some form of ocular disease (spherophakia, lenticonus, myopia, retinitis pigmentosa, other macular lesions, nystagmus, amaurosis, and, most commonly, polar cataracts). Ocular lesions, too, are more frequently and are more severe in males. Families with ocular disease have a higher incidence of renal disease and deafness, but any of the three disorders may appear singly.

Some kindreds have been described with involvement of organs other than the eyes, ears, and kidneys. The disorders include thrombocytopathia, hyperprolinemia, aminoaciduria, cerebral dysfunction, iliac horns, skin changes, polyneuropathies, erythromelalgia, Charcot-Marie-Tooth syndrome, and skeletal abnormalities.

There is probably great clinical and pathological heterogeneity in these various clinical entities, and their relationship with each other is doubtful.

Laboratory evaluations for immunologic or urologic abnormalities are consistently negative, except for C3 degradation factor.

There is an increased incidence of toxemia, prematurity, and spontaneous abortion in affected mothers. Exacerbated nephritis during pregnancy is described.

PATHOLOGY
Gross

Early gross pathologic changes include the absence of pyelonephritic scarring and the presence of yellow linear cortical streaks (foam cells) in cut section. Later shrunken and atrophic kidneys are seen with a decrease in foam cell streaking.

Light Microscopy

Most of the pathologic changes seen by light microscopy are nonspecific. Early in the course of the disease there may be no abnormalities. Principal glomerular features beginning focally and segmentally include mesangial cell proliferation and swelling, increase in mesangial matrix, and thickened glomerular capillary basement membranes. The GBM may thicken up to four times its normal dimension. Silver stains reveal GBM splitting. Capsular adhesions and periglomerular fibrosis occur with progression, as segmental sclerosis advances to diffuse global sclerosis. Crescent formation may be noted, but inflammatory cells and fibrinoid necrosis rarely occur in glomeruli. Red blood cells can be seen in Bowman's space and tubular lumina.

The tubulointerstitium shows changes of varying degrees. Seen earliest are focal tubular atrophy alternating with discrete dilatation and hypertrophy of cortical tubules. These alterations worsen with renal failure and become the predominant lesion, with fibrosis and inflammatory cell infiltration, resembling chronic interstitial nephritis. Tubular basement membrane (TBM) splitting is seen. Small arteries show intimal thickening and arteriosclerosis. This combination of glomerular disease and tubulointerstitial involvement lead to the histopathologic description as a "mixed" nephritis.

Normal tubules are intermixed with tubules composed of parallel rows of lipid-containing foam cells (large cells with pale foamy cytoplasm) which produce the linear streaks seen grossly. The quantity, distribution, and consistency of foam cells, rather than just their presence, make them suggestive of this disorder. They are particularly prominent in the interstitium near the corticomedullary junction, but they may appear anywhere. Their staining properties indicate that they contain neutral fat, mucopolysacchride, phospholipid, cholesterol ester, and phosphatides. Some correlation may exist between TBM thickening and foam cell presence. An abundance of foam cells roughly correlates with extensive GBM alterations. Foam cells are seldom seen in either the very early or endstage disease.

Foam cells have been absent in some cases of hereditary nephritis and have been observed in other nonhereditary nephropathies. Foam cells of Fabry's disease and xanthogranulomatous pyelonephritis appear quite similar. They have also been seen in nephrotic syndrome, chronic glomerulonephritis, pyelonephritis, Fanconi's syndrome, Wegener's granulomatosis, diabetes mellitus, and renal abscess.

The foam cells are thought to be altered tubular epithelial cells, histiocytes, or fibroblasts. It is possible that the glomerular capillary wall abnormality might allow filtration of smaller cholesterol-ester-containing α lipoproteins which are subsequently reabsorbed in the tubule and accumulated in the TBM and foam cells.

Immunofluorescence

Immunofluorescence of renal tissue is negative for immunoglobulins. Occasionally C3 may be focally deposited irregularly in the mesangium.

Electron Microscopy

Electron microscopic examination of capillary and tubular basement membranes is the most reliable method to establish a tissue diagnosis (Fig. 1). The earliest changes are focal, irregularly alternating attentuation and thickening of the GBM. The lamina densa is split and laminated into a heterogeneous network of cloudy material and membranoid strands enclosing clear electron-lucent areas which may contain 500 Å granulations. Similar lesions are seen in the basement membranes of Bowman's capsule and tubular cells. Mesangial cell proliferation is seen, but electron-dense deposits are absent. Focal, but occasionally extensive, foot process fusion is observed even in the absence of significant proteinuria. Accumulation of lipid-like material occurs in tubular cell cytoplasm.

Hill, Jenis, and Goodloe stress that the basement membrane alterations are not unique to hereditary nephritis and are seen to a lesser extent in poststreptococcal glomerulonephritis, IgG–IgA nephropathy, focal glomerulosclerosis, and lipoid nephrosis. GBM attenuation is a frequent finding in benign recurrent familial hematuria, albeit in a different pattern.

These typical electron microscopic lesions have been associated with a poorer prognosis, i.e., progressive nephritis. When they are seen in one family member they are almost always seen in relatives. Since these lesions begin focally, they may be missed in early biopsies. Serial biopsies have shown progression of GBM splitting despite a stable clinical status. Endstage hereditary nephritis has been reported in the absence of these "typical" lesions.

Ear Pathology

Pathological ear changes include degeneration or atrophy of cochlear neuroepithelial structures such as outer hair cells, a decrease in spiral ganglion cells of the basal cochlear turn, spongy vesicular changes involving the spinal ligament, and foam cells in the endolymphatic sac.

DIFFERENTIAL DIAGNOSIS

Variations of hereditary nephritis with other features have been mentioned. Benign recurrent familial hematuria presents in children but is not progressive,

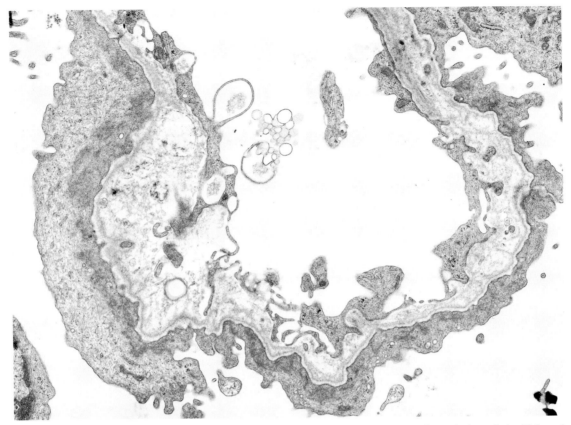

Fig. 1. Glomerular capillary from a patient with hereditary nephritis. The basement membrane is irregularly thickened and split into multiple thin layers separated by electron-lucent spaces containing granular and vacuolar debris. Most endothelial fenestrations are closed, and the epithelial foot processes have collapsed to form a nearly continuous layer over the basement membrane. Original magnification × 14,600.

and attenuation of the GBM is diffuse. Other hereditary conditions associated with hematuria, proteinuria, and azotemia include Fabry's disease, nail-patella syndrome, sickle-cell disease, partial lipodystrophy, polycystic kidney disease, medullary cystic kidney disease, amyloidosis, diabetes mellitus, and familial Mediterranean fever (see the following chapter).

TREATMENT

Recurrent, then persistent hematuria occurs for years before slowly progressive renal failure ensues. No form of therapy slows progression. Prompt aggressive therapy for urinary tract or ear infections is critical. Avoidance of pregnancy may be wise. Renal dialysis and transplantation have been successfully utilized. Stabilization of progressive hearing loss after successful transplantation is reported. Recurrence of disease in the allograft has not been seen. Corneal transplants and lens extraction are available for ocular involvement, but no relief is available for the hearing loss.

REFERENCES

Grünfeld JP, Bois EP, Hinglais N: Progressive and non-progressive hereditary chronic nephritis. Kidney Int 4:216, 1973

Heptinstall RH: Hereditary nephritis, in: Pathology of the Kidney (ed 2). Boston, Little, Brown, 1974

Hill GS, Jenis EH, Goodloe S: The nonspecificity of the ultrastructural alternatives in hereditary nephritis. Lab Invest 31:516, 1974

O'Neill WM, Atkin CL, Bloomer HA: Hereditary nephritis: A reexamination of its critical and genetic features. Ann Intern Med 88:176, 1978

Perkoff GT: Hereditary chronic nephritis, in Strauss MB, Welt LG (eds): Diseases of the Kidney (ed 2). Boston, Little, Brown, 1971

Purriel P, Drets M, Pascale E, et al: Familial hereditary nephropathy (Alport's syndrome). Am J Med 49:753, 1970

Spear GS: Alport's syndrome: A consideration of pathogenesis. Clin Nephrol 1:336, 1973

OTHER HEREDITARY NEPHRITIDES

Charles E. Plamp, III and William M. Bennett

Hereditofamilial diseases are a major cause of endstage renal disease. With inclusion of such disorders as diabetes mellitus and polycystic kidney disease, hereditofamilial disease probably accounts for as much as 20 percent of patients in chronic hemodialysis programs.

Table 1 lists the major inherited renal diseases. This chapter covers those entities which are not discussed in detail elsewhere in this volume.

PRIMARY RENAL DISORDERS
Asphyxiating Thoracic Dystrophy (Jeune's Syndrome)

This syndrome, which is usually lethal in the first years of life, is characterized by hypoplasia of the thorax with short ribs, variable degrees of limb shortening, and polydactyly. Inheritance is autosomal recessive. Some children may survive to develop renal abnormalities including proteinuria, proximal-type renal tubular acidosis, uricosuria, and glycosuria. Tubular abnormalities may precede decreases in glomerular filtration rate. Hypertension is common, and progressive renal disease can be fatal. Histologically, there is interstitial fibrosis, tubular atrophy and dilatation, and focal glomerular sclerosis with mesangial thickening. Pathogenesis is unknown. There is no known treatment, but successful renal transplantation has been reported.

Congenital Nephrotic Syndrome

Congenital nephrotic syndrome is a rare disease accounting for less than 1.5 percent of all cases of childhood nephrotic syndrome. The incidence is higher in Finland and in individuals of Finnish extraction. Inheritance is thought to be autosomal recessive. The disease characteristically presents shortly after birth or in the first 4 months of life with massive proteinuria. Parents are free of disease, and the mother's pregnancy is uncomplicated. The placenta is usually very large, and these children typically have low birthweights. Both sexes are equally affected. Azotemia and hypertension are rare. Laboratory features include microscopic hematuria and changes typical of nephrotic syndrome, except that serum cholesterol remains normal until the terminal stages. Grossly, the renal cortex has a microcystic appearance due to dilatation of proximal tubules, and glomeruli may be normal by light microscopy. Electron microscopy shows only foot process fusion. Immunofluorescence is usually negative, although immunoglobulin and complement deposition have been reported. The pathophysiology is unknown but may involve abnormal glomerular basement membrane metabolism. There is no known treatment for the disease. Steroids and immunosuppressives are of no benefit. The prognosis is poor, with death usually in the first year of life due to complications of nephrotic syndrome, infection, or, rarely, uremia. This entity should not be confused with congenital syphilis, malaria, cytomegalovirus infection, or toxoplasmosis, which may also present with early nephrotic syndrome.

Laurence-Moon-Biedl Syndrome

This is an autosomal, recessively inherited syndrome characterized by retinitis pigmentosa, polydactyly, obesity, hypogonadism, mental retardation, and a high incidence of structural genitourinary tract lesions including hydroureter, hydronephrosis, and hypoplasia. Uremia has been shown to be the cause of death in approximately one-third of cases in recent series, although renal disease has not usually been considered

Table 1
Hereditary Disorders Involving the Kidney

Primary renal disorders
  Alport's syndrome*
  Asphyxiating thoracic dystrophy (Jeune's syndrome)
  Congenital nephrotic syndrome
  Laurence-Moon-Biedl syndrome
  Medullary cystic disease*
  Medullary sponge kidney*
  Nail-patella syndrome
  Nephrogenic diabetes insipidus
  Polycystic renal disease*
Systemic disorders with secondary renal involvement
  Diabetes mellitus*
  Familial mediterranean fever
  Partial lipodystrophy
  Sickle cell anemia
Inborn errors of metabolism with renal involvement
  Fabry's disease
  Fanconi's syndromes†
  Hereditary oxalosis
  Other tubular transport disorders†

*See the chapter so titled.
†See the chapter on *Transport Disorders*.

part of the syndrome. In addition to the structural lesions previously noted, radiologic studies have demonstrated multiple cystic spaces communicating with the collecting system. In addition, nephrosclerosis and chronic glomerulonephritis have been described. The exact pathogenesis of the renal disease is unknown.

Nail-Patella Syndrome (Hereditary Onychoosteodysplasia)

The nail-patella syndrome is transmitted as an autosomal dominant trait closely linked to the ABO blood group locus and is characterized by dysplasia of the nails, absence or hypoplasia of the patella, accessory posterior iliac horns, and elbow deformities. Between 30 and 50 percent of affected individuals display clinical renal involvement with either proteinuria or abnormal urinary sediment. Progression to endstage renal disease occurs in less than 10 percent of patients. The nephrotic syndrome is occasionally seen. Urinary acidification and concentrating ability has been shown to be normal. Light microscopy in endstage disease generally reveals chronic glomerulonephritis. In nonuremic individuals the pathologic findings range from normal to glomerulosclerosis of varying degrees. Electron microscopy in all individuals affected with skeletal abnormalities, regardless of their urine sediments and renal function, shows a characteristic lesion. There is irregular basement membrane thickening and the presence of intramembranous fibrils with the periodicity of collagen which are considered specific for the disease. Immunofluorescence is variable, occasionally showing focal IgG and C'3 staining.

There is no known treatment, but successful dialysis and transplantation have been reported.

Nephrogenic Diabetes Insipidus

Nephrogenic or vasopressin-resistant diabetes insipidus is usually recognized in early childhood by the characteristic features of polydipsia and polyuria. The basic physiologic defect is distal tubular unresponsiveness to vasopressin. Males are much more commonly affected, but severe disease in females has been reported. The mode of inheritance is controversial. The disease appears to be X linked, but since disease of varying degrees is seen in females, autosomal dominance with variable penetrance has also been suggested. Most authors favor X linkage with full expression in males and variable expression in heterozygotic females. The disease may go unrecognized in infancy until severe dehydration develops with associated vomiting and seizures. Other features include mental and growth retardation, felt to be due to repeated bouts of hyperosmolality, and hydronephrosis, thought to be secondary to high urine volumes and prolonged voluntary urinary retention. Other aspects of tubular function are normal, and uremia usually does not occur.

Urine volumes can be reduced up to 50 percent by moderate salt restriction and administration of thiazide diuretics. The major beneficial physiologic effect is to induce mild sodium depletion and thus enhance proximal tubular reabsorption.

SYSTEMIC DISORDERS WITH SECONDARY RENAL INVOLVEMENT

Familial Mediterranean Fever

Familial Mediterranean fever (periodic disease) is a syndrome with protean clinical features including recurrent episodes of fever, serositis, synovitis, and erythema. It is inherited as an autosomal recessive trait and is seen mainly in Sephardic and Armenian Jews. Insidious development of secondary amyloidosis is common. Renal failure is the major cause of death in over 50 percent of cases, and the renal disease can sometimes precede the development of the clinical syndrome. Peak incidence of renal involvement is usually in the third decade of life. Renal abnormalities include proteinuria, the severity of which generally correlates with the degree of renal involvement. Once the nephrotic syndrome or azotemia have developed, the prognosis is poor, with an approximately 50 percent per year survival. In patients without evidence of amyloidosis, persistent hematuria with or without proteinuria is common. Histologic findings include changes typical of amyloidosis. Reddish-pink glomerular deposits in the mesangium, peripheral capillary walls, and blood vessels can be highlighted with Congo red staining. On routine light microscopy the glomeruli may appear solidified with eosinophilic material. Electron microscopy reveals the characteristic presence of fine amyloid fibrils in bundles in the basement membrane.

There is no known treatment for the disease. Management with chronic hemodialysis may prolong life comfortably without major technical difficulties.

Partial Lipodystrophy

Partial lipodystrophy is a syndrome consisting of greatly diminished or absent subcutaneous fat. The face and upper extremities are most involved. The disease is manifested in females with onset of lipodystrophy early in life, hirsutism, hyperpigmentation, splenomegaly, and diabetes mellitus.

There is a tendency toward familial aggregation of cases, but the exact mode of inheritance is unknown. Hypertension can also be associated. In addition to the above constellation of findings, there is a characteristic renal lesion consisting of membranoproliferative glomerulonephritis. The renal lesion is usually associated with persistently low serum levels of the third component of complement (C'3) and the presence in the patient's serum of a factor which cleaves C'3 in vitro (C'3 nephritic factor). Renal functional abnormalities most commonly consist of asymptomatic proteinuria or the nephrotic syndrome. Progression to endstage renal disease can occasionally occur. The exact relationship among the hypocomplementuria, presence of C'3 nephritic factor, and lipodystrophy is unknown. Membranoproliferative glomerulonephritis has been shown to be present on renal biopsy even in the absence of clinically evident renal disease.

There is no known treatment for the disease, but renal transplantation has been successful.

Sickle-Cell Anemia

Both sickle-cell disease and trait are associated with several distinct renal abnormalities. The most common manifestation of renal disease is recurrent gross hematuria, which occurs primarily with sickle-cell trait rather than sickle-cell disease. The exact mechanism of the hematuria is unknown but is thought to relate to intravascular sickling in the hypertonic renal medulla. The sickling results in medullary ischemia and destruction of vasculature. Hematuria is painless and usually resolves spontaneously. Prolonged bleeding is best treated conservatively with bedrest, hydration, alkalinization of urine, and diuretics to decrease medullary tonicity. Epsilon aminocaproic acid has been successfully used in severe cases. Besides hematuria, a reduction in renal concentrating ability and acidification are commonly noted.

Distinct from sickle-cell hematuria is the progressive renal disease associated with sickle-cell disease. As the management of sickle-cell disease has improved, allowing more prolonged survival, endstage renal disease has become more common. The overall incidence of renal failure in sickle-cell disease remains low, however. Mild proteinuria and microscopic hematuria are the most common urinary findings. Nephrotic syndrome can occur. Papillary necrosis is frequent but may be clinically silent without decrease in creatinine clearance. Infection complicating papillary necrosis is high. Renal vein thrombosis has been described.

Histologic findings are quite varied, and proliferative, membranoproliferative, and membranous glomerular changes all have been reported. Immune complex disease with antibody to renal tubular epithelial antigen has been described. In addition, light microscopy reveals an increase in overall glomerular size, capillary bed engorgement, hemosiderin deposition, and patchy interstitial fibrosis with tubular atrophy.

In endstage renal disease hemodialysis can be accomplished with no increased incidence of sickle-cell crisis. Indeed, some investigators have noted a decrease in transfusion requirements after the initiation of hemodialysis in this group of patients.

INBORN ERRORS OF METABOLISM WITH RENAL INVOLVEMENT

Fabry's Disease (Angiokeratoma Corporis Diffusum Universale)

Fabry's disease is an inborn error of glycosphingolipid metabolism resulting from deficiency of ceramide trihexosidase. It is inherited as an X-linked trait, with carrier females displaying no clinically important disease. The enzyme deficiency results in the accumulation of ceramide trihexoside in many tissues, including the kidney. The clinical features of disease include the appearance of punctate red-purple papules by the end of the first decade of life. These skin lesions are clustered on the lower trunk, thighs, and scrotum. Associated symptoms are pain or burning sensations in the extremities. Corneal opacities, posterior capsular cataracts, and retinal abnormalities are common. Renal disease is the rule and becomes evident in the second or third decade of life, with endstage disease by the fifth decade. Premature cerebrovascular disease, coronary artery disease, and hypertension are also found. The earliest laboratory findings include the excretion in the urine of large amounts of ceramide trihexoside, and hematuria with mild proteinuria. The urinary sediment may contain red blood cells, white blood cells, hyaline and granular casts, and lipid-containing "foam" cells which display metachromasia with toluidine blue staining. Hyposthenuria and polyuria are commonly seen.

Pathological examination with light microscopy reveals lipid deposition in blood vessels, glomerular epithelial cells, Bowman's capsule, and in the epithelium of Henle's loop and distal convoluted tubule. Electron microscopic examination displays rounded or ellipsoid electron-dense myelin figures in epithelial cells. Immunofluorescence is negative. There is no known treatment except enzyme replacement, which is difficult to achieve. There have been conflicting reports as to whether renal transplantation leads to correction of the metabolic abnormality. Although some reports have been encouraging, renal transplantation at this point must be considered as a treatment for chronic renal failure rather than a means of enzyme replacement.

Fanconi's Syndrome

Fanconi's syndrome, as defined by complex dysfunction of the proximal tubule, is seen in a wide variety of inherited disorders. These include cystinosis, Wilson's disease, Lowe's syndrome, tyrosinemia, hereditary fructose intolerance, vitamin D dependent rickets, and medullary cystic disease. A detailed discussion of the syndrome can be found in the following chapter.

Hereditary Oxalosis

Hereditary oxalosis or primary hyperoxaluria is an inherited disorder of glyoxylate metabolism leading to an increased synthesis and urinary excretion of oxalic acid. There are at least two distinct metabolic abnormalities leading to hyperoxaluria with similar clinical presentations. Both are inherited as autosomal recessive traits. Clinically, the disease presents as recurrent nephrolithiasis, usually before age 5 years. Both sexes are equally affected. Progression to terminal renal failure usually occurs before age 20 years. An acute arthritis is often associated with hereditary oxalosis. Cardiac arrhythmias due to oxalate deposition in the conducting tissue may occur. Laboratory features include a marked increase in the urinary excretion of oxalate. Examination of the kidneys microscopically reveals widespread deposition of intratubular calcium oxalate, with dilation and destruction of tubular cells, and prominent interstitial fibrosis. There is no effective treatment for the disease, and oxalate deposition tends to recur in transplanted kidneys.

REFERENCES

Alleyne GA, Statius Van Eps L, Adae S, et al: The kidney in sickle cell anemia. Kidney Int 7:731, 1975

Ari JB, Zlotnik M, Oren A, et al: Dialysis in renal failure caused by amyloidosis of familial Mediterranean fever. Arch Intern Med 136:449, 1976

Bennett WM, Musgrave JE, Campbell R, et al: The nephropathy of the nail-patella syndrome. Clinicopathologic analysis of eleven kindred. Am J Med 54:304, 1973

Gruskin AB, Baluarte H, Cote M, et al: The renal disease of thoracic asphyxiant dystrophy. Birth Defects 10:44, 1974

Nadjmi B, Flanagan MJ, Christian JR: Laurence-Moon-Biedl syndrome associated with multiple genito-urinary tract anomalies. Am J Dis Child 117:352, 1969

Perkoff GT: The hereditary renal diseases. N Engl J Med 277:79, 1967

Sissons JGP, West R, Fallows J, et al: The complement abnormalities of lipodystrophy. N Engl J Med 294:461, 1976

Williams HE, Smith L: Primary hyperoxaluria, in S tansbury J, Fredrickson D (eds): The Metabolic Basis of Inherited Disease (ed 3). New York, McGraw-Hill, 1972, p 196

Wise D, Wallace JH, Jellink EH: Angiokeratoma corporis diffusum. A clinical study of eight affected families. Q J Med 31:177, 1962

TRANSPORT DISORDERS

Michael J. Hanley

The overall homeostatic function of the renal tubular epithelium is to reduce the 150 liters of glomerular filtrate formed daily to the 1–2 liters of excreted urine. This complex process is characterized generally by (1) the reabsorption or conservation of necessary water and electrolytes, (2) secretion of various ions, toxic products, and metabolites, and (3) reclamation and regeneration of body buffer.

Despite the great complexity of these functions, isolated disorders of various transport systems are relatively rare and generally possess a variety of eponyms. Although they are rare, recognition of these disorders is important for the insight they provide about tubular function and because preventive therapy is sometimes possible to obviate the progressive loss of renal function which can occur due to secondary glomerular impairment later in the course of the disease.

RENAL GLYCOSURIA

Isolated renal glycosuria (see the chapter on *Glucose*) is a rare abnormality characterized by glucose excretion in the urine at normal concentrations of blood glucose. The glucose excretion patterns (splay and T_m) appear to be variable, suggesting that no single defect characterizes all the subjects with this disorder. The reabsorptive mechanism for glucose illustrates the characteristics of an active transport system of limited transport capacity. Under normal conditions, all filtered glucose is reabsorbed and none is excreted in the urine. As plasma levels of glucose are raised above some critical threshold, increasing quantities of glucose are excreted into the urine. When the filtration rate is stable, the quantity of glucose filtered is a linear function of the plasma level. The quantity of glucose excreted per minute is also a linear function of the plasma concentration once the plasma threshold concentration is exceeded. Over a wide range of plasma concentrations above the threshold a constant amount of glucose is reabsorbed per minute. This amount represents the tubular maximal reabsorptive capacity (T_m). As discussed in the chapter on *Glucose*, the rounding of the reabsorption curve in the neighborhood of the T_m is termed the splay of the titration curve. The splay is explained by the fact that the affinity of the carrier for glucose is not infinite and there may be some glomerulotubular imbalance. The amount of glucose excreted varies widely but usually never greatly exceeds 1 g/24 hours (normal less than 100 mg/24 hours).

Biopsy studies of individuals with this disorder have not consistently disclosed any association anatomic abnormality. Normally glucose is actively absorbed against an increasingly steep gradient in the early proximal tubule, so that by the midpoint of this structure little glucose remains in the lumen.

Glucose reabsorption is sodium dependent, and the current hypothesis projects the existence of a single mobile luminal membrane carrier protein on which there are two binding sites, one for sodium and one for glucose. The most widely held view at the present time is that the specific defect of renal glycosuria involves the sodium dependent glucose transmembrane carrier. A decrease in the number of carrier units present would decrease T_m, while a decrease in the affinity of the carrier for glucose would increase the splay in the glucose titration curve (Fig. 1). Since both defects are seen in this syndrome, a spectrum of abnormalities is responsible for this entity. Coinciding with this spectrum of abnormalities is the quantity of glucose present in the urine. A defect in splay characteristics will yield a relatively small amount of glucose in all urine samples; a defect in T_m will result in relatively large amounts of glucose in the urine, but the glycosuria will be confined to the normal blood glucose elevation following a meal.

This tubular abnormality is a familial autosomal disorder with more than one mode of inheritance. In most patients the total urinary glucose loss is insufficient to cause any symptoms or metabolic disturbance;

therefore no treatment is required. In ususually severe cases the glycosuria may produce polyuria, polydipsia, and ketosis due to increased fat metabolism. The association of this disorder with diabetes mellitus is controversial, but it does not appear to be related to the subsequent development of this disease. Glycosuria is known to occur with normal pregnancy and may be due to the higher filtered load of glucose that occurs as GFR increases, to an abnormality of tubular reabsorption, or to a combination of both. Most authors agree that there is nothing to suggest that the normoglycemic glycosuria of pregnancy is hazardous or a forerunner of diabetes mellitus.

RENAL AMINOACIDURIA

Amino acids are readily filtered by the glomerulus and almost completely reabsorbed by the proximal tubule. Normally less than 200 mg amino acid nitrogen is excreted per 24 hours. A very high protein diet or severe tissue breakdown (leukemia chemotherapy) may be expected to raise this level by a variable amount. It should also be noted that reabsorption of amino acids is less complete in infancy and childhood. There are perhaps five separate amino acid transport systems each specific for a particular class of amino acid, but specific familial defects have only been reported in the three classes indicated: (1) basic (cystinuria), (2) iminoglycine (iminoglycinuria—since this is a defect without disease, it will not be discussed further), and (3) monoaminomonocarboxylic acid (Hartnup's disease) (Table 1). These specific defects are fundamentally different from the general tubular disorders to be discussed later (Fanconi's syndrome).

Cystinuria

Cystinuria (see the chapter on *Renal Stones*) is a genetic amino acid transport disorder affecting the renal proximal tubule and the jejenum characterized by the defective absorption of cystine, lysine, arginine, and ornithine. The disease is expressed by the appearance of these four amino acids in the urine and the formation of renal calculi by the least soluble of these compounds, cystine. The diagnosis can be made by finding the hexagonal crystals of cystine in the urinary sediment or by analysis of the stones formed in the collecting system. This entity must be clearly separated from cystinosis, a cystine storage disease characterized by the abnormal accumulation of cystine in many body tissues, including the kidney. Cystinosis initially produces a generalized protimal tubule reabsorption defect (Fanconi's syndrome) with a progressive deterioration of tubular and glomerular function.

Although it was originally postulated that cystinuria was the result of an aberration of a specific basic amino acid transport protein, recent in vitro studies of renal cortical slices demonstrate a defect for dibasic amino acids but not for cystine. These data conflict with the clearance data, which find increased excretion of cystine and dibasic amino acids. The discrepancy between the in vitro and in vivo studies suggest that increased production or decreased degradation of cystine must occur in the kidney in this entity. The exact mode of

Table 1
Renal Amino Acid Transport Defects

Class of Amino Acids	Recognized Defects	Amino Acid Excreted
Basic	cystinuria	Cystine, lysine, arginine, ornithine
Acidic	—	—
Iminoglycic	Iminoglycinuria	Iminoglycine
Monoaminomonocarboxylic	Hartnup's disease	Asparagine, histidine serine, threonine, phenylalanine, tycosine, tryphoplan
Amino acids	—	—

inheritance of cystinuria is likewise not clear. It appears that the defect is transmitted as an autosomal recessive trait. Use of the intestinal transport system as a sensitive genetic marker has identified three types of cystinuric homozygotes.

Since the only relevant clinical sign of this transport derangement is the formation of renal calculi, treatment of the disorder consists of minimizing the opportunity for cystine precipitation. Diet therapy to reduce amino acid excretion has been uniformly ineffective. Alkalinization of the urine with oral bicarbonate or carbonic anhydrase inhibitors is only minimally effective, since it is necessary to increase the urine pH over 7.5 to be therapeutically useful. Dilution of the urine by a large fluid intake seems to be a simple and effective form of therapy. Those patients who have consistently elevated fluid intake, especially during the evening and night, have achieved considerable benefit. Drug therapy to change cystine into a more soluble form has also proved useful. D-Penicillamine and mercaptopropronglycine have the ability to reduce cystine excretion by reacting with its precursor cysteine to form a more soluble cysteine–drug complex which is excreted in the urine. Drug therapy is not without possible side effects (skin rash, leukopenia, nephrotic syndrome, loss of taste), however, and it must therefore be judiciously prescribed.

Hartnup's Disease

Hartnup's disease is a rare recessive hereditary disorder bearing the surname of the first family studied. Like cystinuria, the primary abnormality involves a specific amino acid (monoaminomonocarboxylic acid) transport defect in the proximal tubule and in the jejunum. The tubular defect results in high renal clearances of flutamine, asparagine, histidine, serine, threonine, phenylalanine, tyrosine, and tryptophan. In general, the urinary losses are nutritionally insignificant (except possibly for tryptophan). The jejunal defect is of more clinical significance, since decreased intestinal absorption of tryptophan (leading to decreased synthesis of nicotinamide) is likely responsible for most of the clinical manifestations of the disease. These manifestations include a pellagra-like skin rash and episodic neurologic disorders (ataxia, tremor, delusions) with probably no intellectual impairment. When studied by paper chromatography a distinctive pattern of aminoaciduria is produced with up to a 15-fold increase in

monoaminomonocarboxylic acid excretion. Treatment consists of oral nicotinamide (200 mg/day), which results in marked improvement in the skin rash and neurologic manifestations. The disease appears to improve with advancing age, symptoms being more common in childhood than in later life.

RENAL PHOSPHATURIA

Renal phosphaturia is a common feature of the Fanconi syndrome (to be discussed below). The prototype of a specific phosphate transport defect is X-linked hypophosphatemic vitamin D resistant rickets. As the name suggests, this is a familial disorder resistant to the usual doses of vitamin D. The diagnostic and radiologic findings of this disorder are the same as those seen in rickets and osteomalacia from other causes.

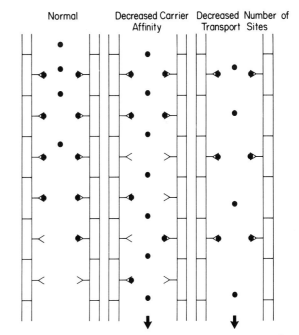

Fig. 1. Proposed defects causing renal glucosuria. Normally no glucose escapes reabsorption by the proximal tubule (left-hand panel). If the membrane carrier has a decreased affinity for glucose, some glucose will appear in the urine before the T_m is reached (middle panel). If there is a decreased number of membrane carriers the T_m will be reduced (right-hand panel).

The hypophosphatemia is a reflection of a defective renal tubular phosphate reabsorption transport system. Studies of gut mucosa indicate that a similar defect exists in this epithelium. The syndrome is resistent to physiologic doses of 1,25-(OH)$_2$-D$_3$, but oral phosphate supplements will restore the serum phosphorus to near normal. The role of PTH in this disorder is more controversial. Reports of exaggerated as well as near-normal response to PTH have appeared.

FANCONI'S SYNDROME

The Fanconi's syndrome is characterized by the urinary excretion of abnormal amounts of proteins, amino acids, glucose, phosphate, bicarbonate, and urate. The inherited defects outlined above have all been postulated to be caused specifically by an abnormal or missing tubular transport protein, but the Fanconi syndrome is the renal response to a nonspecific proximal tubular insult. There is a considerable variation of expression, and not all defects are necessarily present to the same degree. Unlike the genetic defects discussed previously, there are histologic abnormalities present in this entity, variously described as a "swan neck" deformity of the early proximal tubule in some instances and patchy necrosis in other reports. Table 2 gives a classification of the renal Fanconi syndrome. Childhood Fanconi syndrome is most frequently the consequence of cystinosis, while the adult variety is usually either of the idiopathic variety or associated with some type of exogenous toxin.

Cystinosis

Cystinosis is an inherited metabolic disorder characterized by a high intracelluar content of cystine with crystal deposition in cornea, conjunctiva, bone marrow, lymph nodes, leukocytes, kidneys, and other organs. Clinical expression varies widely but usually is manifested by rickets and growth retardation secondary to the Fanconi syndrome induced hypophosphotemia and chronic acidosis. The aminoaciduria of this disorder is generalized and clearly separable from that observed in cystinuria. In addition to the proximal tubule defects,

Table 2
Causes of Fanconi's Syndrome

Metabolic
  Cystinosis
  Lowe's syndrome
  Tyrosinemia
  Galactosemia
  Glycogen storage disease
  Fructose intolerance
  Wilson's disease
  Idiopathic
Exogenous toxins
  Heavy metals
  Creaol burn
  Maleic acid
  Degraded tetraycline
  Multiple myeloma
  Kidney transplantation

distal nephron damage is also common, probably secondary to crystal deposition in the renal medulla. Reduction in the ability to concentrate the urine and a distal type of renal tubular acidosis can result. Treatment consists primarily in correction of the acidosis and rickets by oral alkali and vitamin D therapy, respectively. Since death is usually due to uremia, kidney transplantation has also been employed and is probably an acceptable therapeutic modality, especially if cadaveric organs are used.

Idiopathic (Adult) Fanconi Syndrome

This disorder is different from cystinosis and quite rare. There is no definitive evidence that this entity is an inherited disorder. Cystine deposits have never been found, and the cellular damage appears to be confined to the proximal tubular cells. The disease presents in adult life usually with bone pain secondary to osteomalacia. In addition to the primary proximal tubule defect, there is often some compromise of concentrating ability and variable involvement of the distal nephron. When abnormalities of distal tubular function present they are similar to those encountered in distal renal tubular acidosis. Treatment of the osteomalacia with vitamin D therapy is effective and results in rapid improvement in symptoms. There is no progressive alteration in glomerular filtration as is seen in the childhood cystine deposition disease.

NEPHROGENIC DIABETES INSIPIDUS

Nephrogenic diabetes insipidus is a rare genetic disorder characterized by the failure of the terminal nephron to respond normally to antidiuretic hormone. Normally, plasma osmolality is maintained within narrow limits by an efficient regulatory system involving the thirst mechanism and ADH release (see the chapter on *Water Metabolism*). ADH release is controlled principally by plasma osmolality and blood volume. ADH acts on the collecting tubule where it is initially bound to specific receptor sites on the contraluminal side of the cell (see the chapter on *Antidiuretic Hormone*). The receptor–hormone complex activates adenylate cyclase on the membrane, producing cyclic AMP. By a complex process not fully understood the epithelium then becomes more permeable to water, so that the luminal contents can approach osmotic equilibrium with the normally hypertonic medullary interstitium. The net effect of ADH release is the conservation of solute-free water. While it was originally thought to be an X-linked disorder, recent family studies have indicated a more complicated mode of inheritance for nephrogenic diabetes insipidus. The disorder is probably somewhat different in each of the families carrying the trait. Males are predominantly involved, but affected females are also well described. Recent attempts have been made to characterize the biochemical defect in affected individuals by measurement of urinary osmolality and cyclic AMP production in response to an ADH infusion. Preliminary reports would indicate the expected heterogeneity of results. Nephrogenic diabetes insipidus generally appears shortly after birth with infants presenting with vomiting, recurrent dehydration, and failure to thrive, since polyuria and polydipsia are generally not recognized easily in this population. Older children can usually preserve a normal balance between intake and output, so that the secondary complications are generally absent. The acquired disorders which lead to nephrogenic diabetes insipidus are discussed in the chapter on *Water Balance*. Administration of diuretics such as chlorothiazide has been found to be quite efficacious in the hereditary forms of nephrogenic diabetes insipidus. More recently, prostaglandin inhibitors such as indomethacin have been utilized, but their beneficial effect has not been proved.

RENAL TUBULAR ACIDOSIS (RTA)

Renal tubular acidosis may be defined as a metabolic acidosis generated and maintained by deficient renal acidification. There is a reduction in net secretion of hydrogen ion by the renal tubules at normal plasma bicarbonate concentrations. Although not fully established, the prevailing view is that renal acidification is primarily the result of tubular hydrogen ion secretion (see the chapters on *Hydrogen Ion Transport* and *Disorders of Acid–Base Metabolism*). By far the largest proportion of hydrogen ion secretion is marshalled to reclaim the bicarbonate ion filtered by the glomerulus. With a plasma bicarbonate level of 25 mEq/liter and normal renal function this filtered bicarbonate load is approximately 4500 mEq per day. In addition to reclaiming the filtered bicarbonate the kidney is responsible for the regeneration of bicarbonate titrated by mineral acids (principally acid sulfates and phosphates derived from the metabolism of phospholipids and proteins) released into the extracellular fluid. This bicarbonate loss from the extracellular fluid amounts to approximately 1 mEq/kg per day. If all filtered bicarbonate was reclaimed but none of the decomposed bicarbonate was regenerated, acidosis would develop. The bicarbonate regeneration process involves the formation of titratable acid and the secretion of ammonia. The proximal tubule normally reclaims 85–90 percent of the filtered bicarbonate, while the distal tubule reclaims the remaining 10–15 percent and titrates urinary buffer to regenerate the consumed bicarbonate. The ability of the distal segments to maintain large lumen to peritubular fluid hydrogen ion gradients allows the luminal fluid pH to be brought below 6.0. At this level the bicarbonate concentration is negligible and luminal buffer is titrated as necessary to dispose of the metabolic acid load. In RTA, the acidosis is caused by the disparity between renal bicarbonate reclamation and regeneration on one hand and plasma bicarbonate titration and urinary bicarbonate loss on the other. Net loss of bicarbonate results in a decrease in the serum bicarbonate and metabolic acidosis. Further, this syndrome is usually associated with a normal GFR and is thus presumed to be the consequence of some type of hydrogen ion transport defect.

Classic (Type I, Distal) RTA

This disorder (Table 3) is characterized by bicarbonaturia and inappropriately high urine pH even with severe degrees of metabolic acidosis. When the plasma bicarbonate is increased to normal by alkali administration, neither the pH nor bicarbonaturia increases by a substantial amount. The bicarbonaturia of type I RTA is usually very small, amounting to less than 5 percent of the filtered load of bicarbonate. These characteristics imply that the major bicarbonate reclamation and regeneration mechanisms located in the proximal tubule are intact and the major defect involves the low-capacity distal acidification system. The disorder is generally considered to be due to the inability of the distal nephron to generate or maintain the necessary hydrogen ion pH gradient. The magnitude of the hydrogen ion secretory defect is variable among patients with this disorder, which is paralleled by the amount of exogenous alkali therapy necessary to maintain the plasma bicarbonate in the normal range. The amount of bicarbonate can be calculated by measuring the daily urinary bicarbonate loss and adding to this the difference between necessary bicarbonate regeneration [1 mEq/kg × wt (kg)] and titratable acid plus ammonia formation. In a 70 kg man, if daily urinary bicarbonate excretion is 0.5 mEq/kg and titratable acidity plus ammonia excretion is 0.25 mEq/kg, then the amount of exogenous HCO_3 necessary is [0.5 mEq/kg + (1 − 0.25) mEq/kg] × 70 kg = 87.5 mEq/day = 7.35 g $NaHCO_3$ hr/day. In some infants there is a considerable component of bicarbonate wasting in what otherwise appears to be a classic RTA. Some studies suggest that this massive bicarbonaturia may be the result of a proximal tubule acidification defect in conjunction with a classic distal RTA.

Acidification defect in type I RTA. The exact mechanism of the renal acidification defect in type I RTA has not been clearly defined. One theory proposed was the existence of a persistent bicarbonate leak in the proximal tubule. This would result in a bicarbonate-containing alkaline urine as well as a reduction in titratable acidity and ammonium excretion. An attempt was made to distinguish between this model and a pure hydrogen ion gradient defect in the distal nephron by subjecting a patient with classic RTA to a water diuresis. Since bicarbonate concentration and urine pH was unchanged during a water diuresis, it was assumed that the defect in type I RTA was not a proximal tubular leak but an inability to lower urine pH in the distal nephron. Further studies in other patients with RTA, however, have shown that bicarbonate concentration and urinary pH fell during a water diuresis, indicating that at least in some patients a proximal bicarbonate leak may exist. It is probably not possible to separate the two proposed mechanisms on the basis of studies utilizing water diuresis.

Another experimental technique used to delineate the defect in distal RTA has been the examination of urinary carbon dioxide tension (also see the chapter on *Disorders of Acid–Base Metabolism*). The argument is based on the fact that normal subjects during a bicarbonate diuresis increase the pCO_2 of their urine considerably, while patients with RTA type I do not. The mode of increase was presumed to be hydrogen ion secretion into a bicarbonate-rich fluid giving a high

Table 3
Renal Tubular Acidosis

	Proximal	Distal
Etiology	Familial	Classic type
	Fanconi's syndrome	Incomplete RTA
	Cystinosis	Nephrocalcinosis
	Hereditary fructose intolerance	Amphotericin B toxicity
	Lowe's syndrome	Lithium toxicity
	Renal transplantation	Vitamin D intoxication
		Hyperglobulinemic states
		Renal Transplantation
Diagnosis	Urine pH 5 with low serum bicarbonate	Urine pH>6 at all times
Treatment	Resistant to alkali therapy, some control with diuretics	Alkali therapy usually successful

concentration of carbonic acid in the distal nephron. The delayed dehydration of carbonic acid due to the absence of luminal carbonic anhydrase in this segment together with the unfavorable surface–volume relations in the urinary collecting system for the loss of CO_2 from the newly formed urine yield a fluid of high carbon dioxide tension. Since there was no rise in pCO_2 in the patients with renal tubular acidosis, it was assumed that the secretion of hydrogen ion necessary to generate the high carbonic acid concentrations in the distal nephron was defective.

In addition, the low urinary pCO_2 in the presence of adequate buffer has been offered as evidence that the defect in distal RTA involves the rate of hydrogen ion secretion rather than a limitation of the pH gradient that could be developed. In the presence of adequate bicarbonate buffer the pH of the liminal fluid should never fall to a level which would limit net secretion because of back diffusion; however, the finding of a low urinary pCO_2 indicates only that the luminal concentration of carbonic acid is low. This could come about by alternate means—back diffusion of carbonic acid, or rapid dehydration in the tubular lumen by exposure to carbonic anhydrase. Two recent experimental findings have now raised some serious questions about urinary pCO_2 measurements in patients with distal RTA—(1) the urinary carbon dioxide tension is a function of the bicarbonate concentration, and since patients with distal RTA usually have a concentrating defect, the urinary bicarbonate concentration in these individuals during a bicarbonate diuresis is lower than that found in normals, and (2) it has generally been assumed that the renal pCO_2 is the same as arterial blood, but recent evidence indicates that this is a variable parameter and possibly a function of the degree of bicarbonate reabsorption. The net result of all of these findings is that no clear delineation of the distal RTA defect has been forthcoming. Circumstantial evidence that a permeability defect is the underlying cause for distal RTA is suggested by the occurrence of a typical distal RTA-like syndrome with amphotericin B, an agent known to alter membrane permeability. In vitro acidification studies in the turtle bladder in the presence of amphotericin B support this concept. It has been demonstrated that net hydrogen ion gradient existed. The defect was presumed to be due to back diffusion. This same membrane defect could be used to explain the urinary potassium loss that accompanies amphotericin nephropathy.

Renal tubule abnormality in distal RTA. Type I RTA can be transmitted as an autosomal dominant trait. At present there is no definitive information on whether this is a structural or enzymatic defect, although there is suggestive evidence that either abnormality can be operative in a given case. In a number of patients with distal RTA not of the primary genetic type, the acidification disorder appears to be secondary to nephrocalcinosis. This is true of primary hyperparathyroidism, vitamin D intoxication, hyperthyroidism, and idiopathic hypercalcuria. The distal RTA syndromes which occur in association with hyperglobulinemia appear to demonstrate a female predilection.

Incomplete type I RTA. This variant of distal RTA is characterized by normal net acid excretion and no systemic acidosis. The major abnormality appears to be an inappropriately high urinary pH in response to an ammonium chloride acidosis. These patients appear to excrete a greater than normal portion of their acid load in the form of ammonium compounds. Reports also exist of a transition from incomplete to complete distal RTA which accompanied a general loss of renal function.

Clinical manifestations of type I RTA. Disorders of sodium, potassium, and calcium metabolism are the principal sequelae of distal RTA, yet it is unclear whether the sodium, potassium, and calcium wasting are primary defects or merely secondary to the persistent metabolic acidosis. Reports on individual patients have appeared which support both positions. Alkali therapy in amounts which correct the acidosis has been reported to correct all of these defects in some patients. The abnormal sodium and potassium wasting, at the very least, returns toward normal, and even though nephrolithiasis may persist the frequency of stone passage decreases. Whether the persistent defects after alkali administration are due to tubular damage secondary to nephrocalcinosis remains unclear.

Proximal (Type II) RTA

Proximal RTA (Table 3) is a disorder characterized by bicarbonaturia and inappropriately high urine pH only under conditions of mild to moderate acidosis. The renal response to more severe degrees of acidosis is the disappearance of bicarbonate from the urine and an appropriate lowering of urinary pH. The magnitude of the wasting at normal serum bicarbonate and the appropriate lowering of the urinary pH during severe acidosis localizes the defect in this case to the proximal tubule. As might be expected, proximal RTA is usually associated with the Fanconi Syndrome. Also, some patients may have a combined proximal and distal defect. An incomplete type II RTA has also been described. Analogous to the incomplete Type I RTA, there is no systemic acidosis, since the urinary bicarbonate loss appears to be appropriately matched by increased ammonia production, so that net acid excretion is normal. The role of serum calcium and parathyroid hormone in the genesis of type II RTA has been the subject of many investigations. Parathyroid hormone can suppress proximal tubular bicarbonate reabsorption, but many studies suggest that this is an insufficient modulating effect to be a major consideration in the etiology of the disorder. Hypocalcemia and vitamin D deficiency appear to be pathogenic factors which sensitize the renal tubule to the bicarbonate effect of PTH in patients with proximal RTA. Therefore it can be postulated that in some patients with type II RTA, the impairment in renal bicarbonate reabsorption is in part due to hypocalcemia and vitamin D deficiency. Phosphate depletion has also been found to play a role in a proximal tubular acidification defect. This probably represents no more than a contributing factor in the overall syndrome. Unlike patients with distal RTA, correction of the systemic acidosis with exogenous alkali in patients with the proximal RTA initiates or intensifies potassium wasting. This is due to the delivery of large amounts of sodium bicarbonate to the distal nephron together, at least in some patients, with the persistence of hyperaldosteronism. In this setting bicarbonate can probably behave as a nonreabsorbable anion increasing luminal negativity and enhancing passive potassium entry. Hyperaldosteronism would be expected to augment this effect, but whether type II RTA patients with hyperaldosteronism do indeed waste more potassium than those individuals without elevated hormone levels remains to be determined. Patients with proximal RTA, like those with nephrogenic diabetes insipidus, appear to benefit from thiazide induced extracellular volume depletion. The enhanced proximal tubule reabsorption brought about by this physiologic alteration lessens bicarbonate loss from the early nephron segments and diminishes bicarbonate wasting.

Experimental Type II RTA (Hereditary Fructose Intolerance)

In patients with hereditary fructose intolerance a proximal RTA can be induced by the administration of fructose. In these individuals fructose ingestion causes a generalized proximal tubule disorder. Renal function appears to be completely normal when fructose is eliminated from the diet.

Type IV Renal Tubular Acidosis

In marked contrast to the renal potassium wasting noted in patients with distal and proximal RTA, persisting hyperkalemia is noted in some patients with hyperchloremic acidosis. Other features of adults with this syndrome are (1) some degree of renal insufficiency (usually resulting from a tubulointerstitial disease), (2) an impairment of renal renin secretion and secondary reduction of aldosterone production, and (3) a reduced urinary ammonia excretion rate even when the urine is highly acidic. The hyperkalemic acidosis noted in these patients is disproportionate to the degree of renal insufficiency. Unlike distal RTA, the urine is acidic and bicarbonate free during systemic acidosis; like proximal RTA, the tubular reabsorption of bicarbonate is subnormal when the plasma bicarbonate is raised to normal with exogenous alkali. Yet the magnitude of the defective bicarbonate reabsorption is not sufficiently great to unequivocally implicate a proximal nephron defect. In addition, no other abnormallity of proximal tubular transport is present in this condition. Type IV RTA thus represents a unique defect in renal tubular hydrogen ion and potassium secretion. Since aldosterone is known to stimulate both hydrogen ion and potassium secretion by the kidney, the presence of hypoaldosteronism in this disorder suggests that this may be a major pathophysiologic impairment determined of this syndrome. It has been demonstrated that the oral administration of a mineralocorticoid (1) can diminish the bicarbonaturia in patients with normal plasma bicarbonate (an exogenous oral alkali therapy) and (2) can substantially increase net acid excretion and ameliorate the acidosis in acidotic patients. On the basis of these observations it appears mineralocorticoid deficiency together with some distal defect plays a key role in the development of the syndrome. The defect in ammoniagenesis does not appear to be primary in the disorder as ammonia excretion can be returned toward normal with the correction of the hyperkalemia.

REFERENCES

Glorieux F, Scriver CR: Loss of a parathyroid hormone-sensitive component of phosphate transport in X-linked hypophosphatemia. Science 175:997, 1971

Lee DBN, Drinkard JP, Rosen VJ, et al: The adult Fanconi syndrome. Medicine (Baltimore) 51:107, 1972

O'Doherty PJA, DeLuca HF, Eicher EM: Lack of effect of vitamin D and its metabolites on intestinal phosphate transport in familial hypophosphatemia of mice. Endocrinology 101:1325, 1977

Rodriguez-Soriono J: Renal tubular acidosis, in Edelman CM Jr (ed): Pediatric Kidney Disease, vol. 2. Boston, Little, Brown, Company, 1978

Schneider JA, Schulman JD: Cystinosis: A review. Metabolism 26:817, 1977

Schulman JD, Schneider JA: Cystinosis and the Fanconi syndrome. Pediatr Clin North Am 23:779, 1976

Sebastian A, McSherry E, Morris RC Jr: Metabolic Acidosis with special reference to renal acidosis, in Brenner B,

Rector FD (eds): The Kidney, vol 2. Philadelphia, W.B. Saunders, 1976

Short E, Morris RC Jr, Sebastian A, et al: Exaggerated phosphaturic response to circulating parathyroid hormone in patients with familial X-linked hypophosphatemic rickets. J Clin Invest 58:152, 1976

Stambury JB, Wyngaarden JB, Fredrickson DS (eds): The Metabolic Basis of Inherited Disease (ed 3). New York, McGraw-Hill, 1972

RENAL VEIN THROMBOSIS

H. John Reineck

CLINICAL FINDINGS

The clinical manifestations of renal vein thrombosis may be conveniently divided into those associated with acute thrombosis and those seen with chronic renal venous occlusion. Acute renal vein thrombosis occurs primarily in newborns and young children and is usually associated with profound dehydration or infection. Under these circumstances, the clinical findings are quite dramatic and include fever, grossly bloody urine, severe flank pain and tenderness, and, if bilateral, severe renal failure. In adults, acute renal vein thrombosis, accompanied by the above findings, is virtually limited to neoplastic invasion of the renal veins and trauma.

Chronic renal vein thrombosis was first described in1840 by Rayer, who noted its association with proteinuria. Since that time, a relationship between renal vein thrombosis and the nephrotic syndrome has gained generalized acceptance. Nonetheless, clinical findings often fail to distinguish between nephrotic patients with and without renal vein thrombosis. Recent studies have described a high incidence of microscopic hematuria, pyuria, and hyperchloremic acidosis in the former group of patients. A sudden worsening of proteinuria with deterioration of renal function may occasionally herald the development of renal venous occlusion, especially in amyloidosis. Finally and probably most significantly, the occurrence of pulmonary emboli in nephrotic patients should raise the possibility of renal vein thrombosis.

DIAGNOSIS

Intravenous pyelography may suggest the presence of renal vein thrombosis. Abnormalities may include a significant difference in renal size and/or excretory patterns and "notching" of the proximal ureter caused by the development of an extensive venous collateral circulation (Fig. 1). Renal biopsy findings offer relatively little help in establishing the diagnosis, although glomerular capillary leukocyte accumulation and disproportionate interstitial edema and fibrosis have been described. Definitive diagnosis usually requires selective renal venography.

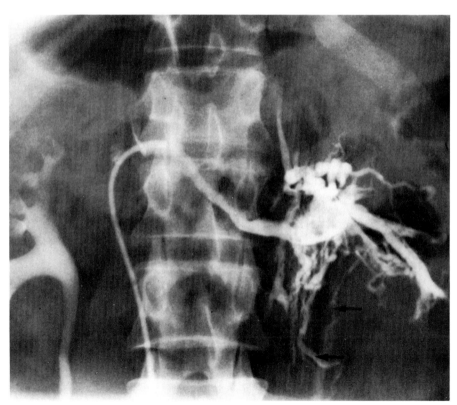

Fig. 1. Selective left renal vein venogram demonstrates extensive venous collaterals which have developed in response to longstanding renal vein thrombosis. These collateral vessels cause ureteral notching.

PATHOGENESIS

Most textbooks of medicine and nephrology list renal vein thrombosis as a cause of the nephrotic syndrome. While this entity may exaggerate or worsen the degree of proteinuria, most observers now agree that renal vein thrombosis is a complication of the nephrotic syndrome rather than a cause. This conclusion is based on the following evidence: First, in the vast majority of patients with renal vein thrombosis, renal biopsy or postmortem findings describe glomerulopathies well known to cause the nephrotic syndrome (e.g., membranous or membranoproliferative glomerulonephritis, amyloidosis). Second, in cases of unilateral renal vein thrombosis, glomerular disease capable of causing proteinuria is found in the contralateral kidney. Third, in some of these cases of unilateral renal vein thrombosis, selective ureteral catheterization reveals quantitatively similar degrees of proteinuria from both kidneys. Fourth, renal vein thrombosis has been described in 20 percent of animals with experimentally induced immune complex nephritis. Finally, initially normal venography has been described in nephrotic patients who have subsequently developed renal vein thrombosis.

The mechanism by which the nephrotic syndrome causes renal vein thrombosis is not yet clear. A so-called hypercoaguable state has long been clinically recognized in nephrotic patients. Recent studies have described increased activity of clotting factors V, VIII, and the VII–X complex. Hyperfibrinogenemia, accelerated thromboplastin generation, and prolonged euglobulin lysis times have also been reported. While it seems likely that these alterations may be operative in the development of renal vein thrombosis, the explanation for these findings remains obscure.

TREATMENT

Anecdotal reports of improvement in proteinuria and renal function following anticoagulation have appeared in the literature; however, to date no long-term control study has evaluated the efficacy of anticoagulation in patients with renal vein thrombosis and nephrotic syndrome. In the presence of documented pulmonary emboli, anticoagulation should be considered as in any other patient with that condition. Finally, it should be mentioned that in chronic renal vein thrombosis the use of surgical thrombectomy has not been adequately evaluated.

REFERENCES

Cade R, Sponner G, Juncos L, et al: Chronic renal vein thrombosis. Am J Med 63:387, 1977

Glassock RJ, Bennett CM: The glomerulopathies, Brenner BM, Rector FC (eds): The Kidney. W.B. Saunders, 1976, p 941 Philadelphia

Llach F, Arieff AI, Massry SG: Renal vein thrombosis and nephrotic syndrome: A prospective study of 36 adult patients. Ann Intern Med 83:8, 1975

Klassyn J, Sugasaki T, Mulgrom F, et al: Studies on multiple renal lesions in Heymann nephritis. Lab Invest 25:577, 1971

Rayer PFO: Traite des Maladies des Reins et des Alterations de la Secretion Urinaire. Paris, J.B. Balliere et Fils, 1840

Rosenmann E, Pollak VE, Pirani CL: Renal vein thrombosis in the adult: A clinical and pathologic study based on renal biopsies. Medicine (Baltimore) 47:269, 1968

Thomson C, Forbes CD, Prentice CRM, et al: Changes in blood coagulation and fibrinolysis in the nephrotic syndrome. J Med 49:399, 1974

OBSTRUCTIVE UROPATHY

Howard M. Radwin

Obstructive uropathy may be considered to be one aspect of the general subject of impaired transport of urine. Such familiar problems as congenital anatomic obstructions, calculus disease, neoplasm, stricture, and prostatic hyperplasia would be included, but equally important would be those aspects of dysfunction without frank anatomic obstruction which may lead to impaired urinary transport. These would include dysplastic conditions, neuromuscular dysfunction, and vesicoureteral reflux. Appreciation of this distinction is central to some of the most significant advances in the understanding of urinary tract pathophysiology in recent years. The recognition that not all that is dilated is obstructed is analogous to the realization that not all that wheezes is asthma. The clinical similarities of these entities may lead to important errors in diagnosis and management, such as attempts to surgically correct ureteral dilatation due to transient ureteritis with impaired peristalsis and no obstruction (Fig. 1). The distinction is not always simple, since problems may coexist, as in obstructive hyperplasia seen as a sequel to distal physiologic dysfunction or in vesical hypotonia resulting from longstanding distal anatomic obstruction (Fig. 2).

This chapter deals with the mechanisms of impaired urinary transport, their sequelae, appropriate diagnostic techniques, and management.

MECHANISMS OF IMPAIRED URINARY TRANSPORT

Congenital anatomic obstruction can occur anywhere in the urinary tract from the renal tubule to the urethral meatus; however, this continuum is not without peaks of probability where lesions are more likely to be found. Obstruction of calyces due to congenital narrowing of the infundibula leading to the renal pelvis is unusual. When such a lesion is noted, it usually is due to acquired inflammatory disease. An exception to this would be compression of an infundibulum by a blood vessel, causing partial obstruction of the dependent calyces. This would appear on urography as an abrupt linear filling defect in the infundibulum distal to a dilated calyx. Calyceal diverticula occur as the result of an anomaly of branching of the ureteric bud without the development of appropriate tubular structures. Stasis may be present within the diverticulum and may con-

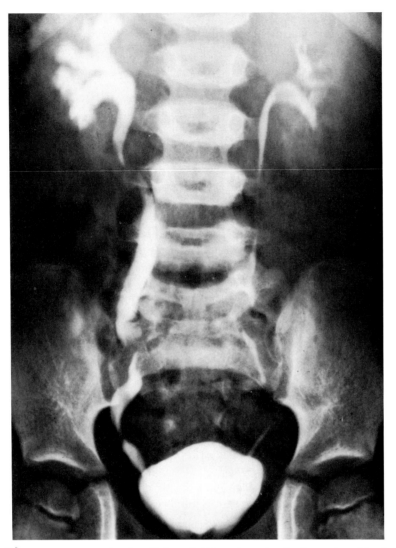

Fig. 1. Intravenous urogram showing dilation of right ureter and collecting system. No obstruction or reflux present. Creatinine and PAH clearance on right, 49 percent of total.

tribute to infection and stone formation, but calyceal diverticula rarely are the cause of functional impairments associated with obstructive uropathy unless the adjacent calyces are compressed.

The most common site of obstruction in the upper urinary tract remains the ureteropelvic junction. This may be caused by extrinsic entities, such as aberrant blood vessels or bands, or it may be caused by intrinsic abnormalities (Fig. 3). At times the two coexist. Normally, the upper ureter and renal pelvis fill simultaneously during a period of diastole. Filling of the upper ureter does not result normally from active contraction of the renal pelvis propelling urine into the upper ureter. Rather, during the filling phase these two structures form a pyeloureteric cone which fills as a unit, and at that time it is impossible radiographically to define a precise ureteropelvic junction. This area appears only subsequently, when the proximal ureter is filled and its most cephalad portion contracts at the beginning of the

propulsion of the first ureteral peristaltic wave into the more distal ureter. This mechanism protects the intrarenal structures from the hydrostatic pressure of ureteral contraction, which exceeds that of normal renal pelvic activity. From the above can be seen that ureteropelvic junction obstruction interferes with the passive filling of the upper ureter. Thus a pyeloureteric cone is not formed. In addition to extrinsic compression, abnormal arrangement of the muscle bundles in the upper ureter, their replacement by fibrous tissue, or an intraureteric lesion such as a neoplasm may be responsible.

Congenital anomalies of the ureter between the ureteropelvic junction and the ureterovesical junction are uncommon. Retrocaval ureter is unusual and results from the infrarenal component of the inferior vena cava developing from the ventral inferior cardinal vein rather than the more dorsal superior cardinal vein. This causes the ureter to be drawn medially around the inferior vena cava or common iliac vein. The anomaly is one of the venous system and of significance only if it is accompanied by hydronephrosis. Congenital ureteral strictures, valves, vascular obstructions, and diverticula may occur but are rare. Neoplasms, calculi, ureteritis, and sloughed renal papillae, as well as retroperitoneal fibrosis, may interfere with transport.

The pathophysiology of ureterovesical junction obstruction is much more complex than was generally recognized when the entire spectrum was encompassed in the all inclusive term "megaloureter" (Fig. 4). These lesions do not necessarily include reduced lumen diameter and may or may not be associated with vesicoureteral reflux. Classification with recognition of these differences has been profitable in terms of understanding the effects on ureteral and renal function, prognosis, and management. Abnormalities in this area also provide an excellent example of the difference between anatomic obstruction as defined by lumen caliber and functional obstruction in which urinary

transport is defective despite adequate ureteral patency. An understanding of this has depended on the clarification not only of the physiology of ureteral function, which is complex, but also of ureteral anatomy, which surprisingly continues to be an area of discovery. While the traditional teaching that the wall of the ureter contains three muscle layers remains valid, it has been found that a given muscle bundle may appear in different strata throughout the course of the ureter and that these muscle bundles are arranged as intertwining helices. At the most superior and inferior ends of the ureter, longitudinal muscle predominates. In the most distal ureter, which traverses the bladder wall, the muscle is almost exclusively longitudinal. These muscle fibers retain their continuity to open fanlike to form a portion of the vesical trigone and then extend into the proximal urethra. Although the subject is beyond the scope of this discussion, this phenomenon is considered important in the prevention of vesicoureteral reflux. One cause of functional impairment of urinary transport

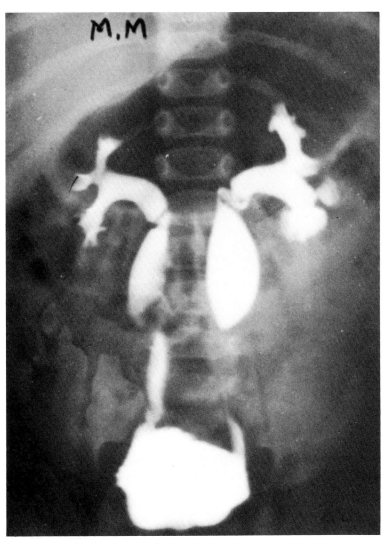

Fig. 2. Ureteral dysplasia and reflux shown on cystogram.

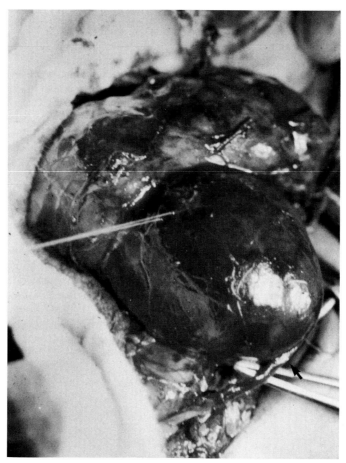

Fig. 3. Ureteropelvic junction obstruction with intrinsic narrowing of ureter.

in the distal ureter is an inappropriate distribution of distal ureteral muscle fibers with a predominance of the circular fibers, resulting in impairment of propulsion of the urine bolus into the intramural ureter and bladder. In this circumstance, distal ureteral caliber is normal but the ureter above it remains dilated. The radiographic appearance of such a ureter may be startling, but at times its dilatation may be disproportionate to the minimal calyceal changes which are observed, together with what may be only slight derangement of nephron function. In this circumstance, the importance of the evaluation of renal function as a guide to the appropriateness of surgical intervention is obvious.

The urinary bladder is also a much more complex structure than is commonly recognized. It not only serves as an organ of convenience, but it also has the properties of preventing reabsorption of undesirable solutes, preventing vesicoureteral reflux, preventing retrograde ejaculation, allowing a nonlinear increase in both vesical pressure and sensation of fullness with urinary filling, and facilitating complete emptying. The bladder derives from both mesoderm and endoderm, is innervated by both the sympathetic and parasympathetic nervous systems, and is influenced by striated as well as smooth muscle along the urethra and external

sphincter. Whereas bladder neck obstruction once was thought to be the most common cause of urologic abnormalities in children, congenital anatomic obstruction at the bladder neck is now considered unusual in the male and almost unheard of in the female; however, it has been supplanted by much greater emphasis on the phenomenon of bladder neck and proximal urethral dysfunction without anatomic constriction. This concept has been augmented by recent increases in recognition of the role of the alpha adrenergic receptors at the bladder neck and the proximal urethra. Thus congenital bladder neck obstruction on the basis of anular constriction is no longer thought a prevalent form of urinary tract abnormality, but physiologic dysfunction has become increasingly so.

The posterior urethra in the male is the site of one of the most serious forms of congenital urinary tract obstruction, resulting in potentially lethal renal changes if uncorrected. The lesion is that of posterior urethral valves, which may exist in a variety of configurations and which may lead to renal failure. The resultant changes in the kidneys are those described by Potter as type IV polycystic disease and are the result of obstructive uropathy. Congenital obstruction at the level of the urogenital diaphragm involving the external urinary sphincter is not generally included in a list of types of congenital uropathy. It usually arises from an abnormality of the central nervous system, leading to spasm of the sphincter and a lack of coordination during micturition. This is exemplified by a failure of the external sphincter to relax while the vesical detrusor contracts, producing the phenomenon of detrusor–sphincter dyssynergia. Simultaneous sphincter electromyography and cystometry as commonly performed clinically today may demonstrate this.

The most usual form of obstructive uropathy seen in the male results from benign prostatic enlargement. This develops from hyperplasia of the periurethral prostatic glands with enlargement of the prostate causing varying degrees of blockage of the urethral lumen. The magnitude of the prostatic enlargement as appreciated on rectal examination correlates poorly with the degree of obstruction to the flow of urine. Thus it is not the size of the overall mass but rather the component which is located intraurethrally which determines the effect on flow. As a response to partial urethral obstruction in BPH, the vesical musculature hypertrophies, forming trabeculations which are visible endoscopically as the enlarged intertwining muscle bundles of the bladder wall. Following this, cellules which appear as outpouchings between the hypertrophied muscle bundles will develop, and these may lead to the formation of pseudodiverticula. The hypertrophy of the bladder musculature may in itself partially obstruct the terminal ureter as it traverses the bladder wall. This, as well as increased intravesical pressure, may lead to ureteral dilatation and hydronephrosis. Carcinoma of the prostate arises from the periphery of that organ and may cause urethral obstruction but is accompanied by early ureteral obstruction more commonly than is the case with BPH. This results from tumor infiltration under the base of the bladder and directly involving the ureter. Thus in the presence of prostatic disease with ureteral dilatation, more pronounced than would be expected in conjunction with low-grade urethral obstruction, the presence of prostatic carcinoma should be suspected.

The urogenital diaphragm, which contains the external sphincter, separates the anterior or distal urethra from the posterior or proximal urethra. In the distal urethra, congenital lesions such as stenosis and diverticula may be found as well as many acquired obstructive processes such as stricture, tumor, and, rarely, calculi.

EFFECTS ON RENAL FUNCTION

The effects of impaired transport of urine and particularly of obstructive uropathy are dependent on a number of variables including whether the lesion is acute or chronic. Among factors to be considered are pressures within the collecting system, impairment of intrarenal circulation, the configuration of the collecting system such as the presence of an intra- or extrarenal pelvis, and the occurrence of complicating factors such as bacterial infection and immunologic injury. In the presence of acute uncomplicated partial ureteral ob-

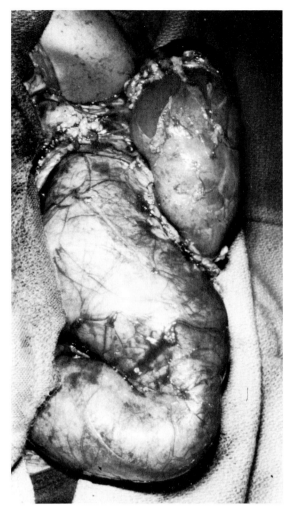

Fig. 4. Hydroureter draining atrophic upper pole of kidney. Normal-appearing renal mass is drained by normal-size ureter crossing upper portion of dilated ureter.

struction, an initial increase in total renal blood flow occurs and is probably mediated by prostaglandins. The composition of the urine demonstrates changes consistent with those seen with medullary vascular hypoperfusion. These include a decrease in urinary flow rate and an increase in osmolality. The concentration of all solutes is increased with the exception of sodium and chloride, which are diminished. It is of interest that these are the same changes which may be found on the side of the lesion in unilateral renovascular hypertension. With complete acute obstruction, pressure relationships proximal to the obstruction are such that a state of stop-flow is achieved at a rate which is proportional to the fluid load and state of renal perfusion. When stop-flow is reached, glomerular filtration continues but reabsorption through the tubules is markedly enhanced. Lymph flow increases, particularly through the capsular lymphatics. As obstructive uropathy becomes chronic, intrarenal pressures decrease. Renal blood flow drops and nephron loss ensues as the result of hypoperfusion. Thus loss of functional renal mass is related to inadequate blood flow rather than to hydrostatic pressure. Chronic hydronephrosis is accompanied by an increase in urinary sodium concentration and excretion, as well as decrease in free water clearance (CH2O). CH2O per 100 ml GFR is increased. It is suggested that this is explained by a combination of reduced nephron population and overperfusion of the residual functioning nephrons. Thus there is postulated increased filtration and diminished fractional reabsorption in the proximal nephron. In addition, ability to concentrate and acidify the urine is impaired.

Animal studies suggest that complete unilateral ureteral occlusion for 7 days is a totally reversible lesion but that obstruction for 28 days is followed after relief of the obstruction by a return of inulin clearance to only approximately 25 percent of control levels. During the initial recovery phase there is a decrease in fractional sodium and water reabsorption. After stabilization in the postobstructive kidney which has recovered to the maximum degree possible, the pattern of function per nephron is similar to that of the control kidney, yet reductions in inulin clearance, transport, and concentration ability and in sodium reabsorption may be noted. Excessive sodium and water loss in the stable, partially damaged postobstructive kidney does not lead to excessive total salt and water loss because of reduction of glomerular filtration. Following relief of obstruction, the phenomenon of postobstructive diuresis may occasionally be observed. This is characterized by voluminous loss of salt and water and is most commonly of clinical importance in those individuals who had demonstrated evidence of hypervolemia prior to relief of the obstruction. The mechanism of postobstructive salt-losing nephropathy is thought to involve an increase in distal delivery of sodium secondary to an increased osmotic load, a sudden elevation in glomerular filtration rate, and persistent inappropriate depression of fractional reabsorption of sodium in the proximal tubule. A role may also be played by abnormal absorption of salt and water in the distal nephron. These phenomena are contributed to by elevation of blood urea during the obstructive phase as well as by fluid administration. Postobstructive diuresis is not ordinarily seen following unilateral obstruction with a normal contralateral kidney. This may be due to the absence of urea accumulation in the presence of the normal kidney as well as perhaps, to lack of accumulation of natriuretic and vasodilatory substances. Increased release of erythropoietin does not commonly result from uncomplicated obstructive uropathy. Hypertension is also uncommon.

There has been recent interest in the observed coexistence of immunologic injury of the glomeruli in the presence of vesicoureteral reflux and obstructive uropathy. This relationship has been observed most commonly in the presence of massive reflux, which is postulated to establish a pathologic process which cannot be reversed by surgical correction of the reflux.

Whether reflux alone in the absence of infection is in itself deleterious to renal function has long been debated. The preponderance of evidence suggests that unless the reflux is massive, significant loss of renal function will not occur. It has been observed that when progressive interstitial nephritis without infection is initiated by vesicoureteral reflux, it is associated with intrarenal reflux extending into the medulla. This entity has been reported in the presence of reflux severe enough to produce marked dilatation of the ureter and collecting system. In addition, under these circumstances the surface of the papilla in the calyx is thought to lose its convexity and so distort the opening of the papillary ducts that intrarenal reflux can occur. In the presence of impaired transport of urine with intrarenal stasis, superimposed infection can be somewhat more difficult to resolve and calculi may form as the result of stasis. That dilatation of the intrarenal collecting system and renal pelvis in the absence of contamination does not usually lead to infection is suggested by the common finding of ureteropelvic junction obstruction which has persisted for years without ever having been associated with infection.

DIAGNOSTIC TECHNIQUES

The evaluation of the various forms of impaired transport of urine involves not only the identification of the lesion but also an appraisal of its effect on renal function as well as the occurrence of complications such as infection and stone formation.

The intravenous urogram remains the primary screening test for identification of these abnormalities. The commonly employed contrast agents require only glomerular filtration and proximal tubular reabsorption of water for their visualization. They are neither secreted nor reabsorbed by the tubules. In the presence of diminished GFR and a large residual of noncontrast-containing urine in the collecting system and ureter, delayed appearance of the contrast agents may be expected. Thus when obstructive uropathy is suspected, delayed films possibly involving reinjection of the contrast agent will often lead to identification of the abnormality, even in the presence of early nonvisualization (Fig. 5). This technique is particularly valuable in the localization of both nonopaque ureteral calculi and those opaque calculi which are difficult to visualize because of relatively low density, small size, and/or overlying bowel gas or bone. In the absence of visualization by excretory studies, retrograde examinations may be performed. These will demonstrate the morphologic status of the urinary tract as well as the presence of radiolucent stones, tumors, blood clots, strictures, and sloughed papillae, all of which may cause obstruction. These studies do not elucidate the functional capacity of the kidney, but films taken at various intervals following injection will suggest the extent of the obstructive process by the degree to which the contrast material is retained proximal to the lesion.

Retrograde studies may be employed to visualize any portion of the urinary tract from the urethral meatus

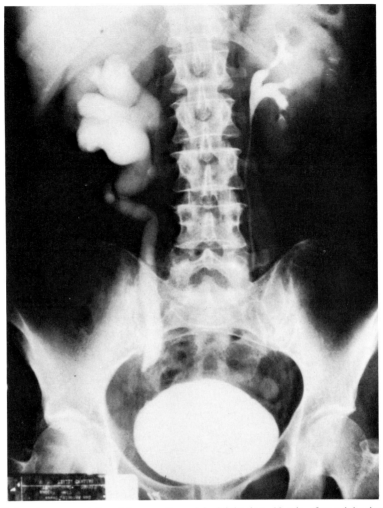

Fig. 5. Delayed urogram taken 4 hours after original injection, 30 min after reinjection. Site of extrinsic obstruction of lower third of right ureter is demonstrated.

to the calyces. Antegrade radiologic evaluation of the urinary tract usually involves the percutaneous puncture of the renal pelvis with the injection of contrast material. This permits the visualization of the system proximal to the obstruction as well as the performance of pressure determinations. Not only the location and degree of the obstructive process may be observed radiographically, but also some estimate may be made of the residual cortical mass. This may be done by evaluation of the nephrogram phase of the intravenous urogram. The contrast material is seen in the compressed tubules of the renal parenchyma following glomerular filtration but prior to its appearance in the collecting system. The arteriogram also can assist in the evaluation of renal mass both by nephrogram demonstration and the appearance of the intrarenal circulation. Scintillation scans with radioisotopes correlate well with the degree of impairment of renal blood flow but have been inconsistent predictors of the recoverability of renal function following relief of the obstructive process. In one series the ability of the abnormal kidney

to acidify the urine correlated well with the recoverability of the kidney. Clarification of the etiology of lower urinary tract processes leading to impaired transport has improved significantly in recent years with the employment of CO_2 cystometry, electromyography, and urethral pressure profilometry. These methods have been particularly useful in clarifying the mechanisms of dysfunctional impairments of urinary transport.

MANAGEMENT

Although discussion of the treatment of the various urinary tract abnormalities which lead to impaired transport of urine on a lesion-by-lesion basis is beyond the scope of this chapter, certain general principles do apply. The first step in successful management is the recognition of the problem, and this is not always simple. Whereas acute ureteral obstruction may present with classical colic, chronic obstruction of the upper urinary tract is often silent and must be suspected. Congenital ureteropelvic junction obstruction severe enough to lead to the destruction of the involved renal unit may be totally asymptomatic. There may be only the occasional experience of discomfort with fluid loading, unless infection or trauma supervene to produce an acute episode. If the lesion is unilateral, there will be none of the stigmata of renal insufficiency. Nevertheless, lesions also are often missed when the evidence is considerably less subtle. Many an aged male with renal failure has had the most likely cause of his problem, BPH, ignored for an inappropriate period of time while more arcane explanations were sought. Thus an awareness of statistical probabilities is as important here as in other areas of medical practice. The acuity of the physician will be enhanced if he is aware of the differences in presentation between acute and chronic lesions, unilateral versus bilateral disease, and upper versus lower urinary tract pathology.

After impaired transport of urine has been suspected, an attempt is usually made to identify the location of the lesion. This may be accomplished by the employment of those diagnostic techniques which were discussed in the previous section. Second, the abnormality should be characterized by type. This involves distinguishing between the anatomically obstructive lesion and dysfunctional states. This is not always a simple process, but the clinician should be aware of certain clues to assist him. An example would be the presence of a palpable or radiologically apparent sacral abnormality in the child with voiding problems, suggesting the presence of a neurogenic bladder. Within each of these broad classifications, the specific etiology should then be sought. The abnormality may be the result of a congenital anomaly, a malignancy, a metabolic defect, infection, or a host of other causes. A third consideration prior to the institution of definitive treatment is the evaluation of the significance of the disease process. Foremost in this area is an accurate evaluation of the effect on renal function. As has been emphasized, radiologic evaluation alone will usually not suffice. Once this has been accomplished, some appraisal should be made of the likelihood of progression and its relationship to the age and overall medical status of the patient. Finally, the effect of those complications which may ensue, such as infection and calculus disease, should be appraised.

The degree of alacrity with which treatment must be instituted will relate to such factors as patient discomfort, extent of renal insufficiency, and—of particularly great significance—the presence or absence of concomitant infection of the urinary tract. The combination of obstruction and infection creates a situation of urgency because of the likelihood of pyonephrosis, gram-negative sepsis, and even gram-negative septic shock if the patient is not treated promptly.

REFERENCES

Gross JB, Kokko JP: The influence of increased tubular hydrostatic pressure on renal function. J Urol 115:427, 1976

Howards SS: Post-obstructive diuresis: A misunderstood phenomenon. J Urol 110:537, 1973

Radwin HM, O'Dell RM, Schlegel JU: The renal response to acute partial obstruction. J Urol 90:243, 1963

Suki W, Eknoyan G, Rector FC, et al: Patterns of nephron perfusion in acute and chronic hydronephrosis. J Clin Invest 45:122, 1966

Vaughan ED, Sweet RE, Gillenwater JY: Unilateral ureteral occlusion: Pattern of nephron repair and compensatory response. J Urol 109:979, 1973

HEPATORENAL SYNDROME

Robert T. Kunau, Jr.

A significant number of patients who die because of cirrhosis have evidence of renal insufficiency prior to their death. Not infrequently, many of these patients fulfill the clinical criteria for what has become known as the hepatorenal syndrome (HRS). The term HRS was initially used to describe the postoperative renal failure seen in patients with biliary tract obstruction. Since that time, the term has frequently been used, in large part incorrectly, to describe any clinical disorder with both hepatic and renal components. Table 1 lists a number of clinical disorders which affect the function of both the kidney and the liver.

Those entities which constitute a pseudohepatorenal syndrome may be differentiated from the classic HRS by recognition of the precipitating event or by certain characteristic clinical and laboratory features with which these patients present. The classic HRS occurs in patients with decompensated cirrhosis, usually of alcoholic origin, and typically presents as functional renal insufficiency in the absence of the usual causes and without significant anatomical lesions within the kidney.

CLINICAL FEATURES

The syndrome occurs primarily in cirrhotic patients, the cirrhosis usually being of alcoholic origin.

The majority, but not all, of the patients have decompensated liver disease characterized by jaundice, hepatosplenomegaly, hypoalbuminemia, and portal hypertension.

Most of the patients have ascites; when present it may be of any degree.

Renal insufficiency may occur suddenly or develop slowly without precipitating factors, but it frequently follows diuretic therapy, paracentesis, gastrointestinal hemorrhage, infection, surgery, etc. Azotemia and oliguria are the usual manifestations of the renal insufficiency, although azotemia may be present in the absence of oliguria.

Hepatic coma and various electrolyte disturbances may precede or accompany the renal insufficiency but are not invariably present.

A modest decrease in systemic blood pressure is often present and is common late in the course of the disease.

Spontaneous recovery is quite unusual although

renal failure is rarely the cause of death; infection, hemorrhage, and hepatic coma are the more frequent causes of the patient's demise. Spontaneous recoveries seem to follow a dramatic improvement in liver function.

The urinalysis is quite nondescript. The urine sodium concentration is usually less than 10 mEq/liter, even in patients who are not oliguric. Urinary osmolality in the early course of the disease is typically two to three times the plasma value but falls toward the plasma osmolality as the oliguric state continues.

PATHOPHYSIOLOGY

Seemingly, the cardinal abnormality responsible for the renal functional impairment in HRS is a decrease in renal blood flow. This may result either from a fall in blood pressure or, more frequently, from an increase in renal vascular resistance. Although several studies using gas washout techniques have suggested that the vasoconstriction was largely limited to the outer cortex, it is difficult to determine the intrarenal distribution of blood flow with this technique, and conclusions based upon it are tenuous.

Evidence that the renal abnormality in HRS is functional in origin is derived from a number of observations. First, there are no consistent morphologic abnormalities noted in kidneys obtained from patients with HRS. Second, tubular function is usually well maintained until very late in the course of the disease. Third, when kidneys from patients with HRS are transplanted into appropriate recipients, renal function returns; likewise, following liver transplantation, renal function improves in patients with HRS. Finally, drugs which alter renal perfusion are frequently effective, at least transiently, in improving the functional state.

A number of factors have been suggested as possible causes of the renal vasoconstriction, e.g., a decrease in effective plasma volume or an alteration in cardiovascular dynamics such that renal perfusion is compromised. In addition, the presence of false neurotransmitters and depletion of renin substrate and of bradykinin have been proposed as having potentially important roles, yet, to date, no clearly definable mechanism has been identified as the cause of the renal vasoconstriction in HRS. It is also important to bear in mind that a number of causative factors may need to interact in order for the syndrome to develop.

Inasmuch as the circulatory degrangements in cirrhotics are so marked, it is not surprising that they have been strongly implicated in causing the decrease in renal perfusion noted in patients with the HRS. Extensive arteriovenous shunting develops between the portal and systemic circulations in the cirrhotic. Whether the shunts develop exclusively as a result of an increase in portal pressure or as a consequence of some humoral agent is unknown. The presence of these shunts, which result in a low resistance circulatory pathway and likely cause a decrease in the effective extracellular volume, necessitates that the cardiac output increase to maintain satisfactory levels of tissue perfusion. Indeed, the meas-

Table 1
Classification of Clinical Disorder With Hepatic and Renal Involvement

Hepatorenal syndrome

Pseudohepatorenal syndromes
  Generalized disorders
    Infectious—leptospirosis, yellow fever, Reye's syndrome
    Circulatory—shock, congestive heart failure
    Genetic—Polycystic disease, sickle-cell anemia
    Collagen vascular—disseminated lupus erythematosus, periarteritis nodosa
    Unknown etiology—toxemia of pregnancy, amyloidosis, sarcoidosis, Waterhouse-Friedrichson syndrome, hyperthermia
  Toxins
    Direct—carbon tetrachloride, copper sulfate, chromium, Toadstool toxins
    Idiosyncratic or mixed—methoxyflurane, tetracyclines, sulfonamides, stretomycin, iproniazid
  Neoplasms
    Metastatic
    Hypernephroma
  Experimental
    Choline deficiency
    Bile duct division

From: Conn HO: Progress in hepatology: A rational approach to the hepatoral syndrome. Gastroenterology 65:321, 1973. Reprinted by permission, © 1973 The Williams and Wilkins Co, Baltimore

ured cardiac output in these patients, although occasionally low or normal, is not infrequently high. It has been suggested that whatever the cardiac output may be in absolute terms, it is inadequate to provide for peripheral requirements. This may be due, in part, to the presence of intrinsic cardiac disease and/or ascites which may impair venous return to the heart. In this schema, renal vasoconstriction may occur as an attempt to maintain adequate circulation to other areas. Precisely how, if at all, these derangements in the systemic circulation induce the renal vasoconstriction is not clear. Infusion of an alpha adrenergic blocking agent into the renal artery of patients with HRS does not improve renal hemodynamics, suggesting, but not proving, that increased sympathetic activity was not responsible for the renal vasoconstriction. Although renin substrate may be diminished in HRS, renin activity is not infrequently increased and, through the generation of angiotension II, the renin-angiotension system appears to play an important role in the maintenance of the arterial blood pressure in these patients. Whether the renal vasoconstriction is the cause of or the consequence of the increased renin activity is not fully established.

TREATMENT

Restoration of the effective plasma volume, closure of arteriovenous shunts, improvement of cardiac function, and dilation of the renal vascular bed are rational goals to which any effective therapeutic modality for the renal insufficiency in HRS might be directed, yet therapy in these patients is notoriously difficult, with few patients surviving in spite of accomplishing one or more of the goals outlined. This, as stated above, is in large part due to the progression of the liver disease, the onset of hemorrhage, or infection in spite of amelioration of the renal complication. For this reason, many of the experimental maneuvers used to increase renal perfusion and water and sodium excretion have failed to provide more than a transient beneficial effect and must be considered to be experimental.

What can be done with patients who either manifest the full-blown picture of HRS or in whom this complication is likely to occur? First, it is important to prevent the occurrence of any known factor capable of precipitating HRS. This includes vigorous diuretic therapy, gastrointestinal bleeding, surgery, excessive paracentesis, etc. Any diuresis, for example, should be done bearing in mind that the rate of ascitic fluid mobilization is limited.

A question which is raised frequently is the necessity for giving the patient with HRS a solution—e.g., colloid—designed to expand the intravascular and/or extracellular volume. Occasionally, a salutory response is derived from such infusions, but a clinical response is rarely sustained, and not infrequently the administration of such solutions results in a greater degree of positive salt and water balance than was present prior to their initiation. The administration of such solutions beyond that required to repair obvious deficits therefore is not warranted.

A variety of pharmacologic agents have been administered, either systemically or into a renal artery, in an attempt to improve renal function. Included in this list are metaraminol, octapressin, phenoxybenzamine, acetylcholine, prostaglandin A, papaverine, aminophylline, isoproterenol, angiotensin, and phentolamine. Although a salutory response may be noted transiently, these drugs appear to do little to alter the ultimate course. The use of portacaval anastomoses or peritoneal–jugular venous shunts have occasionally been used with success and may offer some hope, particularly for the patient with stable liver function. Nevertheless, additional studies will be required for proper evaluation of these techniques.

REFERENCES

Cohn JN: Renal hemodynamic alterations in liver disease, in Suki WN, Eknoyan G (eds): The Kidney in Systemic Disease. New York, J. Wiley & Sons, 1976

Cohn JN, Tristani FE, Khatri IM: Renal vasodilator therapy in the hepatorenal syndrome. Med Ann DC 39:1, 1970

Conn HO: Progress in hepatology: A rational approach to the hepatorenal syndrome. Gastroenterology 65:321, 1973

Fullen WD: Hepatorenal syndrome: Reversal by peritoneovenous shunt. Surgery 82:337, 1977

Groszman RJ, Kotelanski B, Cohn JN, et al: Quantitation of portasystemic shunting from the splenic and mesenteric beds in alcoholic liver disease. Am J Med 53:715, 1972

Papper S: The hepatorenal syndrome. Clin Nephrol 4:41, 1975

Papper S: Renal failure in cirrhosis, in Epstein M (ed): The Kidney in Liver Disease. New York, Elsevier North-Holland, 1978, p 91

Papper S, Belesky JL, Bleifer KH: Renal failure in Laennec's cirrhosis of the liver. I. Description of clinical and laboratory findings. Ann Intern Med 51:759, 1959

THE KIDNEY IN PREGNANCY

Thomas F. Ferris

There are several extraordinary changes in cardiovascular physiology which occur during pregnancy. There is an approximate 50 percent increase in blood volume in late pregnancy, with the rise in both plasma volume and red cell mass beginning in the first trimester. Plasma volume increases more than red cell mass; thus a physiologic anemia or hemodilution occurs with pregnancy. Accompanying the increased blood volume, cardiac output increases in the first trimester and is 30–40 percent above the nonpregnant level at approximately the 24th week of gestation. In spite of the increase in cardiac output, arterial blood pressure falls during pregnancy; thus a striking reduction in total peripheral resistance occurs. This vasodilation is frequently evident clinically in the spider telangiectases and palmar erythema which develop during pregnancy. Renal blood flow increases 30–50 percent during pregnancy as a result of the increase in cardiac output and a decrease in renal resistance. Accompanying the increase in renal blood flow, glomerular filtration rate also increases as early as the second month of pregnancy. The increase in GFR and renal plasma flow remain proportional until late in pregnancy, when a disproportionate increase in glomerular filtration occurs. The increase in GFR in early pregnancy may be due to the increase in renal plasma flow, with the increase in filtration fraction in late pregnancy due to a decrease in serum oncotic pressure. Serum protein concentration falls approximately 1 g/dl in the last trimester, which would diminish plasma oncotic pressure approximately 7 mm Hg. All other factors remaining constant, a fall in oncotic pressure would increase the filtration fraction. It is important to recognize the increase in glomerular filtration rate during pregnancy since mean BUN is 8.7 ± 1.5 mg/dl and mean serum creatinine is 0.46 ± 0.6 mg/dl in pregnant women. Thus a serum creatinine of 1.5 mg/dl or BUN of 15 mg/dl is distinctly abnormal during pregnancy and may represent a 40–50 percent decrease in glomerular filtration rate.

RENAL TUBULAR FUNCTION IN PREGNANCY

Glucosuria and aminoaciduria are frequent during pregnancy, glucosuria occurring in 5–40 percent of pregnant women studied. The glucosuria is due to a reduction in maximal reabsorption of glucose during pregnancy. Urate clearance increases in pregnancy with mean serum urate 3 ± 0.17 mg/dl, compared to 4.2 ± 1.2 mg/dl in nonpregnant women. The increase in GFR with pregnancy necessitates an equal increase in tubular sodium reabsorption. In this regard, pregnant women conserve sodium as well as nonpregnant women on a low sodium intake.

PLASMA RENIN AND ALDOSTERONE IN PREGNANCY

There is an increase in both renin and aldosterone secretion in pregnancy. The increase occurs in the first trimester with plasma renin activity (PRA) 15 times higher than nonpregnant levels because of the rise in both plasma renin and substrate concentration. Plasma angiotensin is also significantly increased and probably maintains arterial pressure, since angiotensin blockage causes a significant fall in blood pressure in pregnant animals. The increase in renin and aldosterone secretion has been postulated to be due to elevated progesterone secretion during pregnancy, since progesterone antagonizes the effect of aldosterone at the renal tubule; however, no consistent relationship has been found between plasma aldosterone and progesterone. This explanation would imply that pregnancy is a salt-wasting state with increased aldosterone secretion needed to maintain sodium balance; however, approximately 900 mEq sodium is retained during pregnancy and, as noted previously, pregnant women conserve sodium normally on extremely low salt intake.

Since renal prostaglandin synthesis is a factor in renin secretion, the increase in renin secretion may be due to increased renal prostaglandin synthesis. An increase in urinary PGE excretion has been noted in pregnant women. An increase in the production of prostaglandin E, which is a vasodilator and antagonist to angiotensin, might explain the insensitivity to angiotensin which occurs early in pregnancy.

TOXEMIA IN PREGNANCY

Toxemia is a disease of late pregnancy characterized by hypertension, edema, and proteinuria. The disease has a bimodal frequency with peak incidence in young primiparous and older multiparous women. When hypertension occurs in the absence of proteinuria, particularly in multiparous women, it may be an early manifestation of essential hypertension induced by pregnancy. The disease has been divided into preeclampsia and eclampsia based upon whether or not a convulsion has occurred. Although eclampsia usually is associated with severe disease, the separation of the disease on the basis of convulsions is probably outdated

and tends to minimize the preeclamptic state. The hypertension and proteinuria in toxemia are unrelated, with hypertension more prominent in some patients and proteinuria in others.

Mechanism of Hypertension in Toxemia

An increase in peripheral resistance occurs in toxemia, the cause of which is unknown. Increased sensitivity to angiotensin has been demonstrated in toxemia which precedes the clinical manifestations of toxemia and has been demonstrated to occur as early as the 20th week of gestation in women destined to develop toxemia (Fig. 1). The cause of the increased sensitivity is unknown, but since toxemia is usually associated with sodium and water retention, arteriolar swelling might be a factor. The salt retention in toxemia occurs with a concomitant reduction in renal blood flow and glomerular filtration rate; thus a natriuresis in response to hypertension is prevented. Also, salt retention occurs in the face of a decrease in venous capacitance which results in exquisite sensitivity to volume expansion.

Since there is clinical evidence that reduction in uterine blood flow occurs with toxemia, explanations for the hypertension based upon uterine hypoperfusion have been made. Renin is present in both animal and human uterus and is released from the uterus with reduction in uterine perfusion. Human amniotic fluid contains high concentration of the larger molecule prorenin, which may also escape into the circulation under certain circumstances; however, the role that uterine renin plays in the hypertension of toxemia is not clear. The high plasma renin of pregnancy does not seem to be of uterine origin, since plasma renin activity responds to changes in sodium intake during pregnancy but uterine renin concentration does not. Uterine renin may act as a local hormone in regulating uterine blood flow; angiotensin increases uterine blood flow in the pregnant animal. Since angiotensin also increases prostaglandin E synthesis, the vasodilation might be caused by increased uterine synthesis of PGE. Toxemia is associated with variable plasma renin and angiotensin concentration, but usually both fall with the development of toxemia; however, since there is increased sensitivity to angiotensin in toxemia, the concentration of plasma renin and angiotensin is not as important as sensitivity. If insensitivity to angiotensin in normotensive pregnancy is dependent upon PGE synthesis, it is tempting to speculate that the increase in sensitivity with the development of toxemia is due to decreased PGE synthesis. Thus the combination of a small but inappropriate release of uterine renin during uterine hypoperfusion in a setting of increased angiotensin sensitivity could cause hypertension. The increased prostaglandin synthesis in pregnancy may be of uterine origin or may represent increased prostaglandin synthesis by all blood vessels.

Renal Function in Toxemia

There is a reduction in both glomerular filtration rate and renal blood flow with toxemia. Although the

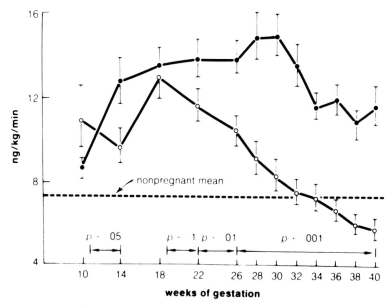

Fig. 1. Angiotensin sensitivity throughout pregnancy. Note the decrease in sensitivity to angiotensin (measured as ng angiotensin/kg/min needed to raise diastolic pressure 20 mm Hg) seen as early as the 10th week. In women who developed toxemia (open circle), a progressive increase in sensitivity began at about the 22nd week. With the development of clinically evident toxemia, after 32 weeks, sensitivity had increased to levels greater than in nonpregnant women.

decrease in glomerular filtration rate increases BUN and serum creatinine, plasma urate is a better criterion than either in assessing the severity of the disease. The cause of the decrease in urate clearance with toxemia is not clear. It has been suggested that increased plasma lactate from an ischemic uterus inhibits urate secretion, but studies have failed to demonstrate a consistent correlation between arterial lactate and urate concentration in toxemic women. Since urate clearance falls with volume depletion or with an increase in filtration fraction caused by angiotensin or norepinephrine, a similar change in intrarenal hemodynamics may cause the decrease in urate secretion with toxemia.

Renal Pathology

Uneven thickening of the capillary basement membrane with striking swelling of the cytoplasm of endothelial cells occurs with toxemia which has been termed "glomerular capillary endotheliosis" (Fig. 2). Immunofluorescent studies have revealed deposits of fibrin without evidence of antigen–antibody complexes in the glomeruli. The absence of an immunologic reaction in toxemia points to a direct glomerular injury. The glomerular pathology correlates with the extent of proteinuria.

Clinical Features of Toxemia

The incidence of toxemia varies widely, from 30 percent in Puerto Rico to approximately 7 percent in Scotland. The incidence depends upon the criteria used for the diagnosis. A significant rise in blood pressure has been reported to occur in 25 percent of women in Scotland during their first pregnancy. The decrease in blood pressure with pregnancy has important clinical implications, since blood pressure considered normal in

nonpregnant women can be elevated in pregnancy. In a large series of pregnant women mean arterial pressure (diastolic pressure plus one-third the pulse pressure) was found to be 72 ± 9 mm Hg at the 22nd week of gestation and rose to 82 ± 8 mm Hg at term. Fetal mortality rises when diastolic pressure is greater than 84 mm Hg. Thus a blood pressure of 120/80, which represents a mean arterial pressure of 93 mm Hg, is elevated in pregnancy, particularly if it was lower earlier in gestation. The failure of physicians to recognize these new values of normal blood pressure has frequently resulted in a failure to detect toxemia at its earliest stage.

Treatment

The initial therapy of mild toxemia is bedrest with mild sedation with either phenobarbital or diazepam. If edema is present, a 2 g salt diet with 50 mg hydrochlorothiazide daily usually brings the blood pressure to normal levels. If the pregnancy is beyond 36 weeks, delivery is indicated. With more severe toxemia (blood pressures greater than 140/90), antihypertensive drugs are indicated. Although it has been the feeling of some obstetricians that reduction in blood pressure reduces uterine blood flow, there are no data to support this opinion. Uterine blood flow autoregulates over a wide range of perfusion pressures in pregnant animals, and in most studies in which antihypertensive drugs have been administered to pregnant animals uterine blood flow either remains the same or increases. Magnesium sulfate has been used for many years for treatment of toxemia, since it has a mild vasodilating effect and is a central nervous system depressant; however, more potent antihypertensive drugs are available. Hydralazine, for example, given orally every 6 hours in 25–50 mg doses is effective, particularly when used in conjunction with a diuretic and with either propranolol or methyldopa (Aldomet). Propranolol can be given in doses of 40 mg every 6 hours or Aldomet 250 mg twice daily. With severe toxemia, in which diastolic blood pressure is greater than 110 mm Hg, parenteral antihypertensive therapy is warranted. Either 500 mg of Aldomet or hydralazine 25 mg intramuscularly or 50 mg in 500 ml glucose in water can be given slowly intravenously with constant monitoring of the blood pressure. If edema is present 40 mg furosemide can also be given. When the diastolic pressure is greater than 120 mm Hg, 300 mg diazoxide can be given intravenously with 40–80 mg of intravenous furosemide. Diazoxide has proven to be an excellent drug to treat severe hypertension with toxemia. One side effect is the cessation of labor, which occurs in about 50 percent of patients due to the generalized smooth muscle relaxant effect of the drug; however, oxytocin can be used to restart labor in these patients. With severe toxemia, once the clinical state has been stabilized and the blood pressure brought under control, delivery is indicated. In rare instances where the decision to continue the pregnancy is made, the patient should remain hospitalized and antihypertensive drugs utilized to control the blood pressure. Daily BUN, serum creatinine, and urate, as well as 24 hour urine collections for protein, are monitored; if proteinuria and azotemia persist, delivery is indicated.

In most circumstances the baby does better in a neonatal intensive care unit than in the uterus of a toxemic woman.

ESSENTIAL HYPERTENSION DURING PREGNANCY

Essential hypertension accounts for approximately one-third of all hypertension occurring with pregnancy. The detection of hypertension can be the result of a woman having her blood pressure taken for the first time during pregnancy or may represent the development of hypertension in pregnancy. The absence of proteinuria, reduced glomerular filtration rate, hyperuricemia, and edema accompanying hypertension point to essential hypertension rather than toxemia. There is a normal increase in blood pressure with increase in angiotensin sensitivity in the last 8 weeks of pregnancy; thus in women with a hypertensive diathesis this might result in the development of hypertension. A proportion of women who develop hypertension during pregnancy either remain hypertensive after the pregnancy or develop essential hypertension in later life. No workup of the hypertension is necessary during the pregnancy, but since pheochromocytoma is associated with a high maternal mortality in pregnancy, symptoms suggestive of such a tumor should be elicited.

The prognosis for a successful pregnancy in women with essential hypertension preceding the pregnancy is good. If blood pressure is below 160/100 the spontaneous abortion rate is no greater than in normotensive

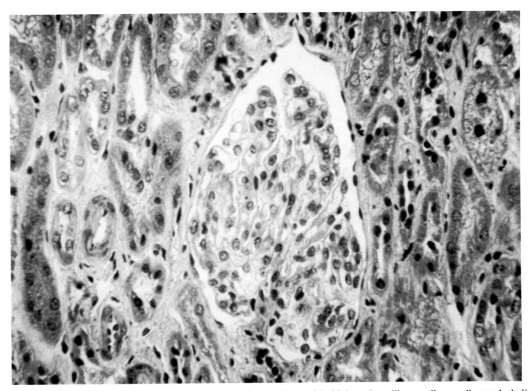

Fig. 2. Glomerulus in toxemia. The glomerulus is relatively bloodless with thickened capillary walls, swollen endothelial cells, and narrowed capillary lumen.

women. In women with higher blood pressure fetal mortality is higher and the incidence of superimposed toxemia is greater; however, with the use of antihypertensive drugs, blood pressure can be maintained normal during pregnancy. Hypertension should be treated similar to the nonpregnant state using antihypertensive drugs to maintain the blood pressure as close to normal as possible. Diuretics can be used throughout pregnancy. They will not interfere with the normal 900 mEq sodium retained in the expansion of maternal blood volume and development of the fetus unless dietary sodium is concomitantly severely restricted. The use of diuretics may cause elevation in serum urate, but seldom to levels in excess of 6.5 mg/dl; higher levels usually indicate superimposed toxemia. If one compares fetal survival today with previous reports of pregnancy in untreated women, antihypertensive agents have increased fetal survival. Since maternal death with toxemia or essential hypertension during pregnancy is usually caused by intracerebral hemorrhage, control of the blood pressure is essential.

RENAL DISEASE DURING PREGNANCY
Glomerulonephritis

Acute glomerulonephritis is a rare complication during pregnancy and frequently results in fetal loss; however, with control of blood pressure and fluid balance, women with acute glomerulonephritis have had normal deliveries. There is an increased incidence of toxemia with chronic glomerulonephritis. Not only is the incidence higher in these women, but the toxemia occurs early, often before the 28th week of pregnancy. When proteinuria is the only manifestation of chronic glomerulonephritis, the incidence of toxemia and fetal loss is not much higher than in normal women; however, when hypertension accompanies the proteinuria, the risk in pregnancy is greater; fetal loss rises to approximately 45 percent, with an incidence of toxemia of about 50 percent. With both hypertension and azotemia there is a worsening of the renal disease with superimposed toxemia in approximatley 75 percent of patients during the pregnancy. There is evidence that these patients should be delivered at about the 34th week of pregnancy, since the incidence of uterine death increases after that. Regardless of cause, women with renal disease must be seen frequently during pregnancy, and any rise in blood pressure or rapid weight gain must be considered significant. Since two or more of the usual features of preeclampsia—i.e., proteinuria, hypertension, edema—may precede the pregnancy, one depends upon a rise in serum creatinine, BUN, or urate concentration to detect the onset of toxemia. Treatment consists of maintaining normal blood pressure with antihypertensive agents and using diuretics as needed. If toxemia occurs in the first or second trimester in a woman with preexisting renal disease, termination of the pregnancy is indicated, since there is little likelihood the pregnancy will be successful and there is some evidence that renal function may be permanently damaged from a prolonged toxemic state.

In women with the nephrotic syndrome and normal renal function, pregnancies are usually successful, although the risk of toxemia is twice normal, about 15 percent. Birthweight of children of nephrotic mothers correlates best with serum albumin levels, and these children frequently are premature. Renal vein thrombosis as a cause of the nephrotic syndrome has been described in pregnant women, possibly secondary to the increase in clotting factors and venous stasis of late pregnancy.

Pyelonephritis

Acute pyelonephritis. The incidence of bacteriuria in pregnancy is not different from nonpregnant women, 4–7 percent. Woman with bacteriuria on the first prenatal visit have a 20–40 percent incidence of acute pyelonephritis during pregnancy. Treatment of the bacteriuria lowers the subsequent incidence of acute pyelonephritis during the pregnancy by approximately 90 percent. Although original reports suggested premature delivery in women with asymptomatic bacteriuria, subsequent studies have not confirmed these findings. If bacteriuria is detected during pregnancy, treatment with either sulfamethoxazole 0.5 g four times daily or a combination of trimethoprim and sulfisoxazole for approximately 7–10 days is indicated. Ampicillin should be used in the last month of pregnancy because of the theoretical danger of hyperbilirubinemia in the newborn from use of sulfonamide drugs.

In chronic interstitial nephritis or chronic pyelonephritis the course of pregnancy is similar to chronic glomerulonephritis, the success of the pregnancy being dependent upon whether hypertension and azotemia are present.

Systemic Lupus Erythematosus

The clinical course in patients with SLE is variable during pregnancy. Perinatal mortality and the incidence of preeclampsia are higher than in normal women, with the risk of clinical exacerbation of SLE being approximately three times greater in the first 20 weeks of pregnancy and eight times greater in the postpartum period. The last half of pregnancy does not seem to be associated with worsening of the disease. The incidence of toxemia and the risk of decreasing renal function during pregnancy are similar to other types of chronic glomerulonephritis.

Diabetic Nephropathy

Most studies have demonstrated that diabetic women can have normal pregnancies with good chance of fetal survival. Even women with significant diabetic nephropathy, proteinuria, and reduction in renal function at the start of pregnancy usually have successful pregnancies. There has been no evidence of a uniform reduction in glomerular filtration rate during pregnancy with diabetic nephropathy, and although the incidence of toxemia is higher in this group of patients, with careful control of blood pressure most diabetics can have a successful pregnancy.

Acute Renal Failure

Acute renal failure is a serious complication of pregnancy and can occur either early in pregnancy, caused by a septic abortion, or in late pregnancy, usually associated with toxemia and a related obstetric complication. *Clostridium welchii* and *Streptococcus pyogenes* are the usual offending organisms following a septic abortion, with the characteristic feature of clostridial infection being intravascular hemolysis, hemoglobinemia, and renal failure. The danger of acute renal failure in late pregnancy is the possibility of cortical necrosis developing in this setting. This is probably caused by intravascular coagulation in the kidney, with the pathologic feature being intimal hyalinization of the arcuate arteries and thrombus formation in interlobular afferent arterioles and glomeruli. Pregnant women are predisposed to intravascular coagulation because of several factors: (1) increase in clotting factors in pregnancy; (2) the increased risk of gram-negative infection during pregnancy which may activate a Schwartzman reaction; (3) toxemia where hypertension and arteriolar constriction may cause endothelial cell injury which may act as a nidus for intravascular clotting; and (4) abruptio placentae during toxemia with release of thromboblastic material from the placenta into the circulation. The diagnosis of cortical necrosis should be considered when oliguria in acute renal failure lasts more than 21 days. The treatment of acute renal failure in pregnancy is similar to that in nonpregnant patients, with attention to control of blood pressure and sodium, potassium, and water balance, with hemodialysis utilized when necessary. Since the development of acute renal failure in pregnancy usually follows either an abortion or obstetrical catastrophe, fetal survival is not usually a consideration.

POSTPARTUM RENAL FAILURE

Rapid development of renal failure 2–10 weeks postpartum with findings at autopsy of malignant nephrosclerosis has been reported. In some patients there is evidence of a microangiopathic hemolytic anemia, and the disease has been called postpartum hemolytic-uremic syndrome. The pathologic changes in the kidney are fibrin deposits in glomeruli and afferent arterioles. The cause of the disease is unknown, but factors predisposing to intravascular coagulation in pregnancy are probably important. In adults, unlike children, the hemolytic-uremic syndrome usually results in permanent renal failure.

PREGNANCY FOLLOWING RENAL TRANSPLANTATION

Most patients on long-term hemodialysis have amenorrhea and are infertile, but resumption of menses occurs following transplantation if renal function becomes normal. Pregnancy is being reported more frequently in women following transplantation, and the chance of a successful pregnancy is excellent. Although cesarean section has been advocated by some, most deliveries are vaginal. The incidence of toxemia may be higher in these women, particularly if renal function is not normal prior to the pregnancy, but its treatment is similar to toxemia in any pregnant woman. The patients are maintained on steroids and immunosuppressive therapy throughout the pregnancy, and careful observation of renal function and blood pressure is made. The incidence of fetal abnormalities does not seem higher in these women than in control populations.

REFERENCES

Burrows GN, Ferris TF: Medical Complications During Pregnancy, Philadelphia, W. B. Saunders, 1975

Ferris TF: The kidney in pregnancy, in Gottschalk C, Earley L (eds): Strauss and Welt's Diseases of the Kidney (ed 3). Boston, Little Brown, 1978

Gant NF, Daley GL, Chand S, et al: Study of the metabolic clearance rate of dehydroisoandrosterone sulfate in pregnancy. Am J Obstet Gynecol 111:555, 1971

Lindheimer MD, Katz AI, Zuspan FP: Hypertension in Pregnancy, New York, J. Wiley & Sons, 1976

RENAL NEOPLASMS

J. Daniel Johnson and Howard M. Radwin

Renal malignancies account for just under 3 percent of all malignant tumors, with an incidence of 3.5 cases/100,000 population/year. Renal cell carcinoma was first described by Grawitz in 1883 and comprises over 85 percent of renal neoplasms. Males predominate 2:1. The peak age of presentation is in the sixth decade, but an increased number of renal cell carcinomas are being recognized in children. Approximately 25–33 percent of patients will have metastases at the time of diagnosis, 10 percent of which may be asymptomatic. The usual sites for metastases are lungs (50 percent), liver (33 percent), and bone (32 percent), but spread to brain and thyroid are fairly common.

The etiology of renal cell carcinoma is unknown, but several carcinogens have been implicated. Dimethylnitrosamine is a known carcinogen present in tobacco smoke which will induce renal cell carcinoma in rats and mice. Tobacco smoking by humans is associated with a rate of renal cell carcinoma 5–12 times greater than is seen in nonsmokers. Other agents inducing renal tumors in animal models include aromatic hydrocarbons and amines, aliphatic compounds, aflatoxins, lead, cadmium, and estrogens. It was the induction of renal cell carcinoma by administration of estrogen to hamsters coupled with the demonstration of tumor regression following progesterone therapy that led to the clinical use of progestational agents. A high incidence of renal cell carcinoma (80 percent) has been associated with Lindau–von Hippel disease. Although an increased incidence of these tumors is found in patients with adult polycystic kidney disease, this may reflect only a population which is studied more frequently.

Two main cell types are seen. Clear cells with cytoplasm full of lipid and glycogen are the most common. Granular cells have little cytoplasmic lipid, but many mitochondria produce the effect of eosinophilic granular cytoplasm. While one cell type may predominate, most tumors are composed of both. Cells may be arranged in solid sheets, primitive tubules, or papillary and cystic patterns without significant correlation to prognosis. The aggressive but rare sarcomatoid pattern has a poorer prognosis. Electron microscopic studies have demonstrated that renal cell carcinoma shares many ultrastructural features with the proximal convoluted tubule. It is distinctly unrelated to other normal renal cell types.

Hypernephromas are often occult and may grow to great size prior to causing symptoms or metastasizing. Hematuria occurs in two-thirds of patients and is typically intermittent, gross, and painless. The complete classical triad of hematuria, flank pain, and palpable mass is a late constellation of findings occurring in only 9-15 percent of the patients, half of whom have evidence of metastatic disease. Other sequelae of renal cell carcinoma may include high-output congestive heart failure caused by large neoplastic arteriovenous shunts, varicocele unrelated to position caused by renal vein occlusion, and signs of inferior vena cava obstruction.

Systemic effects may be produced in a large proportion of patients with renal cancer in the absence of metastatic disease. Apparently localized hypernephroma is associated with elevated erythrocyte sedimentation rate in 56 percent, anemia in 41 percent, fever in 20 percent, and hepatic dysfunction with liver enzyme and bilirubin elevation. These usually resolve after nephrectomy, but they may return to herald clinically undetected metastatic disease. Neuromyopathy, possibly autoimmune in origin, is a rare finding. Amyloidosis may accompany 3–5 percent of renal carcinomas, and it is associated with poor survival despite therapeutic efforts.

Endocrine-like abnormalities are less commonly found. Erythrocytosis may be seen in 4 percent of these patients and appears to lend a more favorable prognosis. Hypercalcemia may also accompany hypernephroma and an immediate threat to life by its unremitting severity. Compounds with effects resembling parathormone, prostaglandins, and erythropoietin have been identified to explain these abnormalities. Hypertension due to compression of the renal artery or the entire renal substance by the tumor mass may be associated with renal cancer. No pressor substance produced by renal cell carcinoma has been demonstrated. Almost 50 percent of patients will have gastrointestinal complaints, possibly caused by glucagon production. Gonadotropin elaboration by the tumor has been reported.

While these nonspecific symptoms and biochemical abnormalities may allow suspicion of renal carcinoma, the diagnosis is usually made radiographically. Nephrotomography will correctly suggest tumor in 80 percent of the patients with malignancy. If the mass is calcified, tumor is more common. Twenty percent of otherwise benign appearing cysts containing peripheral rim calcification and almost 90 percent of renal masses with central calcification will be malignant. Renal masses associated with compression fractures of the spine or pathologic long bone fractures are particularly suspect.

Hypernephroma may be accurately defined in 87–95 percent of patients by the use of selective angiography, although epinephrine or angiotensin assistance, subtraction techniques, or magnification arteriograms may be required (Fig. 1). If the renal vein is not seen on the venous phase films, inferior vena cavography is needed due to the frequent extension of this tumor into the venous system. Computed tomography appears to offer accurate diagnosis with less risk to the patient, but it currently assumes an adjuvant diagnostic role to angiography. Ultrasonography and percutaneous cyst puncture are frequently employed to differentiate cystic from solid masses and characterize their contents as a means of confirming a benign cyst. If all criteria of benignity are not met, the mass must be suspected to be malignant. Occult metastatic lesions should be sought with whole lung tomography, bone scan, liver function studies, and celiac angiography or liver scan.

The natural history of renal cell carcinoma is variable and seemingly at times capricious. In a large series of untreated, inoperable patients, the 5 year survival was 1.7 percent, with an average survival of 5–8 months. Spontaneous regression of hypernephroma has been reported, often following an infectious complication. Metastatic tumor may regress and stabilize without therapy in 0.1 percent of cases, but these responses are limited almost exclusively to pulmonary lesions following nephrectomy. Spontaneous regression occurs almost eight times more frequently in men, supporting a hormonal association with renal cancer. The absence of detectable disease does not eliminate the possibility of indolent growth, since recurrent metastases have been reported up to 31 years following apparently curative surgery. Followup should be of indefinite duration.

Surgical therapy continues to be the only modality with demonstrated effectiveness against renal cell carcinoma. Simple nephrectomy has yielded a 25–32 percent overall 5 year survival rate in those patients without demonstrable metastases. In the early 1960s, Robson introduced the practice of extensive preoperative evaluation coupled with a "radical" en bloc resection of the kidney, Gerota's capsule and fat, the encompassed ipsilateral adrenal gland, and the regional lymph nodes along the great vessels. This approach improved overall 5 year survival to 41–59 percent.

There has been no clearly demonstrated benefit from radiation therapy for renal cell carcinoma either alone or as an adjunct to surgery. Local symptomatic palliation for metastatic lesions may be achieved with radiotherapy in selected patients. No chemotherapeutic agent has shown consistent effectiveness against renal cell carcinoma. Objective response rates of 20 percent for multiple cytotoxic agents, alone and in combination, have never been exceeded. Provera alone has yielded stabilization or regression of metastatic disease in 16 percent. Immune RNA and BCG immunotherapy alone and in combination with other treatment modalities has been used with a few encouraging preliminary responses.

In patients with stage D disease, the value of

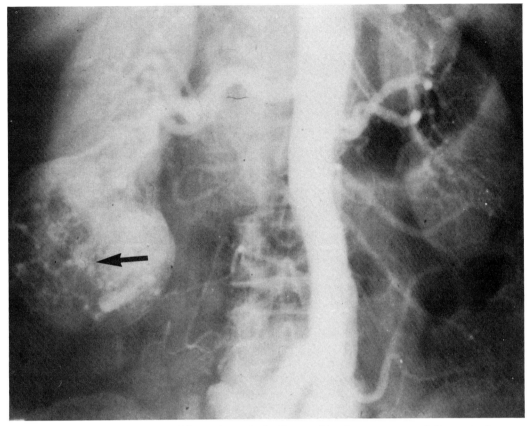

Fig. 1. Renal cell carcinoma demonstrated by angiography is diagnosed by the appearance of disorganized neovascularity within the renal mass.

removing the primary tumor is a matter of dispute. Statistically significant increased survival or palliation has not been shown for most patients with soft tissue metastases who are subjected to nephrectomy. Those with only osseous metastases, however, may benefit from adjuvant nephrectomy by enjoying significantly increased survival.

RENAL CARCINOMAS

Tumors of the renal pelvis account for 12–14 percent of renal cancers and are most commonly transitional cell carcinoma. The tumors occur predominantly in males (4:1), with a peak age of presentation in the sixth decade. Multifocal tumors are common, and associated simultaneous or dyssynchronous bladder tumors occur in up to 93 percent of patients. Even with proper surgical therapy, recurrent tumors afflict up to 30 percent of patients, and 10 percent will arise in the contralateral renal pelvis or ureter.

The etiology of transitional cell carcinoma is unknown, but many environmental factors have been implicated in both clinical settings and animal models. Aniline dyes, certain petroleum intermediates such as β naphthylamine, tryptophan metabolites, phenacetin, and tobacco smoke all have demonstrated statistical association with transitional cell cancer.

Transitional cell carcinomas may be classified by histologic grade based on cellular differentiation, growth pattern (papillary, sessile, polypoid), and depth of invasion. Higher-grade transitional cell tumors often demonstrate adenomatous and squamous metaplasia. The tumors are similar to bladder tumors with the exception that invasive lesions have a poorer prognosis when arising primarily in the kidney. Noninvasive low-grade papillomas have an 80–90 percent 5 year survival, contrasted with 12–30 percent for invasive tumors.

Hematuria is the most common presenting complaint, and colic may accompany passage of clots. Filling defects may be noted on excretory urograms and can be confirmed by retrograde pyelography (Fig. 2). Cytologic examination of urine obtained from both voided specimens and selective ureteral catheterization is helpful, as are brush biopsies of filling defects in the renal pelvis. Angiography is seldom diagnostic with this tumor, since it is generally a hypovascular lesion.

Surgical excision of the kidney and the entire ureter, including a cuff of bladder surrounding the ureteral orifice, is the current treatment of choice for transitional cell tumors in the renal pelvis or ureter. The importance of complete removal of the ureter is emphasized by an observed recurrent rate in retained ureteral stumps of 25–40 percent. Noninvasive lesions occurring in a solitary kidney may be managed by segmental resection.

Radiotherapy has little therapeutic benefit with

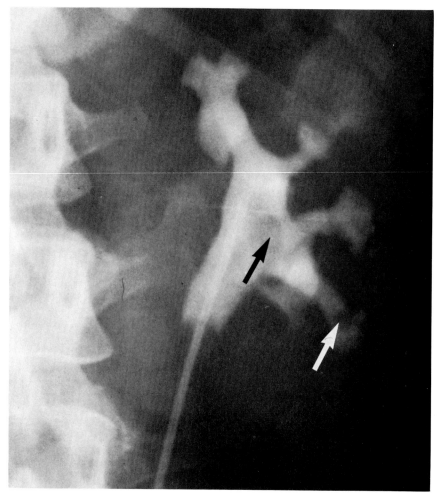

Fig. 2. Transitional cell carcinomas may be detected as filling defects in the renal pelvis on excretory urograms and confirmed with retrograde pyelography as illustrated here.

transitional cell tumors of the renal pelvis. Many moderately effective chemotherapeutic agents have been employed for palliation of transitional cell tumors which are unresectable or which represent surgical failures. Doxorubicin and *cis*-platinum currently appears to be the most effective combination.

Squamous cell carcinoma of the renal pelvis constitutes 2–3 percent of renal tumors overall and 15–25 percent of tumors arising in the renal pelvis. These may occur at any age, and they appear to affect both sexes equally. Approximately one-half of squamous cell carcinomas arise from transitional cell tumors by metaplasia. These have a very poor prognosis, more closely approximating that of pure squamous cell tumors than transitional cell tumors. The only clear etiologic association with pure squamous cell cancer appears to be the presence of renal calculi and squamous metaplasia caused by chronic irritation. The prognosis is uniformly poor, with only a 15–20 percent 5 year survival rate. Radical nephrectomy is recommended, with complete ureterectomy required only when concurrent transitional cell carcinoma is present. Neither radiotherapy nor chemotherapy are effective against these tumors, al-

though newer agents such as bleomycin offer promise.

CHILDHOOD TUMORS

Wilms' tumor is the most common abdominal neoplasm in childhood. It usually presents prior to 7 years of age, with a peak incidence at 3 years. Nephroblastoma, as it is also termed, originates in the nephrogenic blastema prior to differentiation. While the majority of patients have no associated abnormalities, a syndrome of aniridia, hemihypertrophy, hamartomas, and visceral cytomegaly has been linked to an increased incidence of Wilms' tumors. There is some evidence that a complex form of hereditary predisposition is involved.

A palpable abdominal mass, usually detected by a parent, is the presenting complaint in 90 percent of the patients. Bilateral tumor masses may be found in 5–12 percent. Although gross hematuria is rare, up to 50 percent may have microscopic hematuria. Hypertension has been noted in a significant proportion of these patients, and elevated renin levels have been detected in tumor extracts.

Gastrointestinal complaints associated with diarrhea are common and may cause marked dehydration and electrolyte imbalance. Anemia or polycythemia may be present. Hyperuricemia is frequent. Bone marrow examination, bone survey, urinary homovanillic acid (HVA), vanillylmandelic acid (VMA), and carcinoembryonic antigen (CEA) determination will help to differentiate neuroblastoma from Wilms' tumor.

The intravenous pyelogram is the single most productive diagnostic test for Wilms' tumor. Characteristically, this tumor distorts the architecture of the collecting system, in contrast to neuroblastoma, which tends to displace and extrinsically compress the kidney. Large exophytic and encapsulated nephroblastomas can be exceptions to this rule and may cause only an abnormal renal outline. A pattern of calcification which is typically subtle may occur in 15 percent of these tumors. A nonfunctioning renal mass is more consistent with hydronephrosis but may be seen in 20 percent of Wilms' tumor patients.

The tumor spreads by direct infiltration and venous invasion. Lymphatic and pulmonary metastases are common; bone and cerebral metastases are rare. Histologic characteristics are variable, but all tumors contain a mixture of renal blastema with differentiated mesenchymal tissue such as muscle fibers, cartilage, osteoid, fat, primitive glomeruli and tubules. Careful examination is necessary to differentiate Wilms' tumor from the more benign mesoblastic nephroma (fetal renal hamartoma).

Surgical excision is necessary for prolonged survival, since to date no child has survived without undergoing nephrectomy. If resection appears impossible, chemotherapy and radiotherapy may be initiated; if a response is noted, a secondary attempt at resection may be feasible.

Radiotherapy is used postoperatively to control residual local disease and to manage metastatic lesions. Reports of significant antitumor activity with actinomycin D were first reported in 1960. It is now included in multiple drug chemotherapy programs for Wilms' tumor with vincristine and less often with doxorubicin or cyclophosphamide. Chemotherapy is often strikingly effective. With current multidiscipline therapy programs, patients with localized disease achieve an 80–90 percent cure rate. Patients with distant metastases have a poor prognosis, but some series now report 60–80 percent of these patients with disease-free intervals of 2 years.

MISCELLANEOUS TUMORS

Many rare connective tissue and fibrous malignant tumors are discovered arising in the kidney. These include sarcomas, malignant fibrous histiocytomas, lymphoma, and vascular tumors. Tumors metastatic to the kidney are occasionally encountered, most commonly originating from squamous cell cancers of the lung. Testicular tumor in the retroperitoneal nodes rarely may invade the kidney and collecting system.

The benign neoplasms arising in the kidney are of little clinical importance except that they must be differentiated from malignant lesions. The majority of these tumors are found incidentally at autopsy, although some lesions may cause symptoms. The renal cortex may be the site of a renal adenoma. These tumors were historically defined as benign adenomas by virtue of their size (less than 3 cm) and the lack of metastases. No other criterion, such as histology, growth pattern, predominant cell type, or location, can successfully differentiate these tumors from small renal cell carcinoma. Both tumors are related statistically to smoking. Electron microscopic studies show similar ultrastructural characteristics in both tumors, and each appears to have its origin in the proximal convoluted tubule cell. Certainly tumors found ante mortem of less than 3 cm in diameter with angiographic features consistent with renal cell carcinomas must be treated as malignant lesions. The existence of renal adenoma as a benign lesion would seem to be at least controversial.

Renal angiomyolipoma is a benign hamartoma of clinical importance because it mimics hypernephroma radiographically and often causes hematuria or retroperitoneal hemorrhage. This tumor occurs in about 80 percent of patients with tuberous sclerosis and is often bilateral. Angiographic studies reveal a hypervascular tumor with disorganized vessels and often prominent aneurysms in the tumor. Preoperative diagnosis in the patient without tuberous sclerosis may be difficult.

The majority of renal tumors detected in the newborn are benign mesenchymal hamartomas known as fetal renal hamartoma or mesoblastic nephroma. Although frequently confused with Wilms' tumor, correct diagnosis following curative resection will obviate the need for adjuvant irradiation and chemotherapy with their attendant complications. Incomplete resection will lead to local recurrence.

Other benign tumors may be clinically important despite their rare occurrence. Hypertension can be caused by renin producing tumors, presumably arising from the juxtaglomerular apparatus. Oncocytoma is a rare renal tumor which attains large size without causing symptoms and usually cannot be distinguished from hypernephroma without resection and histologic examination.

REFERENCES

Batala M, Grabstald H: Upper urinary tract urothelial tumor. Urol Clin North Am 3:79, 1976

Berdon WE, Wigger J, Baker DH: Fetal renal hamartoma—A benign tumor to be distinguished from Wilms' tumor: Report of 3 cases. Am J Roentgenol Radium Ther Nucl Med 118:18, 1973

D'Angio GT, et al: The treatment of Wilms' tumor: Results of the National Wilms' Tumor Study. Cancer 38:633, 1976

Daniel WW, Hartman GW, Witten DM, et al: Calcified renal masses, a review of 10 years experience at the Mayo Clinic. Radiology 103:503, 1972

Gibbons RP, Montie JE, Correa RJ, et al: Manifestations of renal cell carcinoma. Urology 8:201, 1976

Holland JM: Natural history and staging of renal cell carcinoma. CA 25:121, 1975

Robson CJ, Churchill BM, Anderson W: The results of radical nephrectomy for renal cell carcinoma. Trans Am Assoc GU Surg 60:122, 1968

Skinner DG, Vermillion CD, Colvin RB: The surgical management of renal cell carcinoma. J Urol 107:705, 1972

Treatment of Chronic Renal Failure

CONSERVATIVE THERAPY

Marsha Wolfson

Each year 50–75 people per million population either die from renal disease or require some form of renal replacement therapy. Careful management of patients with chronic renal disease will retard disease progression and lengthen the time period before a patient must undergo definitive renal replacement therapy. The purpose of this chapter is to outline the various metabolic disturbances which are associated with the uremic state and to describe the appropriate management of these disturbances as they appear during the progression to endstage renal disease. Management by dialysis or transplantation is the subject of the following two chapters. Careful attention by the physician to the details incorporated in this chapter will enable the patient with chronic renal failure to enjoy an improved quality of life before renal replacement therapy is required.

CAUSES OF ENDSTAGE RENAL DISEASE

The causes of endstage renal disease are obviously multiple. Many renal diseases have in common progressive nephron destruction even though multiple pathophysiologic mechanisms may be operative. Despite the fact that these diseases have different etiologies, pathological findings, clinical presentation, and natural histories, management in the late stages is similar. Bricker et al. have demonstrated that the diseased kidney responds to the uremic environment in such a manner as to maximize homeostatic mechanisms independent of the underlying disease. These adjustments to reduction in functioning nephron mass produce a characteristic set of signs, symptoms, and physiologic derangements enabling the use of uniform methods to manage most patients.

DEFINITION OF CHRONIC RENAL FAILURE AND NATURAL HISTORY OF DISEASE

Chronic renal failure involves irreversible nephron loss such that the glomerular filtration rate is substantially reduced below normal. Most cases of chronic renal disease are characterized by a variable but somewhat predictable rate of deteriorating renal function. The underlying disease plus the severity of complicating renal disease are characterized by a variable but somewhat predictable rate of deteriorating renal function. factors such as hypertension usually determine the rate of decline in renal function. Acute exacerbations of renal failure are often superimposed on chronic disease. When this occurs, renal function rarely returns. Ideal conservative management of renal failure includes prevention of any acute insult that worsens renal function and thereby hastens the progression to endstage renal failure.

Chronic renal failure may be divided into three somewhat arbitrary stages. The advantage of such a subdivision is that the problems presented in each stage and their management may vary. Early chronic renal insufficiency is said to occur when renal function reaches a reduction in GFR of 25–40 cc/min. Patients are usually either asymptomatic or have only minor nonspecific symptoms. BUN is usually in the normal range and serum creatinine insignificantly elevated. Although patients are complaint free, the introduction of prophylactic management at this stage will often reduce the rate of progression of disease by reversing or modifying those abnormalities which are amenable to therapy.

Moderate chronic renal failure is defined by a glomerular filtration rate between 10 and 25 ml/min. The signs and symptoms noted by the patient are primarily associated with impaired solute excretion. Advanced chronic renal failure is the final stage in which conservative medical management is necessary to maintain the patient. In this stage the GFR is 5–10 cc/min and patients are generally symptomatic and exhibit the abnormalities one associates with uremia.

Division into these stages, although arbitrary, is useful for developing a logical stepwise approach to the management of chronic renal failure. It should be remembered that at any stage, chronic renal failure implies irreversible nephron loss with a corollary of progressive deterioration at a variable rate. Furthermore, division into stages also serves to introduce the clinician to the different types of problems as they appear at various times in the natural history of the patient with chronic renal failure.

MANAGEMENT OF THE VARIOUS STAGES OF RENAL FAILURE
Early Chronic Renal Failure

Because GFR is greater than 25 cc/min, solute excretion is not compromised in early renal failure. Thus the management of this stage involves (1) establishing the diagnosis, (2) estimating the rate of progression of the disease, and (3) preventing acute complications which may exacerbate renal failure. In early renal insufficiency, it is imperative to identify and treat any reversible lesions. The progression of analgesic nephropathy and hypokalemic nephropathy are examples of such lesions which may be reversed by discontinuing the offending drugs or correcting the metabolic abnormality. In this stage, control of hypertension is particularly important, since such therapy may lead to stabilized or even improved renal function. Additional aspects of conservative management, which are emphasized during early chronic renal failure, includes avoidance of potential nephrotoxic agents, maintaining normal salt and water balance, and either avoidance of or reduced dosage of drugs requiring renal excretion.

In pursuing an etiologic diagnosis, a good data base is required for each patient. This includes documentation of renal symptoms and their duration, a complete history and physical examination, and several basic laboratory studies. The urinalysis is essential because it may provide important clues to the underlying disease. A BUN, creatinine, serum electrolytes, calcium, phosphorus, and serum protein are important baselines for future therapeutic manipulations. At this stage, it is important to obtain a 24-hour urine collection to determine creatinine clearance. Both serum creatinine and creatinine clearance are very useful measures of renal impairment when followed serially. Serial clearances, together with knowledge of the natural history of the underlying disease, often enable the physician to predict rate of progression to endstage renal disease, i.e., serum creatine > 10 mg/dl. Although inulin clearance is the most accurate method of measuring glomerular filtration rate, the ease and reasonable correlation between creatinine clearance and glomerular filtration rate make it the clinical standard.

If present, proteinuria in the nephrotic range is characteristic of the earlier stages of glomerular disease. As renal function deteriorates, proteinuria often becomes less prominent and the 24 hour excretion often diminishes as the clearance drops below 10 cc/min. A notable exception is diabetic nephropathy, where severe proteinuria can persist until the terminal stage of renal failure. Nephrotic range proteinuria is defined as protein excretion which exceeds 3.5 g/24 hours. It is usually associated with edema, hypoalbuminemia, and hypercholesterolemia. Indiciations for treatment of the edema include improvement of patient comfort and/or physical appearance. Salt restriction and, if necessary, diuretics are usually successful in the management of this problem, which may be very distressing to the patient. Hypoalbuminemia contributes to the edema and is best managed by assuring adequate dietary protein intake commensurate with clearance. In the early stages of renal failure, protein restriction is not indicated, and adequate nutrition should be promoted. Hypercholesterolemia can, theoretically, contribute to atherogenesis. If levels of cholesterol are very high, clofibrate can be used. This drug is usually effective in lowering serum cholesterol. Since protein binding is decreased in hypoalbuminemic states, dosage adjustment is required to avoid the potential myotoxic side effects associated with this drug. The dose of clofibrate should be altered according to the degree of hypoalbuminemia and degree of renal insufficiency. Usual recommendations are to limit the daily dose to 1 g if the serum albumin is 1 g/dl and to 2 g if the serum albumin is 2 g/dl. It is also advisable to monitor serum CPK and SGOT levels while using this drug in patients with nephrotic syndrome and hypoalbuminemia.

MODERATE AND ADVANCED RENAL FAILURE

In these two stages, creatinine clearance varies between 5 and 25 cc/min. The management of moderate and advanced renal failure can be considered together because the problems that arise are due to the impaired solute excretion seen in diseased kidneys. The difference between these two stages is one of magnitude of the impaired solute excretion. The derangements that occur represent a spectrum of metabolic abnormalities which overlap both stages. Figure 1 is a flow diagram illustrating the various abnormalities that occur when the nephron mass is reduced to such a degree that the solutes which are normally excreted are now retained.

SODIUM REGULATION

The regulation of sodium intake within prescribed limits is critical to the management of most chronic renal failure patients. Depending on the dietary sodium intake, a patient may experience either salt depletion or salt and water overload. Marked salt wasting characterizes patients with tubulointerstitial nephritis and cystic kidney disease.

In addition to the threat of salt depletion, patients with chronic renal failure have a limited capacity to increase their sodium excretion in response to a sodium load. Intake in excess of 7–8 g salt per day often results in fluid overload with edema, congestive heart failure, and elevation of blood pressure. Since the usual American diet contains in excess of 9 g of salt per day, sodium restriction to some degree is required for virtually all patients once GFR falls below 25 ml/min.

In order to avoid either salt overload or salt depletion, a measurement of 24 hour urine sodium excretion with the patient ingesting a known content of dietary sodium can be used to determine the allowable amount of daily salt intake in patients with chronic renal failure.

FLUID BALANCE

Fluid balance is closely linked to sodium balance. Patients with renal disease have compromised diluting and concentrating abilities. Water balance may be difficult to assess clinically, usually requiring serial observations. The impaired diluting ability is due primarily

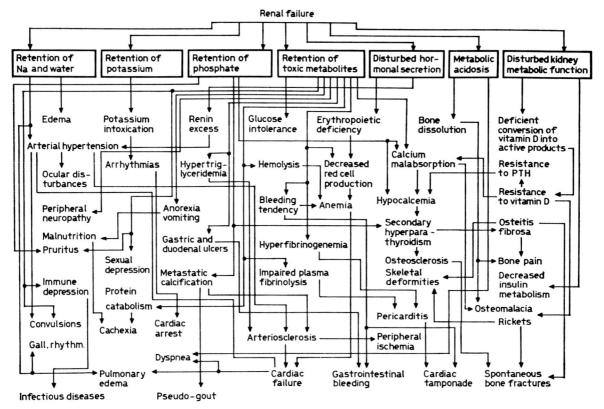

Fig. 1. Retention of solutes in renal failure and derangements that ensue. [Reprinted from Giovanetti S, Berlyne GM: An outline of the uremic syndrome. Nephron 14:119, 1975. By permission of S. Karger AG, Basel.]

to augmented solute excretion in each remaining nephron. Impaired concentrating ability also results from the osmotic diuresis but, in addition, is influenced by distorted nephron architecture. Damage to those nephrons with long loops of Henle and alterations in renal circulation due to disease may diminish meduallary tonicity.

Impaired diluting ability renders the patient susceptible to water overload and hyponatremia as the capacity to adjust clearance is decreased. On the other hand, there is also obligatory water loss due to the solute diuresis, making patients susceptible to dehydration if oral intake is restricted. Most patients with advanced renal insufficiency are unable to concentrate their urine to levels above plasma osmolality. The usual daily solute load is 600 mOsm/day. This necessitates the loss of 2000 cc of water/day to excrete the daily solute load. Sodium depletion and water retention can both present clinically with hyponatremia. Patients with dilutional hyponatremia have normal skin turgor with no evidence of orthostatic hypotension and usually present with peripheral edema. Changes in BUN and hematocrit require prior values for interpretation. Severe dehydration may be associated with hypernatremia where the loss of water is greater than the loss of salt.

Water restriction is the management of choice for water excess with dilutional hyponatremia. The serum sodium will slowly return to normal once output exceeds intake. If edema or hypertension are present, sodium restruction is also indicated. Conversely, if the patient is dehydrated, combined salt and water replacement will be required. This can be accomplished by increasing the sodium intake and allowing free access to water.

POTASSIUM BALANCE

The ability to regulate potassium balance is usually well maintained and hyperkalemia is rarely seen in patients whose GFR exceeds 5 cc/min. Potassium balance is a function of intake, tubular load, and excretion. The normal kidney has a large capacity to excrete potassium. Potassium clearance may exceed inulin clearance two- to fourfold. The filtered load of potassium undergoes nearly complete reabsorption in the proximal tubule, and this urinary potassium represents that secreted in the distal tubule in exchange for sodium and hydrogen ions. In renal failure, one of the adaptive mechanisms responsible for maintaining potassium balance involves progressive utilization of the latent capacity of residual nephrons to secrete potassium in exchange for sodium. This is thought to be mediated, at least in part, by the adrenal hormone aldosterone. A second mechanism involves the marked enhancement of fecal excretion of potassium which characterizes renal failure. Problems in the maintenance of a normal serum potassium arise when intake of potassium suddenly increases or sodium intake suddenly decreases.

In such a setting potassium retention with resulting hyperkalemia may occur, often being compounded by a coexisting metabolic acidosis. The contribution of metabolic acidosis to the hyperkalemia involves potassium translocating from its intracellular stores because of displacement by the inward movement of hydrogen ions.

Hypokalemia occurs much less commonly, but when it is associated with symptoms of muscle weakness and pain it should be treated with oral potassium repletion. Severe hypokalemia can result in changes in the ECG. The causes of potassium deficiency are variable and may be due to renal losses, as in the Fanconi syndrome or in those diseases characterized by excessive sodium wasting. Hypokalemia may also be due to diarrhea, poor dietary intake associated with anorexia, or chronic diuretic therapy.

Hyperkalemia with serum values of 5.5–.0 mEq/liter often responds to dietary potassium restriction alone. The treatment of concomitant metabolic acidosis will aid in the management of hyperkalemia. Achieving significant dietary protein restriction is always associated with a reduced potassium intake. Bananas, citrus fruits, potatoes, and coffee are all high in potassium, and patients can easily be instructed in the avoidance of these substances. Foods of low biologic protein value, such as beans, also contain substantial amounts of potassium. For potassium values between 6.0 and 7.0 mEq/liter, more rigorous therapy is indicated. An ion exchange resin like Kayexalate is quite useful; for oral administration, 60 g/day in divided doses is usually adequate to control this degree of moderate hyperkalemia. The effectiveness of the resin is enhanced by mixing it in a solution of 70 percent sorbitol. This also helps to prevent the constipation which complicates the use of such resins. It should be remembered that the use of these resins causes an increase sodium intake, since their mechanism of action is an exchange of potassium for sodium. Patients who have hypertension or mild CHF may experience worsening of these conditions when ion exchange resins are prescribed.

ACID–BASE BALANCE

The usual nonvolatile hydrogen ion load is about 60 mEq/day. This arises mainly from endogenous protein catabolism. The main plasma buffer is bicarbonate. The kidneys reclaim filtered bicarbonate and excrete hydrogen ion in the form of titratable acid and ammonia. The most important tubular mechanism for precise acid–base regulation comes from ammonia genesis. Acidosis in chronic renal failure is mainly due to the inability of the diseased kidneys to generate sufficient ammonia to titrate the load of nonreabsorbable anions which accumulate in renal failure. Bicarbonate reclamation capacity by the proximal tubule remains almost entirely intact. With each new plateau of progressive nephron destruction comes a transient decrease in hydrogen ion excretion. This, in turn, leads to hydrogen ion retention and decreased plasma bicarbonate. Ammonia excretion should increase if hydrogen ion balance

is to be maintained, but as the nephron population diminishes the ability of the kidney to compensate is further compromised. Titratable acid excretion remains stable as long as phosphate intake continues. While the rate of ammonia production per nephron is high, it is not high enough to completely compensate for the reduction in nephron mass. The progressive acidosis resulting from this is modulated by the buffering of retained hydrogen ions by bone. Plasma bicarbonate levels usually stabilize at 15–18 mEq/liter. There is evidence of a small proximal tubular bicarbonate leak, since bicarbonaturia is seen with plasma levels as low as 20 mEq/liter. Those renal diseases associated with acidosis early in their course often are complicated by a more severe renal osteodystrophy, since plasma buffering by bone leads to calcium mobilization.

Management of acidosis is not difficult. No therapy is usually necessary until the plasma bicarbonate ranges between 15 and 18 mEq/liter. At levels of less than 15 mEq/liter treatment will often improve symptoms of anorexia and lethargy and may improve congestive heart failure by improving acidosis-depressed myocardial contractibility. In addition, acidosis exacerbates hyperkalemia. Thus certain of the signs and symptoms of uremia can be ameliorated by correcting the acid–base status. The usual therapy is sodium bicarbonate. Patients vary widely in their requirements for $NaHCO_3$, and enough should be given to maintain the plasma bicarbonate at about 18 mEq/liter. Sodium bicarbonate can cause unpleasant gastrointestinal side effects; in such cases, Shohl's solution may be substituted. This is a mixture of sodium citrate and citric acid. Both of these bicarbonate supplements will increase the intake of sodium. In those patients in whom sodium restriction is necessary, acid–base status should be corrected with the aforementioned compounds, but diuretic therapy may have to be added. Diuretic therapy may also help to correct acidosis. Calcium carbonate is not as effective in correcting acidosis and causes a risk of hypercalcemia; however, some patients may require calcium supplementation in concert with bicarbonate, as will be discussed below. These patients may improve their metabolic acidosis with calcium carbonate treatment. Use of calcium carbonate requires periodic monitoring of serum calcium.

CALCIUM AND PHOSPHORUS

Phosphorus balance remains well controlled until the GFR falls below 25 cc/min. At this point, regulation persists but serum phosphate rises on a normal diet because intake exceeds excretion. This occurs in spite of the fact that phosphate excretion per nephron rises. The tradeoff for this maintenance of phosphate balance is increased parathyroid hormone secretion and, ultimately, the development of renal osteodystrophy. With each wave of nephron destruction there is a transient decrease in phosphorus excretion and a rise in serum phosphorus. The rise in serum phosphorus causes a reciprocal decrease in serum calcium and thus stimulation of parathyroid secretion. The increase in parathyroid hormone acts to enhance phosphate excretion by tubular reabsorption. As a result, serum phosphorus declines and serum calcium is maintained at a normal or near-normal concentration. Each time this sequence of events occurs, PTH levels stabilizes at a higher level.

Hypocalcemia in renal failure is further aggravated by impaired calcium absorption by the gastrointestinal tract. This calcium absorptive defect is secondary to impaired conversion of cholecalciferol to its most active metabolite, 1,25-dihydroxycholecalciferol. The conversion of the hepatic metabolite 25-OHD$_3$ to 1,25-(OH)$_2$-D$_3$ takes place in kidney mitochondria. Nephron dysfunction thus renders patients functionally vitamin D deficient. Uremia per se also appears to be associated with skeletal resistance to the calcemic action of the parathyroid hormone. This makes hypersecretion of parathyroid hormone a necessity if serum calcium is to be maintained near the normal range. Figure 2 represents a summary of the interrelationship of mechanisms which lead to the development of renal osteodystrophy.

Serum calcium and phosphorus abnormalities appear relatively early in the course of progressive renal failure. Management, if instituted at this stage, can prevent or control these abnormalities and prevent disabling bone disease. Because severe bone disease interferes with successful rehabilitation and can progress after the institution of dialysis therapy, it is essential that the physician managing patients with moderate renal insufficiency actively correct any abnormalities of hyperphosphatemia and hypocalcemia. Control of the serum phosphorus is important to successful management and will modify the lowering of serum calcium. Serum phosphorus may be controlled by decreased phosphorus intake as achieved by a low-protein diet. In patients who do not yet require protein restriction, the use of phosphate binding antacids are quite effective. These antacids contain aluminum, either hydroxide or carbonate, as the major active calcium binder. Magnesium-containing antacids may lead to magnesium accumulation in renal insufficiency. It should also be emphasized, however, that aluminum salts have recently been associated with adverse central nervous system effects in uremic patients. On the other hand, recent work has also suggested that prevention of hyperphosphatemia may prolong the course of chronic renal failure.

As renal failure advances, control of serum phosphorus may not be sufficient to raise serum calcium levels. Calcium supplementation in the form of calcium lactate or calcium carbonate may be needed to return serum calcium levels to normal. Calcium carbonate contains more calcium and, in addition, may aid the therapy of acidosis; it is therefore the agent of choice. Constipation is a frequent adverse effect of both phosphate binder therapy and calcium supplementation, and patients may not tolerate either calcium carbonate or aluminum hydroxide for this reason.

In advanced renal failure some form of vitamin D therapy must be added to enhance calcium absorption from the gut. Dihydrotachysterol (DHT) is useful. It is a synthetic analogue of vitamin D, and smaller doses are more effective than vitamin D$_3$. DHT is not affected by negative feedback inhibition by vitamin D hydroxylase in the liver, as is ordinary vitamin D$_3$. Its short plasma half-life makes it more suitable for use in patients with renal failure. 1,25-Dihydroxycholecalciferol, the active vitamin D metabolite, has proved effective in early clinical trials.

Maintenance of the serum calcium and serum phosphorus in the normal range is the aim of therapy. Both

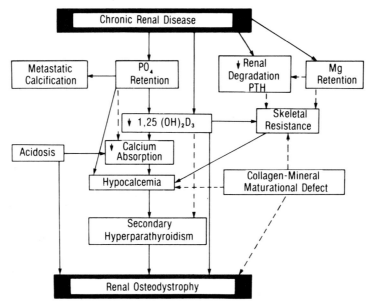

Fig. 2. Pathogenetic mechanisms responsible for the development of renal osteodystrophy. Dashed lines represent hypothetical relationships. PTH, parathyroid hormone.

hypercalcemia and hypophosphatemia are to be avoided. Hypercalcemia may be associated with central nervous system abnormalities and symptoms that can be confused with uremia. In addition, hypercalcemia may reduce the GFR and worsen already impaired renal function. A calcium–phosphorus product greater than 70 is said to lead to metastatic calcification. Calcium phosphate deposition in skin may cause severe itching. Deposition in blood vessels is common and may contribute to the accelerated atherogenesis associated with renal failure. Severe tissue deposition may lead to necrosis and loss of digits. Caldium phosphate may also deposit in the heart and lungs. Death due to intractable cardiac arrhythmias or progressive pulmonary insufficiency has been reported as a consequence of calcium deposition.

Low serum phosphorus is rare in renal failure but, if present, requires treatment. It may lead to osteomalacia with disabling bone disease which may be refractory to conventional therapy. Excessive blood levels of parathormone have been shown to contribute to calcium deposition in both brain and peripheral nerves. The latter probably contributes to the neuropathy of uremia.

ADVANCED RENAL FAILURE

This stage is customarily referred to as "uremia." Although blood urea is markedly elevated, it clearly is not responsible for the metabolic abnormalities manifested in this stage of renal failure. Almost every organ system is involved in the uremic state. Many of the abnormalities can be modified by conservative therapy, but some will improve only after the institution of dialysis or transplantation.

PROTEIN METABOLISM

The elevation of blood urea nitrogen parallels many of the symptoms of uremic patients. When GFR drops below 25 cc/min, blood urea nitrogen rises exponentially. Unlike creatinine, whose rate of production is constant, the production of urea and associated uremic toxins is dependent upon certain dietary factors which may be controlled by dietary adjustments. The symptoms and perhaps the progression to endstage renal failure may be slowed by proper dietary management.

The amount of protein intake is the prime determinant of steady-state BUN level. Thus decreasing protein intake, within certain limits, is very effective in reducing the level of BUN. In addition, many investigators feel that other uremic toxins which are not routinely measured are also lowered by restricting protein intake. Improvement in the patient's sense of wellbeing is associated with a decrease in BUN as well as a reduction in other protein metabolic breakdown products.

Many of the metabolic abnormalities associated with the uremic state cause increased protein catabolism. Carbohydrate intolerance, acidosis, and gastrointestinal bleeding may contribute to the negative nitrogen balance characteristic of uremic patients. Actual nitrogen requirements in the patient with advanced renal failure are difficult to quantitate. Increased protein catabolism is associated with increases in the symptomatology of uremic patients independent of their renal function. If catabolism is avoided, patient wellbeing is improved and the time interval prior to the need for renal replacement therapy may be prolonged.

Negative nitrogen balance should be avoided. Gastrointestinal bleeding and acidosis should be managed appropriately. Once the glomerular filtration rate falls below 10 cc/min, most patients will require reduction in total dietary protein intake. A 40 g/day protein diet has been successfully used in the conservative management of patients with advanced renal failure. It is important that despite reduction of total amount of protein ingested, the diet must contain all of the essential amino acids, i.e., be of high biological value. When the glomerular filtration rate is below 5 cc/min further reduction of protein will be necessary to avoid large increments in the BUN level. At this level a 20 g/day protein diet will be necessary, or dialysis therapy should be supplemented with essential amino acids or the ketoanalogues of essential amino acids. The rationale for so-called renal failure diet therapy is that urea and other nitrogenous waste products are utilized in endogenous protein synthesis, thus recycling them and reducing urea levels. Adequate calories, at least 55 kcal/kg/day, must be incorporated into diets of this type in order to maximize this protein sparing effect.

Dietary therapy may be very effective in reducing urea levels by incorporating urea that is generated and not excreted by the kidneys into usable protein. Many patients have been treated for long periods of time with diets of this type and have experienced symptomatic improvement while remaining adequately nourished, with lengthening of the interval before dialytic therapy is required. The major drawback to this form of therapy is that the diets are for many patients unpalatable and poorly tolerated. Although this limits the usefulness of dietary manipulation to alter the progression of renal failure, a combined effort on the part of the physician, patient, and renal dietitian can prove most rewarding.

ANEMIA

Anemia, usually normocytic and normochromic, is almost inevitable in far advanced renal failure. It develops slowly and insidiously and usually becomes clinically apparent when the GFR is less than 30 cc/min. The anemia is partially caused by decreased erythropoietin production by the diseased kidney. The anemia may be aggravated by gastrointestinal bleeding or uterine bleeding, vitamin deficiencies, or malnutrition. A hemolytic defect has also been described in uremia. Red blood cell lifespan is shortened by uremic plasma. Therapy is usually not necessary before dialysis is instituted, since hematocrit levels of 18–20 percent are usually tolerated easily by most younger patients. Elderly patients with coronary artery disease may require higher hematocrit levels to prevent anginal pain or heart failure. The most effective therapy is transfusion. This is usually carried out with packed red cells to avoid excessive fluid intake. In patients who may be future candidates for cadaveric transplant, transfusion therapy has been shown to improve graft survival; however, most transplant centers recommend the use of degly-cerolized red cells to minimize formation of lympho-cytoxic antibodies. Anabolic steroids also may be useful in the management of the anemic patient with endstage renal disease, while iron supplementation can be guided by serum ferritin levels.

CARDIOVASCULAR ABNORMALITIES

It is well recognized that chronic renal failure is often associated with hypertension and congestive heart failure. These problems are usually related to salt and fluid overload. They can sometimes be managed by dietary sodium restriction, but antihypertensive ther-apy is usually necessary in patients in whom hyperten-sion is secondary to the underlying renal disease. The management of these problems will be outlined below.

Uremic patients appear to have accelerated ather-ogenesis. This is felt to be secondary to carbohydrate intolerance and lipid abnormalities associated with the uremic state.

Pericarditis is a late event in renal failure and is usually considered an absolute indication for dialysis.

The cardiovascular manifestations of uremia are usually ameliorated by dialysis. Antihypertensive re-quirements are lessened by adequate ultrafiltration of salt and water. There are many acceptable antihyper-tensive regimens, but combinations of vasodilators and beta adrenergic blocking drugs have achieved wide acceptance.

NEUROLOGIC ABNORMALITIES

Various neurologic abnormalities are associated with advanced renal failure. A peripheral neuropathy usually develops which is characterized by lower ex-tremity numbness, tingling, and myoclonic jerks. In severe cases, foot drop may occur. Peripheral neuro-pathy may be quite disabling and a major source of morbidity in renal failure patients. The peripheral neu-ropathy is believed by some investigators to be related to the effects of excess parathyroid hormone. No effec-tive therapy is available besides intervention with di-alysis and transplantation. Central nervous system symptoms and signs include lethargy, insomnia, anxi-ety, and behavioral changes. Untreated renal failure may proceed to seizures, stupor, and eventually coma. This is a preterminal event and calls for urgent institution of dialysis.

GASTROINTESTINAL ABNORMALITIES

Gastrointestinal disturbances such as diffuse bleed-ing, peptic ulcer disease, anorexia, nausea, vomiting, and singultus are also common in late renal failure. The gastrointestinal bleeding is felt to be due to the action of gut bacteria on urea leading to the formation of large amounts of ammonia in the gastrointestinal tract. The ammonia causes diffuse mucosal ulcerations, which often have a tendency to bleed.

ACUTE RENAL INSUFFICIENCY SUPERIMPOSED ON CHRONIC RENAL FAILURE

It should be remembered that at any stage of renal failure, acute insults may occur which lead to sudden decrements in renal function. These decrements may be irreversible and may hasten the progression to end-stage renal disease. Therefore it is imperative that the clinician be aware of the types of insults that can occur and be aggressive in their prevention and management. Whenever the decrement in renal function is sudden, as reflected by a serum creatinine rise to greater than 1 mg/dl, a diligent search should be made for an explanation before that decrement is considered to be part of the natural history of the disease. Nephrotoxin administration, dehydration, acute infection, congestive heart failure, acute obstruction, hypercalcemia, hypo-kalemia, and acidosis all may worsen preexisting renal failure. Potentially nephrotoxic drugs should be avoided whenever possible. If their use is necessary, then the lowest possible doses should be used with monitoring of serum level whenever possible. A more complete discussion of drug management in renal failure follows below. Radiographic contrast material may be nephro-toxic in patients who are elderly or dehydrated or who suffer from multiple myeloma or diabetes mellitus. In addition, contrast agents will often induce a transient decline in renal function in patients with GFR less than 25 ml/min. Reactions to contrast agents may lead to oliguric acute renal failure. Thus the indications for intravenous pyelography should include the fact that the information derived will be critical in the manage-ment of elderly patients with preexisting renal failure or diabetes. Often, kidneys can be visualized by plain x-rays with tomography. If obstruction is suspected, renal ultrasound may be helpful in confirming this suspicion. If both renal pelves are not shown to be enlarged by ultrasound, obstruction becomes less likely. If it is necessary to carry out intravenous pyelography for diagnostic purposes in renal failure, the presence of dehydration and volume depletion will magnify the danger to these high-risk patients. Acute infection should be treated immediately to avoid nephron de-struction. Although many antibiotic agents are excreted by the kidneys, dosage rarely has to be altered in early renal failure. Patients with heart disease, especially the elderly, may exhibit worsening of their renal function when heart failure develops. Salt restriction, diuretic therapy, and digitalis can be useful in the management of this problem. Digoxin is excreted by the kidneys, and plasma levels should be monitored for potential accumulation and toxicity.

Hypertension, when uncontrolled, can also exac-erbate renal insufficiency. Persistent hypertension is probably the major contribution to the deterioration of renal function. If sodium restriction alone does not control the elevated blood pressure, diuretic therapy, with or without propranolol or alpha methyldopa, can be successful in regaining control of blood pressure. Malignant hypertension can cause rapid and irreversible deterioration in renal function. Under such conditions, the blood pressure should be returned to normal levels as soon as possible. Potent antihypertensives such as nitroprusside or diazoxide are extremely useful for rapid therapy of malignant hypertension. Although normotension can be associated with transient deterioration in glomerular filtration rate, the function usually returns to its previous level when blood pressure control is achieved.

USE OF DRUGS IN RENAL FAILURE

Drug therapy for concurrent medical problems is often required by patients with varying degrees of renal failure. Antibiotics, antihypertensives, and cardiac drugs are just a few examples of the common classes of drugs used in patients with renal failure. Many drugs are metabolized or excreted by the kidneys. Other characteristics of drug action (e.g., protein binding) may be altered by renal insufficiency. In addition, some drugs are directly toxic to the kidneys. It is important in a discussion of conservative management of renal failure to point out how the action of drugs can be affected by renal disease and how to effectively use drug therapy in patients with renal failure.

The presence of renal disease may affect drug action in several ways. The apparent volume of distribution may be altered by renal failure due to the presence of edema or ascites. Drugs distributed in the extracellular fluid may achieve suboptimal blood levels in patients with edema. Many drugs bind to plasma proteins. In cases of hypoalbuminemia, as can be seen in nephrotic syndrome or malnourished uremic patients, the bound fraction of the drug decreases and the free form, which is pharmacologically active, increases. Adverse reactions can occur with seemingly therapeutic blood levels. There also seems to be a qualitative reduction in albumin affinity for some drugs in renal failure. The net result of decreased binding of the drug is to increase the volume of distribution of the drug or to increase the free fraction. This can result in a faster rate of metabolism or, alternatively, toxic side effects. Analytical methods for drug levels commonly measure both free and bound drug for this reason. Low total plasma level may be quite appropriate for the patient with renal failure and a reduced plasma albumin.

Drug elimination is usually altered in renal failure. The rate of drug elimination is usually expressed in terms of drug half-life. Volume of distribution, glomerular filtration, extent of tissue receptor binding, lipid solubility, and hepatic drug metabolism all affect the drug removal rate. The half-life will be prolonged if the volume of distribution is increased or if the rate of renal excretion is limited due to the renal disease; however, hepatic metabolism may also affect the half-life of certain drugs, and this must be considered before concluding that drug elimination is retarded in renal failure.

Most drugs that are metabolized by the liver have a normal half-life in patients with chronic renal failure; however, certain drugs have accelerated metabolism due to decreased protein binding with resultant increased free drug available for metabolism. Decreased metabolism due to the uremic state occurs with other compounds. Drug dosage must therefore be individualized. Hepatic metabolism converts most drugs into more water soluble and less lipid soluble substances.

The increased water solubility allows drugs to be excreted by the renal tubules. Liver metabolism also converts many drugs into less pharmacologically active metabolites. With other drugs, however, pharmacologically active compounds may be formed which depend on functioning kidneys for their elimination. These metabolites may accumulate in renal failure if dosage of the parent compound is not altered.

GUIDELINES TO DRUG DOSAGE IN RENAL DISEASE

For the most part, patients with renal failure should be given the usual loading dose of a drug in order to attain therapeutic blood levels; however, for those drugs which may accumulate in renal failure, alterations in maintenance dosages will be required. Either a reduction in each subsequent dose or an increase in the interval between doses should be made. Many drugs, especially antibiotics, have been extensively studied, and nomograms exist for their administration in renal failure; however, it should be remembered that the patient's response may vary and therefore drug administration should be carried out taking into account each patient's response. Monitoring of blood levels may be helpful in managing drug therapy in these patients. Even measurements of blood levels may be misleading in patients with altered volumes of distribution or changes in protein binding. In some cases a combination of reduced dose and altered dose intervals may be the most practical approach to drug therapy.

Table 1 summarizes the use of drugs commonly required in the routine management of patients with chronic renal failure. Cardiac, antihypertensive, antibiotic, analgesic, and narcotic drugs are the most commonly used drugs in patients with renal failure. Propranolol is frequently used as an antihypertensive, an antiarrhythmic, and an antianginal drug. In usual doses this drug reaches higher peak plasma levels in patients with renal disease than in normal subjects owing to reduced hepatic extration; however, uremia also induces the hepatic microsomal enzymes which metabolize the drug, and the net effect is that the dose need not be altered in renal failure.

Quinidine dosage does not need to be altered in renal failure, but procainamide is metabolized to a pharmacoligically active compound, n-acetylprocainamide, which accumulates in renal failure. For procainamide, the interval between maintenance doses should be increased to 8–12 hours.

Diuretics may be useful in moderate renal failure, but once the glomerular filtration rate is below 20 cc/min thiazides are ineffective. The potent loop diuretics furosemide and ethacrynic acid may still have an effect at GFRs of 5–10 cc/min; however, large doses may be required increasing the risk of ototoxicity. Furosemide is preferred over ethacrynic acid because the latter agent seemingly has a greater potential for ototoxicity.

Dosages for the usual antihypertensive agents such as methyldopa, guanethidine, hydralazine, prazocin, clonidine, and minoxidil do not require adjustment in

Table 1
Drug Management in Renal Failure

Drug	Effect of CRF on Elimination	Dose Modification Required
Cardiac and antihypertensive drugs		
Propranolol	Cumulative effect is unchanged	None
Digoxin	Reduced	Usual loading dose 0.125 mg 3–5 times/week
Quinidine	None	None
Methyldopa	None	None
Hydralazine	None	None
Furosemide	Efficacy is reduced	Increase dose up to 400 mg
Sedative and analgesic drugs		
Phenobarbital	None	None; usual precautions
Diazepam	None	None; usual precautions
Meperidine	↓ Elimination of active metabolite	Use caution; contraindicated for chronic pain
Antibiotics		
Penicillin G	None	Lower range of usual therapeutic dose
Ampicillin	None	Lower range of usual therapeutic dose
Methicillin	None	Lower range of usual therapeutic dose
Cephalexin	↓ elimination	Depends on level of GFR; 250–500 mg/ 12 hours
Gentamicin	↓ elimination	Depends on level of GFR. Loading dose 1–2 mg/kg; then 0.5–0.3 mg/ kg/8 hours

GFR, glomerular filtration rate; ↑ increased; ↓, decreased.

renal failure. Diazoxide is useful in hypertensive emergencies, but if it is used after ultrafiltation dialysis it may cause severe hypotension. Nitroprusside is metablized to thiocyanate and may accumulate to toxic levels in patients with renal failure. Levels should be monitored and kept below 5–10 mg/dl. The infusion should be terminated within 48 hours.

Digoxin has a prolonged half-life in patients with renal failure. The daily maintenance dose should be equal to the nonrenal losses, which represent 14 percent of body stores, plus an additional percentage related to the glomerular filtration rate. For patients with advanced renal failure, very little is lost via the urine. Therapeutic levels are usually maintained with 0.125 mg three to five times per week; however, the drug response may be variable in patients, and both clinical judgment and plasma levels should be utilized in the decisions regarding drug dosage. Since digitoxin is eliminated mainly by extrarenal routes, its dosage schedule need not be altered for renal failure.

Narcotics are primarily metabolized in the liver to more polar metabolites. Some of these metabolites may have greater pharmacologic activty than the parent compound. Toxicity may develop in patients with renal failure who receive multiple doses. Meperidine is metabolized to normeperidine, which, when accumulated in renal failure, may produce seizures, stupor, and eventual coma with death. Morphine may cause increased respiratory depression in patients with renal failure due to lower protein binding and should therefore be administered at substantially lower dosages. Codeine, petazocine, and nalotone may be used without dose modification.

Benzodiazapines are commonly used drugs in renal failure patients and can be safely administered to most individuals. Excessive sedation, however, can develop but is often avoided by careful dose monitoring.

Antibiotics are also commonly required in patients with renal failure. They frequently depend on renal elimination, and dose modification is therefore needed.

The aminoglycoside antibiotics are nephrotoxic and ototoxic, and serum levels should guide maintenance dosage. Penicillin G, carbenicillin, cephalosporins, tetracyclines, and vancomycin all depend on glomerular filtration for their elimination, and dose modification is necessary. Several extensive reviews are available to aid in therapeutic management.

REFERENCES

Bennett WM: Principles of drug therapy in patients with renal disease. West J Med 123:372, 1975

Bricker NS: On the pathogenesis of the uremic state. An exposition of the "trade-off" hypothesis. N Engl J Med 286:1903, 1972

DeLuca HF: Vitamin D metabolism and function. Arch Intern Med 138:836, 1978

Fabre J, Balant L, Chavoz A: Drug management advances in renal insufficiency. Adv Nephrol 4:223, 1974

Giovanetti S, Berlyne GM: An outline of the uremic syndrome. Nephron 14:119, 1975

Hayes CP Jr, Robinson RR: Fecal potassium excretion in patients on chronic intermittent hemodialysis. Trans Am Soc Artif Intern Organs 11:242, 1965

Mitch W, Walser M, Buffington GA, et al: A simple method of estimating progression of chronic renal failure. Lancet 2:1321, 1976

Morini PV, Hull AR: Uremic pericarditis. Kidney Int 7(suppl 2): 163, 1975

Richards P: Protein metabolism in uremia. Nephron 14:134, 1975

Slatopolsky EA, Rutherford WE, Hruska K, et al: How important is phosphate in the pathogenesis of renal osteodystrophy? Arch Intern Med 138:848, 1978

Walser M, Coulter WA, Dighie S, et al: The effect of ketoanalogues of essential amino acids in severe chronic uremia. J Clin Inest 52:678, 1973

DIALYSIS
Robert A. Gutman

Dialysis is the process wherein small solute molecules pass through a semipermeable membrane in response to a pressure gradient or to a solute concentration gradient between fluids on either side of the membrane. The process is entirely passive and quite unlike the function of the mammalian kidney. Nevertheless, the principle has been adapted widely to provide support and life extension to patients with advanced renal failure. This clinical application, *renal dialysis*, is reasonably effective if there is sufficient exposure of body fluid to the dialysate, whose composition is described later in this chapter. The intervening semipermeable membrane may be manufactured, as is the case in *hemodialysis*, or it may be the peritoneal membrane. Maintenance dialysis treatment is neither uniformly worse nor better than renal transplantation for patients with endstage renal failure. The two forms of therapy are mutually supportive. This chapter will consider the application, complications, and results of dialysis therapy for this group of patients and in less detail for those with acute renal failure and exogenous poisoning. Newer methods of altering blood solute concentration by absorption technology and high flux filtration will be considered briefly.

PERFORMANCE AND PRINCIPLES OF HEMODIALYSIS

Hemodialysis alters the composition and volume of body fluids by two processes (diffusion and convective transport) which may be carried out separately but are generally combined. The rate of transfer of solutes by diffusion depends upon the concentration gradient, the rate of blood flow, the rate of dialysate flow, the permeability and charge of the semipermeable membrane, the thickness of the blood film, and the size and charge of the solutes. Convective transport, often called ultrafiltration, refers to bulk transfer of fluid with its solute and depends on the algebraic sum of the hydraulic and osmotic pressure gradient and on the hydraulic permeability of the membrane. Measurements of these transfer rates are considered in detail by Henderson and Gotch. In general, three terms should be familiar to physicians using these devices. *Clearance,* the apparent volume of blood "cleared" entirely of its solute per unit time, is a mathematical concept borrowed from renal physiology. It is calculated as

$$C = \frac{[B]_i - [B]_o}{[B]_i} Q_B$$

where C is clearance (ml/min), $[B]_i$ and $[B]_o$ are the concentration values for a given solute in the blood entering (i) and leaving (o), and Q_B is the rate of blood flow through the dialyzer (ml/min). Clearance for any solute is usually higher when measured in vitro than when measured in vivo. The clearance of urea, a small uncharged molecule is greater than that of creatinine, a slightly larger and charged molecule; this in turn is cleared faster than substances with molecular weights of 500–5000 daltons. Beyond that range, little or no exchange occurs at all. Since dialyzer clearance is, in part, dependent on the concentration gradient between the two fluids, a phenomenon which is not true to the filtering mammalian kidney, other terms have been used to describe more precisely the function of the membrane. *Mass transfer coefficient* (K) is calculated using a term which considers the concentration gradient as

$$K = \frac{N}{A\,\overline{\Delta\text{CM}}}$$

where N is the measured mass transfer rate (moles/min), A is the surface area of the membrane (cm²), and $\Delta\,\overline{CM}$ is the logarithmic mean concentration gradient. Though this term is a more precise measure of membrane function, for most purposes comparison of clearance values rather than mass transfer coefficients is useful. Comparisons of dialyzer performance is often given in terms of the clearance of urea, representing one of the highest attainable clearance values in clinical practice; of creatinine, uric acid, and phosphate, which are small molecular weight charged molecules of clinical interest; and of vitamin B_{12} and inulin, which are measurable sustances that may be administered to patients and which serve as markers for putative but unidentified uremic toxins whose molecular weight is believed to be between 1000 and 5000 daltons. Table 1 provides some side-by-side comparisons of a few of the popular and clinically effective dialyzers on the market.

Table 1 also contains data for the third term of interest, the *ultrafiltration coefficient* (K_u), which is a measure of the hydraulic conductivity of the membrane. This value is generally expressed as the rate of transfer of water and its solute per unit time per unit transmembrane pressure gradient (ml/hour/mm Hg). The composition, size, and configuration of the membrane all govern the K_u. The transmembrane pressure cannot be measured precisely but is estimated from the measured pressures at the blood ports and, where applicable, the dialysate port. Ultrafiltration rate may be controlled by changing the resistance to blood returning to the body ("venous resistance") or by application of variable amounts of negative pressure to the dialysate. There may be need for several devices of varying K_u in order to manage different patients, but regardless of the choice, ultrafiltration must be reasonably predictable in order to carry out hemodialysis safely.

Commercially available dialyzers may be built as parallel flow devices in which both the dialysate compartment and the blood compartment are contained within the dialyzer and each compartment has its own ports. The blood compartment in these dialyzers is in the form of either a group of flat envelopes arranged in parallel or in the form of a hollow fiber bundle. Dialysate flows around the blood-containing elements at a rate of usually 500 ml/min; as it exists, negative pressure may be applied to generate ultrafiltration losses. An alternative design is the "coil dialyzer," in which one or two envelopes of cellophane, the blood compartment, are wrapped around a supporting core. This device is simply bathed in a constantly renewing pool of dialysate. The materials used to make the semipermeable

membranes for both kinds of dialyzers are cellulose acetate, cuprophane (also a cellulosic substance), and, in Europe, other polymers including polyacrylonitrile. Other, more porous membrane materials are being considered or have been introduced on a small scale because of the possibility that important uremic toxins may have molecular weight in the range of that of vitamins B_{12} or inulin. Better clearance of substances in this weight range may be accomplished also by using a dialyzer with a greater surface area. Regardless of the specific type of dialyzer, they generally employ nearly the same rates of blood flow (200 ml/min), dialysate flow (500 ml/min), and extracorporeal blood volume (150–250 ml).

Blood is circulated through the external circuit usually from a vein, engorged by surgical anastomosis to an artery. This vein allows repeated needle puncture both by the needle which carries the blood to the dialyzer and the needle which returns blood to the patient. An alternative method of acquiring repeated access to the circulation is the use of implanted teflon-silastic cannulas, one in an artery and one in a nearby vein. When not in use, they are interconnected to allow blood to shunt through the tubing. These "shunts," originally developed by Dr. Belding Scribner, made maintenance dialysis possible; however, the internal fistula is far less subject to clotting and infection and has become the preferred system. If a patient's native vein is inadequate for the anastomosis, a vein graft is substituted; it may be an autologous saphenous vein or, more commonly, a treated bovine carotid artery or an entirely artificial material. Heparin is required to prevent clotting within the extracorporeal circuit during dialysis. In general, the administration of between 1000 and 2000 IU per hour suffices and somewhat less can be used. Occasionally, one might attempt to achieve anticoagulation within the dialyzer while maintaining normal clotting function within the patient by simultaneously pumping heparin and protamine into the blood entering and leaving the dialyzer, respectively. This has

Table 1
Performance Characteristics of Representative Hemodialysis Devices

Model	Construction/ Material	Blood Volume (ml)	Surface Area (m²)	K_u (ml/min/mm Hg)	Urea Clearance (ml/min)	Vitamin B_{12} Clearance (ml/min)
C-DAK 1.3	Hollow fiber cellulose acetate	100	1.3	1.9	160	23
C-DAK 2.5	Hollow fiber cellulose acetate	180	2.5	3.6	186	40
COBE PPD	Parallel plate cuprophan	140	1.6	4.1	151	36
RP 6	Parallel plate polyacrylonitrile	150	1.2	27.	145	51
CD 1400	Coil cuprophan	250	1.0	2.7	130	30

Values are approximate and were taken from many sources. Clearances are measured in vitro at 200 ml/ min "blood" flow and 500 ml/min dialysate flow. Blood volume, especially for coil constructed models, depends on transmembrane pressure.

often proved impractical, and since it requires large amounts of heparin and protamine, which may itself impair coagulation, the technique has been used less frequently.

The dialysate is a crystalloid solution containing (with the approximate concentration in mEq/liter) sodium (135), chloride (98), acetate as a bicarbonate source (35–38), potassium (0–4), calcium (2–4), and magnesium (1–3). Acetate is used in the place of bicarbonate because it avoids the problem of coprecipitation with calcium. Acetate is usually well metabolized, but there may be adverse consequences when used with high-efficiency dialyzers. Potassium, calcium, and magnesium concentrations are more variable in order to allow individual prescription. Modern dialysis machines use a commercially prepared dialysate concentrate. The concentrate is diluted 35 to 1, warmed to body temperature, and pumped at a rate which may be prescribed, generally 500 ml/min. The dialysis machine contains, among other things, a conductivity meter which monitors the dilution process and a thermocouple for control of the temperature.

Two processes are taking place during routine dialysis—(1) *ultrafiltration*, the convective transfer of isotonic extracellular fluid, and (2) *diffusion*, which corrects plasma salt concentration and removes waste products including but not limited to urea and creatinine. With conventional dialyzers, ultrafiltration of as much as 1 liter per hour can occur, a process analogous to rapid diuresis. A physician's judgment of the patient's "dry weight" is required in order to carry out this process safely. Excessive ultrafiltration may cause hypotension, violent nausea, muscle cramps, loss of consciousness, and seizures. Occassionally extracellular volume (ECV) contraction may occur between treatments as a result of diarrhea, vomiting, or renal salt wasting. In such cases, saline administration should be initiated early.

Adjustment of plasma concentrations of bicarbonate, potassium, calcium, magnesium, and phosphate is a recurring need of patients with severe renal failure and can be accomplished, at least partly, by the dialysis treatments. Gains or losses of salt and water are usually proportional, and such changes are managed by ultrafiltration for excess or by administration of saline for deficit. Plasma bicarbonate concentration decreases between treatments because of the gain of unmetabolizable acid present in dietary protein or as a consequence of catabolism of endogenous protein. Therefore the available buffer in dialysate is usually set at approximately 35 mEq/liter. The buffer used is acetate rather than bicarbonate for technical reasons. Most patients metabolize acetate effectively, so that by the end of the treatment the rate of generation of bicarbonate from the available acetate exceeds the dialysis losses of bicarbonate and thus the plasma concentration has begun and will continue to rise beyond the treatment; however, the use of efficient dialyzers may cause dialysis-associated acidosis if the rate of bicarbonate loss ex-

ceeds the rate of acetate metabolism. Plasma potassium concentration rises between treatments in most cases. Therefore the concentration in dialysate is set at approximately 2 mEq/liter, although special formulations are available for the treatment of severe hypokalemia or hyperkalemia. Plasma calcium concentration in dialysis patients may be low, normal, or high as a result of the net effect of several influences discussed in the chapter on *Chronic Renal Failure—Pathophysiology*. Most maintenance dialysis patients require an increase of the plasma calcium concentration, a goal which dialysis can help achieve. Therefore the dialysate concentration of ionized calcium is in the range of 3.0–3.5 mEq/liter. Magnesium excess or depletion may occur in patients with renal failure. For this reason the dialysate concentration of magnesium is generally set in the physiological range of 1.0–1.5 mEq/liter. The consequences of hyperphosphatemia are discussed in the chapter on *Chronic Renal Failure—Pathophysiology*, and the maintenance of serum values below 6 mg/dl is considered desirable.

The dialytic removal of dissolved nitrogenous substances which are abnormal or present in abnormally high concentration appears to control many uremic signs and symptoms; however, the nature and identification of the substances responsible for the clinical findings remains elusive. A full discussion of this problem is found in the chapter on *Chronic Renal Failure—Consequences*. Table 2 lists a representative—though incomplete—group of biological processes which improve or become normal following the institution of maintenance dialysis treatments for uremic patients.

Hemodialysis therapy has also been used for the removal of exogenous poisons. Those substances which can be most effectively removed by dialysis treatment are soluble in aqueous solutions, are incompletely protein bound, and have a favorable plasma:intracellular concentration ratio. Most such substances are rather easily excreted by the kidneys, and in the case of some (e.g., phenobarbital and aspirin) renal excretion can be enhanced by physiological or pharmacological means. In contrast, those poisons which are not readily excreted may also be difficult to remove by conventional dialysis. Recent introduction of the technique of hemoperfusion, in which blood is brought into direct contact with activated charcoal or similar absorbing surfaces, will probably allow more effective application of extracorporeal circulation-based removal of toxins.

Complications of Hemodialysis Therapy

Exposure of circulating blood to improperly mixed dialysate or dialysate contaminated with hemolysins, products of bacterial metabolism, or other toxins may cause sudden and severe complications. Hemolysis of blood occurs if salts have been inadvertently omitted or their concentration is too low. Most modern machines have adequately designed safety features to prevent this complication. If it occurs the patient experiences symptoms of cardiovascular instability accompanied by severe generalized muscle pain, loss of

Table 2
Symptoms, Signs, and Processes Which Improve Following
Dialysis Treatment of Uremic Patients

Gastrointestinal	Nutrition
Nausea and loss of appetite	Hypoalbuminemia
Diffuse bleeding	Hyperglycemia
Cardiovascular	Negative nitrogen balance
Peripheral and pulmonary edema	Negative calcium balance
Hypertension	Nervous system
Pericarditis	Peripheral neuropathy
Pulmonary	Confusion
Cilia function	Seizures
Hematopoietic	EEG abnormalities
Anemia	Musculoskeletal
Platelet dysfunction	Weakness
Lymphocyte dysfunction	Bone pain
	Osteomalacia
	Secondary hyperparathyroidism

consciousness, marked air hunger, and, less commonly, convulsions. Treatment consists of control of blood pressure, administration of oxygen, and the reinstitution of proper dialysis treatment. Severe hemolysis and death have been reported as a result of copper contamination of the dialysate. Less dramatic but persistent hemolysis occurs as a consequence of the use of dialysate prepared from water containing chloramine or from water which has come in contact with residual formaldehyde. In addition to hemorrhage, air embolus may occur if blood tubing separates during dialysis. Air embolus may cause sudden death, but in mild cases the patient will complain of some chest discomfort and dyspnea and then spontaneously improve. Hypotension and seizures have occurred as well. Treatment includes oxygen, support of blood pressure, and control of seizures. Any air remaining within the right atrium may be prevented from causing further difficulty by turning the patient to his left side, thus trapping the air bubble against the right side of the atrium away from the outflow tract. Foaming of blood by the agitation associated with pumping and extracorporeal circulation has been reported to cause similar, though usually clinically undetectable, problems.

Acute cardiopulmonary decompensation, including hypotension, cardiac arrhythmias, angina, and myocardial infarction, during hemodialysis treatments has been observed in the absence of blood loss or air embolus. Mild or moderately severe but similar events occur in about 20 percent of dialysis treatments. Such complications often are attributed to excessively rapid filling of the dialyzer and its tubing from the patient's circulation or to excessive ultrafiltration. Several other mechanisms may play a significant role in such symptoms. Most individuals undergoing hemodialysis experience a transient neutropenia which begins within minutes, reaches a nadir about 20 min lates, and returns to normal within 1 hour and which is followed by a transient neutrophilia. Exposure of blood to dialyzer membranes activates serum complement; this, in turn, increases adhesiveness of circulating neutrophils. Evidence in man and animals has suggested that these neutrophils are sequestered in pulmonary capillaries, leading to intravascular microthrombi, hypoxemia, and increased pulmonary artery pressure, phenomena which together may be responsible for cardiopulmonary decompensation. An alternative mechanism of dialysis-associated hypoxemia has been proposed recently. Hemodialysis-induced losses of carbon dioxide occur because of the low partial pressure of this gas in dialysate. In order to avoid reduction of the partial pressure of CO_2, the patient responding to sensitive chemoreceptors may hypoventilate and thus develop hypoxemia. While it is not clear how important this effect is, it has been demonstrated, at least in some patients, that addition of carbon dioxide to dialysate prevents hypoxemia. In those cases in which metabolic acidosis occurs as a consequence of "delayed" metabolism of acetate, dialysis and ultrafiltration appear to precipitate hypotension. Hemodialysis associated hypotension occurs in some patients with dysfunction of the autonomic nervous system, a common complication of chronic uremia. This defect, which appears to be localized to the afferent limb of the sympathetic portion of the system, would account for an inadequate response to the hypotensive influences of a hemodialysis treatment. Obviously all of these phenomena may contribute to morbidity, and any may play a predominant role in individual cases.

Septicemia or endoxemia related to contaminated dialysate are clinically indistinguishable. They present with the sudden onset of chills, followed by fever and hypotension. Treatment consists of stopping dialysis and starting treatment for Gram-negative sepsis while awaiting blood culture results. The symptoms will usually cease within a few hours.

PERFORMANCE AND PRINCIPLES OF PERITONEAL DIALYSIS

The serosal surface of both the parietal and visceral peritoneum is a semipermeable membrane, though somewhat more leaky than the cellulosic membrane used in hemodialysis. The capillaries within the peritoneal membranes provide sufficient blood exposure to allow dialysis exchange when a physiological salt solution is introduced into the abdominal space. The dialysate used is similar to that used in hemodialysis except for the presence of high concentrations of dextrose. In order to avoid resorption of the dialysate, approximately 1.5 g/dl of dextrose, a relatively poorly diffusable, nontoxic, metabolizable, and osmotically active substance, must be present in order to counterbalance the protein oncotic pressure of the blood. As much as 4.25 g/dl may be used safely in order to carry out ultrafiltration. Other osmotically active solutes have been suggested or used, including sorbitol, fructose, and dextran, but none has been as satisfactory as dextrose.

Peritoneal dialysis is carried out by means of a single transabdominal catheter which is used for both introduction and drainage of fluid. It is made of silastic rubber and has attached to it one or two dacron felt cuffs. A section of the catheter is made to lie in a subcutaneous tunnel. This arrangement provides both stability and protection from bacterial contamination of the peritoneal cavity once fibrous ingrowth of the dacron has occurred. The first cuff lies just under the exit site, and the second lies just above the peritoneum if it is used.

When peritoneal dialysis was first introduced, it was common to exchange about 2 liters per hour. Generally treatment sessions were 24–36 hours in length, and two treatments per week was the usual practice. About 1–2 hours of equilibration is required for small molecular weight substances (longer for larger moieties) and faster exchange rates seemed unnecessary and excessively demanding. Automated equipment has allowed consideration of faster exchanges. The peritoneal clearance of urea and creatinine increase by about 50 percent if 4 rather than 2 liters per hour is exchanged. Characteristic values are 25 ml/min for urea and 15 ml/min for creatinine. While these values are less than 20 percent of that with modern hemodialysis, larger molecules are cleared at more nearly the same rate. Current experience in many centers has verified that three or four 10 hour, 4 liter/hour treatments provide the clinical equivalent of three conventional hemodialysis treatments possibly because of the advantage afforded by the leakier peritoneal membrane. Recently, a third tactic has been employed successfully. Continuous peritoneal dialysis with exchanges performed every 4–6 hours throughout the week increases the overall efficiency especially for larger substances. Although there is presently increased incidence of infection as a result of the frequent connections and disconnections, the enhanced effectiveness, the ability to be ambulatory while being dialyzed, and the lack of complicated machinery make the technique very attractive to some patients.

Pharmacological augmentation of the rate of transfer of solutes during peritoneal dialysis has been demonstrated with several classes of compounds. High concentration of glucose in the dialysate increases the clearance of urea, creatinine, and other substances by virtue of its effect on bulk fluid transfer. Vasodilators such as nitroprusside and isoproteronol increase the clearance of small molecular weight substances probably by opening splanchnic capillaries. Preliminary clinical studies suggest this may be a useful technique.

Complications of Peritoneal Dialysis

The early application of routine peritoneal dialysis for long-term maintenance was thwarted by the occurrence of peritonitis and malnutrition. Both problems still occur, but with modern techniques and meticulous attention to detail they are less common. Protein losses with present techniques are usually between 10 and 20 g per 10 hour treatment but may be as high as 200 g, especially in the presence of peritonitis. Losses of amino acids and other nutrients may be appreciable as well. With the use of the implanted catheter and careful technique, bacterial peritonitis occurs less than once per patient-year. If the problem is recognized early, 48–72 hours of continuous abdominal lavage with dialysate containing an appropriate antibiotic, and systemic use of the same drug for an additional 2 weeks, usually is effective. If pain and symptoms resolve quickly, the catheter seldom needs to be removed. Cellulitis surrounding the catheter may occur either alone or accompanying infectious peritonitis. It may require catheter removal. Sterile peritonitis occurs with approximately the same frequency as infectious peritonitis and is hard to distinguish at the outset. Mechanical irritation, acid pH of the fluid, and, on occasion, the presence of endotoxin in the fluid are some of the recognized causes of sterile peritonitis. In either case, the patient may present with pain, abdominal distention, constipation, purulent fluid (white cell count exceeding 50,000/mm^3), and catheter dysfunction. Lavage of the abdomen is indicated. Repeated bouts of peritoneal inflammation may lead to reduction of the efficiency of dialysis.

Late catheter failure may be due to peritonitis, to distention of the surrounding hollow viscous, or to the growth of a fibrous sheath around the tip. If stimulation of large bowel function does not improve the flow, the catheter needs to be replaced.

Patients on maintenance peritoneal dialysis may do poorly because of the long hours required, the psychological disturbance caused by the catheter, or the long-term effects of slightly inadequate dialysis. A few patients complain of unrelieved thirst stimulated by each treatment, which may be improved by the use of dialysate with a concentration of sodium as low as 110 mEq/liter. Among diabetic patients, hyperglycemia may be severe and is difficult to control even with the use of supplemental insulin. Very mild but persistent pelvic discomfort may render rehabilitation difficult to achieve; catheter repositioning or replacement may resolve this difficulty.

NONDIALYTIC ADJUSTMENT OF BLOOD COMPOSITION

Newer techniques to adjust the solute concentration of the circulating blood of uremic or poisoned patients have been demonstrated in small groups of patients. Solution of some technical problems may lead to wider application in the near future.

Hemodiafiltration is, in principle, most similar to dialysis treatment. Blood is circulated through a hollow fiber bundle with a dialysate solution outside the fibers. In contrast to conventional dialysis devices, the hemodiafilter has a far more leaky membrane which allows transmembrane convection of large amounts of plasma water. In this case, the transfer of the water is used as the principal driving force for solute removal. Simultaneous administration of balanced salt solution is required. Preliminary experience suggests that patients experience fewer hypotensive episodes with this technique. Until large amounts of sterile fluid can be produced reliably at the bedside, it is unlikely that this system will enjoy wide application.

Hemoperfusion, the in-line exposure of circulating blood to activated charcoal in order to remove solutes by adsorption, is currently available and has been used for the treatment of acute drug intoxication. More general use has been limited by the tendency of blood exposure to charcoal to cause significant thrombocytopenia and hypocalcemia.

INDICATIONS FOR DIALYSIS THERAPY

Acute intoxication by exogenous poisons or drugs is a relative indication for the use of hemodialysis. In many cases, perhaps most, the risks and the inconvenience of this therapy, when weighed against the importance of sound physiological management of the patient in coma, would justify the decision to omit it; however, in severe poisonings, in patients with limited ability to excrete or metabolize the ingested substance, or in institutions where dialysis is a part of a coordinated effort to care for poisoned patients, dialysis can be valuable adjunctive care. There is great variation in the effectiveness of dialysis to remove certain classes of substances. Low molecular weight, water solubility, and low binding to plasma proteins favor the dialytic removal of phenobarbital and aspirin. It should be noted that these are also characteristics which facilitate renal excretion. Agents such as diphenylhydantoin (Dilantin) which are water soluble but highly protein bound can be removed by dialysis, though somewhat less effectively. Drugs which are lipid soluble, including etchchlorvynol (Placidyl) and glutethemide, are not well removed by conventional dialysis, and when removal does occur there is a tendency for the clinical condition of the patient to relapse as body lipid stores gradually return the drug to the circulation. The use of lipid in the dialysate or the use of charcoal or resin hemoperfusion probably facilitates the removal of these and many other substances, including most of the barbiturates, many sedatives and antidepressants, digoxin, and several herbicides and insecticides. Before using hemoperfusion, the physician should acquaint himself with specific experience with the agent and be aware of the potential additional hazards of this technique. Peritoneal dialysis for the removal of exogenous poisons and drugs is usually inefficient; however, it may be of some value

in special cases where, for example, there is accompanying renal failure or where albumin is added to the dialysate.

Dialysis of patients with acute renal failure may be required for several reasons. Prior to the advent of maintenance dialysis programs and the associated staffing and technology, the indications for dialysis of patients with acute renal failure were limited to immediate life-threatening circumstances. For example, initiation of treatment after sudden cessation of effective glomerular filtration would often await the appearance of severe pulmonary edema in the presence of metabolic acidosis and/or marked hyperkalemia. While such complications require dialysis, it is best to use other indications so as to prevent their appearance. Injury, sepsis, or recent major surgery increases gluconeogenesis and the rate of generation of urea and other nitrogenous substances. The uremia which follows impairs normal recovery processes, including functions of while cells, bone marrow progenitors, fibroblasts, respiratory tract cilia, the gastrointestinal tract, and the central nervous system. In addition, the absence of ability to form urine reduces the opportunity to provide the large amounts of caloric intake such patients require. These and related considerations have lead to the conclusion that dialysis treatments of patients with acute oliguric renal failure should begin soon after the diagnosis is established and certainly when there is reason to suspect that the patient's condition may be related, at least in part, to uremia.

Both hemodialysis and peritoneal dialysis are useful in acute renal failure. The decision to use one and not the other often rests on their relative convenience within a given institution or on considerations of the ease of attaining a reliable access to either the peritoneal cavity or to the blood stream in an individual patient. Recent abdominal surgery is not an absolute contraindication to the use of peritoneal dialysis, but it may make placement or function of the catheter difficult. In the presence of severe injury or sepsis, peritoneal dialysis has been unable to control uremia, hyperkalemia, and acidosis, even if used continuously. It is also likely that peritoneal dialysis is ineffective in patients with marginal circulatory status, since splanchnic blood flow is often quite low in this circumstance. Unfortunately hemodialysis may be difficult to accomplish as well in such patients.

Patients with endstage chronic renal failure may present initially with far advanced signs and symptoms of uremia including intractable pulmonary edema, pericarditis, hyperkalemia, severe metabolic acidosis, mental clouding, myoclonus, seizures, gastrointestinal hemorrhage, and accelerated hypertension. Dialysis is required under these conditions.

Ideally, patients with chronic renal failure should be identified and prepared for the eventual need for renal placement therapy well before the onset of these life-threatening uremic complications. When referral is made early, there may be an opportunity to prevent or delay further deterioration. Even if this is not possible, early referral does allow time for patient and family to consider the alternative forms of therapy and play an active role in the selection of maintenance hemodialysis, maintenance peritoneal dialysis, or transplantation. The most common initial therapeutic choice is hemodialysis. Since this regimen requires the development or creation of a usable vein for repeated placement of large-gauge needles, it is generally useful to perform the necessary arteriovenous anastomosis well ahead of time. As renal function gradually deteriorates, a judgment must be made as to when to initiate regular repetitive dialysis or to perform renal transplantation. The overriding consideration in making this judgment is to prevent the severe complications which threaten life and require extensive hospitalization. Therefore less dramatic, perhaps more subtle manifestations of uremia are reasonable indications for initiation of dialysis treatments for patients with chronic renal failure. Evidence of peripheral neuropathy in an individual with severe filtration rate reduction is an indication for dialysis. Return of peripheral nerve function is slow or may not occur at all in maintenance dialysis patients, although recovery may be prompt after successful renal transplantation. Reduction of appetite accompanied by recurrent nausea and vomiting, especially if there is evidence of recent loss of body fat and muscle, is now considered a strong indication of the need to initiate maintenance dialysis for any patient whose glomerular filtration rate has fallen below 5 ml/min.

CHOICE OF DIALYSIS TREATMENT TECHNIQUE, LOCATION, FREQUENCY, AND DURATION

It is unclear that either hemodialysis or peritoneal dialysis provides a better maintenance treatment regimen. Those who favor hemodialysis point to its widespread availability, shorter hours, higher efficiency, more certain ultrafiltration, and better developed technology. Those who favor peritoneal dialysis, at least for some patients, underscore its potential for self-care without the need for assistance and its usefulness for patients whose vascular access fails repeatedly or for those who develop angina or severe hypotension with hemodialysis treatments. It has been suggested without evidence that maintenance peritoneal dialysis will help maintain higher hematocrit values, reduce the risk of peripheral neuropathy, and decrease the risk of vitreous hemorrhage among diabetic dialysis patients. All these considerations notwithstanding, the choice is often made on the basis of experience and availability within a given environment.

Both home-based and center-based, assisted dialysis regimens have strong advocates. The fraction of dialysis patients receiving the bulk of their treatments at home varies from place to place. It is likely that home dialysis is cheaper, but there are hidden costs. Data which suggest less morbidity and mortality among home dialysis patients are based largely on retrospective analysis of selected patients. Nevertheless, in an environment which includes strong family support, ad-

equate space, and ready contact with a center, home dialysis is preferred for many patients since it increases the flexibility of scheduling, possibly reduces dependency, and therefore enhances the opportunity for rehabilitation.

Selection of dialysis frequency and duration for maintenance has been based on limited scientific observations, practical considerations, and developing consensus. Initially, most patients were dialyzed twice a week, but since general experience with thrice-weekly treatment seemed to improve patients' sense of wellbeing, result in better marrow function, and reduce nervous system abnormalities, this regimen has become commonplace. Even more frequent treatments remain impractical for most patients. There is some evidence that the duration of therapy safely may be as little as 4 hours per hemodialysis treatment or even less in spite of the fact that 6–8 hours per treatment was common until the mid 1970s. Preliminary studies suggested that larger surface area dialyzers are necessary to provide adequate removal of uremic toxins in a short dialysis, but this also is debated. Mathematical models which consider urea generation rate and residual renal function have been used to predict the minimal amount of dialysis required, and this appears to be a promising approach. Until it is more clear precisely why dialysis treatments improve uremia, selection of dialysis type and tactics will remain largely empiric.

MEDICAL PROBLEMS OF MAINTENANCE DIALYSIS PATIENTS

Initiation of a maintenance dialysis regimen for the treatment of patients with severe renal failure clearly prolongs life and reduces the severity of many uremic signs and symptoms (Table 2). It is just as clear that these patients are not spared the consequences of a chronic—in some cases debilitating—illness. Many are undernourished, weak, intermittently hypertensive, and chronically anemic. Many seem to age quickly with early manifestations of atherosclerosis, generalized muscle weakness, cardiac abnormalities, loss of libido, drying and thinning of skin, capillary fragility, loss of bone structure, disturbance of bowel function, and mental depression. Those patients whose renal failure is due to diabetes mellitus are especially likely to acquire these problems very early in their course. The severity of the problems varies with the patient's age, initial degree of associated illness, psychological motivation, and perhaps the adequacy of the dialysis regimen. Traditionally, the adequacy of chronic dialysis, or, conversely, the severity of unrelieved uremia, in patients on maintenance dialysis was thought to be reflected by the serum concentration of nitrogenous substances known to be excreted by normal kidneys; however, it is unlikely that urea and creatinine are toxic per se. Ordinarily, the serum urea concentration is five to ten times the normal level in dialysis patients, and serum creatinine may be more elevated. Since more muscular chronic dialysis patients produce larger amounts of creatinine than cachectic patients, it is not unusual for the "healthier" dialysis patients to have the greater serum creatinine values, an apparent paradox. Ingestion of usual quantities of meat found in American diets is no longer considered unwise for dialysis patients in spite of the slight tendency for this practice to increase the blood urea concentration. For these and other reasons, neither measurement has proved of overriding value in determining the need for more or less dialysis unless experience with an individual patient has shown that a given urea or creatinine concentration is associated with a decline in health.

Fluid and Electrolyte Abnormalities

Abnormal blood concentrations of bicarbonate, potassium, calcium, and phosphorus are common, especially at the end of an interdialytic period of more than 1 day. In addition, isotonic overhydration with accompanying hypertension and edema occurs during this interval. These abnormalities are discussed in detail elsewhere. In part, the remarkable tolerance to these perturbations is the result of known adaptive mechanisms including bowel secretion of potassium and the development of hyperparathyroidism; however, the possible relations of these recurring abnormalities to the morbidity of dialysis treatment is poorly defined. It seems likely that provision of daily or constant dialysis would correct most electrolyte abnormalities and thus improve the long term results of chronic dialysis.

Hematopoietic System

Anemia is almost universal among chronic dialysis patients. Their red cells are normal in size and hemoglobin content; production rate is slow for the degree of anemia, and survival is short. The reduced erythropoiesis is due in part to end-organ failure, perhaps attributable to uremic "toxins," and in part to a relative failure of erythropoietin production. Iron absorption is comparable to that of normal people but may be reduced in comparison to nonuremic iron-deficient persons. In any case, iron deficiency occurs in up to 25 percent of chronic uremia patients, perhaps because of unrecognized gastrointestinal losses and blood losses in the dialyzer. The anemia is generally more severe in surgically anephric patients because of the loss of residual renal erythropoietin production. Most dialysis patients with intact native kidneys respond to androgenic steroids with a modest increase in hematocrit. Three times per week dialysis, combined with good nutrition, provision of water-soluble vitamins, and adequate supplemental iron, also appears to improve the hematocrit. Nevertheless, it is unusual to achieve a value of 35 percent or greater, and values in the range of 25 percent are considered satisfactory. Routine transfusions are unnecessary and expensive, increase the risk of hepatitis, and may lead to iron overload. The fear that the practice will sensitize the patient to a later renal graft has not been realized. In fact transfusion appears to improve the chance of graft survival.

Granulocyte concentration and function are normal or near normal except for the transient reduction in number associated with pulmonary margination during the first hour of hemodialysis. Leukocytic response to infection is usually normal. Most patients have a slight lymphopenia, and several abnormalities of "uremic" lymphocytes in vitro have been described. The number of platelets is usually normal, but tests of platelet function reveal defects in most hemodialysis patients; however, the demonstrable defects are appreciably improved by dialysis treatment. Active capillary bleeding may cease within 1–2 hours of a uremic patient's first dialysis even while heparin is being infused.

Cardiovascular System

Among dialysis patients, hypertension is common and is associated with increased risk of stroke and heart disease. Expanded extracellular volume (ECV) which would otherwise be undetectable may be the principal cause of elevated blood pressure. Approximately 80 percent of hypertensive dialysis patients will become normotensive following stepwise reduction of ECV by ultrafiltration. Among the remaining patients, it is likely that disordered regulation of cardiac output, the autonomic nervous system, the renin–angiotensin system, and other factors contribute to the hypertension. These latter patients require antihypertensive drugs in addition to control of their ECV, and there is no specific contraindication to any of those in common use; however, some, most notably alpha methyldopa and guanethidine, may seriously impair cardiovascular reflexes and lead to episodic hypotension during hemodialysis treatments. Rarely a patient may remain extremely hypertensive despite adequate sodium and water control and the use of so much antihypertensive medication that hemodialysis causes severe hypotension. Some of the patients become quite cachectic and may acquire ascites. For such patients, bilateral nephrectomy has been performed and hypertension and cachexia has improved. Nevertheless, this operation should be avoided because the patient usually will become severely anemic. Minoxidil, a potent new vasodilator, appears to be a very useful alternative.

Clinical evidence of cardiac failure may appear in any dialysis patient, usually in association with an obvious expansion of ECV. Generally, ultrafiltration dialysis will provide complete relief, and cardiac glycosides are unnecessary. Most nephrologists prefer to avoid digitalis because of the risk of toxicity during dialysis-induced decline in serum potassium concentration; however, in rare cases, manifestations of congestive heart failure or inadequate peripheral circulation appear to improve after low-dose digitalization. In a small number of documented cases, closure or modification of a patient's arteriovenous fistula was necessary to achieve clinical improvement. Regardless of the contribution of the AV fistula, cardiac output in dialysis patients is usually 50–70 percent higher than normal, and, in most cases, temporary occlusion of the fistula will cause a slight reduction.

Chronically uremic patients have a high incidence of atherosclerotic complications resulting in stroke, peripheral ischemic disease, myocardial infarction, and angina. Angina may become especially severe during hemodialysis presumably because the combination of anemia, hemodialysis-associated hypoxemia, and blood pressure instability adversely affects myocardial oxygen demand–delivery ratio. Blood transfusion, treatment of hypertension, and use of long-acting vasodilators may help control angina. Coronary artery bypass surgery has been successfully applied in the management of a few selected dialysis patients.

Pericarditis occurs in about 10–30 percent of otherwise well dialyzed patients. The cause is obscure, though it is likely that the incompletely controlled uremic condition is at least partially responsible. Evidence for tuberculosis or cancer is not found generally, and most attempts to identify a viral etiology have failed. The usual manifestations include typical pericardial pain, a friction rub, and, in some cases, the development of pericardial tamponade. Typically, the pericardial fluid has the characteristics of a bloody exudate. The natural history is variable. It is not unusual for resolution to occur without a change in either dialysis schedule or technique. Indomethacin seems to hasten this recovery and does provide pain relief. Nevertheless, many nephrologists recommend the routine use of more frequent dialysis employing regional heparinization. One or two weeks of high-dose oral glucocorticoid therapy has been suggested. Should these more conservative measures fail and the patient continues to have pain, unresolved effusion, or evidence of impaired cardiac function, more intensive therapy may be required. Pericardiocentesis, either with or without steroid injection or pericardectomy, has been recommended. It is not clear which is the best choice. Constrictive pericarditis may follow, but this seems to be a rare complication.

Cardiac arrhythmias, often in association with symptomatic coronary artery disease or with pericarditis, may be noted in dialysis patients. Episodic supraventricular tachyarrhythmias may be especially troublesome but will respond to conventional drug therapy including cardiac glycosides. Ventricular ectopic beats also may cause symptoms during dialysis. Quinidine in usual doses or procainamide in reduced amounts may be effective.

Neuromuscular System

Abnormalities of peripheral or central nervous system function may be noted in underdialyzed patients before it is otherwise manifest. Some of the demonstrable abnormalities may be partially improved by increasing the frequency or duration of dialysis; others may remain stable at best.

Peripheral neuropathy begins with distal dysesthesia, hypoesthesia, and paresthesias which may progress to motor weakness. In presymptomatic cases, vibratory sense and ankle reflexes are reduced or absent, and nerve conduction velocity is impaired. These abnormalities are more likely to develop in patients as they lose the small amount of residual renal function which is usually present when maintenance dialysis is initiat-

ed. Abnormalities of motor nerve conduction velocity are somewhat more common among functionally anephric patients who are dialyzed twice a week than among similar groups who are dialyzed three times a week.

Similar observations of the effects of increased frequency of dialysis on central nervous system function have been made. The predominant slow wave (3–7 Hz) electroencephalographic (EEG) activity of uremic patients, characteristic of metabolic encephalopathy, is partially corrected with twice a week dialysis and, in most cases, normalized by treatments three times per week. These changes are paralleled often by improvement of patient alertness and response to detailed psychological testing.

Central nervous system disorders of uremic patients which are unrelated to dialysis scheduling may mimic the effects of underdialysis. Subdural hematoma occurs presumably because of the combined risk of the platelet defect and the repeated use of heparin. Dialysis patients appear to be more susceptible to the toxic effects of mood altering drugs or their metabolites. Recently a distinctive syndrome designated "dialysis dementia" or, more properly, "dialysis-associated encephalopathy" has been described. It is characterized by the stereotypic onset of myoclonic activity, a stuttering dysarthria, followed in weeks to months by episodic myoclonic seizures, dementia, bizarre behavior, and finally death. Although the myoclonus and dysarthria may respond dramatically to small amounts of diazepam early in the patient's course, treatment does not prevent progression of the disease. The disease is probably caused by aluminum accumulation in the central nervous system, perhaps as a result of the continued use of aluminum-containing phosphate binders, but the use of water with substantial amounts of aluminum for dialysate preparation probably plays a larger role.

Dialysis dysequilibrium is a constellation of transient behavioral and central nervous symptoms and signs which are precipitated by dialysis. Manifestations include headache, nausea, decreased alertness, and, in severe cases, coma, seizures, and psychosis. These phenomena are related to highly efficient dialysis, especially when performed in cases of severe uremia. Although normal in uremia, cerebrospinal fluid pressure rises in this disorder. Brain accumulation of water as a result of temporary dysequilibrium of osmotic pressure across the blood–brain barrier is the principal cause of the spinal fluid pressure elevation. Although delayed urea transfer from cerebrospinal fluid probably contributes to the osmotic dysequilibrium direct evidence suggests that the brain tissue temporarily develops new, unidentified, osmotically active particles under these conditions.

Proximal muscle weakness out of proportion to the patient's general condition has been reported to respond to active forms of vitamin D or to parathyroidectomy. Intracellular electrode recording of muscle cell resting potential, abnormal in untreated uremic patients, returns to normal with thrice weekly dialysis but often fails to normalize with less frequent treatments.

Skeletal and Articulating Surfaces

The pathophysiology, histology, and recognition of the several forms of uremic bone disease are discussed in the chapters on *Chronic Renal Failure (Pathophysiology; Consequences)*. Management of these problems in chronic dialysis patients includes administration of intestinal phosphate binders to maintain serum phosphorus below 6 mg/dl; calcium to maintain concentration between 9 and 11 mg/dl; and use of an active form of vitamin D to help sustain serum calcium and induce osseous healing. Parathyroidectomy may be required where disease progresses, but the precise criteria for surgery have not been defined.

There are several causes of the acute and chronic arthritides observed among dialysis patients. Although elevated serum uric acid concentration is common, gout is rare presumably because of a reduced inflammatory response. Most authorities agree that allopurinol need not be used routinely for hyperuricemic dialysis patients unless acute gouty arthritis or tophi are found. Similar attacks of pain (pseudogout) may occur in response to the deposition of calcium pyrophosphate crystals in joints, a syndrome which probably occurs more frequently in a uremic population. Both syndromes will respond to indomethacin, phenylbutazone, or large doses of colchicine. Acute arthritis without crystals in the fluid may be caused by hydroxyapatite deposits in periarticular tissues. Symptoms of this disorder are generally more mild and may respond to rest. Patients on dialysis are probably somewhat more susceptible to some problems requiring specific therapy, including joint infection and ischemic necrosis of periarticular bone.

Gastrointestinal System

The most common complaints of dialysis patients are referrable to the gastrointestinal system, including nausea, vomiting, and constipation. Often there are persistent but nonspecific disorders of taste and appetite. Reduced gastrointestinal tract motility occurs in dialysis patients. Constipation is often exacerbated by the use of the phosphate binders. Judicious use of stool softeners and bowel stimulants is necessary for most patients.

Gastric and duodenal ulceration may occur more frequently than in the general population. This has been ascribed to the finding of elevated gastrin levels and some evidence of gastric hyperacidity.

Because of the hepatitis B virus exposure, described below, a few dialysis patients become ill with chronic active or occassionally chronic persistent hepatitis. The prognosis is guarded, and steroid therapy may be indicated.

Ascites out of proportion or in the absence of other manifestations of ECV excess occurs in a minority of dialysis patients. Usually there is associated cachexia. The fluid has the characteristics of an exudate and generally is bloody. With few exceptions no cause is found.

Endocrine System

Many examples of renal or apparent endocrine disorders are known to exist among uremic patients being maintained on dialysis. Those that are of greatest general concern are related to diabetes mellitus, reduced sexual function, and thyroid status.

It has been estimated that with continued evolution of acceptance criteria, as many as 10,000 patients with diabetes mellitus will be undergoing maintenance dialysis by 1982. Excess morbidity is characteristic of this group. The management of the hyperglycemic tendency has not been satisfactory. In general, the goal in the management of insulin-dependent diabetics has been to avoid severe hyperglycemia (e.g., over 500 mg/dl) rather than to try to exercise tighter control. There are several reasons for this. Many of these same patients suffer also from autonomic insufficiency and lapse into severe hypoglycemia with very little sympathetic activity as an early warning. Urine sugar testing can no longer be considered reliable, and the lack of ability to undergo an osmotic diuresis actually affords some protection against the immediate consequences of hyperglycemia. Because of reduced renal catabolism, insulin requirements usually decrease in advanced uremia. The long-range adverse consequences of hyperglycemia may progress rapidly under this type of management. Nondiabetic patients with uremia have a mild, probably insignificant, glucose intolerance.

Measurable abnormalities of thyroid function are common in clinically euthyroid dialysis patients. Iodine metabolism of these patients differs from study to study, probably because of variations of dietary iodine, iodine content of dialysate, and use of iodine-containing antiseptics. Thyroid stimulating hormone levels are usually normal, but reduction of serum T_3 has been reported. Euthyroid goiter is common among dialysis patients in at least one region of the U.S.

Sexual function is generally reduced in dialysis patients. Male impotence and secondary amenorrhea occur in up to 80 percent of patients. Plasma testosterone concentration is low, but luteinizing hormone (LH) and follicle stimulating hormone (FSH) levels are usually normal. Successful pregnancy has occurred in a few dialysis patients.

Gynecomastia is found in up to 20 percent of male dialysis patients. It appears to be related to the height of LH and FSH but probably is more common with the use of certain drugs including alpha methyldopa and digitalis.

Common Infectious Complications of Dialysis Patients

Endophlebitis of a native vein, an engrafted vein, or some other vascular prosthesis used for hemodialysis may be followed by sepsis, endocarditis, or vascular rupture. Occasionally the first sign of endophlebitis is the development of a thrombus within the vascular access site. The infecting organism is usually *Staphy-*

lococcus aureus, though *S. albus,* several Streptococcus species, and Gram-negative organisms have been implicated. Routine scrubbing of the skin overlying the vein before each needle puncture and after removal of the needle probably reduces the frequency of this complication. Similarly, regular care of cannula exit sites by gentle debridement of accumulated serum and blood and application of an effective antiseptic is important. Treatment of established infection should begin promptly, usually with a penicillinase-resistant penicillin. Removal of a shunt cannula, engrafted vein, or prosthetic is usually necessary. Patients with endophlebitis of a native vein may require closure of the fistula or partial removal of the vein itself but often will effect cure.

Among chronic peritoneal dialysis patients, infectious peritonitis occurs about once a year. *S. aureus* is the most common agent, but Gram-negative organisms may be responsible in up to 40 percent of all cases, and others, including *Candida sp.,* have been noted. Good catheter techniques, care of the exit site, and use of properly prepared dialysate are necessary to prevent frequent infections. Signs and symptoms vary considerably. Typical peritoneal pain with fever is present in over half the cases, but in some the only symptoms are constipation, catheter occlusion, or vague pelvic pain. The fluid is usually frankly purulent, and organisms often may be seen with Gram stain. White cell counts in the range of 10^2–10^4 may be found in the fluid in the absence of infection. Cellulitis surrounding the catheter tunnel or exit site may occur with or without peritonitis. The management of these infections was discussed earlier.

Maintenance dialysis patients acquire other bacterial infections more readily than nonuremic individuals. Urinary tract infections, either with or without symptoms, are present in the majority regardless of the nature of the original renal disease. In some cases, pyocystitis develops presumably because of the combination of intractable infection and oliguria. Radical cystectomy and bilateral nephrectomy may be required for this complication. A few reports suggest that *Streptococcus pneumoniae* and *Mycobacterium tuberculus* infections are also more common than in the normal population; while this seems to be true, it may be the result of chronic illness alone. There does not appear to be an excess chance of acquiring fungal and other opportunistic infections unless the patient has been exposed to glucocorticoid agents or other immunosuppressive drugs.

With the important exception of hepatitis B infection, dialysis patients show little evidence of special clinical problems associated with viral disease. Influenza and herpes zoster seem to attack this group more often and with more severe consequences, much as they do any group with chronic illness. Routine vaccination of all dialysis patients with the appropriate influenza monvalent or polyvalent vaccine is recommended by the United States Public Health Service, but many nephrologists have avoided this practice because of the morbidity experienced by the majority of their patients.

Hepatitis B infection in some dialysis units has reached endemic and occassionally epidemic proportions. The infection is far less severe in the dialysis patients than in nonuremic people (staff members and family) in their environment; however, the biological circumstances which blunt the severity of the infection in most dialysis patients appear to allow them to become chronic carriers. Thus a reservoir for a very contagious disease tends to develop. Most dialysis patients who become infected acquire the virus from contact with other patients. The original infection in a dialysis unit may come from a visiting patient, a staff member, or transfused blood. Evidence for the infection often comes from the results of routine testing of blood for hepatitis B surface antigen or antibody in an asymptomatic individual. Among the fewer than 25 percent who become ill at all, the disease is usually mild, though a few deaths have been reported. There may be a brief period of anorexia, arthralgia, myalgia, and malaise. Jaundice is even less frequent. Serum glutamic oxalic transferase (SGOT) concentration may rise, but rarely more than two- or threefold. The illness may linger or wax and wane for several months. Only about 25 percent will develop antibodies, more commonly women than men. It has proved very difficult to avoid spread of the infection unless susceptible patients are separated entirely from the carriers. The administration of hyperimmune gamma globulin prepared from normal humans with high-titer antibody will protect nonuremic contacts for about 6 weeks. Recent reports suggest that a practical and approved vaccine is only 2 years away from being available. It seems likely that antibody response in dialysis patients to a vaccine will also be attenuated and that vaccination will not entirely control the hepatitis B problem in dialysis treatment areas.

Nutrition and Metabolism

Many dialysis patients are clearly undernourished as judged by their appearance, muscle mass, and skin thickness and turgor. There are accompanying reductions of serum concentrations of transferrin, albumin, and other proteins. Plasma amino acid profiles are abnormal. Some of these patients experience episodic hypoglycemia the mechanism of which is unclear.

Gluconeogenesis may be accelerated, especially in the presence of infection, pericarditis, or other acute illnesses. Hypertriglyceridemia is common and is generally type IV in character. Neither a clear cause nor treatment has been defined, though there is evidence of both rapid lipolysis and inadequate hepatic lipid metabolism.

DRUGS FOR DIALYSIS PATIENTS

Detailed review of drug usage for dialysis patients is beyond the scope of this chapter (see the preceding chapter). A few drugs have been chosen for brief discussion because of their common usage as well as to elucidate certain principles. The rate of drug disappearance from body stores is affected not only by loss of renal function but also by the decreased plasma protein binding and altered volume of distribution which occur in uremia. The fate of active metabolites or coexisting substances similarly may be altered even if the metabolism of the principal drug is not. Moreover, dialysis patients are unusually sensitive to some drugs.

Penicillin and its congeners depend on renal function, but hepatic clearance becomes important in its absence. For this reason and because the therapeutic–toxic ratio is high, no modification of the usual penicillin dosage is required; however, very high dosage, as might be used for the treatment of endocarditis, must be modified in order to avoid neurotoxicity. High-dosage penicillin may be associated with sodium or potassium excess as well. Gentamicin and other aminoglycosides rely exclusively on renal excretion and have a low therapeutic index; however, these important drugs can be used with appropriate dose modification. Chloramphenicol is not appreciably excreted by the kidney, but its potentially toxic metabolites are. Therefore it is best to avoid use of the drug in dialysis patients.

Diphenylhydantoin is much less protein bound in patients with uremia than in normals. This probably explains both its faster metabolism and relatively low effective plasma drug concentration. Diazepam and other centrally acting substances are metabolized by the liver, but mildly uremic patients seem to be more sensitive to them.

Digitoxin is also metabolized in the liver. Thus while drug dose modification may not be necessary, the risk of digitalis intoxication occasioned largely by shifts of body potassium make its use hazardous. Digoxin dosage requires modification because normally it relies, in part, on renal excretion. Procainamide dosage should be reduced because renal handling is normally important, but quinidine metabolism is less affected.

Most commonly employed antihypertensive agents are normally cleared because few of them rely exclusively on renal excretion. Therefore dose selection is not appreciably altered for propanolol, hydralazine, clonidine, alpha methyldopa, guanethidine, and others.

Most dialysis patients are given several water soluble vitamins, iron, phosphate binder, calcium, some form of vitamin D, and usually an antipruritic agent, a sleeping pill, and often an antihypertensive. Compliance is uncertain, and there is opportunity for complex or untoward drug interaction. Frequent review of the drug regimen is well advised.

SURGERY FOR DIALYSIS PATIENTS

Virtually no surgical procedure is contraindicated. Indeed circumstances generally require several operations during the years a patient may be undergoing dialysis. The most common are vascular access, peritoneal catheter placement, transplantation, nephrectomy, pericardectomy, and parathyroidectomy. Aortic aneurysm repair, coronary bypass, and major gastrointestinal and neurosurgery have been done in many dialysis patients.

In order to reduce the risk of general surgery, serum potassium must be well under 5.0 mEq/liter. Most experienced physicians and surgeons agree that the hematocrit value should be above 25 percent, but a normal value is probably not necessary. Bleeding is probably best controlled by performing dialysis the day before and 1–2 days after surgery. Fluids may be administered as long as adequate ultrafiltration is planned and carried out. Under these conditions the risk of surgery is probably not much different than in other chronically ill patients.

FUTURE OF DIALYSIS

At best dialysis will probably remain a halfway therapy capable of prolonging useful life for many but associated with significant morbidity for more than half. Innovations will continue to provide some improvements. The most promising is the portable slow but continuous dialysis devices which currently exist in prototype. A large amount of new knowledge about the uremic state is being gathered and will provide practical assistance in patient management.

REFERENCES

Anderson RJ, Gambertoglio JG, Schrier RW: Fate of drugs in renal failure, in Brenner BM, Rector FC (eds): The Kidney, vol 2. Philadelphia, W.B. Saunders, 1976, p 1911

Blagg CR, Scribner BH: Dialysis, medical, psychosocial, and economic problems unique to the dialysis patient, in Brenner BM, Rector FC (eds): The Kidney, vol 2. Philadelphia, W.B. Saunders, 1976, p 1705

Gotch FA: Hemodialysis: Technical and kinetic considerations, in Brenner BM, Rector FC (eds): The Kidney, vol 2. Philadelphia, W.B. Saunders, 1976, p 1672

Massry SG, Sellers AL (eds): Clinical Aspects of Uremia and Dialysis. Springfield, Ill., Charles C. Thomas, 1976

Winchester JF, Gefland MC, Knepshield JH, et al: Dialysis and hemoperfusion of poisons and drugs—Update. Trans Am Soc Artif Intern Organs 23:762, 1977

RENAL TRANSPLANTATION

L. H. Banowsky and P. C. Chauvenet

For hundreds of years men have harbored the dream of modifying or curing disease by replacing pathologic organs with normal ones. This dream is as old as recorded civilization and has been documented in both oriental and occidental literature and art. Ancient Chinese folklore credits one of its legendary surgeons with successfully transplanting a heart. Saints Cosmos and Damian were reported to have transplanted the leg of a dead Ethiopian to a white patient whose led had required amputation. In order for the transplantation of organs to be more than a medical fantasy, however, significant technical and scientific problems had to be solved.

A prerequisite for the grafting of vascular organs such as the heart and kidney was a reliable technique for arterial and venous reconstruction. This formidable technical barrier was removed when Alexis Carrel described a procedure for vascular anastomosis. Within a few years of Carrel's breakthrough several surgeons tested the clinical application of organ transplantation. Initially animals were the most frequent donors. Ullman attempted to save the life of a woman dying of uremia by anastomosing a pig's kidney to the brachial artery and vein. A small immediate output of urine was rapidly followed by the destruction of the graft. Other attempts at renal transplantation using a variety of donors, including a mother who donated a kidney to her dying child, all met with failure. The lesson was rapidly learned that although the grafting of certain organs— e.g., skin and kidney—was technically feasible, an unknown biological barrier consistently prevented success.

Several early experiments involving animals hinted at an immunologic basis for the failure of transplanted organs. Clear definition of the cause of graft failure awaited the classical experiments of Sir Peter Medewar. His studies of skin grafts during the 1940s firmly established an immunologic basis for graft rejection.

At this point the stage was almost set for the clinical transplantation of organs to begin in earnest. All that was lacking was an agent or agents that would allow pharmacologic suppression of the recipients immune response. In 1952, 6-mercaptopurine (6MP) was discovered, and in 1960 this agent was found to prolong renal allograft survival in experimental animals. Its imidazole derivative, azathioprine, was found to possess similar immunosuppressive properties and to have a wider margin of safety. The availability of azathioprine encouraged several institutions to begin serious programs to study the efficacy of renal transplantation in man.

Great scientific and clinical advances in renal transplantation were made during the 1960s. Rarely has any decade seen such a rapid proliferation of information and such an admirable display of cooperation between basic scientists and clinicians. Problems observed at the bedside were pursued in the laboratory, and advances in the laboratory were rapidly but responsibly applied to the care of sick patients.

Improved clinical skills, a better understanding of the use and abuse of immunosuppressive agents, and increased knowledge of transplantation immunobiology and histocompatibility testing have allowed renal transplantation to evolve from experimental surgery to the preferred mode of therapy for most patients with chronic renal insufficiency. Lessons learned from renal transplantation and the success it has enjoyed have stimulated clinical trials at transplanting a variety of other organs, including liver, heart, lung, bowel, pancreas, and testicle. At selected centers, the results of liver and cardiac transplants are most encouraging and approach the allograft survival of cadaver kidneys. In order for clinical organ transplantation to move significantly forward, however, safer, more effective, and more specific forms of immunosuppression must be found.

The impact of clinical transplantation on the field of medicine has gone far beyond improved care for the patient with chronic renal insufficiency. Organ transplantation has been the catalyst that allowed immunology to blossom as a basic science in its own right rather than function as a little notice appendage of microbiology. New scientific fields such as histocompatibility testing have been born. More complete knowledge of the immune system has already lead to a more thorough understanding of neoplastic disease, infections, the aging process, and immunodeficiency diseases.

RELATIONSHIP BETWEEN RENAL TRANSPLANTATION AND CHRONIC HEMODIALYSIS

Prior to the early 1960s, there was no treatment for the patient with endstage renal disease. Death automatically followed the onset of uremia in a short period of time. At the present time, because of renal transplantation and chronic hemodialysis most patients with endstage renal disease not only have their lives significantly prolonged for many years but also enjoy a reasonable level of rehabilitation.

Renal transplantation and chronic hemodialysis should be viewed as complementary and *not* competitive forms of treatment. While both forms of therapy have demonstrated their effectiveness, neither represents the optimal solution to the problem of chronic renal insufficiency. Chronic hemodialysis offers the advantages of widespread availability, low mortality rates, and for most patients satisfactory rehabilitation. Its disadvantages are cost, dietary restriction, and inability to halt some of the important complications of uremia (anemia, neuropathy, bone disease, etc.), and patient noncompliance.

A successful renal transplant removes many of the limitations of chronic hemodialysis. Following the first post-transplant year the cost of treatment is less. Most dietary restrictions are removed, and many of the complications of chronic renal failure are arrested or reversed. The most telling argument favoring renal transplantation, however, is that even under the best of circumstances the level of rehabilitation achieved with chronic hemodialysis cannot match that achieved in the patient with a normally functioning renal allograft. The disadvantages of renal transplantation are as follows: not all transplants are successful, major surgical procedures are necessary, there is a lack of sufficient numbers of cadaveric kidneys, and the side effects of immunosuppressive therapy can be devastating. Since the optimal treatment for the patient with chronic renal failure is currently not available, each patient's specific problems and desires must be considered and the most appropriate form of therapy for that patient selected. The goal of prolonging patient survival with maximum rehabilitation can best achieved currently by careful integration of maintenance hemodialysis and renal transplantation.

SELECTION OF PATIENTS FOR RENAL TRANSPLANTATION

During the 1970s, one of the most significant trends in clinical renal transplantation has been a relaxing of the criteria for patient selection. Initially most centers had strict selection criteria because of the high morbidity and mortality associated with transplantation and a shortage of adequate facilities and personnel. In some instances, patients were excluded on the basis of the etiology of their renal disease because of the fear that the original disease would rapidly recur in the renal allograft. The vast majority of patients selected were low-risk candidates. Such a restrictive policy is no longer reasonable or justified, and the potential benefits of transplantation can be offered to a much larger number of patients.

Renal transplantation has become a much safer procedure. Recipients of related living donor allografts have a 1 year patient survival of 90 percent or more. Many centers currently report 1 year patient survival of more than 85 percent in recipients of cadaver allografts. Both of these patient survival figures compare favorably with patient survival on chronic hemodialysis. These lower mortality figures have been achieved in spite of selecting higher-risk candidates for transplantation and reflect an absolute increase in safety and not a more rigid process of selection.

Transplant surgeons and nephrologists have also become aware of the concept of relative risk. Certain groups of patients do represent a higher than normal risk for transplantation—e.g., the juvenile onset diabetic—but this same group of patients may be at even greater risk if left on maintenance hemodialysis. The form of therapy with the lower relative risk should be offered to the patient. A partial list of factors that increase risk to the patient undergoing renal transplantation are as follows:

1. Age—greater than 44 years or less than 16 years
2. Significant disease in other organ systems, especially coronary artery and cerebrovascular disease
3. Diabetes mellitus.
4. An abnormal lower urinary tract
5. History of peptic ulcer disease
6. Serious psychiatric problems that may cause noncompliance in the postoperative period

Several of the diseases that cause chronic renal failure are known to recur in the renal allograft—e.g., focal glomerulosclerosis, membranoproliferative glomerulonephritis, diabetes mellitus, lupus erythematosus, cystinosis, and oxalosis. In selecting patients for renal transplantation the crucial question is not whether or not the primary disease will recur in the allograft but rather the *rate* of recurrence. If the primary disease recurs at a slow enough rate, this does not exclude transplantation as a practical means of treatment. At the present time only primary oxalosis recurs with sufficient rapidity and vigor to warrant excluding patients with this diagnosis as potential transplant recipients.

The current policy of selection employed by most transplant centers is one that stresses flexibility and considers each patient individually. An effort is made to avoid arbitrary exclusion of groups of patients by age, primary disease, and so on unless absolutely necessary. It should be remembered that some factors placing patients at increased risk can be corrected with adjuvant operations in the pretransplant period (e.g., peptic ulcer disease). Patients should be selected for transplantation after thoughtfully balancing potential risks versus potential benefits, modifying the above equation when appropriate with the patients' own desires.

HISTOCOMPATIBILITY TESTING

Those cell surface structures responsible for rejection of tissues transplanted within a species are known as histocompatibility antigens. While weaker antigenic systems may contribute to graft rejection, a group of strong antigens, called major histocompatibility antigens, are primarily responsible for rejection of intraspecies transplants. A complex of closely linked genetic loci code for the major histocompatibility antigens in all species studied thus far. This segment of chromosome is called the major histocompatibility complex (MHC) and in man is referred to as the HLA region. The human MHC has been assigned to the sixth chromosome, and it codes for the major histocompatibility antigens, known in man as HLA antigens. The HLA region contains three loci which code for three corresponding allelic series of antigens detectable with serological reagents (A, B and C) and one locus which codes for a corresponding series of antigens recognized by lymphoid cells in the mixed lymphocyte reaction (D).

Historical Background

The importance of HLA antigens in transplantation was first realized when it was found that HLA incompatible grafts were rejected in an accelerated manner if the recipient serum had antibodies specifically reactive with the donor HLA antigens. This was the basis for deducing that serologically detected HLA specificities were transplantation rejection antigens. Early serological typing reagents, obtained primarily from multiparous women, were multispecific, thus making characterization of HLA specificities exceedingly difficult. With the introduction of χ^2 contingency tests coupled with computerization of serological reactivities against cell panels, these complex arrays or reactivity were translated into definitive groups of HLA specificities. Through a series of international workshops, the HLA-A, -B, and -C allelic series of specificities was delinated and given standard nomenclature under supervision of the World Health Organization (WHO). A "w" is used to designate provisional (workshop) specificities which have not received official approval by the WHO.

In 1963 it was discovered that when lymphocytes from two HLA incompatible individuals are cocultivated, they undergo blastogenesis and division. It was subsequently noted that genes controlling these mixed lymphocyte reactions (MLR) are associated with the HLA region. At first there was a tendency to associate mixed lymphocyte stimulation with disparity at HLA-A and -B, but exceptions were found wherein lymphocytes from siblings serotypically identical at HLA-A and B nevertheless exhibited mutual strong stimulation in MLR. This led Yunis and Amos to postulate the existence of an MLR-stimulating locus separate from HLA-A and -B. Their hypothesis that the genetic locus responsible for MLR—now designated HLA-D—was separate from the HLA-A, -B, and -C gained support through identification of additional recombinant haplotypes.

Genetics of the Major Histocompatibility Complex

The HLA region has been assigned to the sixth human chromosome on the basis of family and cell hybridization studies. A schematic representation of chromosome 6 is shown in Fig. 1. The HLA gene complex, together with its neighboring genes, is referred to as the HLA linkage group. The intragenetic distances between loci in the HLA linkage group are given in centimorgans (Fig. 1) and are computed from frequencies of genetic recombination obtained through study of a large number of families. Genetic loci controlling approximately half the known factors of the complement system (C2, C4, C6, C8, and Bf) map in or near the HLA region. Structural genes for three enzymes, PGM3, PG5, and G10, are located in close proximity to HLA. Also associated with the HLA complex are the red cell antigens Rodgers and Chido, and recent evidence suggests that these are antigenic components of C4.

The HLA-A, -B, -C, and -D gene products are expressed codominantly on the surface of somatic cells. Since chromosomes are paired, it follows that each individual can express two different A, B, C, and D antigens, for a total of eight HLA gene products. HLA alleles located together on the same chromosome are called haplotype, and except for the rare event of genetic recombination within the HLA complex (0.80 percent), those alleles located together on the same chromosome are inherited as a unit. Each individual thus has two HLA haplotypes, which together form his HLA genotype. [The important distinction between HLA genotype and phenotype must be understood. A phenotype merely lists the HLA specifications as determined by serotyping (HLA-A, -B, -C) or MLR typing (HLA-D) without regard to which alleles are linked together on the same haplotype. The only method available for determining HLA genotype is by deduction, usually from maternal and paternal HLA phenotypes.]

An example of HLA inheritance in a single generation is shown in Fig. 2. Since HLA inheritance follows simple Mendelian genetics, segregation of maternal and paternal HLA haplotypes (barring genetic recombination) results in four possible sibling genotypes. A parent and child therefore will always share one haplotype. Since a parent has two haplotypes, each of which segregate independently, there are four possible sibling genotypes. The probability that two siblings will be HLA identical, i.e., inherit the same haplotypes from each parent, is one in four. The probability that two siblings will be haploidentical or share one haplotype is one in two, while the probability that two siblings will have no haplotype in common is one in four.

An unusual feature of the HLA system is the fact that certain HLA alleles are found associated together in a haplotype more often than would be expected based on gene frequencies. This phenomenon, called linkage disequilibrium, results in frequent haplotype association in white populations of, for example, A1 and B8, A3 and B7, A29 and B12, and A1 and B17. Striking linkage disequilibrium also occurs for certain alleles of HLA B with C, D, and DR.

Detection of HLA Antigens and Antibodies

Since 1964, serotyping for HLA-A, -B, and -C antigens has been routinely accomplished through the cytotoxicity test. In this procedure, lymphocytes are incubated with typing sera in the presence of rabbit complement. If the lymphoid cell surface expresses an HLA specificity recognized by antibodies in the typing sera, the lymphocytes are lysed. Vital stains are used to distinguish nonviable from viable cells, and the

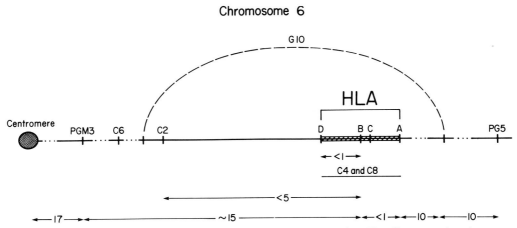

Fig. 1. Current map of the sixth human chromosome, including the HLA region. Map distances, where known, are expressed as centimorgans (cM).

INHERITANCE OF HLA

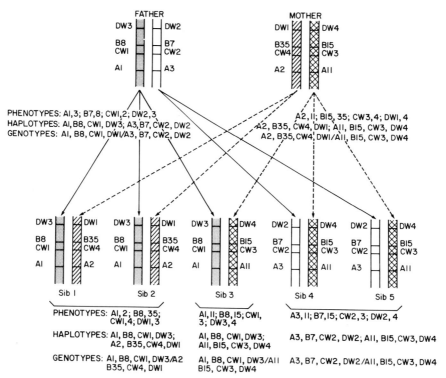

Fig. 2. Segregation of maternal and paternal haplotypes results in four possible sibling genotypes. In this family, HLA-identical siblings 1 and 2 share no haplotypes with HLA-identical siblings 4 and 5. Sibling 3 shares one haplotype with siblings 1 and 2 and the other haplotype with siblings 4 and 5.

degree of cytolysis is assessed by simple counting of stained cells. Precise identification of HLA-A, -B, and -C antigens relies on a series of "monospecific" serological reagents, or antisera that recognize only a single HLA antigen.

Antibodies directed against HLA antigens do not occur naturally but instead are formed as a result of pregnancy or sensitization by grafting or transfusion. Sera from such donors are made operationally monospecific by absorption with cells expressing the undesirable specificities. When an individual is serologically typed for HLA antigens and less than two each of the A, B, and C specificities are detected, "blanks" are said to occur. Such blanks can be due to either (1) homozygosity or (2) presence of antigens for which corresponding serological reagents are not available. Homozygosity can generally be established by determining whether the antigen in question is shared by maternal and paternal haplotypes.

The cytotoxicity test is also used to monitor sera of transplant candidates for anti-HLA antibodies. If serum from a transplant candidate reacts positively with a potential donor's lymphoid cells, this is considered a positive antibody crossmatch. Of the current methodology available, the crossmatch when positive is the most powerful gauge for predicting transplant

failure, and a positive crossmatch between donor and recipient is universally accepted as an absolute contraindication to transplantation. One recent study suggests that a positive crossmatch attributable to anti-B-lymphocyte reactivity, rather than to conventional anti-HLA, -B, -C, reactivity, may not be a contraindication to transplantation.

Routine monitoring of serum for anti-HLA reactivity can be accomplished through the use of a cell panel. Such a panel is compiled from a select series of previously typed lymphoid cells, at least one of which expresses each of the currently established serologically detectable HLA specificities. By use of properly chosen cell panels, sera from patients awaiting transplants as well as potential reagent sera (obtained, for example, from multiparous women) can be screened for HLA reactivity. When the degree of serological activity or percentage reactive antibody (PRA) against the cell panel is narrow, specific anti-HLA antibodies can be identified.

Serological reagents which detect antigens of the HLA-D series are as yet not available. Among living related donors and recipients, disparity at HLA-D is commonly measured by the degree of lymphocyte stimulation in reciprocal MLR tests. As essment of disparity at HLA-D between cadaveric donors and recipients is not feasible except in retrospect due to the length of time involved (approximately 7 days) in the MLR assay. Eleven distinct HLA-Dw specificities have been identified by the use of reagent cells homozygous at HLA-D. A responder cell is considered positive for a given HLA-D allele when low or undetectable levels of MLR are induced by stimulation with the corresponding homozygous HLA-D typing cell. An abridged version of HLA-D typing employs previously sensitized lymphocytes as typing reagents, but even this test is impractical for use in matching cadaveric donors and recipients at HLA-D, since it generally requires 48–72 hours.

Considerable effort on the part of many investigators has been aimed at development of serological reagents which discriminate the HLA-D determinants. A number of serologically detected allelic determinants have been defined with antisera directed against B (bone marrow derived) lymphocytes. The DR locus which controls this series of antigens is apparently distinct from, but located in close proximity to, HLA-D. Whether or not serological reagents which detect HLA-DR specificities can be used to discern the HLA-D determinants is a matter under intensive investigation.

HLA System and Transplant Prognosis

Aside from HLA, ABO is the only well defined antigen system in man known to exert a strong influence on graft survival. Kidneys transplanted between HLA-identical siblings have a better than 90 percent 2 year survival. For kidneys transplanted between siblings identical at only one HLA haplotype, the survival rate is significantly inferior, and for transplants between HLA-mismatched siblings the 2 year survival rate is less than 50 percent. In the majority of cases, these results are based on matching for specificities of the HLA-A and -B series. Where living related transplants are concerned, this implies (with few exceptions) matching at the closely linked HLA-C and -D loci as well. These results provide unequivocal support for the importance of HLA in determining transplant failure or success among living related donor recipient pairs; however, matching of serologically detected HLA-A, -B specificities has not generally improved transplant survival in unrelated donor–recipient pairs. With the possible exception of blood type A, B, or AB recipients, the degree of HLA-A, -B matching is not considered to be considered to be a contributing factor in cadaveric transplant survival.

The current nomenclature for alleles of the HLA complex as established by the Seventh International Workshop is shown in Table 1. During the last decade the number of A and B specificities has increased tremendously, in large part due to the "splitting" of former broad specificities into narrow ones. Moreover, even for the best studied racial group, i.e., Caucasoid, there remain A and B specificities for which serological reagents are as yet unavailable. To complicate this matter further, many antigenic specificities of the HLA-A and -B series are prone to cross-reactivity (Table 2), the basis of which has not been explained. The HLA-C series of antigens may also have relevance in transplantation. Owing to the location of the C locus (between B and A), HLA-C incompatibilities could occur in HLA-A, and -B phenotypically identical unrelated individuals but not between HLA-A, and -B–identical siblings. At the present time, serotyping for HLA-C specificities is not a commonly used prognostic tool in transplantation. Further unraveling of the cross-reactive and polymorphic complexities of the HLA system will presumably contribute to the success of necrodonor transplants.

Posttransplant Immunological Monitoring

While the basis of graft rejection is immunological, ctntroversy exists regarding the relative importance of cellular and/or humoral components. Hyperacute rejection, which occurs when transplant recipients have performed donor-reactive cytotoxic antibodies in their sera, has largely been avoided by pretransplant cross-matching of patient sera with donor cells. Posttransplant formation of cytotoxic antibodies directed against donor T or B lymphocytes is generally associated with poor graft prognosis. The appearance of cytotoxic antibody in sera of transplanted patients has frequently accompanied acute rejection, although acute rejection is thought to be mediated predominantly by cytotoxic T (thymus derived) lymphocytes. Recent findings suggest that detection in transplant recipients of antibodies which mediate antibody dependent cell-mediated cytotoxicity (ADCC) against donor target cells may be associated with chronic rejection.

Neither the posttransplant level of circulating T cells nor the lymphocyte responsiveness to phytohermagglutinin (PHA) or donor cells (MLR) has been found to correlate with transplant prognosis. Recent studies indicate that suppression of donor-reactive cytotoxic T lymphocytes (CTL) in transplant recipients is associated with long-term graft survival. To summarize, posttransplant monitoring of immunological responsiveness would serve to augment and facilitate the diagnosis and management of clinical rejection. Specific inhibition of host immune reactivity to donor histocompatibility antigens, through, for example, induction of specific enhancement or tolerance, remain viable alternatives toward long-term prolongation of survival of incompatible transplants in the future.

SELECTION OF DONORS

One of the many unique aspects of organ transplantation is that the operation cannot be performed until a healthy donor organ is available. Thus the timing of the operation is dictated not by the need or convenience of the recipient but by the availability of a suitable donor. The source of the donor organ is one of the most important factors in determining the ultimate success or failure of the renal allograft (Fig. 3).

Most centers perfer to use a related living donor (RLD) if one is available. This preference is based on both significantly higher immediate and long-term pa-

Table 1
Nomenclature and Frequency of Factors of the HLA System

Locus A	Antigen Frequency (%)*	Locus B	Antigen Frequency (%)	Locus C	Antigen Frequency (%)	Locus D	Antigen Frequency (%)
A1	32	Bw4	—	Cwl	10	Dw1	19
		B5	11				
A2	49	Bw6	—	Cw2	15	Dw2	15
		B7	23				
A3	22	B8	20	Cw3	26	Dw3	16
A9	17	B12	24	Cw4	20	Dw4	16
A10	13	B13	6	Cw5	14	Dw5	15
A11	8	B14	11	Cw6	—	Dw6	11
Aw19	—	B15	7			Dw7	—
Aw23(9)	6	Bw16	12			Dw8	—
Aw24(9)	16	B17	7			Dw9	—
A25(10)	7	B18	9			Dw10	—
A26(10)	11	Bw21	4			Dw11	—
A28	11	Bw22	5				
A29	7	B27	10			Locus DR	
Aw30	5	Bw35	17				
Aw31	7	B37	5			DRw1	
Aw32	8	Bw38 (16)	0			DRw2	
Aw33	3	Bw39 (16)	—			DRw3	
Aw34	0	B40	12			DRw4	
Aw36	0	Bw41	1			DRw5	
Aw43	—	Bw42	0			DRw6	
		Bw44 (12)	—			DRw7	
		Bw45 (12)	—				
		Bw46	—				
		Bw47	—				
		Bw48	—				
		Bw49 (21)	—				
		Bw50 (21)	—				
		Bw51 (5)	—				
		Bw52 (5)	—				
		Bw53	—				
		Bw54 (22)	—				

Nomenclature according to the Seventh International Workshop in Histocompatibility Testing, 1977. Broad specificities are shown in parentheses following particular splits (such listing is optional).

*Antigen frequencies are those determined for whites at the Sixth International Histocompatibility Workshop.

tient and allograft survival. An available RLD also gives the patient the assurance that a transplant can be done and allows the operation to be done at the most advantageous time for the recipient. When a RLD is identified early in the course of the patient's disease, the time on maintenance hemodialysis can be minimized. This not only reduces dialysis-related complications but also results in a significant reduction in cost.

Histocompatibility testing of the recipient's family is the initial step in determining the availability of a suitable RLD. If no HLA-identical sibling is found, haplotype-matched siblings, parents, or children can be further screened by the use of the mixed lymphocyte culture (see the section on Histocompatibility Testing). Medically suitable RLD need not be perfect physical specimens, but their overall health should be such that a major operation will not represent excessive risk and their renal function must be normal. Unwilling RLDs

should be excluded from evaluation in such a way that family pressure or resentment is minimized.

If the physical examination, history, and screening laboratory and x-ray examinations are normal, a renal angiogram should be performed. The renal angiogram defines the number and integrity of the renal arterial supply. It should be mentioned that anatomical abnormallities that do not reflect disease—e.g., ureteral duplication or multiple renal arteries—should not exclude an otherwise suitable RLD.

Over 70 percent of potential renal transplant recipients in this country do not have a willing or medically acceptable RLD. If these patients are to be transplanted, the kidney must be obtained from a cadaver (CAD) donor. A nationwide shortage of CAD donors exists. This shortage is most obviously manifested by the waiting list of recipients found at all transplant centers. Depending on the particular center and area of the

Table 2
Common Cross-reactive HLA-A and -B Specificities

HLA-A Antigens	Cross-Reactive Specificities	HLA-B Antigens	Cross-Reactive Specificities
A1	A3, A11, Aw36	B5	B15, B17, B18, Bw21, Bw35
A2	A28	B7	Bw22, B27, B40, Bw42
A3	A1, A11	B8	B14
A9	A2, Aw23, Aw24	B12	B17, Bw21, Bw44, Bw45
A10	A11, A25, A26, Aw32, Aw34	B13	B7, B40
A11	A1, A3, A26	B14	B8, B18
Aw23	A2, A9, Aw24	B15	B5, B17, B18, Bw21, Bw35
Aw24	A2, A9, Aw23	B16	Bw22, Bw38, Bw39
A25	A10, A26, Aw32, Aw33	B17	B5, B12, B15, B18, Bw21, Bw35
A26	A10, A11, A25	B18	B5, B14, B15, B17, Bw35
A28	A2	Bw21	B5, B12, B15, B17, Bw35
A29	Aw30, Aw31, Aw32, Aw33	Bw22	B7, Bw16, B27, Bw38, B40, Bw42
Aw30	A29, Aw31, Aw32, Aw33	B27	B7, Bw22, B40
Aw31	A29, Aw30, Aw32, Aw33	Bw35	B5, B15, B17, B18, Bw21
Aw32	A25, A29, Aw30, Aw31, Aw33	B37	No strong associations
Aw33	A25, A29, Aw30, Aw31, Aw32	Bw38	B16, Bw22, Bw39
Aw34	A10, Aw26	Bw39	B16, Bw22, Bw38
Aw36	A1	B40	B7, B13, Bw41
Aw43	No strong associations	Bw41	Bw40
		Bw42	B7, Bw22

country, patients can wait from 8 to 24 months before a suitable donor organ is available. This shortage of CAD organs is not due to a lack of suitable donors but rather to inadequate public and professional awareness of the need for CAD kidneys.

Not all agonal patients are suitable CAD donors. Commonly used criteria for selecting CAD donors are as follows:

1. Age—less than 55 years and more than 1 year
2. No transmissible disease, i.e., infections or malignancy (excluding primary central nervous system tumors)
3. No diastolic hypertension
4. Normal renal function at the time af admission
5. Urine output exceeding 100 cc/hour
6. If vasopressors have been used, their effects should be reversed with agents such as chlorpromazine or phenoxybensamine
7. Warm ischemia time of less than 15 min
8. Consent of next of kin

Once a CAD kidney is obtained, two methods of short-term (24–48 hours) renal preservation are available. The simplest method of short-term preservation consists of flushing the kidney with a cold hyperosmolar electrolyte solution having a composition similar to intracellular fluid (low in sodium and high in potassium and magnesium). After the initial flushing the kidney is immersed in sterile iced saline. The kidney is cooled by this method to a core temperature of 7°–10°C. This simple technique provides excellent renal preservation

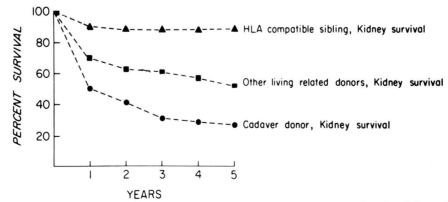

Fig. 3. Renal allograft survival according to the source of donor organ. Data based on information from the Human Renal Transplant Registry.

for up to 24 hours. It offers the advantages of simplicity and low cost. When compared with pulsatile perfusion, however, the incidence of postoperative acute tubular necrosis is higher, although renal function at 1 month is comparable to kidney preserved with pulsatile perfusion.

Pulsatile perfusion remains the most popular form of renal preservation. Using this technique, cadaver kidneys can be safely preserved for up to 48 hours. Cryoprecipitated plasma, plasma protein fraction, or modified albumin solution can be used as the perfusate. The basic principals of this form of preservation are (1) continuous *pulsatile* perfusion, (2) hypothermia (renal core temperature of 4°–7°C), and (3) oxygenation of the perfusate. Pulsatile renal preservation units now exist that are battery operated and small enough to sit on a car or airplane seat. Pulsatile perfusion offers the advantages of a lower postoperative incidence of acute tubular necrosis, longer periods of preservation, and by assessment of the perfusion characteristics of the kidney (i.e., pressure and flow) some means of monitoring the viability of the organ during preservation. Either form of renal preservation allows sufficient time to do histocompatibility testing, prepare the recipient, or distribute the kidney to another transplant center in the absence of a suitable local recipient.

PRETRANSPLANT PREPARATION OF THE RECIPIENT

Pretransplant preparation of the potential recipient contributes a great deal to the ultimate success or failure of the renal allograft. Unrecognized or uncorrected problems are very likely to surface during the postoperative period and either threaten the patient's life or cause an otherwise unwarranted reduction in immunosuppressive therapy. Preoperative preparation should focus on improving the general status of the patient, identification and correction of renal or potential medical or surgical problems, and institution of any measures that will make immunosuppression safer or more effective.

Patients starting on maintenance hemodialysis have severe metabolic, hematologic, and nutritional derangements secondary to the uremic syndrome. Virtually all patients benefit from a 6–12 week period of hemodialysis before transplantation. This allows time to correct metabolic and nutritional problems, identify patients with non-volume-dependent hypertension, partially correct the associated anemia, improve platelet function, and give the patient some time to emotionally adjust to the reality of the disease. The most notable exception to the above policy is the patient with juvenile onset diabetes mellitus. The ophthalmologic complication associated with diabetes mellitus are aggrevated by both uremia and chronic hemodialysis. In order to minimize the occurrence of blindness, transplantation should be performed approximately 1 year before the patient would be normally started on maintenance hemodialysis when the creatinine is 4.5–6.0 mg/dl.

Patients should be carefully screened to detect existing or previous gastrointestinal disease. Of particular concern are patients with a history of peptic ulcer disease. These patients are in great jeopardy in the posttransplant period. Active peptic ulcer disease should be initially treated medically and when the ulcer has become inactive a vagotomy and pyloroplasty should be done. In one series, failure to perform prophylactic ulcer surgery in patients with a recent history of active peptic ulcer resulted in an 80 percent incidence of posttransplant gastrointestinal hemorrhage. Even patients with an inactive ulcer of long standing benefit from prophylactic pretransplant ulcer surgery. The posttransplant reactivation rate of patients who were asymptomatic but had a documented ulcer in the past has been 47–67 percent. Posttransplant patients who sustain gastrointestinal heorrhage from a peptic ulcer have had reported mortality rates of as high as 60 percent.

Colonic complications are not common in the posttransplant period but are significant because of the extremely high mortality rate (50–100 percent) associated with perforation. Patients awaiting transplantation who have a history consistent with diverticulitis should be sigmoidoscoped and have a barium enema. Some centers advocate routine barium enemas on all patients over 44 years of age. If significant disease is found, a preoperative colectomy should be seriously considered.

Infection with hapatitis B virus is common in chronic hemodialysis patients. Transplantation should be deferred in patients with active hepatitis or in those who have recently become HBsAg positive until sufficient time has elapsed to determine the activity of the disease. The fate of the HBsAg positive patients and patients who have HBsAg antibodies after transplantation is controversial. Pirson reported a fivefold increase in mortality from liver disease in patients transplanted who were HBsAg positive; other centers have refuted this report. There are also data that suggest that patients who have HBsAg antibodies have a significantly lower 1 year allograft survival than either HBsAg positive patients or HBsAg and HBsAg antibody negative patients. This area awaits further documentation. In any event, patients who are HBsAg positive should be identified so that dialysis and operating room personnel can take appropriate precautions.

Other obvious problems, such as parathyroid disease, gall bladder disease, and significant peripheral or cardiovascular disease, should be identified and dealt with appropriately. The oral cavity deserves special mention because it is frequently overlooked. Poor oral hygiene, dental caries, and abscessed teeth are not uncommon sources of posttransplant fever and sepsis. A dental examination and Panorex film of the mouth should be a routine part of the pretreatment evaluation.

Blood Transfusions

During the last 6 years, many transplant centers' policies on blood transfusions have undergone complete reversal. In the early 1970s, dialysis and transplant centers tried to minimize or completely eliminate blood transfusions in their dialysis patients. Most of the known facts about blood transfusions in the dialysis population were negative; transfusions had no real impact on the anemia, the transmission of viral particles was likely (hepatitis virus, cytomegalovirus, etc.), and sensitization of the patient to the HLA cell surface antigens on leukocytes was possible. Sensitization of the patient to HLA antigens with the resultant formation of performed circulating cytotoxic antibodies posed a dual threat to the potential renal transplant recipient. If the sensitized patient formed cytotoxic antibodies to a wide range of HLA antigens, the likelihood of finding a donor against whom the recipient had a negative crossmatch became remote. Since the titer of cytotoxic antibodies waxes and wanes, a false negative crossmatch in a previously sensitized recipient could result in hyperacute rejection with immediate loss of the allograft.

Coincident with the minimal or no transfusion policy was a significant reduction in CAD renal allograft survival. Opeltz and Teraski were the first to note a beneficial or protective effect of blood transfusions on CAD renal allografts. This protective effect of blood transfusions on renal transplants was also reported to occur in several strains of experimental animals. Virtually all transplant centers that have examined the effect of pretransplant blood transfusions on renal allograft survival have noted a positive correlation. The improvement in allograft survival in transfused patients has varied from 15–50 percent.

Although the mechanism by which this protective action occurs is unknown, several possibilities exist. The HLA cell surface antigens present on leukocytes have the potential of stimulating either cytotoxic or blocking antibodies. Blocking antibodies do not fix complement and can coat antigen sites on target cells, thereby potentially reducing the effectiveness of both the afferent and efferent limbs of the host's immune response. There is scanty evidence to support this theory.

Pretransplant blood transfusions could also improve allograft survival by selecting out a more favorable donor and recipient population. Some patients respond to the HLA antigen stimulation be forming circulating cytotoxic antibodies to virtually *all* HLA antigens. This group of "overresponders" is effectively removed from the transplant waiting list, since they will have a positive crossmatch against almost all potential donors. Other patients respond to foreign HLA antigens by forming cytotoxic antibodies to only some HLA antigens. Theoretically, then, the pretransplant crossmatch will select out and exclude donors that the recipient would react strongly to. Thus pretransplant exposure to the foreign HLA antigens in blood may exclude some recipients (the overresponders) and may also exclude some donors that might be capable of stimulating an unusually strong immune response in a particular recipient. The net result of the above would be a much more favorable donor–recipient population.

Evidence against this theory is that transfused recipients who develop *no* circulating cytotoxic antibodies to any HLA antigens also have improved renal allograft survival.

While the majority of transplant centers accept as fact the protective effect of blood transfusions on renal allografts, many pertinent and practical clinical questions remain to be answered: the type of blood product to use (whole blood, packed cells, or frozen washed red cells), the amount of blood transfused, the optimal time schedule for giving transfusions in the pretransplant period, and the number of transfusions. In spite of the many unanswered questions, a careful policy of pretransplant blood transfusions for recipients of CAD kidneys is being followed by most centers.

ADJUVANT OPERATIONS

While adjuvant operations can cover a wide spectrum of clinical problems, only the two most commonly performed, bilateral nephrectomy and splenectomy, will be discussed here.

Bilateral nephrectomy was a routine pretransplant procedure until the early 1970s. Removal of the diseased kidneys had been considered mandatory to eliminate a real or potential source of infection, to correct hypertension, to minimize the recurrence of the original disease in the allograft, and in some instances to enable use of the recipient's own ureter to establish urinary continuity of the allograft via uretero-or pyeloureterostomy. Documentation of the morbidity and mortality of the procedure, combined with the knowledge that even endstage kidneys contributed to the wellbeing of the patient, led to the discontinuation of bilateral nephrectomy as a routine procedure.

Maintaining patients on chronic hemodialysis has allowed a significant body of knowledge to be gathered on the various functional capabilities of endstage kidneys. Many of these functions contribute in a positive way to the patients' life on hemodialysis. Most endstage kidneys maintain the ability to excrete some urine. Whatever amount of urine is made allows the patient to liberalize fluid intake by a like amount. The anemia associated with chronic renal failure is one of the more disabling aspects of life on dialysis. Bilateral nephrectomy always makes the anemia worse. While anabolic steroids have been found to partially alleviate the anemia of uremia, they have no effect in the anephric patient. The effect of bilateral nephrectomy on the patient with polycystic disease is especially pronounced, since many of these patients will have a hematocrit greater than 30 percent. Calcium metabolism may also be less efficient in the anephric patient, since the kidney is necessary for the production of 1,25-dihydrocholecalciferol, which is the most active form of vitamin D_3 in promoting calcium absorption from the gut.

Several centers have examined factors that place a patient undergoing bilateral nephrectomy in a high-risk group—(1) age greater than 44 years, (2) severe or uncontrolled hypertension, (3) diabetes mellitus, (4) active urinary tract infection, (5) polycystic kidney disease. It is ironic that while uncontrollable hypertension and active urinary tract infection place the patient in a high-risk group, they still represent absolute indications for pretransplant bilateral nephrectomy.

The common indications for pretransplant bilateral nephrectomy are (1) severe or uncontrolled hypertension, (2) active urinary tract infection, (3) significant anatomical abnormalities of the urinary tract, and (4) patients with polycystic kidney disease who have a history of infection or serious renal bleeding. While there is general agreement that routine bilateral nephrectomy is ill advised, the pendulum should not be allowed to swing too far in the opposite direction. Many patients receive a substantial benefit from pretransplant bilateral nephrectomy and have a safer and smoother posttransplant course. It must also be remembered that renal allograft survival is slightly higher in the anephric patient for up to 3 years posttransplant regardless of the etiology of the primary disease. Judicious patient selection and thoughtful surgical technique allows bilateral nephrectomy to be a beneficial tool in the pretransplant preparation.

Splenectomy

In spite of the large number of splenectomies performed at a variety of transplant centers, the value of splenectomy is still a debatable issue. A variety of indications for performing splenectomy have been suggested: prophylactic splenectomy to gain an immunologic advantage, specific splenectomy to correct pretransplant hypersplenism, and therapeutic splenectomy to correct unexplained leukopenia in the posttransplant period.

Prophylactic pretransplant splenectomy has been advocated to gain an immunologic advantage in the posttransplant period, i.e., to make immunosuppression more effective and/or safer. The spleen represents the largest lymphoid organ in the body and houses a large number of B lymphocytes and some T lymphocytes. For vascularized organ grafts the spleen serves as a site for both recognizing and responding to foreign antigens. In addition, the WBC count is the limiting factor in determining the dose of azathioprine, one of the pharmacologic cornerstones of posttransplant immunosuppressive therapy. Several investigators have demonstrated that splenectomized patients tolerate a higher dose of azathioprine. When considering the above, one can make an attractive argument that splenectomy would not only rid the body of its largest lymphoid organ but also increase the patient's tolerance to azathioprine.

Unfortunately, the effect of prophylactic splenectomy has not yielded consistently improved renal allograft survival in either experimental animals or human beings. It should be pointed out, however, that many of the clinical studies showing splenectomy had no effect on allograft survival suffered from being retrospective studies or from using historical controls, small numbers of patients, or pooled data. Recent clinical studies by Kaufman and experimental animal studies by Fabre have supported splenectomy as a successful adjunctive immunologic tool in improving renal allograft survival.

Berne and associates found that approximately 10 percent of their chronic hemodialysis population suffered from clinical hypersplenism. Patient white blood counts (WBC) were less than 4500, platelet counts were less than 125,000, and patients required at least one blood transfusion per month. Transplantation of these patients usually resulted in failure because of the patient's intolerance to even low doses of azathioprine. Pretransplant splenectomy seems to correct this problem and allows adequate doses of azathioprine to be given posttransplant.

Some patients develop a severe and protracted posttransplant leukopenia. These patients are not able to tolerate even low doses of Imuran and frequently lose their allografts because of uncontrollable rejection. Frequently the leukopenia cannot be explained on the basis of overdosage with azathioprine, sepsis, or a concomitant viral infection. These patients respond favorably to therapeutic splenectomy even when the bone marrow is hypocellular and can tolerate a therapeutic dose of azathioprine within the first 3–4 days postsplenectomy.

Thus there seem to be two reasonable indications for splenectomy in the transplant recipient: the patient identified pretransplantation as having hypersplenism and the posttransplant patient who has an inappropriate response to azathioprine. The value of prophylactic pretransplant splenectomy still needs to be demonstrated in a controlled, prospective study with adequate numbers of patients.

TECHNIQUE OF OPERATION

The transplantation of vascularized organ grafts became technically feasible in the early 1900s when Carrel perfected the technique of anastomosing blood vessels. This surgeon and his co-workers subsequently described a method for renal transplantation that is essentially the same as used today. The kidney is placed extraperitoneally in the right or left iliac fossa. This area has the advantages of easy accessibility, protection afforded by the pelvic bones and the muscles of the anterior abdominal wall, appropriate vessels to accomplish revascularization of the kidney, and proximity to the bladder for reestablishing continuity of the urinary tract. The goal of the transplant surgeon is to perform an operation that will heal primarily, be free of infection, and allow normal immediate and long-term function of the allograft.

Revascularization of the kidney is achieved by first anastomosing the renal vein end to side to the external iliac vein and anastomosing the renal artery end to end with the hypogastric artery. While variations in anatomy or preexisting arterial disease in the recipient may require changes in the above technique, this type of revascularization is achievable 70 percent of the time.

Continuity of the urinary tract can be achieved by

either ureteroneocystostomy, ureteroureterostomy, or ureteropyelostomy. Ureteroneocystostomy is the preferred technique, having the lowest incidence of fistula formation. The urinary bladder is placed at rest by providing drainage via a urethral catheter for 2–7 days.

SURGICAL COMPLICATIONS

While rejection accounts for the vast majority of failed renal allografts, approximately 10 percent are lost due to surgical complications. The immunosuppressed state of the host removes the surgeon's oldest and ablest ally, nature. Owing to the compromised state of the recipient, surgical imperfections are magnified and poorly tolerated. When evaluating impaired function of a renal allograft, the mechanical integrity should be proved, not assumed. Surgical complications will be broken down into vascular, urologic, lymphatic, and wound categories.

Vascular

Thrombosis of the renal artery is a catastrophic complication that virtually always results in permanent allograft failure. Fortunately, it is a rare complication, occurring in only 1–2 percent of patients. While rejection can be implicated as the origin in some patients, a technically unsatisfactory anastomosis is the most common cause. Clinically the patient becomes anuric, the allograft bruit vanishes, and the patient may become hypertensive. When renal artery thrombosis is suspected, the diagnostic evaluation should be rapidly and vigorously pursued. A rapid diagnosis is not only necessary for successful revascularization but also will spare the patient needless exposure to high-dose steroid therapy. A renal scan with ^{99}Tc is helpful only if it deomonstrates renal blood flow. The absence of renal blood flow in the scan indicates the prompt need for renal angiography. A renal angiogram is the only means of making a definitive diagnosis and should be done *as soon as* the diagnosis is suspected. The only treatment is usually transplant nephrectomy.

Significant renal artery stenosis has been reported to occur in 4–15 percent of transplant recipients (Fig. 4). The actual incidence is unknown, since many lesions are probably never diagnosed because they are low grade and have no functional significance. Four types of renal artery stenosis occur: (1) preexisting arteriosclerosis in the recipient's iliac arterial system that becomes worse, (2) suture line stenosis, (3) torsion or kinking of the renal artery due to excessive arterial length, and (4) immunologic injury to the donor artery. Immunologic injury to the donor artery is usually multifocal and pathologically represents intimal proliferation. Of the four different types of renal artery stenosis, immunologic injury is the most common. Regardless of the etiology, the patient may present with persistent, severe hypertension that is exceedingly difficult to control. Renal function usually but not always shows some degree of deterioration. An arterial bruit heard over the allograft in itself has no significance, but a change in character of the bruit, especially if it is high pitched with a diastolic component, is very character-istic of renal arterial narrowing. If renal artery stenosis is suspected, it can be confirmed or excluded only by performing a renal angiogram. An intravenous pyelogram or renal scan is not helpful. If the stenotic lesion is high grade, the allograft should be revascularized even if the elevated blood pressure can be controlled. This avoids the possibility of the stenosis progressing to thrombosis.

Renal vein occlusion is exceedingly rare, having an incidence of less than 1 percent. It usually occurs in conjunction with an iliofemoral venous thrombosis or nephrotic syndrome. Swelling of the allograft, significant proteinuria, and altered renal function are the usual signs.

Urologic

Ureteral obstruction can occur either early or late in the posttransplant period and should be excluded any time renal function begins to deteriorate without an adequate explanation. The diagnosis is made by either intravenous or retrograde pyelography. Early ureteral obstruction is most commonly due to ureteral torsion but can also be caused by intraureteral blood clots or extrinsic compression by a hematoma or abscess. Postoperative edema is rarely a cause of significant ureteral obstruction.

Chronic ureteral obstruction can be due to devascularization of the ureter, rejection, lymphocele, encasement of the ureter with retroperitoneal scar tissue, or stenosis at the ureterovesical junction. It may be entirely asymptomatic, manifesting only by a decline in renal function. Significant ureteral and calyceal ectasia associated with a decline in allograft function should be surgically corrected. One should avoid the pitfall, however, of operating on an ectatic ureter with normal calyces and stable renal function.

Urinary fistulas can initiate from any portion of the drainage system but most commonly involve the distal ureter and bladder. Fistulas of the ureter usually occur as a result of excessive stripping and devascularization of the ureter during donor nephrectomy. Bladder fistulas occur as the result of a faulty closure of the cystotomy. Urinary fistulas place both the allograft and patient in great jeopardy. Urinary fistula is commonly associated with a deep wound infection that can lead to sepsis and death of the patient.

While urinary fistulas frequently present in a straightforward way with decreasing urinary output the fluid draining from the wound, such is not always the case. Urinary fistula should be suspected and excluded any time the patient has unexplained alterations in renal function, fever, ileus, positive blood cultures, or significant alterations in urine output. The diagnosis can be best made by using standard diagnostic tools, i.e., intravenous pyelogram, cystogram, and intravenous injection of indigo carmine.

The key to successful treatment is early diagnosis and prompt surgical repair of the fistula. Surgical repair of these lesions should be considered an emergency if contamination of the wound is to be avoided or mini-

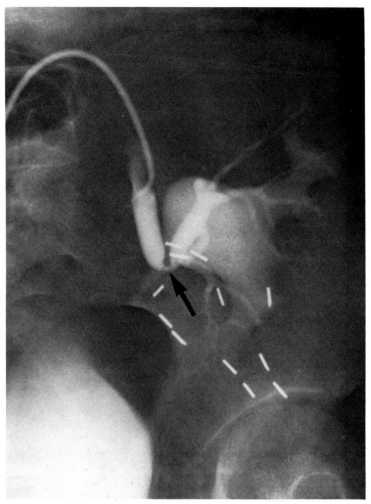

Fig. 4. Renal artery stenosis occurring at the suture line. Patient presented with severe hypertension 16 months after renal transplantation.

mized and morbidity and mortality to the patient decreased.

Lymphatic

Lymphatic complications may occur as either a lymph fistula or lymphocele. Excessive lymphatic drainage in the wound may be the result of inadequate ligation of the lymphatic tissue on the recipient's iliac artery and vein or inadequate ligation of lymphatic tissue on the surface of the donor kidney. Significant lymphatic regeneration does not usually begin until 21 days postoperative. During this period of time many events occur that promote increased lymphatic flow, including rejection and the use of diuretics, anticoagulants, and steroids.

A lymph fistula may occur any time before the wound is completely healed. It manifests as the seepage of large or small amounts of clear fluid from the incision. It is significant in that it can be confused with a urine leak and/or serve as a source of contamination. Definitive diagnosis can be easily made by analyzing some of the fluid for sodium, potassium, creatinine, and urea.

The concentration of these elements should be comparable to that found in a serum sample obtained at the same time. No treatment is necessary, since the fistula will close spontaneously in 7–21 days. Precautions should be taken, however, to avoid contamination of the wound.

A lymphocele represents an undrained collection of lymph in the retroperitoneal space between the allograft and the bladder. Lymphoceles can be multiocular. Lymphoceles usually present between 3 and 24 months postoperative. Lymphoceles are capable of reaching a large size and causing significant pressure on the allograft, ureter, renal artery, and renal vein. As a result of this pressure, the patient can develop hypertension, hydronephrosis, altered renal function, ipsilateral lower extremity edema, and a palpable mass. Definitive diagnosis can be made with sonography, cystography, or intravenous pyelogram. Simple aspiration of the lymphatic fluid not only always results in reaccumulation of the lymphocele but also creates the risk of contaminating the fluid with bacteria. If the lymphocele is causing any alteration in renal function or significant symptoms, it should be surgically drained.

Wound

Wound infections have been reported to occur as rarely as 1.6 percent and as often as 25 percent. In primary operations the rate of wound infections should not exceed 2–4 percent. Steps that can be taken to minimize contamination of the wound with bacteria are good surgical technique, use of local antibiotics in the wound, appropriate preoperative identification and handling of staphylococcal carriers, aseptic care of the wound during the postoperative period, and minimal preoperative hospital stay.

MEDICAL COMPLICATIONS

Medical complications following renal transplantation are usually either related to the immunosuppressed state of the recipient or represent the unresolved and lingering problems of urema or chronic hemodialysis. The two most common causes of posttransplantation death, infection and cerebro- or cardiovascular disease, are vivid examples of each of these two broad groups of complications. Since the problems associated with uremia and chronic hemodialysis have been dealt with in detail in other sections of this book (see the preceding chapter), they will not be reviewed here. Mention will be made only of the more common or important problems associated with the immunosuppressed state. The two most common complications seen in an immunosuppressed host are a reduced ability to combat infection and an increased tendency to develop malignant neoplasms.

Infectious complications account for approximately 70 percent of all transplant deaths. Eighty percent of infections originate in the genitourinary system, respiratory tract, transplant wound, or the blood. While the genitourinary tract is most commonly involved, these infections rarely result in patient death (mortality rate of 3–5 percent). Pulmonary, central nervous system, and wound infections are the most lethal.

While early postoperative infections (first 2 weeks) are usually bacterial and have portals of entry similar to nonimmunosuppressed patients, late infections (beyond 6 weeks) have several distinctive characteristics. A multiplicity of infectious agents may be involved. In addition to the usual bacterial pathogens, opportunistic infections are common. Microorganisms have the ability to penetrate and colonize organ systems which are usually resistant to their efforts, e.g., gram-negative bacteria causing pneumonia. One should expect a large number of late infections, especially in the lung (50 percent), to be *mixed*, i.e., multiple bacteria, a bacteria and fungus, two fungi, etc. A partial list of common infectious agents causing infection in the immunosuppressed patient is as follows:

1. Bacteria—usually gram-positive and gram-negative bacteria
2. Fungi—candida, cryptococcus, nocardia, aspergillius

3. Viral agents—herpes simplex, cytomegalovirus (CMV), varicella Zoster
4. Protozoa—Pneumoncystis carinii

Several general principles have been found to be helpful in the management of late infections. Diagnostic evaluation must be absolutely complete and unusually prompt. Procrastination or taking shortcuts may result in death of the patient. Owing to the variety of potential infectious agents all reasonable efforts should be made to obtain material from the suspected site of infection—e.g., bronchoscopy, biopsy, aspiration, etc. for smears and cultures. When possible, antimicrobial therapy should be specific and based on the results of smears and cultures. Broad antimicrobial therapy based on incomplete or inaccurate data usually fails. If the infection is serious, immunosuppressive therapy should be reduced to a minimum until the infection is resolved.

Viral infections occur in 40–90 percent of recipients following renal transplantation. The most common viral infections are cytomegalovirus (CMV), herpes simplex, varicella zoster, and hepatitis B virus. At the present time, no consistently effective antiviral agents or vaccines are available. Recognition of these infections is important, especially in the case of CMV, to avoid confusion with other problems and to be alerted to the possibility of associated complications.

Cytomegalovirus can occur as either a primary or secondary infection. In primary infections the more common vectors for transmission of the viral particles are blood transfusions and the renal allograft. Secondary infections occur as latent viral particles in the recipient and are reactivated by immunosuppression or perhaps rejection reactions. Primary infections tend to be more severe and are associated with a higher incidence of viremia, bacteremia, and renal allograft loss. Clinical findings that may be found in conjunction with CMV infection are diverse and include fever, leukopenia, pneumonia, pericarditis, hepatitis, central nervous system disease, and renal allograft dysfunction that can mimic mild to moderate rejection.

Malignant neoplasms develop in renal transplant recipients at a frequency 100 times greater than would be expected in the general population. The absolute incidence of malignant neoplasms occurring in renal transplant recipients is 6 percent. Tumors may develop de novo or in some instances may have been transplanted from the renal donor. The most common de novo tumors in renal transplant recipients are skin tumors, carcinoma of the cervix, lymphomas, and carcinoma of the lung. Reticulum cell sarcomas are the most frequent type of lymphoma and occur with a much higher rate in the central nervous system than is seen in nonimmunosuppressed patients.

While aspetic necrosis of the femoral head occurs in renal dialysis patients, the incidence is much higher in recipients of renal transplants. The etiology of this disease is unknown, but both total steroid dosage and fat emboli to the femoral head secondary to fatty change in the liver have been implicated. This very debilitating complication can be treated safely and effectively with total hip replacement.

CLINICAL PATTERNS OF REJECTION

Not all renal transplants are successful. The most common reasons for failure are surgical complications, recurrence of the primary renal disease in the allograft, death of the patient, and immunologic rejection of the allograft. Rejection accounts for at least 70 percent of the allografts that fail, and attempts to modify the rejection reaction account for a significant number of patient deaths. Although there has been a tremendous increase in understanding the rejection process, less significant strides have been made in clinically altering its course.

Hyperacute Rejection

Hyperacute rejection of renal allografts is a humorally mediated process that arises from presensitization of the host. Presensitization occurs when the host has had prior exposure to foreign HLA antigens. This most commonly occurs following pregnancy, blood transfusions, or previous organ transplantation. Cytotoxic antibodies are formed by the host that may either be specific for the HLA antigens involved or may be more generalized against a wide variety of HLA antigens. When the performed cytotoxic antibodies come in contact with foreign antigen, a catastrophic reaction occurs that invariably results in immediate allograft destruction. This lesion is not treatable and is avoided by performing the crossmatch between donor cells and recipient serum.

When the performed cytotoxic antibodies come in contact with the foreign HLA antigens and some cell-specific antigen present in the wall of the vascular enthothelium, the complement system is activated. This activation causes endothelial cell distruption, exposure of basement membranes, adherence of neutrophils and platelets, and activation of the clotting mechanism. The predominant histopathology involves the vascular tree of the kidney with fibrin deposition and fibrin thrombi present in the glomeruli and small vessel (Fig. 5). Polymorphonuclear leukocytes and platelets are also noted to be adherent to the walls of small- and medium-sized vessels. These pathologic lesions produce very low blood flow in the kidney. Grossly the kidney is blue and swollen. While good pulsations may exist in the arterial tree, the renal vein is poorly filled, and even when the vein is occluded it fills very slowly. If this clinical picture is identified in the operating room, it should be confirmed with a biopsy and then treated by immediate transplant nephrectomy.

In some instances, the hyperacute reaction is not obvious in the operating room. Postoperatively these patients are anuric or make very small amounts of

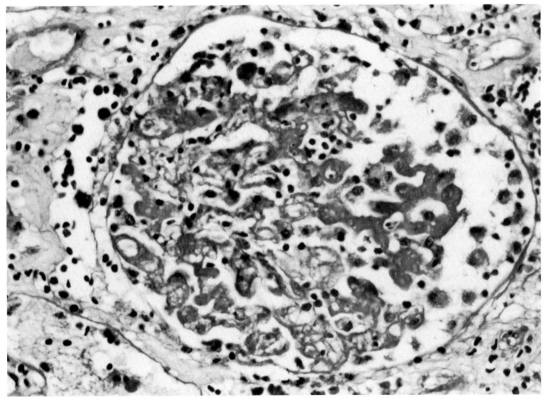

Fig. 5. Histopathology of hyperacute rejection in a renal allograft. Note prominence of fibrin thrombi and polymorphonuclear leukocytes.

bloody urine. Fever and hyperkalemia are common. The diagnosis can be suspected clinically and confirmed by either renal angiography or renal biopsy. Nephrectomy should be done promptly, since no other treatment options are available.

Accelerated Rejection

Accelerated rejection represents a combination of humoral and cellular response. Clinically it resembles a milder form of hyperacute rejection. Circulating preformed cytotoxic antibodies are thought to be present but are undetected by the standard crossmatch test. Either the decreased virulence of this reaction is due to the low concentration of the antibody, or these antibodies may have less ability to activate complement. This lesion will not be recognized in the operating room, and for 1–3 days the patient may produce varying amounts of urine. A marked rejection reaction usually occurs between days 3 and 5, and the need for dialysis is common. While the 1 year survival of allografts with this reaction is very low, some patients do respond to immunosuppressive therapy and treatment should not be arbitrarily discontinued.

Acute Rejection

Acute rejection is the primary reaction observed in the unsensitized host and is mainly cellularly mediated. While it can occur at any time following the transplant, it most commonly occurs 1–3 weeks postoperatively in the patient receiving standard (no antilymphocyte globulin) immunosuppression. The predominant features microscopically are a cellular infiltrate composed mainly of immature lymphocytes and neutrophils with some plasma cells and macrophges (Fig. 6). As the reaction progresses, round cells predominate and tend to cluster or be especially prominant in the pervascular space of small- to medium-sized vessels. Interstitial edema is common and striking. In more severe lesions platelet thrombi can be observed in small vessels, and varying degrees of damage to the intima and media of these vessels is noted. Most striking can be frank fibrinoid necrosis.

The above-described reaction leads to a marked reduction in renal blood flow. This decreased renal blood flow can produce tubular lesions (flattening of tubular epithelial cells and a decrease in cell size) secondary to the decreased availability of O_2 and resultant ischemia. Progressive vascular damage produces thrombosis, infarction, and intarenal hemorrhage. Grossly these kidneys are swollen and hemorrhagic.

Clinically the signs and symptoms of acute rejection can be broken down into those caused by altered renal function and those produced by the systematic nature of the reaction. The primary pathophysiologic component of rejection is decreased renal blood flow and depressed renal function. Excretion of water and

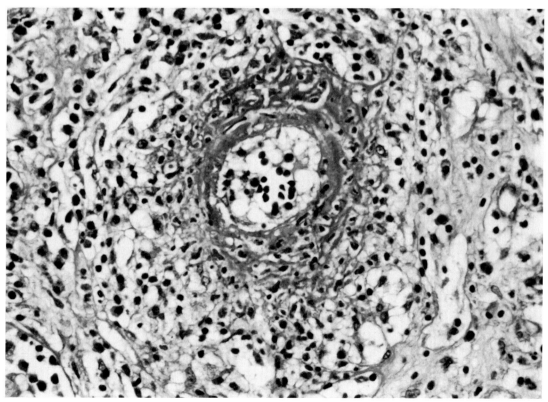

Fig. 6. Histopathology of acute cellular rejection in a renal allograft. The most significant features are round cell infiltrate, interstitial edema, and moderate vasculitis.

salt is diminished (urinary sodium is usually less than 30 mEq/liter). Weight gain, edema, and hypertension are common. Serum creatinine and blood urea nitrogen are elevated. Proteinuria may be increased. Urine osmolality is frequently 400–600 mOsm.

The area around the allograft may become tender, and the allograft itself may become markedly increased in size. If a bruit was present it frequently becomes decreased or absent. Fever is a common component of acute rejection and may be as high as 103°–104°F, although it is usually low grade (100°–102°F). Malaise with vague muscular aching is usually associated with the fever.

Unfortunately, all of the signs, symptoms, and laboratory data that are significantly altered in rejection are *nonspecific* and can also be altered in the other significant clinical problems that must be differentiated from rejection—e.g., acute tubular necrosis, sepsis, pyelonephritis, urinary obstruction or fistula, renal artery thrombosis, etc. The diagnosis of rejection must be made by carefully assembling a variety of pieces of clinical, laboratory, and radiologic data. Often of extreme importance is the degree of experience of the physician analyzing the data. If there is any doubt about the diagnosis, either open or percutaneous biopsy of the allograft should be done to confirm the clinical findings. Treatment of acute cellular rejection centers

around increased corticosteroid therapy. Azathiorpine doses are not raised, and if significant impairment of renal function is present the dose of azathioprine may be reduced.

Chronic Rejection

Chronic rejection is thought to be mediated primarily via a humoral response. Microscopically there is a lack of significant cellular infiltrate. The predominant lesion is one of vascular occlusion of small arterioles (Fig. 7). Intimal proliferation occurs with associated degeneration of the media. This process progresses to thrombosis. As a secondary effect of the thrombosis one sees tubular atrophy and interstitial scarring. Glomerula changes are also present with an increase in the mesangial cells and thickening of glomerular basement membranes. Renal function slowly but progressively declines.

No specific signs or symptoms are present, and the symptoms are predominantly those associated with chronic renal insufficiency from any cause. Hypertension, proteinuria, and increasing serum creatinine are the early findings. As the process progresses, more fulminant symptoms, such as anemia, acidosis, lethargy, etc., are present. Unfortunately there is no specific treatment available to alter this lesion. One should always, however, exclude mechanical causes such as ureteral obstruction or renal artery stenosis which can

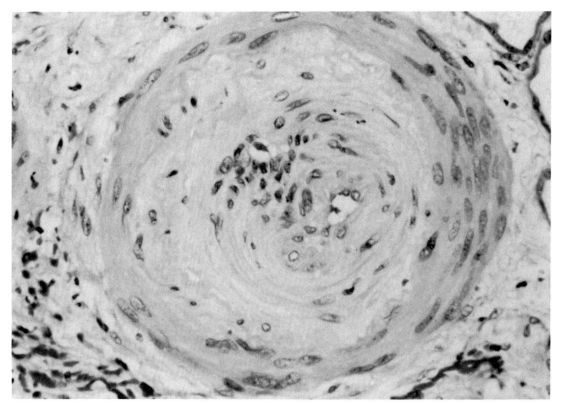

Fig. 7.   Histopathology of chronic rejection in a renal allograft. The prominent lesion is intimal proliferation leading to occlusion of small arteries.

either be responsible for or contribute to the decline in renal function.

IMMUNOSUPPRESSIVE DRUGS
Corticosteroids

At the present time corticosteroids represent the cornerstone of immunosuppressive therapy to avoid or modify the rejection reaction of renal transplant recipients. While other agents are also used (antilymphocyte globulin, azathioprine, cyclophosphamide, etc.) in combination with corticosteroids, no successful immunosuppressive regimen has been used in man that does not include corticosteroids. Corticosteroids influence both the afferent and efferent limbs of the immune response and primary effect cell-mediated immunity.

While the exact mechanisms for modyfing the rejection reaction are not known, several have been postulated. Corticosteroids are capable of both decreasing lymphocyte proliferation and causing lymphocyte death. Lympholysis is caused by inhibiting DNA and RNA synthesis. In high doses corticosteroids both are capable of decreasing antibody synthesis and have anticomplement properties. Inhibition of the inflammatory response also serves to protect the renal allograft. In addition to altering the host's immune response, corticosteroids protect the allograft in a variety of ways—e.g., membrane stabilization. The most common complications of corticosteroid therapy are sodium retention, hypertension, gastric or intestinal ulceration, pancreatitis, cataracts, glaucoma, diabetes mellitus, hyperlipidemia, Cushingoid appearance, acne, increase capillary fragility, myopathy, and psychosis.

Numerous regimens are used to achieve posttransplant immunosuppression. One of the more common is to begin oral prednisone in a dose of 2 mg/kg/day 24–36 hours before the transplant. This initial dose is tapered to arrive at a total daily dose of 30 mg/day by 3 months and 20 mg/day by 1 year. Rejection episodes are treated by either giving an intravenous bolus of methylprednisolone (pulse therapy) or by raising the oral prednisone dose to 3 mg/kg/day. Most centers limit pulse therapy to a cumulative total of 6–8 g. The oral prednisone dose is usually tapered 10 mg/kg/day until a dosage is reached just above where the rejection reaction began; then the standard cuts in dosage are made every 4–5 days.

Corticosteroid therapy should be significantly reduced in the event of infectious complications or other serious signs of corticosteroid toxicity. At 6 months, children should be converted to alternate day steroid therapy to allow maximum growth. Some centers advocate alternate day therapy for adults as well, but opponents of this policy claim that rejection episodes are more common and steroid complications are not signficantly reduced.

Purine Antagonists

Azathioprine and 6-mercaptopurine (6MP) are two purine antagonists that have demonstrated immunosuppressive properties in both man and experimental animals. These agents work by affecting DNA synthesis and are much more effective against T cells than B cells. Azathioprine has less toxicity than 6MP and has been the most commonly used agent in conjunction with corticosteroids.

This drug is usually most effective against sensitized cells after the introduction of antigen. An initial loading dose of 3–5 mg/kg/day is given and maintenance doses of 0.75–1.50 mg/kg/day are used. All doses must be modified with regard to the patient's WBC and platelet count. Splenectomized patients are usually capable of taking larger maintenance doses. In adjusting the dose one must be more attentive to the trend of the WBC count than to the actual numbers. When counts go below 3500, Imuran should be sharply curtailed or discontinued. The more common complications of azathioprine therapy are leukopenia, thrombocytopenia, hepatic dysfunction, and alopecia.

Alkylating Agents

Cyclophosphamide has likewise proven to be an effective immunosuppressive agent in both experimental animals and man. For routine use in man it has not been shown to be more effective than azathioprine. This drug has a profound effect on dividing cells and inhibits ribonucleic acid and protein synthesis. Deoxyribonucleic acid synthesis is also impaired. Cyclophosphamide causes more severe damage to B cells and also hampers the inflammatory response. In order for cyclophosphamide to be active it must first be converted in the liver. The dose of cyclophosphamide is usually 75 percent of an equivalent dose of Imuran.

Cyclophosphamide exerts toxic effects on the bone marrow, and leukopenia is the limiting factor in adjusting the dose. The WBC count usually nadirs more rapidly than with the azathioprine. This drug also has an adverse effect on fertility and can cause severe hemorrhagic cystitis.

Some centers have used intermittent intravenous cyclophosphamide in the immediate posttransplant period or in treating acute rejection episodes in an effort to take advantage of its effect on rapidly proliferating cells. Other centers have converted patients from azathioprine to cyclophosphamide if liver dysfunction is present and thought to be due to azathioprine toxicity. Inspite of the fact that cyclophosphamide must be activated by the liver, the liver is capable of providing this function even in the presence of severe intrinsic disease.

Irradiation

Irradiation has a profound effect on lymphoid cells and is capable of destroying both lymphocytes and stem cells. Total body irradiation was one of the first means used to provide immunosuppression in clinical renal transplantation. As used at the time the side effects, toxicity, and related mortality were too great and its use was discontinued.

Local graft irradiation is still used by many centers either prophylactically or in the treatment of acute rejection, yet there has been little documentation of its value. At best it is an adjunctive form of immunosuppression, and at worst it poses little threat of harm to either allograft or patient. The usual course of therapy consists of 150 rads given every other day for three doses. This course may be repeated. Variations of this regimen are numerous, but the total dose should not exceed 900–1000 rads so that radiation nephritis is avoided.

Antilymphocyte Globulin (ALG)

Antilymphocyte globulin has been shown to be a potent immunosuppressive agent in both man and experimental animals. ALG is usually prepared by injecting human thymocytes or lymphoblasts into a horse, rabbit, or pig. After a suitable period of immunization the anti–human ALG is recovered from the animal.

The potency, safety, and efficacy of ALG are determined by the purity of the antigen source, methods of refinement of the ALG after recovery, dosage, and degree of histoincompatibility between donor and recipient. The ALG used in the pioneer work by Starzl was limited by its purity and could not be given intravenously. This not only caused local problems at the site of intramuscular injection but also limited the dose that could be given. Present ALG can be given safely intravenously, but there is still the possibility of a great deal of discrepancy in potency between batches made at the same center.

In spite of the widespread use of this agent, its clinical efficacy still awaits proof in a controlled, prospective study involving sufficient numbers of patients. While there is no doubt that the frequency and severity of rejection episodes are decreased during the first 2 months posttransplant, a beneficial effect on the long-term survival of the allograft awaits better documentation.

Thoracic Duct Drainage

Thoracic duct drainage removes circulating lymphocytes. This method, used without benefit of other forms of immunosuppression, has prolonged human renal allograft survival from 19 to 78 days. After several successful trials this technqiue was discarded primarily because of the fear of infection and because it was logistically cumbersome. Several centers are currently reevaluating this technique, and in the future it may gain wider acceptance.

REFERENCES

Advisory committee to the Renal Transplant Registry: The thirteenth report of the human renal transplant registry. Transplant Proc 9:9, 1977

Banowsky LH: The role of adjuvant operations in renal transplantation. Urol Clin North Am 3:527, 1976

Lee DBN, Prompt CA, Upham A, et al: Medical complications of renal transplantation: I. Graft and infectious complications in recipient. Urology [Suppl] 9:7, 1977

Opelz G, Terasaki PI: Factors influencing effect of HLA matching on cadaver kidney transplants. Transplant Proc 9:1795, 1977

Penn I: Development of cancer as a complication of clinical transplantation. Transplant Proc 9:1121, 1977

Proceedings of the Fourth Annual Meeting of the American Association for Clincial Histocompatibility Testing: Clinical histocompatibility testing. Transplant Proc 10:4, 1978

Prompt CA, Lee DBN, Upham AT, et al: Medical complications of renal transplantation: II. Noninfectious complications in recipient. Urology [Suppl] 9:32, 1977

Index